Case Studies in
NURSE ANESTHESIA

EDITED BY

SASS ELISHA, EdD, CRNA
Kaiser Permanente School of Anesthesia
Pasadena, California

JONES AND BARTLETT PUBLISHERS
Sudbury, Massachusetts
BOSTON   TORONTO   LONDON   SINGAPORE

World Headquarters

Jones and Bartlett Publishers
40 Tall Pine Drive
Sudbury, MA 01776
978-443-5000
info@jbpub.com
www.jbpub.com

Jones and Bartlett Publishers
Canada
6339 Ormindale Way
Mississauga, Ontario L5V 1J2
Canada

Jones and Bartlett Publishers
International
Barb House, Barb Mews
London W6 7PA
United Kingdom

Jones and Bartlett's books and products are available through most bookstores and online booksellers. To contact Jones and Bartlett Publishers directly, call 800-832-0034, fax 978-443-8000, or visit our website, www.jbpub.com.

Substantial discounts on bulk quantities of Jones and Bartlett's publications are available to corporations, professional associations, and other qualified organizations. For details and specific discount information, contact the special sales department at Jones and Bartlett via the above contact information or send an email to specialsales@jbpub.com.

The authors, editor, and publisher have made every effort to provide accurate information. However, they are not responsible for errors, omissions, or for any outcomes related to the use of the contents of this book and take no responsibility for the use of the products and procedures described. Treatments and side effects described in this book may not be applicable to all people; likewise, some people may require a dose or experience a side effect that is not described herein. Drugs and medical devices are discussed that may have limited availability controlled by the Food and Drug Administration (FDA) for use only in a research study or clinical trial. Research, clinical practice, and government regulations often change the accepted standard in this field. When consideration is being given to use of any drug in the clinical setting, the health care provider or reader is responsible for determining FDA status of the drug, reading the package insert, and reviewing prescribing information for the most up-to-date recommendations on dose, precautions, and contraindications, and determining the appropriate usage for the product. This is especially important in the case of drugs that are new or seldom used.

The views expressed in this book are those of the author and do not necessarily reflect the official policy or position of the Department of the Navy, Department of Defense, or the United States Government.

Production Credits

Publisher: Kevin Sullivan
Aquisitions Editor: Emily Ekle
Associate Editor: Patricia Donnelly
Editorial Assistant: Rachel Shuster
Production Editor: Amanda Clerkin
Marketing Manager: Rebecca Wasley

V.P., Manufacturing and Inventory Control: Therese Connell
Composition: DDC/ASI
Cover Design: Kristin E. Parker
Cover Image Credit: © Arbi Babakhanaians/Dreamstime LLC
Printing and Binding: Malloy, Inc.
Cover Printing: Malloy, Inc.

Library of Congress Cataloging-in-Publication Data
Case studies in nurse anesthesia / [edited by] Sass Elisha.
   p. ; cm.
   Includes bibliographical references and index.
   ISBN-13: 978-0-7637-6387-9 (alk. paper)
   ISBN-10: 0-7637-6387-X (alk. paper)
   1. Anesthesia—Case studies. 2. Nurse anesthetists—Case studies. I.
Elisha, Sass.
   [DNLM: 1. Anesthesia—methods. 2. Anesthesia—nursing. 3.
Perioperative Nursing—methods. 4. Surgical Procedures, Operative—nursing. WY 151 C337 2010]
   RD82.45C38 2010
   617.9'6—dc22
                                        2009033394

6048

Printed in the United States of America
14 13 12 11 10   10 9 8 7 6 5 4 3 2

Contents

Acknowledgments

I would like to thank my family; all of the authors; John Nagelhout, CRNA, PhD, FAAN; Sandy Bordi, CRNA, MSN; Ed Waters, CRNA, MN; Retta Smith; Steve Bebe; Karen Plaus, CRNA, PhD; and Chuck Biddle, CRNA, PhD, for their support of this academic endeavor.

Foreword

Nurse anesthetists have contributed in myriad ways to the practice of anesthesia. These include involvement in research, education, and the many technological advances that are the cornerstone of modern surgery and anesthesia practice. However, the most important contribution has come in the realm of patient care. For many decades, nurse anesthetists have been an integral part of the evolution of clinical practice. Our observations and innovative methods related to clinical care have been essential to the remarkable safety record associated with current anesthesia practice. The complexity and diversity of surgeries performed today were unthinkable just a few years ago and their success in part is due to the excellence of nurse anesthesia practice. The approach to patient care and critical assessment tools used by nurse anesthetists are a model that can be widely applied in many patient care situations. These are the concepts that are the foundation for this book.

This is the first book written by nurse anesthetists to use the case study format for describing an array of procedures and disease states encountered in modern anesthesia practice. In order to properly care for our patients, the perioperative period must be viewed on a continuum within the total surgical experience. This book presents clinical case studies in anesthesia which mirror the thought processes required for successful clinical practice. Each case and patient scenario is discussed from the preoperative, intraoperative, and postoperative perspective. Pathophysiology, pharmacology, surgical intervention, anesthesia case management, and postoperative considerations are thoroughly discussed and evaluated. Key points, suggested readings, and review questions are presented, which further enhance the effect of the educational material.

Dr. Elisha has gathered together a wide variety of national experts to share their knowledge and suggestions on the most current clinical practices. The easily readable case based format will feel familiar to student registered nurse anesthetists and anesthetists in clinical practice. This book is an invaluable resource for the practicing clinician. I am confident that you will enjoy reading and rereading this textbook and that it will become a permanent part of your medical library.

John J. Nagelhout, PhD, CRNA, FAAN

Contributors

Paul Aguiar, CRNA, MSN
Staff Nurse Anesthetist
Kaiser Permanente Medical Center
Harbor City, California

Travis Allen, CRNA, MSN
Lead Nurse Anesthetist
Seattle Children's Hospital
Seattle, Washington

Jessica Bair, CRNA, MSA
Staff Nurse Anesthetist
Kaiser Permanente Medical Center
West Los Angeles, California

Deborah T. Bergstein, CRNA, MSN
Staff Nurse Anesthetist
Kaiser Permanente Medical Center
Panorama City, California

Tatiana Bevans, CRNA, MSN
Nurse Anesthesia Faculty
Rush University Medical Center
Chicago, Illinois

Pamela Binns-Turner, PhD, CRNA, APN
Program Director
School of Nursing, Nurse Anesthesia Track
Union University
Jackson, Tennessee

Sandra K. Bordi, CRNA, MSN
Academic and Clinical Educator
Kaiser Permanente School of Anesthesia
Pasadena, California

Greta Bray, CRNA, MSN
Staff Nurse Anesthetist
Kaiser Permanente Medical Center
Santa Clara, California

Gayne Brenneman, MD
Cardiac Anesthesiologist
Kaiser Permanente Medical Center
Los Angeles, California

Joseph F. Burkard, CRNA, DNSc
Associate Professor
University of San Diego
San Diego, California

John Cavitt, CRNA, MSN
Staff Nurse Anesthetist
Kaiser Permanente Medical Center
Portland, Oregon

Michael Churchin, CRNA, MS
Staff Nurse Anesthetist
Kaiser Permanente Medical Center
Irvine, California

Gary D. Clark, EdD, CRNA
Associate Professor
Department of Biological Sciences
Webster University
St. Louis, Missouri

Joan Cornachio, CRNA, MSNA
Staff Nurse Anesthetist
Virginia Commonwealth University
Richmond, Virginia

Nicholas C. Curdt, CRNA, MS
Staff Nurse Anesthetist
DePaul Health Center
St. Louis, Missouri

Veronica Davis, CRNA, MSN
Staff Nurse Anesthetist
Kaiser Permanente Medical Center
Fontana, California

Matthew D'Angelo, CRNA, DNP
R. Adams Shock Trauma Center
University of Maryland
Baltimore, Maryland

Sass Elisha, EdD, CRNA
Assistant Director
Kaiser Permanente School of Anesthesia
Pasadena, California

Mark Gabot, CRNA, MSN
Staff Nurse Anesthetist
Kaiser Permanente Medical Center
Fontana, California

Marjorie A. Geisz-Everson, CRNA, PhD(c)
Instructor
Louisiana State University Health Science Center
School of Nursing
New Orleans, Louisiana

Sarah E. Giron, CRNA, MS
Senior Staff Nurse Anesthetist
University of California, Los Angeles
Los Angeles, California

Mark Goelz, CRNA, MSNA
Staff Nurse Anesthetist
Virginia Commonwealth University
Richmond, Virginia

Charles Griffis, PhD, CRNA
Assistant Clinical Professor
Department of Anesthesiology
University of California, Los Angeles
Los Angeles, California

C. Wayne Hamm, CRNA, MSN, APN
Staff Nurse Anesthetist
Medical Anesthesia Group
Memphis, Tennessee

Jeremy S. Heiner, CRNA, MSN
Academic and Clinical Educator
Kaiser Permanente School of Anesthesia
Pasadena, California

Yoo Eun Emily Hwang, CRNA, MSN
Staff Nurse Anesthetist
Dallas, Texas

Donna Jasinski, PhD, CRNA
Nurse Anesthesia Program Director
Georgetown University
Washington, District of Columbia

Vickie S. Jordan, CRNA, DNP
Educator Louisiana State University
Nurse Anesthesia Program
Hattiesburg, Mississippi

Joseph A. Joyce, CRNA, BS
Staff Nurse Anesthetist
Wesley Long Community Hospital
Greensboro, North Carolina

Mary C. Karlet, PhD, CRNA
Chair, Department of Nurse Anesthesia
Samford University
Birmingham, Alabama

Loretta Kitabjian, CRNA, MA, MSN
Staff Nurse Anesthetist
Kaiser Permanente Medical Center
Panorama City, California

Lynn L. Lebeck, PhD, CRNA
Program Director
University of Michigan, Flint
Hurley Medical Center
Flint, Michigan

Hamid Mahmood, CRNA, MSNA
Staff Nurse Anesthetist
Virginia Commonwealth University
Richmond, Virginia

Erica J. McCall, CRNA MSN
Senior Staff Anesthetist
University of California, Los Angeles Medical Center
Los Angeles, California

Shaun Mendel, CRNA
Staff Nurse Anesthetist
Pediatric Anesthesiologists, P.A.
LeBonheur Children's Medical Center
Memphis, Tennessee

Nancy A. Moriber, CRNA, MS, APRN
Program Director
Fairfield University Nurse Anesthesia Program
Bridgeport Hospital
Bridgeport, Connecticut

Sandra E. Morris, CRNA, MSN, CDR, NC, USN, retired
Staff Nurse Anesthetist
Kaiser Permanente Medical Center
Fontana, California

Greg Nezat, PhD, CRNA
Commander
Navy Nurse Corps Anesthesia Program
Portsmouth, Virginia

Lisa Osborne, PhD, CRNA
Site Director, Uniformed Services University
Nurse Anesthesia Program
Bethesda, Maryland

Timothy Palmer, CRNA, MS
Anesthesia Education Coordinator
Surgical Services Education
William Beaumont Hospital
Royal Oak, Michigan

Garrett Peterson, CRNA, DNP
Associate Director, Nurse Anesthesia Area of Study
University of Minnesota School of Nursing
Staff Anesthetist, Minneapolis Veterans Affairs
   Medical Center
Minneapolis, Minnesota

Rachel Polazzi, CRNA, MSN
Staff Nurse Anesthetist
Pinnacle Anesthesia Group
Delray Beach, Florida

Michael Rieker, CRNA, DNP
Director, Nurse Anesthesia Program
Wake Forest University Baptist Medical Center
Winston-Salem, North Carolina

Cliff Roberson, CRNA, MS
Assistant Director, Nurse Anesthesia Program
University of New England
Portland, Maine

Bernadette T. Higgins Roche, EdD, CRNA
Assistant Professor
School of Nurse Anesthesia, De Paul University
Administrative Director
North Shore University Health System
Evanston, Illinois

Becky Rubin, CRNA, MSN
Staff Nurse Anesthetist
Asheville Anesthesia Associates
Asheville, North Carolina

Michael Rubin, CRNA, MSN
Staff Nurse Anesthetist
Asheville Anesthesia Associates
Asheville, North Carolina

Allan Schwartz, CRNA, DDS
Dentist-Certified Registered Nurse Anesthetist
ProDental, affiliate of Heartland Dental Care
Columbia, Missouri

Dennis Spence, PhD, CRNA
San Diego, California

Henry Talley, CRNA, PhD
Program Director
College of Nursing
Michigan State University
East Lansing, Michigan

Edward Waters, CRNA, MN
Academic and Clinical Educator
Kaiser Permanente School of Anesthesia
Pasadena, California

Dawn C. Welliver, CRNA, ARNP, MS
Nurse Anesthetist, Independent Contractor
President, Welliver Anesthesia Corp.
Yulee, Florida

Mark D. Welliver, CRNA, ARNP, DNP
Associate Professor of Professional Practice
School of Nurse Anesthesia
Harris College of Nursing and Health Sciences
Texas Christian University
Fort Worth, Texas

Molly Wright, MS, CRNA, APN
Union University
Jackson, Tennessee

Otolaryngology

1

Tonsillectomy

1

Sandra K. Bordi

KEY POINTS

- Tonsillectomy, with or without adenoidectomy, is one of the most commonly performed surgeries on children in the United States.
- Indications for tonsillectomy include: chronic tonsillitis, recurrent peritonsillar abscess, enlarged tonsils that cause upper airway obstruction, tonsil asymmetry with suspected malignancy, and recurrent tonsillar hemorrhage.
- Patients having a tonsillectomy are at high risk for postoperative nausea and vomiting (PONV).
- Postoperative hemorrhage remains the most serious complication following tonsillectomy.
- Postoperative pain management is vitally important to reduce prolonged recovery and hospitalization.

CASE SYNOPSIS

A 7-year-old female presents with a 3-year history of recurrent tonsillitis. Her symptoms became significantly worse, resulting in difficulty breathing at night and snoring. She has been treated with antibiotic therapy that ended 1 week ago and her situation has not improved. Currently, she is scheduled for a tonsillectomy.

PREOPERATIVE EVALUATION AND DEMOGRAPHIC DATA

Past Medical/Surgical History

- Chronic tonsillitis

List of Medications

- No medications

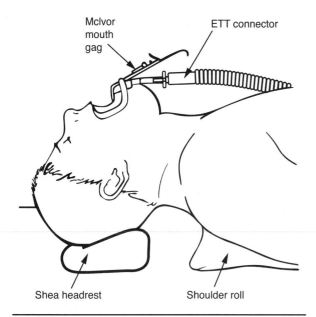

Figure 1-1   *Representation of patient position for tonsillectomy.*

5. Discuss the type of anesthesia most often administered during a tonsillar resection.

General anesthesia with an endotracheal tube is the optimal technique and airway management strategy for a tonsillectomy. The type of anesthetic induction is dependent on the cooperation of the child. If intravenous access is accomplished, then an intravenous induction can be initiated. Otherwise, an inhalation induction is acceptable for most patients and intravenous access is established after the patient loses consciousness and an adequate depth of anesthesia is achieved. The intraoperative goals are to ensure unconsciousness, inhibit sympathetic reflexes, obtund oropharyngeal reflexes during direct laryngoscopy and placement of the oral gag, and prevention of patient movement during the surgical procedure. These objectives can be achieved by administering inhalation agents alone or in combination with neuromuscular blocking agents, propofol, and/or opioids. Unfortunately, upon induction of anesthesia, relaxation of the pharyngeal muscles and tissues may cause airway obstruction in those patients

who present with facial anomalies, severe tonsillar hypertrophy, and other medical conditions, resulting in partial or complete airway obstruction.

6. Discuss the intraoperative anesthetic management during a tonsillectomy.

The average surgical time required for a tonsillectomy is approximately 30 minutes. Even though this is a short procedure, a high degree of physiologic stimulation occurs due to manipulation of the airway and removal of the tonsils. Therefore, a deeper plane of anesthesia is required to adequately blunt the sympathetic reflexes that may elicit hypertension, tachycardia, and arrhythmias. This can be accomplished by increasing the inhalation agent alone or in combination with propofol and/or narcotics. Hypertension will also increase the volume of blood loss.

Figure 1-2   *View of hypertrophied tonsils and surgical resection of the tonsils.*

Tonsillectomy

1

Sandra K. Bordi

KEY POINTS

- Tonsillectomy, with or without adenoidectomy, is one of the most commonly performed surgeries on children in the United States.
- Indications for tonsillectomy include: chronic tonsillitis, recurrent peritonsillar abscess, enlarged tonsils that cause upper airway obstruction, tonsil asymmetry with suspected malignancy, and recurrent tonsillar hemorrhage.
- Patients having a tonsillectomy are at high risk for postoperative nausea and vomiting (PONV).
- Postoperative hemorrhage remains the most serious complication following tonsillectomy.
- Postoperative pain management is vitally important to reduce prolonged recovery and hospitalization.

CASE SYNOPSIS

A 7-year-old female presents with a 3-year history of recurrent tonsillitis. Her symptoms became significantly worse, resulting in difficulty breathing at night and snoring. She has been treated with antibiotic therapy that ended 1 week ago and her situation has not improved. Currently, she is scheduled for a tonsillectomy.

PREOPERATIVE EVALUATION AND DEMOGRAPHIC DATA

Past Medical/Surgical History

- Chronic tonsillitis

List of Medications

- No medications

Diagnostic Data

• No preoperative lab tests

Height/Weight/Vital Signs

• 120 cm, 21 kg
• Blood pressure, 112/62; heart rate, 88 beats per minute; respiratory rate, 22 breaths per minute; temperature, 36.9°C; room air oxygen saturation, 100%

PATHOPHYSIOLOGY

Tonsillitis occurs most often in children 4 to 7 years of age and it is an infection that involves the pharyngeal tonsils. This pathologic process is caused by a virus or a bacterial pathogen. A viral tonsillitis is usually self-limiting whereas a bacterial pathogen will require antibiotic treatment and can produce more severe systemic complications. Bacterial tonsillitis is primarily caused by group A beta-hemolytic streptococcus (GABHS). The type of tonsillitis (acute, recurrent, or chronic) is determined by the symptomatology and the frequency by which the infection reoccurs. Acute tonsillitis is characterized by fever, dysphagia, lymphadenopathy, red or exudative tonsils, and sore throat. Mouth breathing, snoring, and obstructive sleep apnea may also occur due to tonsillar enlargement. Recurrent tonsillitis is diagnosed when there are 7 episodes of acute tonsillitis in 1 year, 5 episodes in 2 consecutive years, or 3 episodes per year in 3 years. When tonsillitis is recurrent or chronic, a definitive treatment such as a tonsillectomy

is recommended. Relative and absolute indications associated with a patient having a tonsillectomy is outlined by the American Academy of Pediatrics and is listed in Table 1-1.

SURGICAL PROCEDURE

Surgical removal of the tonsils, with or without adenoidectomy, can be accomplished using a variety of techniques. The method that is used may be determined by the extent of the surgery (partial tonsillectomy or complete tonsillectomy) and preference of the surgeon. Partial tonsillectomy is performed in patients with tonsillar hypertrophy resulting in obstructive sleep apnea or airway obstruction. This procedure involves excising approximately 90% of the tonsillar tissue. In a complete tonsillectomy, the entire tonsillar tissue is excised, exposing the underlying pharyngeal constrictor muscle of the throat. Tonsillectomy techniques involve excising the tonsils through the mouth by use of a scalpel, scissors, or curettes. Other techniques include the use of monopolar or bipolar cautery, radiofrequency ablation, harmonic scalpel, carbon dioxide laser, and microdebrider coblation. The results from numerous studies have been compared to determine the superiority of a specific method that decreases postoperative pain and the incidence of postoperative bleeding risks. Presently, there is no conclusive data to support an advantage of a distinct technique. Therefore, the surgeon's preference remains the major determinant of the instruments and methods that are used during tonsillectomy.

Table 1-1 Relative and Absolute Indications for Tonsillectomy	
RELATIVE INDICATIONS	**ABSOLUTE INDICATIONS**
Recurrent tonsillitis	Adenotonsillar hypertrophy resulting in obstructive sleep apnea syndrome
Recurrent peritonsillar abscess	High suspicion of malignancy
	Recurrent hemorrhagic tonsillitis

ANESTHETIC MANAGEMENT AND CONSIDERATIONS

Preoperative Period

1. Describe the important elements of the preoperative evaluation for a tonsillectomy.
Preoperative evaluation for the patient undergoing a tonsillectomy depends on physical assessment and history. Upper respiratory tract infections (URI) are commonly associated with patients who present with chronic tonsillitis, recurrent tonsillitis, or a peritonsillar abscess. This may result in airway hyperactivity and potentially increase the incidence of perioperative laryngospasm. Depending on severity of URI symptoms, surgery may be postponed approximately 7–14 days until its resolution. There is controversy whether a URI in pediatric patients increases the incidence of adverse airway reactions during anesthesia.

Adult patients who have tonsillar enlargement may display signs of obstructive sleep apnea (OSA). If OSA is severe, further diagnostic studies are warranted, such as an electrocardiogram and chest radiograph, in order to determine if cardiac involvement exists. An oral examination may reveal that the tonsils encroach on airway structures which can potentially cause difficulty with mask ventilation and/or direct laryngoscopy. Patients having a tonsillectomy should be asked if they have bleeding disorders/tendencies. Evaluating a complete blood count, prothrombin time, and/or activated partial thromboplastin times is justified if there is a reason to believe that a coagulopathy is present. Patients with coexisting medical conditions and facial abnormalities, specifically Down syndrome (trisomy 21) and Treacher Collins syndrome, are of concern due to the increased risk of airway obstruction, difficult intubation, and presence of coexisting disease states.

2. Explain the blood supply and the sensory innervation of the palatine tonsils.
The blood flow to palatine tonsils arises via the external carotid and its branches: ascending pharyngeal artery, facial artery, dorsal lingual artery, and palatine branch of the maxillary artery. Sensory innervation to the palatine tonsils is supplied by the glossopharyngeal and lesser palatine nerves.

3. Discuss premedication for a patient having a tonsillectomy.
Premedication for a child undergoing tonsillectomy should be aimed at decreasing anxiety and providing analgesia. Depending on the child's age and cooperation, an oral anxiolytic (most frequently midazolam) may be administered 30 minutes prior to surgery to alleviate anxiety and to provide sedation. Premedication should be administered sparingly or not at all for patients who have a history of obstructive sleep apnea, facial anomalies, or anticipated difficult mask ventilation and/or intubation. Postoperative analgesia can also be initiated preoperatively by administering rectal or oral analgesic medication (acetaminophen). Lastly, an antisialagogue may be considered to assist with drying of secretions in the pharynx during the intraoperative period, to improve visualization of oral structures due to a decrease in the amount of secretions, and to inhibit vagotonic reflexes.

Intraoperative Period

4. Discuss anesthetic considerations regarding positioning for a tonsillectomy.
Patients are positioned supine with shoulders elevated (with a rolled towel), and head extended. Over extension of the neck may cause postoperative neck pain and can potentially result in atlantoaxial subluxation and displacement of the C1–C2 vertebrae. The head of the operating table is most frequently turned 90 degrees away from the anesthetist. A mouth gag is inserted by the surgeon to open and suspend the mouth for visualization. Special attention to the airway during insertion, positioning, and removal of the mouth gag is imperative as the endotracheal tube may become kinked, dislodged, or inadvertently advanced into the right main stem bronchus. Figure 1-1 depicts a mouth gag and its relationship to the endotracheal tube.

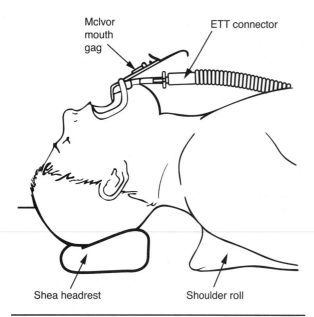

Figure 1-1 *Representation of patient position for tonsillectomy.*

5. Discuss the type of anesthesia most often administered during a tonsillar resection.

General anesthesia with an endotracheal tube is the optimal technique and airway management strategy for a tonsillectomy. The type of anesthetic induction is dependent on the cooperation of the child. If intravenous access is accomplished, then an intravenous induction can be initiated. Otherwise, an inhalation induction is acceptable for most patients and intravenous access is established after the patient loses consciousness and an adequate depth of anesthesia is achieved. The intraoperative goals are to ensure unconsciousness, inhibit sympathetic reflexes, obtund oropharyngeal reflexes during direct laryngoscopy and placement of the oral gag, and prevention of patient movement during the surgical procedure. These objectives can be achieved by administering inhalation agents alone or in combination with neuromuscular blocking agents, propofol, and/or opioids. Unfortunately, upon induction of anesthesia, relaxation of the pharyngeal muscles and tissues may cause airway obstruction in those patients who present with facial anomalies, severe tonsillar hypertrophy, and other medical conditions, resulting in partial or complete airway obstruction.

6. Discuss the intraoperative anesthetic management during a tonsillectomy.

The average surgical time required for a tonsillectomy is approximately 30 minutes. Even though this is a short procedure, a high degree of physiologic stimulation occurs due to manipulation of the airway and removal of the tonsils. Therefore, a deeper plane of anesthesia is required to adequately blunt the sympathetic reflexes that may elicit hypertension, tachycardia, and arrhythmias. This can be accomplished by increasing the inhalation agent alone or in combination with propofol and/or narcotics. Hypertension will also increase the volume of blood loss.

Figure 1-2 *View of hypertrophied tonsils and surgical resection of the tonsils.*

7. During surgical manipulation of the mouth gag, the anesthesia machine alarms "low tidal volume." What action(s) should be taken by the anesthetist?

A diagnosis to confirm or exclude the potential causes of the situation is essential.

The following information is gathered during the assessment of the problem.

- Assessment of bilateral, equal, and clear breath sounds: no breath sounds present
- Assessment of chest rise and fall: no chest rise and fall present
- Assessment of end tidal carbon dioxide ($ETCO_2$): no $ETCO_2$ present
- Assessment of anesthesia bag compliance: no compliance present, large air leak present with bag ventilation
- Assessment of tidal volume: no tidal volume present
- Assessment of the depth of the endotracheal tube (ETT): The ETT was placed at a depth of 17 cm after intubation and breath sounds were bilaterally equal and clear. The ETT depth is currently at 12 cm.
- The anesthetist smells the odor of inhalation anesthetic agent

The anesthetist has determined that the patient has been inadvertently extubated.

The anesthetist should immediately ensure mask ventilation with 100% oxygen and prepare for reintubation. Since the operating room table is positioned 90 degrees away from the anesthetist, the anesthetist will initially maintain the mask seal while a second provider ventilates the patient, while the table is repositioned. After assurance of adequate mask ventilation, the anesthetist can deepen the patient with inhalation agent and/or an intravenous induction agent to help attenuate the sympathetic effects associated with direct laryngoscopy.

8. Discuss the prophylactic treatment strategies used to decrease the incidence of postoperative nausea and vomiting.

Patients having a tonsillectomy are at increased risk for postoperative nausea and vomiting due to the ingestion of blood that occurs during excision. The administration of serotonin antagonists (ondansetron or dolasetron) and/or corticosteroids (dexamethasone) have been shown to alleviate nausea and vomiting postoperatively. Even though dexamethasone has the added benefit of reducing swelling and inflammation in the region of the surgical site, controversy exists as to the anti-inflammatory benefits and increased susceptibility to postoperative hemorrhage due to poor wound healing.

9. Discuss the anesthetic management for emergence.

In preparing for emergence, gentle suctioning of blood and secretions from the mouth and oropharynx minimizes laryngospasm with extubation. Suctioning is preferably accomplished while the patient is in a deep plane of anesthesia. The main goal for emergence is to minimize bucking, coughing, or straining of the patient in order to reduce postsurgical bleeding.

The most commonly utilized emergence technique is to extubate the patient when fully awake and the protective airway reflexes are intact. A smooth emergence can also be accomplished with a deep extubation. Lidocaine 1 ml/kg can be administered 60–90 seconds prior to extubation to attenuate the airway responses while maintaining spontaneous respirations. The disadvantage in performing a deep extubation is that there is the potential for aspiration due to obtunded protective airway reflexes. Also, a deep extubation is not recommended in those patients that were difficult to ventilate or intubate or those with facial anomalies.

Postoperative

10. Discuss the most serious complication associated with tonsillectomy.

The most serious complication associated with tonsillectomy is postoperative hemorrhage. Posttonsillectomy bleeding occurs in 0.1–3% of patients and 75% of those patients hemorrhage within 6 hours postoperatively. The remaining 25% have bleeding 24 hours after surgery and up to 6 days postoperatively. Posttonsillectomy bleeding occurs insidiously due to oozing of the tonsillar bed site; an immeasurable large amount of blood can be swallowed. Often, signs of hypovolemia such as tachycardia and hypotension are evidence of posttonsillectomy hemorrhage. Other postoperative complications regarding tonsillectomy are summarized in Table 1-2.

11. Explain the anesthetic management of the patient with a posttonsillectomy hemorrhage.
If attempts are made to maintain hemostasis by nonsurgical means (with pharyngeal packs) have failed, the patient will return to the operating room for exploration of the site and surgical control of bleeding. The initial concern for the anesthetist should focus on restoring intravascular volume in those patients exhibiting signs of hypovolemia. Intravenous access should be obtained and hydration given prior to induction. A hemoglobin and hematocrit count is warranted for patients with immeasurable blood loss as well as a type and screen with the possibility of blood transfusion. These patients are considered to have a full stomach due to the blood that they have swallowed. Therefore, a rapid sequence intubation with cricoid pressure is recommended. However, in patients with difficult airways or facial anomalies, an awake fiberoptic intubation (to maintain airway reflexes) is an alternative method.

12. Discuss the postoperative pain management for tonsillectomy.
Postoperative tonsillectomy is associated with a high incidence of pain. Unrelieved posttonsillectomy

Table 1-2   Postoperative Complications Associated with a Tonsillectomy

- Hemorrhage
- Infection
- Dehydration
- Aspiration of blood/mucus
- Airway obstruction due to:
    1. Retained throat pack
    2. Laryngospasm
    3. Bronchospasm
    4. Edema of the uvula
    5. Hematoma
- Pulmonary edema
- Glossopharyngeal nerve injury
- Subcutaneous emphysema
- Pneumomediastinum
- Pneumothorax
- Atlantoaxial subluxation
- Nasopharyngeal stenosis (more common with adenotonsillectomy)
- Velopharyngeal insufficiency (VPI; more common with adenoidectomy)

pain may result in a prolonged recovery and subsequent hospitalization due to dehydration from limited oral intake. Strategies that can be used to relieve postoperative pain include local infiltration of local anesthetics and administering opioid analgesics, nonsteroidal anti-inflammatory drugs (NSAIDs), antibiotics, and *N*-methyl-D-aspartate (NMDA) receptor antagonists (ketamine). NSAIDs such as ibuprofen and ketorolac are effective analgesics; however, their use in treating posttonsillectomy pain are controversial due to their potential for increasing risk of bleeding. Commonly, severe pain is treated with intravenous opioid analgesics (fentanyl, hydromorphone, or morphine). Unfortunately, nausea, vomiting, and respiratory depression are common side effects following opioid administration.

Once patients are able to drink liquids postoperatively, moderate to severe posttonsillectomy pain can be treated with oral opioid analgesics (codeine or oxycodone) or an oral opioid combined with acetaminophen. This regimen is routinely started in the recovery room prior to discharge and it is the most common practice of pain management posttonsillectomy.

The administration of local anesthesia (bupivacaine or lidocaine) may be injected in the peritonsillar fossas at the end of the surgical procedure to alleviate posttonsillectomy pain. The risks that are associated with localization of the peritonsillar fossa include loss of pharyngeal reflexes and intravascular injection.

Other adjuvant medication that may decrease posttonsillectomy pain includes antibiotics. It is believed that after tonsillectomy the exposed tonsillar fossas allow oral bacterial flora to colonize, causing a severe localized inflammatory reaction resulting in pain.

The NMDA antagonist ketamine, when administered at a subanesthetic dose (0.2–0.5 mg/kg intravenous), has been used to decrease postoperative analgesic requirements and postoperative pain. Ketamine is not routinely used prophylactically for posttonsillectomy pain because it can cause emergence delirium. Ketamine is advantageous because it does not depress laryngeal protective reflexes or respirations. However, it does increase salivary gland production, and an anticholinergic (glycopyrrolate) should be administered in conjunction with ketamine to decrease oropharyngeal secretions.

REVIEW QUESTIONS

1. Bacterial tonsillitis is most commonly caused by:
   a. influenza A.
   b. Epstein–Barr.
   c. group B streptococci.
   d. group A beta-hemolytic streptococci.
2. The initial concern for a patient with posttonsillectomy hemorrhage includes:
   a. obtaining a hemoglobin and hematocrit.
   b. administering of an antiemetic medication.
   c. fluid administration.
   d. preparing for an awake fiberoptic intubation.
3. The primary intraoperative goal for a patient having a tonsillectomy is to:
   a. obtund oropharyngeal reflexes and to prevent patient movement.
   b. maintain a light plane of anesthesia.
   c. prevent kinking of the endotracheal tube by hyperextension of the patient's head.
   d. administer an antiemetic prophylactically.
4. An absolute indication for tonsillectomy includes:
   a. recurrent hemorrhagic tonsillitis.
   b. recurrent tonsillitis.
   c. recurrent peritonsillar abscess.
   d. recurrent otitis media.
5. Which postoperative pain medication has been associated with increased bleeding when repeated doses are administered?
   a. Fentanyl
   b. Acetaminophen with codeine
   c. Ketamine
   d. Ketorolac

REVIEW ANSWERS

1. **Answer: d**
   Bacterial tonsillitis is most commonly caused by group A beta-hemolytic streptococci.

2. **Answer: c**
   Fluid administration is the initial concern with a patient presenting with posttonsillectomy hemorrhage. Patients often present with hypovolemia due to the immeasurable amount of blood that has been oozing from the tonsillar bed site.

3. **Answer: a**
   The primary goal of intraoperative management during a tonsillectomy is to obtund the oropharyngeal reflexes and to prevent patient movement. Tonsillectomy is very stimulating; therefore, a deep plane of anesthesia must be maintained in order to prevent patient movement during the surgical procedure.

4. **Answer: a**
   An absolute indication for a tonsillectomy is recurrent hemorrhagic tonsillitis. Recurrent bleeding from prominent vessels of the tonsils or from the parenchyma due to recurrent tonsillitis or tonsillar hyperplasia can result in anemia and is indication for tonsillectomy.

5. **Answer: d**
   Ketorolac, an NSAID, inhibits platelet aggregation, thereby potentially increasing the risk of bleeding. The potential for bleeding is increased when subsequent doses are administered.

SUGGESTED READINGS

Aydin O, Ozgun S, Eyigor H, Copcu O. Pain with intraoperative ketamine in outpatient children undergoing tonsillectomy or tonsillectomy and adenotomy. *J Clin Anesth* 2007;19:115–119.

Clark GD, Stone JA. Anesthesia for ears, nose, throat, and maxillofacial surgery. In: Nagelhout JJ, Plaus KL eds. *Nurse Anaesthesia,* 3rd ed. St. Louis, MO: Elsevier Saunders, 2005:872–874.

Discolo CM, Darrow DH, Koltai PJ. Infectious indications for tonsillectomy. *Pediatr Clin North Am* 2003;50: 445–458.

Gigante J. Tonsillectomy and adenoidectomy. *Pediatrics in Review* 2005;26(6):199–203.

Levin B, Sacks R. Post-tonsillectomy bleeding. *Otolaryngology Head and Neck Surgery* 2007:136;S56–S58.

Piltcher OB, Scarton FB. Antibiotic use in tonsillectomies: therapeutic or prophylactic? Required or excessive? *Brazilian Journal of Otorhinolaryngology* 2005;71(5);686–690.

Pop RS, Manworren RC, Guzzetta CE et al. Perianesthesia nurses' pain management after tonsillectomy and adenoidectomy: pediatric patient outcomes. *J PeriAnesth Nurs* 2007;22(2):91–101.

Schmidt R, Herzog A, Cook S, et al. Complications of tonsillectomy. *Archives Otolaryngology Head and Surgery* 2007;133(9):925–928.

Tsui B, Wagner A, Cave D, et al. The incidence of laryngospasm with a "no touch" extubation technique after tonsillectomy and adenoidectomy. *Anesth Analg* 2004;98:327–329.

Walker P, Gillies D. Post-tonsillectomy hemorrhage rates: are they technique-dependent? *Otolaryngology Head and Neck Surgery* 2007;136:S27–S31.

Radical Neck Dissection

Yoo Eun Emily Hwang

2

KEY POINTS

- Lymph node metastasis reduces the survival rate of patients with squamous cell carcinoma by half, and the survival rate is less than 5% in patients who previously underwent surgery and have a recurrent metastasis in the neck.
- The greatest risk in an RND is damage to nerves, muscles, and veins in the neck.
- The outcome of neck dissection depends on the stage of cancer, type of metastasis, and quality of the surgery.
- Patients undergoing RND often present with difficult airway management challenges. Physical examination before the surgery may reveal minor or even no distortions to the airway. A meticulous airway examination must be performed, and any abnormal findings should heighten the concern for difficult ventilation and intubation.
- Assurance of adequate analgesia is essential, as RND procedures are performed on highly reflexogenic areas. An opioid-based technique may increase intraoperative hemodynamic stability and reliably blunt the physiologic reaction to the endotracheal tube (ETT).
- A timely and smooth anesthetic emergence must be accompanied by hemodynamic stability and enables the anesthetist to assess the presence of neurologic deficits.
- Antihypertensive medications may be warranted in order to avoid postoperative hemorrhage and to minimize hemodynamic variability.

CASE SYNOPSIS

A 75-year-old man had been diagnosed with squamous cell carcinoma of the neck and suspected lymph node metastasis. Four years after undergoing a left RND and radiation therapy, the patient presents with a recurrence of the cancer. He is scheduled by his otolaryngologist to have a right RND procedure.

PREOPERATIVE EVALUATION AND DEMOGRAPHIC DATA

Past Medical/Surgical History

- Tobacco smoking with 50 pack/year history
- Hypertension
- Left-sided RND and radiation therapy for squamous cell carcinoma of the neck 4 years prior to surgery

List of Medications

- Hydrochlorothiazide

Diagnostic Data

- Hemoglobin, 11.1 g/dl; hematocrit, 33.2%
- Electrolytes: sodium, 139 mEq/l; potassium, 4.5 mEq/l; chloride, 106 mEq/l

Height/Weight/Vital Signs

- 170 cm, 70 kg
- Blood pressure, 130/81; heart rate, 61 beats per minute; respiratory rate, 14 breaths per minute; temperature 36.8°C; room air oxygen saturation, 97%
- Electrocardiogram (ECG): normal sinus rhythm, 62 beats per minute, no abnormalities

PATHOPHYSIOLOGY

Squamous cell carcinoma can invade the upper aerodigestive tract resulting from dysfunction in cellular proliferation and differentiation. The primary sites most commonly involved include the mucosal areas of the upper aerodigestive tract, particularly the larynx, oropharynx, hypopharynx, and oral cavity. Metastasis into the regional lymph nodes and vascular channel invasion can occur and seed other parenchymal sites if tumor invasion is not controlled at the lymphatic level. The most likely sites for metastasis to occur include the lungs, liver, bone, brain, and adjacent as well as other sites, depending on the tumor histology.

Furthermore, the most important prognostic factor in patients with squamous cell carcinoma of the head and neck is the status of the neck nodes. The extent of cervical lymphadenopathy is also the strongest and most dominant predictor for the overall prognosis, rate of recurrence, and potential for metastasis in head and neck squamous cell carcinoma. Lymph node metastasis reduces the survival rate of patients with squamous cell carcinoma by half, and the survival rate is less than 5% in patients who previously underwent surgery and develop a recurrent metastasis in the neck.

The risk of lymph node involvement by metastasis varies depending on the site of origin, the size of the primary tumor, the histologic grade of the primary tumor, perineural and perivascular invasion, and extracapsular spread. Poorly differentiated tumors at the primary site are also more aggressive and associated with a higher risk of neck metastasis. Moreover, the prognosis is poor when multiple levels of neck nodes are involved. The cervical lymph nodes are divided into superficial and deep chains. Superficial lymph nodes are involved in a late stage of cancer; therefore, they have less oncologic importance. Deep cervical lymph nodes receive drainage from areas of the oral cavity, pharynx, larynx, salivary glands, thyroid, and skin of the head and neck. These deep cervical lymph nodes accompany the internal jugular (IJ) vein and its branches. The greater number of lymph nodes that are involved (greater than four) results in a decreased rate of survival. In addition, posterior triangle and contralateral involvement and node fixation to the carotid artery or a muscle are indications of poor prognosis.

The degree and invasiveness related to the disease process must be discussed collaboratively with the surgeons because the type, size, location, and the presence of impingement on other anatomic structures will influence the anesthetic management. Advances in surgical techniques, radiation therapy, and chemotherapy have allowed for more aggressive treatment of advanced head and neck cancers. Current therapeutic trends attempt to preserve organ function using either primary radiotherapy, or concurrent chemotherapy and radiotherapy with surgery reserved for oncologic salvage. The outcome of an RND is dependent on the stage of cancer, type of metastasis, and quality of the surgery. Advanced deeply attached neck metastasis, recurrence after radiation or chemoradiation, and metastatic neck abscess pose several technical challenges for the head and neck surgeon in the salvage operation. Conversely, no single standardized treatment for cervical metastasis exists. It has been observed repeatedly that management of the same medical or surgical condition varies enormously between physician, institution, and even geographic region, often without evidence of better outcomes.

SURGICAL PROCEDURE

An RND is performed for the surgical control of metastatic neck disease in patients with squamous cell carcinomas of the upper aerodigestive tract, salivary gland tumors, and skin cancer of the head and neck. Surgical time averages 1.5 to 3 hours for primary resection and 3 to 6 hours for reconstruction. The resection consists of a complete cervical lymphadenectomy, together with resection of the sternocleidomastoid muscle, the IJ vein, the spinal accessory nerve (cranial nerve XI), and the submandibular gland. In attempting to remove as much cancerous tissue as possible, much of the local lymphatic system and some muscles, arteries, veins, and glands are removed.

Neck dissections are seldom performed as isolated surgical procedures and are frequently combined with resection of the primary lesion, which may involve the tongue, pharynx, larynx, etc. As depicted in Figure 2-1, an apron incision is made along the posterior border of the sternocleidomastoid muscle, curving medially above the clavicles and extending to the contralateral side. Transection of the sternocleidomastoid muscle at its sternal attachment occurs and the IJ vein is isolated, cut, and tied. The inferior portion of the dissection includes the identification and preservation of the carotid arteries, the vagus nerve, the hypoglossal nerve, the brachial plexus, and the phrenic nerve. As the dissection specimen is swept superiorly, the cervical sensory branches are divided.

In order to maximize oncologic efficacy and to minimize morbidity, modifications to the classic neck dissection occur. One such modification is the preservation of one or more nonlymphatic structures (e.g., spinal accessory nerve, IJ vein, sternocleidomastoid muscle). The spinal accessory nerve (cranial nerve XI), the hypoglossal nerve (cranial nerve XII), and the lingual nerve are preserved. The defect is closed either primarily, with a split-thickness skin graft, or with a chest flap (pectoralis major or deltopectoral). More recently, free flaps may be created for closure and revascularized using the facial artery or superior thyroid artery.

Figure 2-1 *Apron incision along the posterior border of the sternocleidomastoid muscle, curving medially above the clavicles and extending to the contralateral side. (See Color Plate.)*

Figure 2-2   *A modified neck dissection. (See Color Plate.)*

Although common in the 1950s and 1960s, simultaneous bilateral neck dissections are rarely done because of the associated complications, including facial edema, laryngeal edema, blindness, and cerebral edema stemming from the removal of both IJ veins. The operation should not be performed if the cancer has spread beyond the head and neck region, when surgery will not control the primary tumor, or if the cancer invaded the bones of the cervical vertebrae or skull. This is particularly true when invasive cancers such as squamous cell carcinoma, a slow-growing malignant tumor with cells of a distinctive shape, are involved. A modified neck dissection removes less tissue, and a selective neck dissection even less as is shown in Figure 2-2. Depending on the extent of the cancer, these variations on neck dissections exist as depicted in Table 2-1.

Table 2-1 Types of Neck Dissection	
Radical neck dissection	• Tissue is removed from an area in front of the trapezius muscle at the side of the neck. Included in this tissue, which extends from the clavicle inferiorly to the mandible superiorly, are dozens of lymph nodes.
	• The submandibular gland, sternocleidomastoid muscle, internal jugular vein, and spinal accessory nerve are also removed.
Modified radical neck dissection	• Refers to anything that is less than a radical neck dissection.
	• The sternocleidomastoid muscle, jugular vein, spinal accessory nerve, or even all three structures can be safely preserved.
Selective neck dissection	• Preservation of the sternocleidomastoid muscle, the spinal accessory nerve, and the jugular vein.
	• Removes less extensive amounts of lymph nodes and surrounding tissue.

ANESTHETIC MANAGEMENT AND CONSIDERATIONS

Preoperative Period

1. Describe the patient population who may likely present for an RND procedure.

Tumors of the head and neck are most commonly discovered in elderly patients and are frequently associated with tobacco smoking and alcohol consumption. Organ pathology in these patients includes pulmonary and hepatic dysfunction respectively. The presentation of a patient for an RND procedure often includes a high incidence of coronary artery disease, hypertension, bronchitis, pulmonary emphysema, chronic renal insufficiency, and chronic obstructive pulmonary disease. If the tumor interferes with the person's ability to eat, then weight loss, malnutrition, anemia, dehydration, and electrolyte imbalance can be significant. Thus, a careful history and physical must be performed to assure that no current exacerbations of preoperative morbidities exist and the patient's functional status is optimized.

2. Discuss the lab studies, imaging techniques, and other tests completed in order to collect appropriate data for patients presenting for an RND.

- *Laboratory studies*: In cases of malignancy or chronic disease, anemia or coagulopathies may be present. Therefore, a complete blood count with differential and coagulation studies are useful tests, as patients with advanced cancers of the head and neck may present with preexisting anemia. Prothrombin time (PT), activated partial thromboplastin time (aPTT), and international normalized ratio (INR) measures are also especially important in patients with preexisting bleeding diathesis, with hepatitis, or who are on anticoagulation drug therapy. Furthermore, many patients present with other medical problems or take medications that affect their electrolyte status. Squamous cell carcinoma may cause paraneoplastic syndromes; most

commonly syndrome of inappropriate secretions of antidiuretic hormone (SIADH). In addition, liver function tests, glucose tests, BUN, and creatinine testing are useful. Moreover, a blood type and screen may be beneficial. Although refinements in the surgical techniques has significantly reduced blood loss in these procedures, either typing and screening or typing and cross-matching for two units of packed red blood cells are necessary in situations in which blood loss is expected to be significant.

- *Imaging techniques*: Imaging is an integral part of clinical diagnosis and staging, and the results are helpful in deciding treatment. Extensive tests are done before the operation to try to determine the location and the degree of metastasis. Among these techniques are computed tomography (CT) scanning, magnetic resonance imaging (MRI), lymph node biopsies, and barium swallows. CT scanning and MRI scanning provides information as to the presence of lymph node abnormalities which will help to guide further treatment. This diagnostic data may be crucial in delineating the extent of body structures, deep cervical musculature, and carotid artery circumferential involvement. MRI reveals tumor necrosis and extracapsular spread of the nodal capsule with less precision than CT scan, but MRI is better for assessing enlarged lymph nodes that are not metastatic. Some institutions also use ultrasonography and ultrasound-guided aspiration cytology to determine if metastasis to the cervical region of the neck has occurred. Further, positron emission tomography (PET) has recently emerged as an adjunct in the diagnosis of lymph node metastasis. Providing information about the metabolic activity of the tissues, PET scanning has shown the ability to differentiate active tumors from chronic fibrotic changes. Thus, PET scan results can provide early diagnosis of recurrent head and neck cancer, as well as indicate the status of the neck after chemoradiotherapy.

- *Histologic examination*: The standard to detect lymph node metastasis in the neck is the histologic examination of all nodes. Biopsies of the primary site reveal the etiology of the initial mass and the characteristics of the tumor involved, such as squamous cell carcinoma of the upper aerodigestive tract, nasopharyngeal carcinoma, thyroid carcinomas, and skin cancer of the head and neck. Fine needle aspiration cytology of the neck confirms the pathologic conclusions of the primary tumor. Detection and accurate staging of neck metastasis are extremely important because staging has major implications for prognosis and treatment.

- *Balloon occlusion test*: Since the development of newer surgical procedures minimizing surgical morbidity, the treatment of patients undergoing carotid vessel management remains controversial. Many have advocated for preoperative evaluation of these patients by a balloon occlusion test which includes a balloon occlusion test and a four vessel cerebral angiography to evaluate the status of the contralateral carotid, intracerebral circulation, and carotid back pressure.

  Patients who are able to tolerate the occlusion of the ipsilateral carotid artery without any evidence of neurologic dysfunction may be candidates for carotid resection Further, if tumor involvement of the carotid artery is possible, a complete preoperative evaluation assessing the patency of the carotid arteries is indicated.

- *Miscellaneous tests*: A chest radiograph may be performed to exclude metastatic disease. A complete physical examination is mandatory and includes evaluation of neurologic, cardiovascular, and respiratory status. A thorough airway assessment includes palpation of the patient's neck to define size, location, mobility, and degree of softness or hardness of any mass. An ECG is also performed as determined by the patient's condition. A preoperative arterial blood gas analysis in patients with advanced chronic obstructive pulmonary disease, carbon dioxide retention, and oxygen dependence is indicated. Pulmonary flow-volume loops may also be helpful in patients with symptoms associated with obstructive lung disease.

3. Discuss the physical examination and findings that should be noted on the patient's record before performing surgery.

- Physical examination of the head and neck and the findings should be noted. Evaluation of the airway and dentition is essential. A meticulous airway examination must be performed, and any abnormal findings should heighten the concern for difficult ventilation and intubation.
- Medical history (e.g., hypertension, diabetes, cardiopulmonary disease, and other chronic illnesses; previous surgeries; radiation therapy). A thorough assessment of cardiac risk factors and functional status, identification of asymptomatic carotid bruits or existing carotid artery stenosis, and assessment of neurovascular integrity is vital.
- All diagnostic data including those from imaging studies.

4. Describe the importance of the airway examination and specific concerns with airway planning and management in the patient presenting for RND.

Patients undergoing RND often present with the potential for difficult airway. The preoperative physical examination may not reveal the presence of a significant neck mass or other tracheal abnormality. The anesthetist should evaluate the ability of the patient to open the mouth adequately for intubation, reports of airway edema, indications of difficulty with breathing, evidence of tracheal deviation, or changes in the quality of his voice. A history of stridor and hoarseness suggests airway narrowing and possible vocal cord dysfunction. Further, patients with head and neck cancer often have had previous surgery or radiation therapy, and these treatments may further complicate airway management by significantly decreasing tissue compliance.

Radiation therapy alters tissue structure and diminishes the flexibility of native tissues. The cervical spine range of motion may be limited due to prior surgery and radiation scarring. Prior radiation therapy may cause extensive fibrosis of tissues, increased intraoperative bleeding, and ankylosis of the temporomandibular joint, rendering tracheal intubation extremely difficult or impossible.

One must diagnose alterations in the anatomy of the upper airway because of a tumor. Inflammatory or neoplastic growths of the upper aerodigestive tract can occur anywhere within the airway and may achieve significant size with little evidence of airway penetration or obstruction. In 15% of these patients, a metastatic neck mass is present without a distinct primary lesion. These tumors may cause fixation of tissues secondary to expansion and are often fragile and bleed readily even during atraumatic airway management maneuvers. Thus, issues of the pathology must be discussed through effective communication and collaboration with the surgeon. Consultation with a surgeon as to parameters, such as the type, nature, extent, and location of the tumor, potential bleeding, together with the review of appropriate radiographs and prior therapy administered (e.g., radiation or chemotherapy), has a strong influence on outcome and remains important in determining techniques for airway management.

Multiple plans must be devised to decrease the possibility of a "failed airway." The anesthetist must have experience with the alternative airway management techniques and devices Establishing a sequence of interventions is also imperative.

- Extra-glottic device: Laryngeal mask airway
- Fiberoptic devices: GlideScope (Verathon, Bothell, WA), adult fiberoptic scope
- Surgical airway options: Cricothyrotomy, tracheostomy
- A rigid ventilating bronchoscope should be present and assembled.

Prevention and planning prior to induction are mandatory. If the anesthetist decides to proceed with the conventional means of securing the airway by performing an orotracheal intubation, the patient's head positioning should be optimized carefully, and intubating aids (e.g., stylets, gum elastic bougie), as well as ETTs of different sizes, should be available. If a difficult intubation is foreseen, an awake fiberoptic intubation or tracheostomy under local anesthesia before induction of general anesthesia may be the necessary technique.

Additional considerations include that the patient's airway and operative field is not only shared with the surgeon, but immediate access to the airway is difficult because the patient is turned 180 degrees away from the anesthetist as shown in Figure 2-3. Further, the ETT must be secured, and its positioning should be monitored carefully during surgery to avoid supraglottic of endobronchial migration. Nasal intubation may be desirable to facilitate surgical access, and a surgeon should be consulted. In the difficult airway, good communication and understanding between the surgeon and the anesthetist is a priority.

5. Explain the anesthetic concerns associated with patients who have had a previous RND.

Although operation for head and neck cancers carry an increased likelihood for airway obstruction immediately after surgery, this complication can occur after RND and during surgery for another reason. Bilateral RND, even when staged over a period of years, may pose a significant risk to the patient. For patients with previous neck dissection, lymphatic drainage patterns are altered, creating the potential for postoperative edema. This diminishes the ability of tissues within the larynx to tolerate an iatrogenically induced insult that produces edema and swelling, thereby placing this patient at a heightened risk for postoperative airway compromise. Therefore, significant postoperative laryngeal edema and neuronal imbalance may ensue, necessitating a tracheostomy.

In addition, one cause of delayed awakening and failure to breathe is associated with cephalic venous obstruction (e.g., significant facial edema, facial cyanosis despite normal pulse oximetry reading,

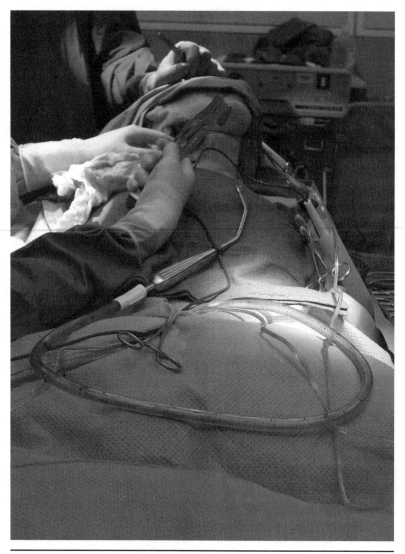

Figure 2-3 *Patient positioning 180 degrees away from the anesthetist. (See Color Plate.)*

rhinorrhea). Cerebral venous congestion may be a result of central apnea secondary to acutely elevated intracranial pressure (ICP). The treatment if this situation were to arise is to employ measures aimed at reducing ICP and to protect cerebral blood flow.

Intraoperative Period

6. Describe the monitoring to be utilized in an RND.

In an RND, the required monitors include standard intraoperative measures, such as ECG, pulse oximetry, end-tidal carbon dioxide monitoring, and body temperature. An arterial line may be indicated in patients with severe cardiopulmonary disease, chronic renal insufficiency, symptoms of cerebrovascular insufficiency, the location of a tumor near the carotid artery, or in patients presenting for lengthy procedures, including any microvascular flap reconstruction. In addition, a nerve integrity monitor may be used by the surgeons to aid in identifying and preserving specific nerves in the neck.

7. Recognize the physiologic considerations associated with patient positioning during RND.
Patients are placed in the supine position with the upper half of the operating table elevated to a 30-degree angle. The head is turned to the opposite side of the surgical site, and a shoulder roll extending the neck is placed. It is important for the anesthetist to ensure that the patient's head is adequately supported and padded in order to avoid hyperextension which can result in postoperative neck discomfort, brachial plexus injury, and pressure sores. The head-up tilt during such procedures is not done simply to improve the surgical field and expedite the procedure, but it is an important measure to ameliorate the effects of jugular venous ligation, increasing the venous return and decreasing blood loss. Thus, elevation of the head should continue into the postoperative period.

8. Discuss relevant nonlymphatic structures in the neck. Investigate the incidence and significance of intraoperative damage to nerves and vasculature in an RND.
The greatest risk associated with RND is damage to nerves, muscles, and veins in the neck. The neck region has multiple sensory nerves that are sacrificed during an RND. Therefore, nerve damage can result in numbness and loss of sensation to different regions on the neck and a temporary or permanent loss of function to multiple parts of the neck, throat, posterior occiput, external ear, mandibular region, lateral shoulder, deltoid area, and upper pectoral area. For instance, it is common following RND for a person to have stooped shoulders, limited ability to lift the arm, and limited head and neck rotation and flexion as a consequence of the removal of nerves and muscles during surgery. Therefore, neuromuscular relaxation must be omitted in order to isolate the nerves and avoid surgical trauma. On occasion, formation of a neuroma at the end of a nerve that has been dissected may cause chronic paresthesias and pain. Sacrifice of the cervical sympathetic chain can produce Horner syndrome, which involves ptosis, anhydrosis, and miosis. The phrenic nerve may also pass into the surgical field, and respiratory problems may develop if diaphragmatic paralysis occurs.

Many arteries and veins are encountered during an RND, including the jugular veins, superior and inferior thyroid artery, and carotid artery. Although the region is highly vascular, major vessel trauma, laceration, tear, or transaction is a rare occurrence. When hemorrhage occurs, the vessel injury is immediately ligated or repaired.

- *Spinal accessory nerve (SAN)*: Surgical trauma to the SAN results in painful "shoulder syndrome." And signs and symptoms include shoulder drop or shrug weakness, limitations in active shoulder abduction or flexion, limited range of motion of the arm, lateral scapular winging at rest, and local pain, typically across the upper border of the trapezius muscle. Since electrophysiologic integrity of the SAN does not completely correlate with clinical outcome measures for "shoulder syndrome," trapezium weakness can occur even when the SAN is preserved.
- *Hypoglossal nerve*: Unilateral resection of the hypoglossal nerve is usually well tolerated without serous sequelae. However, bilateral hypoglossal nerve resection causes serious difficulties with eating, swallowing, and speaking.
- *Facial nerve*: The superficial origin of the facial nerve is located at the level of the tragus of the ear. A small branch of the facial nerve is encountered and preserved when performing a neck dissection. Transection of the marginal mandibular branch of the facial nerve produces lower lip weakness.
- *Vagus nerve*: The vagus nerve in the neck is closely approximated to the carotid sheath and may be injured during the dissection and division of the lower portion of the IJ vein. During RND, dissection around the carotid

bulb or surgical manipulation affecting the carotid sinus may elicit a vagal reflex, inducing profound bradycardia, hypotension, or cardiac arrest. The afferent neural pathway involved with carotid sinus or carotid baroreceptor stimulation involves transmission from the carotid sinus to Hering's nerve to the glossopharyngeal nerve (CN IX) and then to the brain. Parasympathetic nervous system predominance to the heart results from efferent stimulation via the vagus nerve (CN X) which causes vagotonic effects.

The treatment for severe bradycardia or cardiac arrest includes having the surgeon stop carotid sinus manipulation. For persistent severe bradycardia, atropine should be administered. The reflex can also be diminished by injection of local anesthetic in the region of the carotid sinus. Additionally, postoperative hypertension and a loss of hypoxic drive following a bilateral neck dissection may indicate denervation of the carotid sinuses and bodies. The lower or middle neck of the vagus nerve also carries motor and sensory branches to the larynx and pharynx, and resection will cause vocal cord paralysis and sensory dysfunction.

- *Carotid artery*: The carotid artery rarely needs to be resected or reconstructed. In addition, careful dissection around the carotid arterial system in the neck with gentle retraction, ligation, and manipulation may help to prevent the dislodgment of arteriosclerotic plaques from the internal carotid system decreasing the potential for a stroke.
- *Internal jugular vein*: The IJ vein is frequently nonfunctional, either due to invasion or compression resulting in blockage by the mass. Ligation or transfixation-ligation is feasible because drainage is provided by other veins in the neck. However, injury to the IJ veins at the upper or lower ends may cause significant bleeding postoperatively and may

require surgical reintervention. Occasional uncontrollable bleeding requires assistance of a thoracic surgeon to enter the superior mediastinum. Furthermore, major disruptions in venous flow during surgery and venous stasis may result in laryngeal edema and obstruction. Therefore, venous thrombus is commonly seen in patients who are undergoing RND.

- *Venous air embolus*: An air embolism can occur when a large vein in the neck is inadvertently opened. A large volume of air enters rapidly into the open vein by negative pressure and passes directly into the right atrium, causing an airlock at the level of the superior vena cava and the right atrium, leading to decreased or total cessation of blood flow through the heart. Clinically, cyanosis, hypotension, dysrhythmias, a decrease in end-tidal carbon dioxide, an increase in end-tidal nitrogen, ST segment elevation, and a loud churning mill wheel murmur over the precordial area may appear suddenly. If a venous air embolus is suspected, the surgeon must be notified immediately to compress the open neck veins, flood the field with normal saline, and to pack or clamp the offending vein to stop the entrainment of air. The anesthetist must administer 100% oxygen, turn the patient onto the left side with the head down, and provide circulatory support with intravenous fluids and vasopressors, as indicated. In addition, a disappearance of peripheral pulses may indicate cardiac arrest, requiring aspiration of air from the heart via a central venous catheter, cardiac massage, and standard resuscitation procedures.

9. Discuss factors that affect the estimated blood loss during an RND.

The duration of an RND frequently lasts for more than 6 to 8 hours, but the procedure is rarely associated with significant blood loss. Partly due to the benefits of hemostasis with the electrocautery unit or bipolar forceps and the use of clamps and suture ligation, the average estimated blood loss (EBL) is 150 to 200 ml. The total blood loss, however, is highly variable and is related to the patient history and possible events during the procedure. For instance, patient who have had radiation therapy are likely to lose 200 to 400 ml of blood. If a primary tumor is also resected, the EBL may be 400 to 700 ml. Although rare, uncontrolled bleeding of the IJ vein at the skull base can result in a sudden large amount of blood loss, but this can be controlled by the surgeon with digital pressure, allowing the anesthetist to administer fluid or blood as needed.

10. Examine additional considerations and clinical techniques to optimize operating conditions during head and neck surgery.

- *Anesthetic technique*: The anesthesthetic that is provided for a patient who is undergoing RND must be individualized depending on the surgical procedure and the degree of pathophysiology. A balanced technique using intravenous and inhalational agents is commonly used for RND. Maintenance of general anesthesia is frequently includes an inhalational agent blended in air and oxygen. Inspired gases should be humidified to minimize a decrease in temperature and incidence of mucous accumulation. Deep and superficial cervical plexus blocks, as well as a cervical epidural anesthetic, have been used. The doses of anesthetic and hypnotic agents frequently must be reduced due to the patient's age and preexisting medical conditions.
- *Opioid-based technique*: Assurance of adequate intraoperative and postoperative analgesia is an essential anesthesia requirement, as RND procedures are performed on highly reflexogenic areas. Omission of muscle relaxation is necessary in order for the surgeon to assess nerve function during resection. Therefore, an opioid-based technique may be

especially advantageous and is acknowledged to more easily maintain hemodynamic stability, to reliably blunt the patient reaction to the ETT, and to facilitate emergence from anesthesia. Due to the invasive nature of the surgical procedure and the degree of postoperative pain that is experienced, opioids such as fentanyl or sufentanil are ideal choices. A continuous infusion of opioids may offer potential advantages over intermittent boluses, resulting in a decrease in total dose, greater hemodynamic stability, more rapid recovery of consciousness, less pain in the immediate postoperative period, and a decreased time to discharge.

- *Hypotensive anesthesia*: Maintaining relative hypotension (systolic blood pressure 80–100 mm Hg and mean arterial pressure 60–70 mm Hg) reduces blood loss, resulting in faster surgery and less patient morbidity. This controlled decreased blood pressure is widely employed unless contraindicated secondary to concomitant medical conditions such as cardiovascular or neurovascular disease. Deliberate decreased blood pressure can be accomplished by using a variety of anesthetic and sympatholytic agents such as inhaled anesthetics; narcotics; beta-blockers and vasodilators.

11. Analyze the specific concerns related to airway management and emergence from anesthesia following an RND. Compile a list of recommended standard safe practice in order to promote a safe and smooth anesthetic recovery. Airway protection and maintenance is the primary concern for the anesthetist. Most importantly, the patient must have an intact airway, adequate respiratory function, and must be well oxygenated prior to extubation. The recovery of spontaneous ventilation and airway reflexes is required. In addition to standard extubation criteria, patient characteristics that must be considered prior to tracheal extubation following an RND procedure include the patient's preoperative physiologic status and airway assessment and existing comorbidities require a close evaluation. Following a major surgical procedure, the need for a prompt emergence and the patient cooperation with an immediate postoperative neurologic exam is intended to help assess for the presence of a hematoma formation, cerebral ischemia, and nerve injuries. Under these circumstances, residual anesthesia may give the false impression of neurologic deficit. Therefore, the patient must be awake, follow verbal commands, and demonstrate appropriate neurologic function prior to extubation. The patient must be able to sustain spontaneous respirations and maintain normal arterial blood gas values. Additionally, vocal cord inspection prior to anesthetic emergence through laryngoscopy or a fiberoptic scope should prove unremarkable.

The anesthetist must be familiar with the surgeon's preferences, and the surgical procedure that was accomplished prior to extubation. Surgical determinants of requirement for postsurgical mechanical ventilation include the duration and difficulty of surgery and the degree of edema that has developed. Any intraoperative complications, such as swelling, injury to cranial nerves, hematoma formation, ischemia, or bradycardia associated with operative manipulation can have a deleterious effect of the patient's outcome. Airway edema due to retraction, surgical trauma, and intravenous fluid administration can result in postoperative respiratory distress.

Of all patients undergoing general endotracheal anesthesia for RND, 2 to 22% will develop some form of increased laryngeal resistance after extubation. The reduction of airflow results from either anatomic narrowing (e.g., edema) of the glottis (e.g., epiglottis and aryepiglottic folds) or neuronal imbalance of the abductor and adductors of the vocal cords. However, several factors may contribute to laryngeal dysfunction despite an apparently intact vocal cord function. Radiation therapy alters tissue structure and diminishes the flexibility of native tissues. Macroglossia (swelling of the tongue) is a potentially fatal complication of premature extubation. Surgical patients with an unprotected airway are even at greater risk for airway obstruction, hypoxemia, hypercapnia, and aspiration. Reintubation may be impossible, and attempts to secure the airway may cause airway collapse.

A smooth emergence from anesthesia is essential, and every attempt should be made to avoid or minimize the patient's reaction to the ETT. Straining, bucking, coughing, or gagging during emergence will cause an increase in venous pressure that may provoke postoperative bleeding or disruption of delicate suture lines. Prompt emergence and hemodynamic stability are imperative. Excessive bucking or coughing can result in cerebral venous congestion.

Delayed anesthetic recovery has been advocated to limit airway risks linked to awakening from anesthesia. In some patients, elective postoperative ventilation is indicated because of existing neurologic deficits, intraoperative complications, respiratory or hemodynamic alterations, or swelling. By generating a comprehensive list of criteria for early extubation, anesthesia providers can make an educated decision on whether a particular patient would benefit from immediate extubation.

Hematoma formation in the neck most often occurs within the first few hours after surgery has been completed. The mass can impinge upon the trachea and adjacent airway structures and can cause complete airway obstruction. Immediate intervention is necessary and includes the surgeon evacuating the hematoma and achieving hemostasis followed by airway maintenance. Hematoma evacuation is a definitive treatment and must occur expeditiously. The materials, equipment, and ability to perform an emergency tracheostomy are essential.

Strategies that can be used to decrease the possibility of postoperative respiratory distress caused by airway edema include examination of the degree of edema or tracheomalacia using fiberoptic examination, deflating the ETT cuff to determine if a leak occurs during positive pressure ventilation, and inserting a pediatric ETT exchange device and temporarily leaving it in place after tracheal extubation.

An elective tracheostomy may be accomplished prior to the end of surgery, in which the patient may be subject to a reintervention procedure in order to avoid edema. Postoperative sedation and prolonged mechanical ventilation is warranted only in patients with physiologic or pathologic disturbances requiring correction before recovery. This decision is contingent on such prominent factors such as the nature and duration of surgery, the patient's prior physical condition, concurrent respiratory disease, and the degree of edema generated intraoperatively.

12. Recognize the specific physiologic and hemodynamic changes during emergence from anesthesia and tracheal extubation.

Anesthetic drugs which are compatible with the surgical procedure must be selected. If muscle relaxants medications were administered, residual neuromuscular blockade must be completely reversed, anesthetic drugs discontinued, and no further respiratory depressant drugs administered. The incidence of nausea and vomiting following a radical neck dissection is high. Thus, routine antiemetic prophylaxis most commonly is achieved by the intravenous administration of a 5-HT3 blocker.

Postoperative Period

13. List the potential postoperative complications that can occur following RND.

The postoperative complications associated with RND are present in Table 2-2. An RND is associated

Table 2-2   Postoperative Complications Associated with RND

COMPLICATION	PRESENTATION	PREVENTION AND TREATMENT
Hematoma formation	1. A hematoma is usually evident in the first few hours after the operation and is best found with inspection. 2. Blood under the flap accumulates rapidly. 3. If the hematoma is recognized and treated early, no adverse consequences occur. However, if the hematoma is found late, airway compromise, infection, or flap necrosis may occur.	1. Meticulous hemostasis during the surgical procedure is mandatory. 2. Suction drains are used to avoid blood accumulation under the skin flap. Ensure that the Hemovac or drains are functioning properly and maintained on continuous suction until they drain less than 20 ml in 24 hours. 3. With unilateral neck dissections, some surgeons use a floppy, moderately compressive dressing. The disadvantage is that the dressing leaves the flaps unavailable for inspection. 4. Treatment requires urgent reintubation, which comprises taking the patient to the operating room, opening and elevating the neck flaps, and evacuating the hematoma. 5. Any source of bleeding is found, ligated, sutured, or electrocauterized.

(continues)

Table 2-2   Postoperative Complications Associated with RND (continued)

COMPLICATION	PRESENTATION	PREVENTION AND TREATMENT
Facial edema	1. Unilateral RND may result in ipsilateral swelling of the lower face and neck. 2. Bilateral RND performed simultaneously with ligation or resection of both IJ veins results in facial edema, cerebral edema, or both. 3. There is some argument that edema to the face and neck is as much, if not more, a result of lymph stasis as inadequate venous drainage from removal of the IJ vein. 4. Mechanical obstruction of venous drainage and the increase of ICP can cause neurologic deficit and coma. 5. Facial edema commonly appears in patients with previous irradiation and can lead to chemosis. 6. Lid edema may be sufficient to prevent eye opening.	1. Airway management with a tracheotomy is required. 2. Maintain head elevation at a 30-degree angle in order to promote venous drainage.
Electrolyte disturbances	1. Patients undergoing RND are frequently hypovolemic with electrolyte imbalances. 2. The most common electrolyte disturbance is hyponatremia, usually dilutional; however, it may be related to the secretion of antidiuretic hormone. 3. Occasionally, hypernatremia, hypokalemia, hypercalcemia, and hypophosphatemia are also associated with RND.	1. Obtain serum electrolyte values, and correct abnormal values as deemed necessary. 2. Some fluid replacement and electrolyte balance intraoperatively may be required to maintain cardiovascular stability.
Carotid artery rupture	1. The incidence ranges from 3 to 7%. 2. The precipitating factors include radiation therapy, infection, and salivary fistula; suction catheters that cause erosion of the vessel wall; exposure by dehiscence of the suture line or necrosis of the dermis. 3. Most patients have prodromal bleeding (i.e., sentinel bleed) within 48 hours of the carotid rupture.	1. Apply direct, firm pressure to the affected area while the operating room is prepared for neck surgery. 2. Start two large-bore peripheral intravenous catheters for administration of isotonic crystalloid fluids. Controlling blood pressure and blood volume before the ligation is important. 3. The airway should be adequate and stable. If the patient does not undergo a tracheotomy, orotracheal intubation may be necessary.

Table 2-2 Postoperative Complications Associated with RND (continued)

COMPLICATION	PRESENTATION	PREVENTION AND TREATMENT
		4. Type blood and cross-match for 4 to 6 units.
		5. If the bleeding cannot be controlled, emergently clamp the common carotid artery after the blood pressure and pulse are within the reference range.
		6. Definitive treatment includes ligation of the carotid artery with a silk suture that is reinforced distally and proximally.
Hypertension and tachycardia	1. May be secondary to carotid sinus denervation or pain. 2. Up to 10% of patients may develop sustained hypertensive response early postoperatively, increasing the risk of stroke.	1. Treat this aggressively. Consider beta-blockers. 2. Pain management with patient-controlled analgesia and intravenous opiates.
Lymphatic leak via chylous fistula	1. Major lymph channels are encountered at the lower aspect of the neck, especially on the left side. 2. Apply positive pressure to reevaluate if further leaking occurs.	1. Ligating the thoracic duct is mandatory. 2. A return to the OR may be required for repair.
Pneumothorax	1. Involves a sudden compromise of the respiratory and circulatory system and causes difficult breathing, bronchospasm, and a decrease on oxygen saturation. 2. The pressure of the anesthetic bag does not cause normal expansion of the thorax.	1. Listen to bilateral breath sounds. 2. Obtain a chest radiograph. 3. A large pleural leak with a tension pneumothorax requires the immediate aspiration with a no.14 or no.16 needle in the upper anterior thorax and chest tube placement with an underwater drain.

ICP, intracranial pressure; IJ, internal jugular; OR, operating room; RND, radical neck dissection.

with low morbidity and mortality rates; however, associated composite resection and ablation of a large surface of mucosal area adjacent to the neck markedly increases the rate of complications. Other factors, such as poor health, chronic malnutrition, alcoholism, diabetes mellitus, advanced age, systemic illness, and radiation therapy also increases the likelihood for postoperative complications such as wound infection, fistula, flap necrosis, osteoradionecrosis, and carotid artery rupture.

REVIEW QUESTIONS

1. The most important factor that is associated with long term survival in patients with squamous cell carcinoma of the head and neck is:
   a. advanced age of the patient.
   b. positive history of tobacco and alcohol abuse.
   c. prior surgical history of tonsillectomy and adenoidectomy.
   d. status of the neck lymph nodes.

2. Which is the most common electrolyte disturbance that occurs for patients undergoing RND?
   a. Hyponatremia
   b. Hypernatremia
   c. Hyperkalemia
   d. Hyperphosphatemia
3. Shoulder drop or shrug weakness, limited range of motion of the arm and shoulder, scapular winging, and local pain are associated with:
   a. internal jugular vein ligation.
   b. retraction to the sternocleidomastoid muscle.
   c. surgical trauma to the spinal accessory nerve.
   d. vagus nerve compression.
4. Of all patients undergoing general endotracheal anesthesia for RND, _____ percent will develop increased laryngeal resistance after extubation.
   a. 1–2
   b. 2–22
   c. 30–50
   d. 50–75
5. During which period is the formation of a neck hematoma most likely to occur following an RND procedure?
   a. During surgical wound closure
   b. First few hours after the operation
   c. Four to 8 hours postoperatively
   d. Twenty-four hours after the operation

REVIEW ANSWERS

1. **Answer: d**
   Lymphatic metastasis is the most important mechanism of the recurrence, survival rates, and spread of head and neck squamous cell carcinoma from the primary sites. The risk of cervical lymphadenopathy varies depending on the site of origin, the size of the primary tumor, the histologic grade of the primary tumor, perineural invasion, perivascular invasion, and extracapsular spread.

2. **Answer: a**
   The most common electrolyte disturbance for a patient undergoing RND is hyponatremia. This abnormality is usually dilutional. However, a subgroup of squamous cell cancers may result in paraneoplastic syndromes; the most common is the syndrome of inappropriate secretions of antidiuretic hormone (SIADH).

3. **Answer: c**
   Although trapezium weakness can occur even when the spinal accessory nerve is preserved, these collective signs and symptoms are associated with surgical trauma to the spinal accessory nerve, resulting in the shoulder girdle mechanism deformity associated with painful "shoulder syndrome."

4. **Answer: b**
   It is estimated that between 2 and 22% of patients undergoing general endotracheal anesthesia for RND will develop a reduction of airflow postextubation as a result of either anatomic narrowing of the glottis or neuronal imbalance of the abductor and adductors of the vocal cords.

5. **Answer: b**
   A hematoma is usually evident in the first few hours after the RND operation. Since blood under a flap accumulates rapidly, inspection is the best way to assess for hematoma formation.

SUGGESTED READINGS

Burkle CM, Walsh MT, Pryor SG, Kasperbauer JL. Severe postextubation laryngeal obstruction: the role of prior neck dissection and radiation. *Anesth Analg* 2006;102(1):322–325.

Clark GD, Stone JA. Anesthesia for ear, nose, throat, and maxillofacial surgery. In: Nagelhout JJ, Zaglaniczny KL, eds. *Nurse Anesthesia*, 3rd ed. St. Louis, MO: Elsevier Saunders, 2005:858–880.

Craig JR, Power K. Apnoea and delayed emergence following staged bilateral radical neck dissection. *Anaesthesia* 2006;61(9):914–915.

Crosher R, Baldie C, Mitchell R. Selective use of tracheostomy in surgery for head and neck surgery. *Br J Oral Maxillofac Surg* 1997;35:43–45.

Fee WE, Vaughan WC, Roberson JB, et al. Otolaryngology—head and neck surgery. In: Jaffe RA, Samuels SI, eds. *Anesthesiologist's Manual of Surgical Procedures*, 3rd ed. Philadelphia: Lippincott Williams & Wilkins, 2004:140–173.

Ferrari LR, Gotta AW. Anesthesia for otolaryngologic surgery. In: Barash PG, Cullen BG, Stoelting RK, eds. *Clinical* Anesthesia, 5th ed. Philadelphia: Lippincott Williams & Wilkins, 2006:997–1011.

Gendon EM, Ferlito A, Shaha AR. Complications of neck dissection. *Acta Otolaryngology* 2003;123:795–801.

Kido K, Shimoda H, Takahashi, M. Bronchoconstriction induced by carotid sinus stimulation during radical neck dissection. *Anesth Analg* 2005;100:1214–1223.

Magrin J, Kowalski L. Bilateral radical neck dissection: results in 193 cases. *J Surg Oncol* 2000;75:232–240.

Witt RL, Rejto L. Spinal accessory nerve monitoring in selective and modified neck dissection. *Laryngoscope* 2007;117(5):776–780.

Laryngectomy

3

Mark Goelz

KEY POINTS

- Squamous cell carcinoma is the primary cause of laryngeal cancer.
- Tobacco use and alcohol abuse combine to cause the vast majority of laryngeal neoplasms.
- Glottic cancer is the most common form of laryngeal malignancy, followed by supraglottic and subglottic cancer.
- TNM (tumor, node, metastasis) cancer staging largely dictates the form of cancer treatment and surgery.
- Thorough diagnostic information and airway assessment determines whether the patient can be safely intubated or whether the preferred technique for definitive airway management.
- The anesthetist's primary concerns during the intraoperative period are airway protection and massive hemorrhage.

CASE SYNOPSIS

A 62-year-old white man saw his primary care physician with a complaint of hoarseness for the past 2 weeks. The patient was scheduled to have a diagnostic laryngoscopy with an otolaryngologist. It was discovered that the patient has stage II laryngeal cancer. The patient has received preoperative radiation therapy, and he is currently scheduled for a total laryngectomy.

PREOPERATIVE EVALUATION AND DEMOGRAPHIC DATA

Past Medical/Surgical History

- Hypertension
- Chronic obstructive pulmonary disease (COPD)
- History of smoking 2 packs of cigarettes per day for the past 45 years
- Daily alcohol consumption averages 2 to 3 beers
- No past surgical history

List of Medications

- Metoprolol
- Hydrochlorothiazide

Diagnostic Data

- Complete blood count (CBC): white blood cells, 5.5/mm³; hemoglobin, 17g/dl; hematocrit, 51%; platelets, 150,000/mm³
- Electrolytes: sodium, 142 mEq/l; potassium, 4.5 mEq/l; chloride, 102 mEq/l; carbon dioxide, 28 mEq/l; calcium, 9.0 mg/dl; magnesium, 2.0 mEq/l
- Blood urea nitrogen (BUN), 22 mg/dl; creatinine, 0.7 mg/dl
- Liver function tests (LFTs), prothrombin time (PT)/partial thromboplastin time (PTT), and basic metabolic panel (BMP) are normal, revealing no sign of hepatorenal disease
- Electrocardiogram: sinus bradycardia (heart rate, 58 beats per minute) with left atrial enlargement
- Chest x-ray (CXR): mild hyperinflation consistent with emphysema
- Arterial blood gas (ABG), pH 7.36; PaO_2, 95 mm Hg; $PaCO_2$, 45 mm Hg; HCO, 28 mEq/l; O_2 saturation, 99%
- Type and screened for two units blood of packed red blood cells

Height/Weight/Vital Signs

- 180 cm, 81 kg
- Blood pressure, 128/74; heart rate, 62 beats per minute; respiratory rate, 20 breaths per minute; temperature, 36.8°C; room air oxygen saturation, 99%

LARYNGEAL ANATOMY AND PHYSIOLOGY

The larynx performs the following physiologic functions: provides structural support and protection for airway structures. The larynx consists of three unpaired (epiglottis, thyroid, cricoid) and three paired (two arytenoid, two corniculate, and two cuneiform) cartilages. Anatomically, the larynx is divided into three regions: supraglottic, glottic, and subglottic. The supraglottic region encompasses the epiglottis, arytenoids, and false vocal cords. The glottic region consists of the true vocal cords and glottic opening. The subglottic area extends from beneath the glottic opening to the base of the cricoid cartilage.

The cartilaginous bodies of larynx are held together by four different ligaments: the thyrohyoid, cricotracheal, cricothyroid, and hyoepiglottic ligaments. Identification of the cricothyroid membrane is the most important landmark for the anesthetist because it is the site where cricothyroidotomy can be performed.

The muscles of the larynx, which are included in Table 3-1, are divided into the extrinsic and intrinsic muscle groups. The extrinsic muscles shift the larynx upward and downward. The intrinsic muscles are involved in vocal cord tension and relaxation, which is necessary for phonation and extreme exhalation and inhalation.

The recurrent laryngeal nerve and the superior laryngeal nerve supply innervate the airway structures that are housed within the larynx. The recurrent laryngeal nerve provides all sensory innervation below the level of the vocal cords. The internal branch of the superior laryngeal nerve provides sensation the larynx above the vocal cord level. Motor innervation to the larynx is primarily provided by the recurrent laryngeal nerve, except for the cricothyroid muscle, which is supplied by the external branch of the superior laryngeal nerve. Both the recurrent laryngeal nerve and superior laryngeal nerve are branches of the vagus nerve.

The arterial blood supply to the larynx comes from the superior laryngeal artery, derived from the external carotid artery, and the inferior laryngeal artery, which branches from the subclavian artery. Venous return from the larynx occurs via the superior and inferior laryngeal veins.

Table 3-1 Musculature of the Larynx	
EXTRINSIC MUSCLES OF THE LARYNX	**INTRINSIC MUSCLES OF THE LARYNX**
Sternothyroid	Posterior cricoarytenoid
Thyrohyoid	Lateral cricoarytenoid
Inferior constrictor of the pharynx	Interarytenoid Thyroarytenoid Vocalis Cricothyroid

PATHOPHYSIOLOGY

Laryngeal cancer most frequently affects men between 50 and 70 years of age. Laryngeal cancer accounts for 1% of all malignancies and it is the 11th most prevalent carcinoma among men. Men are 10 times more likely to develop this disease as compared to women. Squamous cell cancer accounts for 95% of all laryngeal carcinoma, and the overall incidence of laryngeal neoplasm is 3.7 per 100,000.

There are multiple risk factors that predispose patients to developing laryngeal cancer, and these are listed in Table 3-2. Tobacco use and alcohol

Table 3-2   Risk Factors Associated with Laryngeal Cancer
• Tobacco
• Alcohol
• Environmental exposure (exposure to wood dust, paint fumes, asbestos)
• Viral infection (oncogenic types of human papilloma virus)
• Dietary factors (lack of A and B vitamins)
• Weaken immune system (AIDS)
• Gender (male > female)
• Gastroesophageal reflux disease
• Advanced age (> 50 years old)
• Race (African Americans > Caucasians)

consumption are the two most common etiologies for laryngeal malignancy, accounting for 95% of laryngeal carcinoma. The combination of these two risk factors increases the incidence of laryngeal cancer by 15.5 times.

The assessment of laryngeal malignancy depends primarily on its location and the TNM staging of the tumor. Glottic tumors are the most common and comprise 60% of all laryngeal neoplasms. Additionally, 35% of laryngeal cancers involve the supraglottic structures and 5% invade the subglottic region. The TNM system for cancer staging is defined by the following:

- T is *t*umor size.
- N is lymph *n*ode involvement.
- M is the degree of *m*etastasis.

A complete list of the nomenclature that comprises the TNM staging system is present in Table 3-3.

TREATMENT OPTIONS

Radiation therapy is the primary form of treatment for stage I and stage II laryngeal malignancy. The rate of successful treatment ranges from between 80 to 90% for stage I disease and 70 to 80% for stage II disease. A patient will commonly receive radiation 5 days a week for a 7-week duration.

Chemotherapy, radiation treatments and surgery, are strategies that are commonly utilized to treat patients who have developed advanced stage III or stage IV cancers. Cisplatin and 5-fluorouracil

Table 3-3   TNM System for Cancer Staging

- Tis: Cancer in situ, cancer is completely limited to epithelial layer
- T1: Tumor confined to site of origin
- T2: Tumor is growing into adjacent area
- T3: Tumor is limited to larynx, but vocal cords do not move
- T4a: Tumor extends to tissue beyond larynx
- T4b: Tumor extends into region of cervical spine and chest
- N0: No nodular involvement
- N1: Single lymph node involvement < 3 cm in diameter
- N2: Single lymph node involvement of < 6 cm or multinode involvement size between 3–6 cm
- N3: Multinodular involvement > 6 cm
- M0: No distant metastasis
- M1: Distant metastasis present
- Stage 0: Tis, N0, M0
- Stage I: T1, N0, M0
- Stage II: T2, N0, M0
- Stage III: T3, N0, M0; T1, T2, or T3, N1, M0
- Stage IVA: T1, T2, or T3, N2, M0 or T4a, N0, N1 or N2, M0
- Stage IVB: T4b, any N, M0, or any T, N3, M0
- Stage IVC: Any T, any N, M1

are the most common chemotherapeutic agents that are administered. Chemotherapy is associated with more severe side effects (leukocytopenia, fatigue secondary to anemia, nausea and vomiting) as compared to radiation therapy. These side effects are often accentuated when chemotherapy and radiation therapy are combined. Surgery is rarely performed as the sole form of treatment, and it is often combined with radiation and/or chemotherapy for treating laryngeal carcinoma. There are several surgical treatment options for laryngeal cancer which are listed in Table 3-4.

Table 3-4   Surgical Treatment Options for Laryngeal Cancer

- Vocal cord stripping: used in Stage 0 cancer to strip away epithelial cells
- Cordectomy: removal of all or part of vocal cords, used to treat superficial cancers
- Laser surgery: used to vaporize Stage 0 and T1 carcinomas
- Partial laryngectomy: excision of various portions of the larynx to maximize normal laryngeal function
- Total laryngectomy: involves the complete removal of the larynx and the creation of a stoma to provide airway patency

SURGICAL PROCEDURE

The goal of laryngeal surgery includes the removal of diseased tissue, preservation or creation of a pathway for air exchange, and maintaining vocal cord function if possible. The definitive surgical procedure that is performed is dependent on the degree invasion of the tumor and these variant surgical techniques include:

Microlaryngeal surgery is performed for laryngeal cancers that are present in their early stages can be removed by utilizing an operating microscope, microlaryngeal dissecting instruments, and a carbon dioxide laser. The resection is limited to the diseased tissue which allows for preservation of adjacent laryngeal structures and superior postoperative laryngeal function.

Hemilaryngectomy involves the removal of one vertical half of the larynx. Unilateral vocal cord reconstruction can be accomplished by using a portion of the strap muscle can be created.

Supracricoid laryngectomy includes the removal of supraglottic structures, true and false vocal cords, and thyroid cartilage while the cricoid and arytenoid cartilages remain. It is performed for lesions that are located in the proximity of the anterior glottis.

Preservation of vocal function may be achieved; however, as many as 50% of these patients will continue to be dependent on a tracheotomy.

Supraglottic laryngectomy can be done using an endoscopic approach or a traditional open technique. During this procedure, supraglottic structures including the false vocal cords, epiglottis, arytenoids, and a portion of the laryngeal cartilage is resected.

Total laryngectomy is accomplished for patients who have extensive cancerous involvement of the larynx (T3 or T4) and entails the complete removal of the larynx, thyroid cartilage, cricoid cartilage, hyoid bone, and potentially several upper tracheal rings. Total or partial thyroid gland resection may be involved. A permanent tracheostomy is created by connecting the tracheal stump to the lower portion of the neck.

The postoperative course is most dependent of the extent of the cancerous lesion, the type of laryngectomy that was performed, and the physical state of the patient. Potential complications that are associated with a laryngectomy include: difficultly with speech, airway complications, diminished sense of taste and smell, pharyngoesophageal stenosis, fistula development between the trachea and

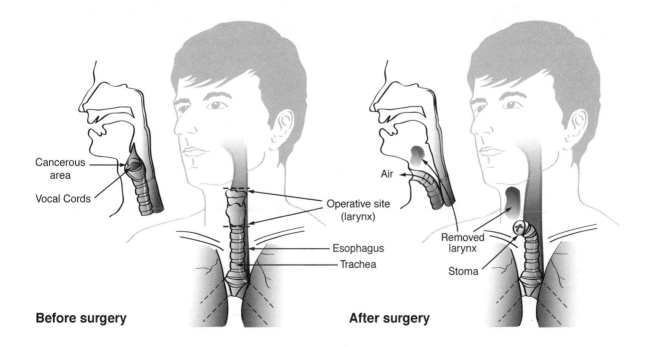

Before surgery   **After surgery**

esophagus, infection, decreased range of motion caused by fibrosis, hematoma formation, and cranial nerve injury. The intraoperative time period for a laryngectomy is highly variable and is dependent of the type of procedure being performed. If a radical neck dissection is to occur in conjunction with a laryngectomy, operative times can exceed 10 hours. The anesthetist's primary initial concern is securing a patent airway (discussed later). Transfusion of packed red blood cells is frequently unnecessary during a laryngectomy because the blood loss is usually less than 300 to 400 ml.

ANESTHETIC MANAGEMENT AND CONSIDERATIONS

Preoperative Period

1. Describe the signs and symptoms associated with laryngeal carcinoma.

This patient had complained of hoarseness to his primary care physician. Hoarseness is a classic sign of laryngeal carcinoma with glottic involvement. Other common signs of laryngeal carcinoma include difficult or painful swallowing, persistent coughing, and dyspnea. A comprehensive list of the signs and symptoms that are associated with this disease is included in Table 3-5. Many of these signs and symptoms do not appear until the disease process is extensive. This is particularly true in cases of supraglottic and subglottic cancer. Approximately 80% of subglottic tumors are diagnosed in late stages (T3 or T4). Careful examination of the neck should be performed to evaluate the patient for the presence of lymph node metastasis and to create a strategy for airway maintenance.

2. Discuss the comorbidities that are associated with laryngectomy.

This patient has a history from both hypertension and COPD. Many of the diseases associated with laryngectomy are a result of the constellation of diseases associated with cigarette smoking and advanced age. The most common comorbidities that are associated with patients having a laryngectomy are listed in Table 3-6. This patient's hypertension (preoperative blood pressure, 110/64) is well controlled with metoprolol (a beta-blocker) and amlodipine (a calcium channel blocker). His

Table 3-5	Signs and Symptoms Associated with Laryngeal Cancer

- Hoarseness
- Muffled voice
- Dysphagia
- Odynophagia (painful swallowing)
- Otalgia (earache)
- Cough
- Airway obstruction
- Fixation of the thyroid cartilage
- Neck mass
- Stridor
- Hemoptysis
- Anorexia
- Weight loss

Table 3-6	Comorbidities Associated with Patients Having a Laryngectomy

- COPD: a combination of emphysema, chronic bronchitis, and/or asthma
- Cerebrovascular accident
- Lung cancer
- Intermittent claudication
- Coronary artery disease
- Myocardial infarction
- Atherosclerosis
- Hypertension
- Alcohol abuse
- Hepatic failure
- Renal failure
- Tobacco use

COPD is managed by using an ipratropium inhaler (an anticholinergic), which is administered four times a day, and an albuterol inhaler (a beta-2 agonist), which he uses as a rescue inhaler.

3. Describe the preoperative diagnostic testing performed for laryngectomy.

The definitive diagnostic test that is used to assess the presence and degree of laryngeal carcinoma is laryngoscopy and evaluation of tissue removed for biopsy. Upon visual inspection with the laryngoscope, this patient's cancer, although primarily a glottic mass, began to spread to the supraglottic region. Computed tomography (CT) scan was used to identify tumor size and lymph node involvement and a positron emission tomography (PET) scan allows for the assessment metastatic disease. Based on these findings, this patient's carcinoma was identified as a stage II cancer: T2, N0, M0. Diagnostic tools that can be used to detect laryngeal cancer are included in Table 3-7. Although a CXR is not used to identify laryngeal malignancy, it can help the physician identify lung metastasis.

4. Discuss the preoperative laboratory evaluation that is associated for patient's having a laryngectomy.

There are no laboratory tests that are diagnostic for laryngeal cancer. However, given the treatment

options and the comorbidities associated with laryngectomy, several lab tests should be performed preoperatively. These tests include the CBC, type and screen (T&S), LFTs, coagulation tests (PT/PTT), electrolyte panel, and an ABG. A list and explanation of laboratory tests are included in Table 3-8. Polycythemia is a common finding caused by COPD. This compensatory change increases the oxygen carrying capacity that occurs due to chronically decreased PaO_2 that is associated with pulmonary pathology. The bradycardia is likely due to his beta-blocker therapy with metoprolol, and the left atrial enlargement is a common result of chronic hypertension.

Table 3-8   Laboratory Testing Associated with a Laryngectomy
• CBC: test used to diagnose pancytopenia caused by radiation or chemotherapy; establishes a baseline blood count in case transfusion is required
• T&S/T&C: the potential for excessive bleeding due to the highly vascular nature of the neck requires preparation for transfusion
• LFTs: assessment of liver function due to the potential for alcohol abuse in this patient population
• PT/PTT: liver function tests are relatively insensitive to liver failure. The PT and PTT are quantitative measure of coagulability. If an abnormality exists, then liver disease may be present. Additionally, the patient's coagulation status should be optimized prior to surgery.
• Electrolytes: assessment would identify hyperkalemia and renal insufficiency from hepatorenal failure
• BUN/creatinine
• ABG: drawn to establish baseline pH, $PaCO_2$, and PaO_2.

ABG, arterial blood gas; BUN, blood urea nitrogen; CBC, complete blood count; LFTs, liver function tests; PT, prothrombin time; PTT, partial prothrombin time; T&C, type and screen.

Table 3-7   Diagnostic Tools for Detecting Laryngeal Cancer
• Laryngoscopy with biopsies: diagnostic gold standard of laryngeal neoplasm
• CT scan: uses cross-sectional x-rays to identify tumor size and lymph node involvement
• PET scan: uses radioisotopes to identify metastasis
• Magnetic resonance imaging (MRI): utilizes electromagnetic waves to produce a three-dimensional image; rarely used to diagnose laryngeal cancer

5. Identify the importance of a comprehensive airway assessment and plan for airway management.

Airway evaluation is an essential preoperative assessment performed by the anesthetist. In addition to standard airway assessment parameters, such as Mallampati class and thyromental distance, it is essential that the anesthetist performs a thorough airway examination. In the event of any preexisting airway obstruction, a decision will be made as to whether the patient can be safely intubated under general anesthesia, whether an awake intubation needs to be performed, or whether the patient requires an awake tracheostomy under local anesthesia prior to start of the laryngectomy surgery. A strong indicator of the degree of airway obstruction that will be encountered after the induction of anesthesia is the patient's ability to lie in the supine position. If the patient is unable to lie flat without dyspnea, this is highly suggestive of the presence of significant airway obstruction. This patient was able to sleep in the supine position while laying his head on a single pillow. In addition, his diagnostic laryngoscopy and his CT scan revealed that it was possible to perform an intubation under general anesthesia.

Diagnostic testing such as CT scan and laryngoscopy will dictate whether or not the patient can be safely intubated or whether an awake tracheostomy with local anesthesia is required. If there are any concerns of impingement and airway distortion that has the potential to cause upper airway obstruction, further, definitive investigation should be performed.

Performing an awake intubation or tracheostomy should be considered when there is preexisting obstructive pathology. The anesthetist and surgical team must be prepared to have all necessary equipment available to perform an emergency tracheostomy. In the specific case of laryngeal cancer, a supraglottic device such as a laryngeal mask airway (LMA) may not be helpful in an emergency situation due to the airway pathology. If the patient

Table 3-9	Regional Anesthetic Techniques for Laryngectomy

- Deep cervical plexus block: local anesthesia is injected into the bilateral transverse processes of C4
- Superficial cervical plexus block: local anesthesia is infiltrated into the area surrounding **Erb's point** on both sides of the neck
- Superior laryngeal nerve: local anesthesia is injected bilaterally 1 cm below the greater cornu of the hyoid bone
- Translaryngeal block: local anesthesia is injected through the cricothyroid membrane

is considered to be a potentially difficult intubation, or if massive unremitting airway obstruction is judged to be a likely consequence of induction, then an awake tracheostomy is the treatment of choice. Tracheostomy can be performed under several regional anesthetic techniques, which are listed in Table 3-9. Tracheostomy can also be performed with or without conscious sedation, using regional anesthetic techniques alone or in combination.

Intraoperative Period

6. Discuss important factors involved in patient preparation for laryngectomy.

The patient is placed in the supine position unless there is preexisting airway obstruction, in which case semi-Fowler or even side-lying positions might be required. The considerations necessary for placing the patient in the supine position includes the potential for brachial plexus or ulnar nerve damage. Supine positioning reduces functional residual capacity in a patient who may already be suffering from partial airway obstruction. Thorough preoxygenation, prior to any attempt at intubation is vital.

During laryngoscopy and intubation, trauma to the tissues results in catastrophic swelling or bleeding in the airway. Pressure exerted on cancerous tissue or patients who have received radiation therapy are at high risk of bleeding. Once ventilation is established, the patient is intubated with an appropriate sized endotracheal tube (ETT). The surgeon may wish to perform a direct laryngoscopy or upper airway exam under anesthesia prior to ETT placement. Several sizes of ETT should be available in the event of difficulty with intubation. The ETT will be secured in a manner that has been discussed with the surgeon in advance (taped midline or to one side, may be sutured). The operating table will be turned to a 90- or 180-degree angle away from the anesthetist. Since the anesthetist will not have ready access to the patient's airway, extension tubing for intravenous lines and the breathing circuit will be needed. In many cases, consideration should be given to using a reinforced ETT to further protect the airway. This should also be discussed with the surgeon in advance of the induction.

The patient's arms will be tucked at his side. The difficulty of accessing the patient's arms during surgery, and the need for secure access for drug and fluid therapy, necessitates the need for two large bore IVs (no. 16 or no. 18). A central line is not necessarily required for laryngectomy, but if central line placement is indicated due to the patient's condition, it should be placed in the femoral vein to avoid disruption of the surgical field.

The patient may be placed on a pillow or shoulder roll depending on the surgeon's preference to create head and neck extension to achieve good operative exposure. The patient's head should be adequately supported. The final position of the patient's head should be discussed in advance with the surgeon. Careful attention to safely covering and protecting the eyes should be a priority.

7. Describe the importance of patient monitors.

Standard monitors (ECG, noninvasive blood pressure monitoring, pulse oximetry, end-tidal carbon dioxide monitoring, peripheral nerve stimulator, temperature) are required. Arterial line placement is recommended because it will provide for a continuous assessment of the patient's blood pressure to detect hemodynamic changes that are associated

with this patient population. Although the surgery takes place in a highly vascular area (close proximity to the carotid and jugular vasculature), blood loss has the potential to become excessive. The average amount of blood loss is estimated to be 200 to 500 ml of blood. The anesthetist must be aware of the potential for hypotension caused by hemorrhage or vagal stimulation caused by baroreceptor or recurrent/superior laryngeal nerve stimulation.

The placement of an esophageal stethoscope allows for accurate core temperature monitoring and simultaneous auscultation of lung and heart sounds. The average duration of this surgical procedure is variable and lasts between 2 and 6 hours. Patient warming should be provided via a lower body or underbody Bair Hugger (Arizant Healthcare Inc., Eden Prairie, Minnesota) and intravenous fluids should be heated via a fluid warming device.

8. Discuss intraoperative complications of laryngectomy.

Intraoperative complications are related to hemorrhage and surgical stimulation of the vagus nerve. Hypotension can be the result of massive blood loss or vagal stimulation. Vagal stimulation can also produce bradycardia. Pulmonary and airway complications of laryngectomy include pneumothorax, airway obstruction, and air embolism. All patients must be carefully evaluated for the presence of surgical complications upon emergence from anesthesia and prior to extubation. The 5-year survival rates published by the American Cancer Society are included in Table 3-10.

Table 3-10	Laryngeal Cancer 5-year Survival Rates		
STAGE	**SUPRAGLOTTIC**	**GLOTTIC**	**SUBGLOTTIC**
I	83%	65%	54%
II	70%	62%	68%
III	57%	55%	53%
IV	43%	37%	36%

Postoperative Period

9. Describe significant postoperative complications associated with laryngectomy.

There are several postoperative complications that are associated with a laryngectomy. The inability to phonate (temporary or permanent), dysphagia, and increased risk of aspiration (with partial laryngectomy) are direct results of laryngectomy. The most common postoperative complications are pharyngocutaneous fistula and wound infection. Other postoperative complications include bleeding, hematoma, pneumonia, airway obstruction, chyle leak, and death.

REVIEW QUESTIONS

1. Which characteristics most accurately describe the comorbidities that are associated with a patient having a laryngectomy?
   a. A 42-year-old female, 50 pack-year smoking history, blood pressure 190/110
   b. A 67-year-old male, nonsmoker, drinks 3 glasses of wine daily
   c. A 65-year-old male, 40 pack-year smoking history, drinks a fifth of vodka daily
   d. A 34-year-old male, history of cocaine abuse, drinks one 6-pack of beer daily

2. Which is the correct sequence indicative of the incidence of laryngeal cancer by region from the greatest to the least?
   a. Supraglottic, glottic, subglottic
   b. Glottic, supraglottic, subglottic
   c. Glottic, subglottic, supraglottic
   d. Supraglottic, subglottic, glottic

3. TNM cancer staging is an abbreviation for which of the following?
   a. Tumor, nodule, mass
   b. Tumor, node, mass
   c. Tumor, neoplasm, metastasis
   d. Tumor, node, metastasis

4. Which diagnostic tests best determine the staging associated with laryngeal carcinoma?
   a. CBC and laryngoscopy with biopsies
   b. PET scan and CXR
   c. CXR and CT scan
   d. Laryngoscopy with biopsies and CT scan

5. What are the most important concerns during the intraoperative period?
   a. Airway protection and massive hemorrhage
   b. Airway protection and bradycardia
   c. Hypotension and bradycardia
   d. Hypotension and massive hemorrhage

REVIEW ANSWERS

1. **Answer: c**
   The risk factors that put this patient choice at highest risk for developing laryngeal cancer include history of smoking, alcohol abuse, gender (male > female) and advanced age (> 50 years old).

2. **Answer: b**
   The incidence of laryngeal cancer by region from the greatest to the least includes glottic to supraglottic to subglottic.

3. **Answer: d**
   The assessment of laryngeal malignancy depends primarily on its location and the TNM staging of the tumor. The letters TNM represent tumor, node, and metastasis.

4. **Answer: d**
   A combination of laryngoscopy with biopsies and CT scan are the diagnostic tests that best determine the staging of laryngeal carcinoma.

5. **Answer: a**
   While the anesthetist should be alert to all of the listed potential complications, the most important factors include airway protection and massive hemorrhage.

SUGGESTED READINGS

BuSaba NY, Schaumberg DA. Predictors of prolonged length of stay after major elective head and neck surgery. *Laryngoscope* 2007;117(Oct):1756–1763.

Cousins VC, Milton CM, Bickerton RC. Hospital morbidity and mortality following total laryngectomy. *J Laryng Otol* 1987;101:1159–1164.

Hall FT, O'Brien CJ, Clifford AR, et al. Clinical outcome following total laryngectomy for cancer. *ANZ J Surg* 2003;73:300–305.

Marioni G, Marchese-Ragona R, Cartei G, et al. Current opinion in diagnosis and treatment of laryngeal carcinoma. *Cancer Treat Rev* 2006;32:504–515.

Mastropietro C. The anesthetic considerations for the patient undergoing total laryngectomy. *J Am Assoc Nurse Anesth* 1987;55(3):237–244.

McKenna JP, Fornataro-Clerici LM, McMenamin PG, et al. Laryngeal cancer: diagnosis, treatment and speech rehabilitation. *Am Fam Physician* 1991;44(1):123–129.

Noordzij JP, Ossoff RH. Anatomy and physiology of the larynx. *Otolaryngol Clin North Am* 2006;39: 1–10.

Prasad KC, Shanmugan VU. Major neck surgeries under regional anesthesia. *Am J Otolaryngol* 1998;19(3): 163–169.

Rinaldo A, Ferlito A. Open supraglottic laryngectomy. *Acta Otolaryngology* 2004;124:768–771.

Young VVN, Mangus BD, Bumpous JM. Salvage laryngectomy for failed conservative treatment of laryngeal cancer. *Laryngoscope* 2008;118(Sept): 1561–1568.

Vocal Cord Polyp Removal with Laser

4

Mark D. Welliver and Dawn C. Welliver

KEY POINTS

- Vocal cord polyps usually do not compromise airway patency.
- Gastroesophageal reflux disease (GERD) may be a concomitant condition.
- A laser (light amplification by stimulated emission of radiation) is an intensified beam of energy that can ignite fires.
- Perioperative complications that are associated with vocal cord polyp removal with laser include airway laceration, laryngospasm, burns, and eye injury.

CASE SYNOPSIS

A 33-year-old female singer is scheduled for laser removal of a left-sided vocal cord polyp.

PREOPERATIVE EVALUATION AND DEMOGRAPHIC DATA

Social History

- Cigarette smoker 1/2 pack per day for 15 years

Past Medical/Surgical History

- Patient denies any past medical or surgical history

List of Medications

- Multivitamin supplement daily

Diagnostic Data

- Hemoglobin, 15 g/dl; hematocrit, 45%
- Glucose, 90 mg/dl
- Blood urea nitrogen, 10 mg/dl; creatinine, 0.5 mg/dl
- Electrolytes: sodium, 140 mEq/l; potassium, 4.2; chloride, 99 mEq/l; carbon dioxide, 25 mEq/l
- Electrocardiogram, normal sinus rhythm (heart rate, 70 beats per minute)

Height/Weight/Vital Signs

- 170 cm, 80 kg
- Blood pressure, 128/88; heart rate, 74 beats per minute; respiratory rate, 18 breaths per minute; room air oxygen saturation 98%; temperature, 36.8°C

PATHOPHYSIOLOGY

Vocal cord polyps, nodules, and cysts have a similar clinical presentation and a slight histologic difference. Vocal cord polyps, nodules, and cysts are most often benign, well defined, hyperplastic tissue. It has been suggested that vocal cord polyps may represent a chronic response to airway stress as compared to an acute pathologic process associated with vocal cord nodules. There is a higher incidence of vocal cord polyps in people who are smokers and those who use their voice in a strenuous manner. Singers and orators may be at greater risk for developing these lesions due to frequent stress that is placed on the vocal cord.

The incidence of vocal cord polyps has been found to be evenly distributed between the sexes. Vocal cord polyps usually do not interfere with vocal cord movement, but larger polyps may alter phonation. Laser ablation of vocal cord polyps is most successful when it is a part of therapy that includes vocal therapy (retraining) and if present, treating GERD. Figure 4-1 illustrates a view during laryngoscopy of this patient's left-sided vocal cord polyp.

SURGICAL PROCEDURE

Laser removal of a vocal cord polyp is accomplished using a low intensity energy laser directed onto the tissue to be ablated. A low intensity laser beam is able to ablate the polyp with minimal transfer of energy to deeper and surrounding tissues. Polyp removal by laser is conducted under direct laryngoscopy or microlaryngoscopy to focus the energy beam. Laser ablation is most often accomplished adjacent to an endotracheal tube (ETT) during mechanical ventilation. A rigid bronchoscope can

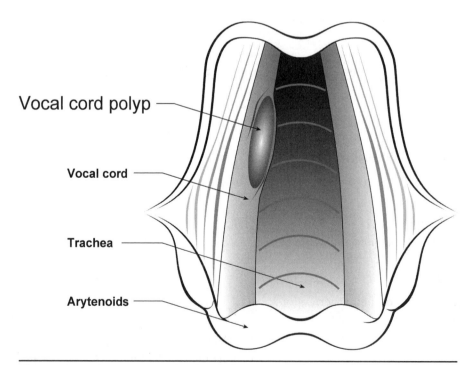

Figure 4-1 *Laryngoscopic view of airway and vocal cord polyp.*

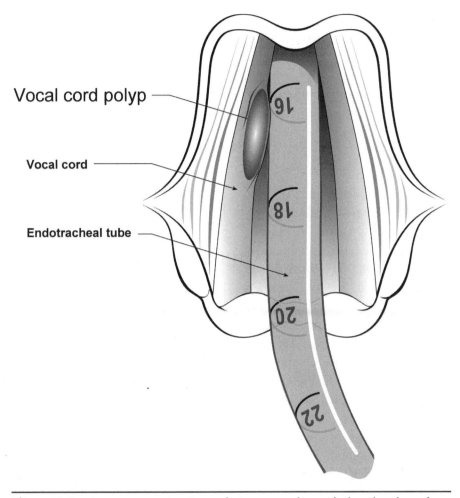

Vocal cord polyp

Vocal cord

Endotracheal tube

Figure 4-2   *Laryngoscopic view of airway and vocal chord polyp after intubation.*

be used along with jet ventilation. The ETT may be removed during the use of the laser to prevent possible ignition and then reinserted. The surgical view of the airway during laser removal of a vocal cord polyp is depicted in Figure 4-2.

ANESTHETIC MANAGEMENT AND CONSIDERATIONS

Preoperative Period

1. Describe the concerns regarding airway assessment for a patient who has a vocal cord polyp.
Performing a standard airway assessment is essential. Unlike tumors, polyps remain relatively small. Polyps are not usually associated with difficult

mask ventilation or intubation. Vocal cord polyps may alter phonation and possibly be irritating but do not interfere with ventilation. Polyps are not usually excessively large and infrequently displace or obstruct the trachea. However, the anesthetist should be prepared for a difficult airway in the event that the polyp is large, multiple polyps are present, edema formation has occurred, or other pathologic conditions exist.

2. What preoperative medications are beneficial for a patient scheduled for laser airway surgery?
Midazolam can be administered to decrease anxiety during the preoperative period. Anticholinergics, such as atropine or glycopyrrolate, should be

given intravenously to decrease airway secretions. Airway secretions may impair a thorough visualization of the vocal cords, and water molecules in the secretions absorb laser energy. Less vocal cord moisture (mucus, phlegm, saliva) improves the ability of the surgeon to focus and control the laser beam during intraoperative ablation.

Intraoperative Period

3. Analyze the need for general endotracheal anesthesia for laser vocal cord polyp removal surgery.
An ETT maintains a patient's airway during the surgical procedure, which includes placement of throat packs, airway manipulation, focused laser energy, and tissue destruction. The ETT protects the airway from debris and secretions while isolating the glottic opening; higher inspired oxygen concentrations increase the potential for ignition caused by the laser. All three components of general anesthesia—amnesia, analgesia, and immobility—are required for laser surgery on the vocal cords. Analgesia is required to attenuate the sympathetic discharge associated with airway stimulation and manipulation. Short-acting and ultra–short-acting narcotics (remifentanil) are beneficial to blunt the stimulation from the airway manipulation during the procedure. Longer acting narcotics will cause narcosis after the procedure has concluded, which may contribute to hypoventilation and bradypnea. Immobility is essential to decrease the possibility of injury to other tissues or disruption of the ETT by the endoscope and laser.

4. Discuss alternatives to placing an ETT for airway management.
The surgeon may want the ETT removed before the laser is used. Mask ventilation, or reintubation and ventilation, may be done between intermittent laser applications. This approach allows for complete vocal cord visualization, but leaves the airway unprotected. Manual or high frequency ventilation may also be done via a supraglottic

small bore ETT, or high frequency jet ventilation through a transtracheal catheter. A side stream ventilation port on the surgical endoscope may also be used for ventilation. There is an increased risk of fire if the airway management technique does not employ the use of a cuffed ETT due to the presence of supraphysiologic concentrations of oxygen that comes into contact with the laser. The surgeon and operating room personnel will also be exposed to anesthetic waste gasses. The fraction of inspired oxygen concentration (FiO_2) should be maintained between *21 and 30%*. Heliox, a mixture of helium and oxygen, has been successfully employed to lower the potential for combustion. A total intravenous anesthetic technique can also be used.

5. Explain the associated risks during laser ablation.
Fire, burns, eye injury, and noxious laser plume are all risks that are associated with the use of a laser. Lasers are a highly focused beam of intense energy that is able to ablate biologic tissues as well as ignite combustible materials. Fire is always a risk when lasers are in use. Burns to the patient or operating room staff may occur directly from the laser beam, or by fire ignited by the laser. Surgical drapes, sponges, many prep solutions, and ETT are flammable. The oxygen rich environment administered during anesthesia increases the risk of fire. Anesthetists must always remain cognoscente of these risks, and be prepared to respond in the event of a fire, as shown in Figure 4-3.

Eye injuries can occur to the patient or staff when the laser's beam is directed toward an unprotected face. The byproducts of tissues ablated with a laser can contain contagious, mutagenic, and carcinogenic substances. Transmission of viruses such as human papilloma can occur. Methods that are used to protect operating room personnel for inhaling the byproducts of tissue ablation include each member wearing a small micron particulate facemask (laser mask) and having the surgical

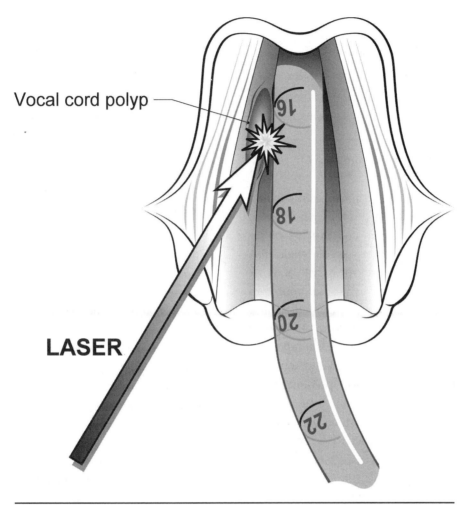

Vocal cord polyp

LASER

Figure 4-3 *Surgical view of airway during laser ablation of vocal chord polyp.*

assistant suction the laser plume exhaust with a vacuum system.

6. Describe appropriate preparations an anesthetist can make for a laser vocal cord polyp removal case.

All personnel that are present during surgical cases that utilize a laser should be trained in its safe operation. Signs warning "laser in use" and "protective eyewear required" should be displayed at all entrances to the operating room. All operating room personnel must wear appropriate laser glasses for the type of laser in use. Saline soaked eye patches, with or without laser goggles, should

be placed on patient to protect their eyes from the laser's beam.

Preparation to prevent and treat fires and burns are necessary. A liter bottle of saline, or water, should be kept immediately available to saturate flames in case of fire. The lowest possible concentration of oxygen should be used. It is preferential to administer a blend of air and oxygen *to maintain the FiO$_2$ between 21 and 30%*. Helium, which is nonflammable, is useful as a carrier gas to decrease the FiO$_2$ when mixed with oxygen. Helium also has a lower density which promotes laminar flow as demonstrated by Reynolds equation. Oxygen and nitrous oxide are both oxidizers and they are associated with rapid combustion of flammable materials. Delivered carrier gases may collect under surgical drapes and may be ignited by a laser placed in close proximity. The laser should be switched into the standby mode or the off position when not in use. It should never be placed on the patient or surgical drapes.

7. Provide a rationale for considering the use of Heliox for ventilation.

Heliox is a mixture of helium and oxygen. Helium is nonflammable and possess a lower density than nitrogen and oxygen, the main constituents of air. Helium allows the use of lower oxygen levels during laser surgery thus lowering the risk of combustion while improving flow dynamics. Improved laminar flow is described by a lower calculated Reynolds number as shown in Equation 4-1. A calculated Reynolds number greater than 2000 reflects a predominantly turbulent flow. A calculated Reynolds number less than 2000 will reflect predominantly laminar flow. The lower the value, the greater the degree of laminar air flow which can also be described as decreased resistance to airflow.

8. Describe special precautions necessary for airway management during a general endotracheal anesthetic for laser airway surgery.

The close proximity of the laser's beam to the ETT and the oxygen enriched environment of ventilation increase the potential for fire. Oxygen supports combustion, and if the integrity of the ETT becomes breached, explosive ignition may occur. Lower FiO_2 levels lessen the explosive potential of laser fire ignition but do not remove it all together. Many anesthetists fill the ETT cuff with saline and a dye to be able to visually identify

---

Equation 4-1

Reynolds number = vpd/η

v is the linear velocity of fluid, p is density of fluid, d is diameter of tube, and η is viscosity

---

perforation of the ETT cuff if it occurs. Frequently, specially manufactured "laser tubes" are used which are covered in a reflective material to lessen the chance of ignition by the laser energy. In addition, some anesthetists use adhesive backed aluminum foil that is wrapped around the ETT providing a reflective surface for the laser's energy.

Maintenance

9. Construct an organized systematic response for treatment of an airway fire.

A quick systematic response to this medical emergency is an absolute necessity to limit injury.

1. *Immediately discontinue ventilation and oxygen flow*
2. *Douse the airway with sterile saline*
3. *Extubate patient*
4. *Verify that the fire is extinguished*
5. *Mask ventilate*
6. *Perform DL, remove any remnants of the ETT or throat packs*
7. *Reintubate*
8. *Perform fiberoptic bronchoscopy to visualize and document degree of injury*
9. *Corticosteroids and antibiotics will likely be required along with continued intubation*

10. Discuss choice of volatile anesthetic agents.

The desirable pharmacokinetic and pharmacodynamic profile associated with sevoflurane make it desirable to use as the main anesthetic during laser polyp removal because it does not cause irritation to the airway and it is easily titrated. Isoflurane and desflurane cause airway irritation that may contribute to excessive coughing during emergence. Laser surgery on the airway for vocal cord polyp removal is usually a short procedure (15 minutes), and therefore saturation of the muscle and fat compartments with inhalation agent does not significantly delay emergence. The low blood–gas solubility of sevoflurane along with its lack of pungency promotes quick and smooth emergence during these procedures.

11. Provide rationale for total intravenous anesthesia during laser polyp removal surgery.

Total intravenous anesthesia (TIVA) using propofol is an appropriate choice for maintenance of anesthesia especially if intermittent ventilation or a significant leak during mechanical ventilation exists intraoperatively. Interrupting the administration of the inhaled agent during periods of extubation and laser ablation makes controlling the anesthetic depth difficult. Providing TIVA is also beneficial to decrease the exposure of the operating room personnel to anesthetic gases.

12. Discuss the use of neuromuscular blocking agents during laser surgery on the airway.

Immobility is absolutely necessary, and therefore neuromuscular blocking agents may be administered. The patient must not move during the use of a rigid endoscope in order to prevent injury. Coughing or "bucking" during laser surgery of the airway can be disastrous as laceration, perforation, and inadvertent laser injury to normal tissues may occur. Short- or intermediate-duration muscle relaxants are best as laser surgery of vocal polyps is a relatively short procedure. The ability to reverse muscle relaxants with cholinesterase inhibitors requires a degree of spontaneous recovery of neuromuscular blockade. Care should be taken to assure adequate depth of anesthesia to prevent patient movement yet maintain the ability to effectively reverse the neuromuscular blockade.

13. Describe the nervous system innervation to the larynx.

The larynx is innervated by two branches of the vagus nerve. The superior laryngeal nerve (SLN) bifurcates into the internal superior laryngeal nerve (sensory) and the external superior laryngeal nerve (motor). The internal superior laryngeal nerve provides sensory innervation above the vocal cords. The external superior laryngeal nerve provides motor innervation to the cricothyroid muscle, a vocal cord tensor. The recurrent

Table 4-1 Sensory and Motor Nerve Innervation to the Larynx
SUPERIOR LARYNGEAL NERVE (SLN)
1. Sensory function: internal branch of the SLN-sensation between the epiglottis and vocal cords
2. Motor function: external branch of the SLN-cricothyroid muscle (tenses vocal cords)
RECURRENT LARYNGEAL NERVE (RLN)
1. Sensory function: sensation below the level of the vocal cords
2. Motor function: innervation of seven intrinsic laryngeal muscles
a. Posterior cricoarytenoid (opens vocal cords)
b. Lateral cricoarytenoid (closes vocal cords)
c. Thyroarytenoid (shortens/relaxes vocal cords)
d. Transverse arytenoid (closes vocal cords)

laryngeal nerve (RLN) innervates all other intrinsic laryngeal muscles to provide motor function and sensory innervation below the level of the vocal cords. The sensory and motor innervation to the larynx is listed in Table 4-1.

14. Discuss the reason that the surgeon may request visual confirmation of vocal cord movement after removal of the vocal cord polyp.

It is possible that the surgeon may request to visualize the vocal cords using direct laryngoscopy or a fiberoptic method. This assessment is done to confirm that the recurrent laryngeal nerve, which is primarily responsible for vocal cord movement, remains intact. In order to accomplish this task, the patient is allowed to spontaneously breathe and then extubated while in a surgical plane of anesthesia in order to avoid laryngospasm and sympathetic nervous system hyperreactivity.

Injury to the SLN is possible with laser surgery on the vocal cords. Unilateral or bilateral injuries to the SLN may cause hoarseness and fatigue during phonation. Since the motor function of the SLN results in vocal cord tension via the cricothyroid muscle, denervation should not result in airway compromise. Injury to the RLN is unlikely during vocal cord laser polyp removal. The motor function of the RLN innervates all other intrinsic muscles of the larynx. If unilateral injury to the RLN occurs, paralysis of that vocal cord will result. Airway patency is rarely compromised, but vocal function and tone would be affected. Bilateral RLN injury causes bilateral vocal cord paralysis and unopposed cricothyroid tension closes the glottic opening. Negative inspiratory pressure pulls the vocal cords together, further occluding the glottic opening. The vocal cords would remain in the midline position and airway obstruction, stridor, and eventual respiratory distress will occur. Intubation or tracheostomy is required to maintain a patent airway with bilateral vocal cord paralysis.

15. Describe the anesthetic goals during emergence and extubation.

The goals for emergence and extubation include maintaining adequate analgesia, decreasing airway irritation, and avoiding laryngospasm and airway compromise. Extubation that occurs while the patient is deeply anesthetized will help decrease the risk of laryngospasm. Lidocaine administered intravenously has been used successfully to attenuate laryngeal reflexes.

Postoperative Period

16. Analyze the physiologic mechanism and causes responsible for laryngospasm.

Sensory stimulation of the internal branch of the SLN causes an afferent reflex arc at the level of the spinal cord. The efferent reflex from the brain travels via the external branch of the laryngeal nerve to the cricothyroid muscle causing contraction. The cricothyroid muscle is attached to the cricoid and thyroid cartilages. When contracted, this muscle tenses (adducts) the vocal cords. Laryngospasm is a spasm (sustained contraction)

of the cricothyroid muscles. Vocal cord stimulation by the laser, irritation, inflammation, and light anesthesia during the emergence phase all contribute to the increased risk of laryngospasm.

17. Construct a systematic plan to treat a laryngospasm.

Light anesthesia (stage II), inadequate analgesia, and airway stimulation contribute to the incidence of laryngospasm. Application of positive pressure (10–20 cm H_2O) via mask pushes on the vocal cords and stretches the cricothyroid muscle. Stretching a muscle in spasm allows the contraction to be relaxed. Additionally, manual digital pressure on the pressure point in front of the mastoid process by the angle of the mandible aids in attenuating laryngospasm. The exact mechanism is unknown, but may be related to an acupressure or pain reflex. Delay in treating laryngospasm allows persistent cricothyroid contraction and may be resistant to positive pressure maneuvers. Succinylcholine 10–20 mg intravenously will relax the cricothyroid muscle when positive pressure does not relieve the laryngospasm. It is important to note that succinylcholine given after cholinesterase inhibitor reversal of nondepolarizing neuromuscular blocking agents will have an extended duration of action due to inhibition of pseudocholinesterase. Prolonged paralysis from inhibited succinylcholine metabolism will require assisted ventilation.

18. Discuss postoperative care for a patient after vocal cord polyp removal.

Adequate pain control and relieving airway irritation are important postoperative considerations. Intravenous narcotics titrated to patient comfort and respiratory adequacy attenuates irritation, coughing, and laryngospasm. Postoperative delivery of humidified oxygen, aerosolized racemic epinephrine, and intravenous corticosteroids help to treat airway hyperreactivity. Stridor is indicative of airway narrowing and may be caused by edema, vocal cord nerve injury, or laryngospasm.

REVIEW QUESTIONS

1. Which is true regarding vocal cord polyps?
   a. Frequently malignant
   b. Contribute to a high incidence of airway obstruction
   c. Usually do not interfere with airway patency and ventilation
   d. Occur from an acute response to airway stress
2. Which is not a risk associated with the use of lasers in the operating room?
   a. Fire
   b. Burns
   c. Eye injury
   d. High dose radiation exposure
3. Which is not a necessary component for fire to occur?
   a. Oxidizer
   b. Carbon dioxide
   c. Ignition source
   d. Fuel
4. Which precautions should be taken during laser surgery that involves the airway?
   a. Eye protection for the patient and the operating room personnel
   b. Administering the highest possible FiO_2
   c. Administering nitrous oxide
   d. Having suction available
5. Which is not a treatment for laryngospasm?
   a. Positive airway pressure
   b. Digital pressure at the angle of the ramus and mastoid process
   c. Cricothyrotomy
   d. Intravenous succinylcholine

REVIEW ANSWERS

1. **Answer: c**
   Vocal cord polyps usually do not interfere with airway patency. Vocal cord polyps may interfere with vocal cord movement (vibration) causing changes in phonation. Vocal cord polyps are benign lesions caused by chronic exposure to stresses.
2. **Answer: d**
   Lasers may cause burns, eye injury, and ignite fires. The frequency of lasers are close to the visible light band and therefore does not expose operating room personnel to ionizing radiation such as gamma or x-rays.
3. **Answer: b**
   Fire requires three components to occur: an ignition source, oxidizer, and fuel. A laser is an excellent ignition source; oxygen and nitrous oxide are oxidizers; and surgical drapes, alcohol disinfectants, and gauze sponges are all fuels. Carbon dioxide is not an ignitor, oxidizer, or fuel source.
4. **Answer: a**
   Precautions to take during laser surgery include using the lowest concentration of oxygen (an oxidizer), avoiding nitrous oxide (an oxidizer), use of proper eye shields and protection, and being prepared to extinguish a possible fire.
5. **Answer: c:**
   Positive airway pressure, digital pressure with jaw thrust, and succinylcholine administration are all treatment for laryngospasm. Cricothyrotomy is not indicated for a laryngospasm that can be treated with less invasive interventions.

SUGGESTED READINGS

American Society of Anesthesiologists. Practice advisory for the prevention and management of operating room fires. *Anesthesiology* 2008;108:786–801.

Barker S, Polson JS. Fire in the operating room: A case report and laboratory study. *Anesth Analg* 2001;93:960–965.

Bigony L. Risks associated with exposure to surgical smoke plume: a review of the literature. *AORN Journal* 2007;86:1013–1023.

Bourgain JL, Desruennes E, Fischler M, et al. Transtracheal high frequency jet ventilation for endoscopic airway surgery: a multicentre study. *Br J Anaesth* 2001;87:870–875.

Johns MM. Update on the etiology, diagnosis, and treatment of vocal fold nodules, polyps, and cysts. *Curr Op Otolaryngol Head Neck Surg* 2003; 11:456–461.

Spiess BD, Ivankovich AD. Anesthetic management of laser airway surgery. *Semin Surg Oncol* 1990;6:189–193.

Werkhaven JA. Microlaryngoscopy-airway management with anaesthetic techniques for CO2 laser. *Pediatr Anesth* 2004;14:90–94.

Visvanathan T, Kluger MT, Webb RK, et al. Crisis management during anaesthesia: laryngospasm. *Qual Safe Health Care* 2005;14:e3.

Uvulopalatopharyngoplasty

Dennis Spence

5

KEY POINTS

- Obstructive sleep apnea (OSA) is characterized by chronic, frequent episodes of upper airway obstruction during sleep which results in hypoxia and hypercarbia and it is associated with increased risk of cardiovascular, neuropsychologic, endocrine disorders, and impaired quality of life.
- It is estimated that up to 93% of women and 82% of men with moderate to severe OSA are undiagnosed.
- Obstructive sleep apnea is associated with increased perioperative morbidity and mortality because of an increased risk of difficult intubation, coexisting diseases, and life-threatening apnea.
- Perioperative risk is based on severity of OSA, invasiveness of surgery, and requirements for postoperative opioids.
- Anesthetic considerations for patients presenting for uvulopalatopharyngoplasty (UPPP) include identifying and managing potential difficult airways, closely observing for airway obstruction and bleeding, and carefully titrating opioids in the postoperative period.

CASE SYNOPSIS

A 45-year-old man with a history of OSA is scheduled by his ear, nose, and throat (ENT) surgeon to have a UPPP.

PREOPERATIVE EVALUATION AND DEMOGRAPHIC DATA

Past Medical/Surgical History

- Severe obstructive sleep apnea
- Obesity
- Non–insulin-dependent diabetes
- Hypertension
- Smoked 1 pack a day for 10 years
- Bilateral myringotomy age 3; no anesthetic complications

List of Medications

- Atenolol

Diagnostic Data

- Hemoglobin, 15 g/dl; hematocrit, 42%
- Blood urea nitrogen, 15 mg/dl; creatinine, 1.1 mg/dl
- Glucose,160 mg/dl
- Electrolytes: sodium, 140 mEq/l; potassium, 3.9 mEq/l; chloride, 104 mEq/l; carbon dioxide, 24 mEq/l
- Sleep study
  - Precontinuous positive airway pressure (Pre-CPAP): apnea–hypopnea index (AHI), 50 events/hour; lowest oxygen saturation (LSAT), 75%
  - Post-CPAP: AHI, 38 events/hour; LSAT, 83% at 10 cm H_2O. The titration of CPAP was stopped due to patient intolerance.
  - Electrocardiogram (ECG): normal sinus bradycardia (heart rate 58 beats per minute), left ventricular hypertrophy

Height/Weight/Vital Signs

- 175 cm, 113 kg
- Body mass index (BMI), 36.6; blood pressure, 152/80; heart rate, 59 beats per minute; respiratory rate, 20 breaths per minute; room air oxygen saturation, 95%; temperature, 36°C

Airway Examination

- Mallampati (MP) class 3; +3 tonsillar hypertrophy; thyromental distance and mouth opening 3 fingerbreadths; short, thick neck (18 inches); and teeth intact

PATHOPHYSIOLOGY

Obstructive sleep apnea is a significant problem that is associated with serious physical consequences. It is characterized by chronic, frequent episodes of upper airway obstruction during sleep that results in hypoxia and hypercarbia and significant morbidity. It is estimated that 2% of

women and 4% of men in the United States have OSA. However, surveys suggest that as many as 21% of women and 31% of men may be at risk for OSA, and that up to 93% of women and 82% of men with moderate to severe OSA are undiagnosed. Additionally, patients with moderate to severe OSA have higher incidence of difficult intubation, postoperative respiratory complications (e.g., severe oxygen desaturation, $SaO_2 \leq 90\%$), unplanned intensive care admission, and prolonged hospital stay.

SURGICAL PROCEDURE

The gold standard treatment for OSA is CPAP or bilevel positive airway pressure (BiPAP). Even though it is extremely effective, tolerance and compliance of the device is difficult for some patients. Patients who cannot tolerate CPAP may be candidates for surgery to alleviate anatomic sites of the obstruction with UPPP. UPPP involves surgical enlargement of the retropalatal airway by trimming and reorienting the posterior and anterior lateral pharyngeal pillars as shown in Figure 5-1. The procedure may be combined with adenotonsillectomy or combined with advancement, limited resection or radiofrequency ablation of the tongue base to achieve maximal enlargement of the retrolingual and retropalatal airway.

ANESTHETIC MANAGEMENT AND CONSIDERATIONS

Preoperative Period

1. Describe the mechanism that causes airway obstruction and diagnostic criteria for OSA.

Obstructive sleep apnea is a syndrome associated with periodic, partial, or complete obstruction of the upper airway during sleep that leads to episodes of apnea–hypopnea, frequent arousals, oxygen desaturation, and daytime hypersomnolence. Apnea is defined as a cessation of airflow for longer than 10 seconds. The event is obstructive if there is effort to breathe during apnea. Hypopnea is an abnormal respiratory event with at least $\geq 30\%$

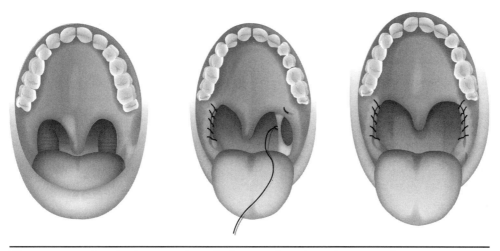

Figure 5-1   *Surgical correction during uvulopalatopharyngoplasty.*

reduction in thoracoabdominal movement or air-flow as compared to baseline lasting at least 10 seconds, and with $\geq$ 4% oxygen desaturation. The formal diagnosis of OSA is made by polysomnography and the severity is based on the AHI (number of times apnea + hypopnea occurs per hour of sleep). The criterion that is based on the AHI is present in Table 5-1. Patients with OSA have significantly higher arousal index, lower SaO_2, and decreased slow wave sleep, respectively, when compared to non-OSA patients. The typical patient with OSA is a loud snorer who has a BMI > 35 kg/m², age > 50, neck circumference > 17 inches, and is male.

2. Describe the pathophysiologic factors and physiologic consequences associated with OSA.
The pathophysiology of OSA is multifactorial, involving upper airway anatomy, motor control of the pharyngeal dilator muscles, ventilatory con-

trol stability, and arousal threshold. The upper airway contains three segments: the nasopharynx, the oropharynx, and the hypopharynx. The inspiratory patency of these segments is controlled by contraction of the tensor palatini, the genioglossus, and the hyoid muscles respectively. The three segments are prone to collapse because of the lack of boney support in the anterior and lateral walls. During wakefulness, the action of these pharyngeal dilator muscles are important in keeping the airway patent. However, during deep non-rapid eye movement (NREM) and rapid eye movement (REM) sleep there is a generalized loss of muscle tone, which may result in airway collapse in susceptible patients as is depicted in Figure 5-2.

Several factors contribute to the pathophysiologic changes that are present with OSA.

- When OSA is associated with obesity, there is a larger deposition of adipose tissue in the uvula, tonsils, tonsillar pillars, tongue, aryepiglottic folds, and lateral pharyngeal walls, and possibly externally, which can contribute to airway obstruction during sleep.
- There is poor upper airway motor control during sleep in patients with OSA, which is associated with substantial decrements in pharyngeal dilator muscle activity; over time these

Table 5-1 Severity of Obstructive Sleep Apnea	
SEVERITY OF OSA	**APNEA–HYPOPNEA INDEX**
None	0–5
Mild	6–20
Moderate	21–40
Severe	> 40

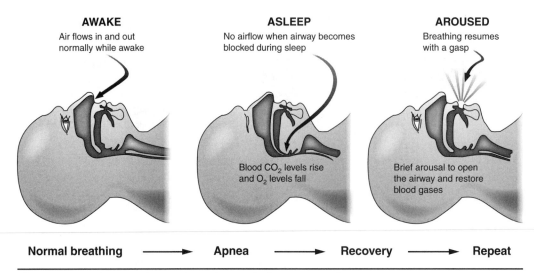

AWAKE
Air flows in and out
normally while awake

ASLEEP
No airflow when airway becomes
blocked during sleep

Blood CO_2 levels rise
and O_2 levels fall

AROUSED
Breathing resumes
with a gasp

Brief arousal to open
the airway and restore
blood gases

Normal breathing ⟶ Apnea ⟶ Recovery ⟶ Repeat

Figure 5-2   *Comparison of awake and obstructive sleep apnea.*

muscles may develop neural/muscle damage which further exacerbates airway obstruction.

• Instability in the control of ventilation results in increases and decreases in respiratory output to pharyngeal dilator muscles which, when combined with increased fat deposition in the airway and poor upper airway motor control, may further contribute to episodes of obstruction.

During episodes of apnea, hypoxemia and hypercarbia develop and lead to progressive increases in respiratory effort. This triggers increased neural stimulation into the reticular activating system, which arouses the individual to a lighter stage of sleep, which then activates the pharyngeal dilator muscles to open the airway. Upon arousal, there is increased electroencephalogram activity and patients may demonstrate vocalization, extremity twitching, turning, gasping, or snorting on airway opening. Ventilation resumes and the hypoxemia and hypercarbia are corrected. However, relief of the obstruction is associated with a short period of hyperventilation, which may significantly decrease the CO_2 and respiratory drive, and may contribute to episodes of apnea that are followed by hyperpnea. These repeated obstructive and hypoxemic/hypercarbic events cause sleep fragmentation, sympathetic hyperactivity, systemic inflammation with higher C-reactive protein (CR-P) and interleukin-6 (IL-6) levels, endothelial dysfunction, and metabolic dysregulation—all of which can increase the risk for cardiovascular, neuropsychologic, and endocrine disorders.

3. Discuss the coexisting diseases that are associated with patients presenting for UPPP and OSA. Ostructive sleep apnea affects the cardiovascular, neuropsychologic, and endocrine systems because of the repeated cycles of apnea and airway obstruction during sleep. Systemic vasoconstriction results in hypertension and may contribute to left ventricular failure. In fact, OSA has been found to be an independent risk factor of essential hypertension after controlling for age, sex, BMI, and antihypertensive agents. Arrhythmias that are caused by hypoxia and hypercarbia such as atrial fibrillation, bradycardia, and atrioventricular block can occur. Sympathetic hyperactivity, inflammation, and endothelial dysfunction contribute to an increased incidence of nocturnal angina and myocardial infarction (MI).

Cerebrovascular disease (CVD) and stroke is associated with OSA. Pulmonary hypertension

Table 5-2   Coexisting Diseases/Symptoms Associated with Obstructive Sleep Apnea

CARDIOVASCULAR	NEUROPSYCHOLOGIC	ENDOCRINE/OTHER
• Hypertension	• Daytime somnolence	• Glucose intolerance and diabetes
• Arrhythmias:	• Cognitive impairment	• Obesity
• Atrial fibrillation	• Accident proneness	• Gastroesophageal reflux disease
• Bradycardia	• Anxiety	
• Atrioventricular block	• Depression	
• Coronary artery disease		
• Nocturnal angina		
• Myocardial infarction		
• Congestive heart failure		
• Pulmonary hypertension		

secondary to frequent hypoxia over many years may lead to right-sided heart failure. Neuropsychologic symptoms include daytime somnolence, impaired cognitive function, increased accidents because of decreased vigilance, depression, and anxiety. The endocrine system manifestations include obesity, glucose intolerance and diabetes, and decreases in testosterone and growth hormone. Table 5-2 summarizes coexisting diseases associated with OSA.

4. Describe the preoperative evaluation and preparation for a patient with OSA presenting for UPPP.

Patients with OSA require a thorough preoperative evaluation to identify and minimize perioperative complications. A complete history and physical examination should be performed, with special attention to the airway examination because patients with OSA have a higher incidence of difficult intubation. Anatomic factors that can complicate direct laryngoscopy and intubation are included in Table 5-3. A history of difficult intubation associated with previous anesthetic experiences, as well as any other complications, should be elicited. Review of systems should focus on the presence, severity, and effectiveness

of current management of coexisting diseases associated with OSA. Preoperative testing is dependent on the individual patient's situation and may include ECG, stress testing, chest x-ray, electrolyte, complete blood counts, and a coagulation panels.

Table 5-3   Risk Factors Associated with Difficult Intubation

- Mallampati Class III or IV
- Long upper incisors
- Prominent overbite
- Mandibular incisors anterior to maxillary incisors
- < 3 finger breadths thyromental distance
- > 3 cm interincisor distance
- Retrognathia or micrognathia
- Macroglossia
- High arched or very narrow palate
- Stiff, indurated, occupied by mass, or nonresilient mandibular space
- Short, thick neck; neck circumference > 40–42 cm
- Limited neck range of motion
- Apnea–hypopnea index > 40
- Obesity

Sleep study results, if available, should be reviewed and documented. If a sleep study is not available, such patients should be treated as having moderate OSA. They should be considered to have severe OSA if they have markedly increased BMI or neck circumference, episodes of apnea, or if the patient falls asleep within minutes if unstimulated. CPAP settings should be documented and patients should be instructed to bring the machines on the day of surgery.

The suitability for inpatient or outpatient surgery, extended postoperative monitoring (i.e., monitored settings vs routine hospital wards) and duration of stay (extended stay in postanesthesia care unit [PACU] vs no extended stay in PACU; hospital admission vs no admission) should be determined prior to surgery. These decisions should be based on severity of the OSA, anatomic or physiologic abnormalities, status of coexisting diseases, type of anesthesia, need for postoperative opioids, patient age, adequacy of postdischarge observation, and capabilities of the facility.

5. Utilizing the American Society of Anesthesiologists (ASA) Practice Guidelines for OSA, predict the perioperative risk for the above patient.

The ASA Practice Guidelines for OSA estimates risk of perioperative complications based on:

- **(A) Severity of OSA**: none, 0 points; mild, 1 point; moderate, 2 points; and severe, 3 points—subtract 1 point if CPAP or BiPAP preop and postop, + 1 point if $PaCO_2 > 50$ mm HG
- **(B) Invasiveness of surgery**: superficial surgery under local or peripheral nerve block anesthesia without sedation, 0 points; superficial surgery with moderate sedation or general anesthesia, 1 point; peripheral surgery with spinal or epidural anesthesia (with no more than moderate sedation), 1 point; peripheral surgery with general anesthesia or airway surgery with moderate sedation, 2 points; and

major surgery or airway surgery with general anesthesia, 3 points
- **(C) Requirements for postoperative opioids**: none, 0 points; low-dose oral opioids, 1 point; high-dose oral, parental, or neuraxial opioids, 3 points.
- Estimation of the overall risk is based on the sum of A + B + C (range 0–6). Patients with a score of 4 may be at increased perioperative risk from OSA; scores of 5 or 6 significantly increase the perioperative risk from OSA.

This patient has severe OSA (3 points), is having airway surgery under general anesthesia (3 points), and has a low-dose opioid requirement postoperatively (3 points). The patient has been using CPAP preoperatively and it is anticipated he will use it postoperatively (subtract 1 point). The overall score is 5, which indicates the patient may be at significantly increased perioperative risk from OSA.

Intraoperative Period

6. Summarize the effects of anesthesia on the airway and respiratory function.

Patients who have OSA are extremely sensitive to the airway and respiratory depressant effects of anesthetic agents and opioids. Anesthetic agents such as propofol, thiopental, midazolam, opioids, small doses of neuromuscular blockers, and nitrous oxide diminish the pharyngeal dilator muscle action and promote upper airway collapse. Additionally, most anesthetics and opioids alter the control of breathing by affecting the chemical, metabolic, or behavioral control of respiration. Propofol has been shown to produce a dose-dependent decrease in genioglossal muscle, which results in greater airway collapsibility. Nasopharyngeal anesthesia with 4% lidocaine is associated with decreased genioglossal muscle function and increased pharyngeal airway collapsibility. Dexmedetomidine is associated with anxiolytic, sedative, and analgesic effects without causing significant respiratory depression.

7. Describe the effects of anesthesia and surgery on postoperative sleep patterns.

Patients with OSA who use opioids during the postoperative period for pain relief are at increased risk of life-threatening apnea for approximately a week after surgery. Sleep architecture is altered after surgery with suppression of stage 3 and 4 REM and NREM sleep. Postoperative pain is greatest in the first several days after surgery and these patients are at increased risk for life-threatening obstructive apnea secondary to respiratory depressive effects of opioids. After the third postoperative day, deep REM sleep rebounds and patients who have OSA are at risk for life-threatening deep sleep-induced apnea.

8. Formulate an anesthetic plan for a patient presenting for UPPP with severe OSA and a potential difficult airway.

The patient's airway exam, obesity, and severe OSA increase the risk that the patient may be a difficult mask ventilation and intubation, respectively. Given this information, an awake fiberoptic intubation is recommended. Table 5-4 lists considerations for performing an awake fiberoptic intubation. Important points to consider when a fiberoptic intubation is planned include:

- Administration of an antisialagogue such as glycopyrrolate in the preoperative area
- Carefully administering sedation to maintain meaningful contact with patient
- Adequately anesthetizing the patient's airway
- Utilizing proper technique when manipulating the fiberoptic scope
- Ability to troubleshoot problems

Sedation for the procedure may include anxiolytics such as versed titrated to effect, and opioids such as fentanyl or alfentanil. Extreme caution should be used when determining to give opioids to patients with severe OSA while in the preoperative area. Other sedatives include dexmedetomidine and ketamine. Once the patient is intubated fiberoptically an intravenous and/or inhalation induction may be performed. Agents chosen should be based on the patient's coexisting diseases. Placement of a mouth gag that is used to keep the jaw in the open position is stimulating and boluses of propofol or an opioid may be needed to blunt the airway response. Dexamethasone is frequently given to decrease the degree of edema formation in the oral cavity.

The anesthetic can be maintained by administering short-acting agents such as desflurane with or without nitrous oxide, remifentanil, or alfentanil and subtherapeutic doses of intermediate-acting neuromuscular blockers. Since blood that enters the stomach is highly emetogenic, antiemetics such as odansetron or dolasetron should be considered. Based on surgeon preference and the presence of adequate hemostasis, ketorolac may be given for postoperative analgesia. This patient was identified as having a difficult intubation and the fiberoptic scope and airway cart/adjuncts should be immediately available if the need for emergent reintubation should arise. The patient should respond to commands appropriately and meet other extubation criteria prior to removal of the ETT. Hemostasis should be confirmed prior to extubation. The patient may need to be extubated over a tube changer if there was difficulty or concern with the airway. Extubation should occur in the semi-recumbent or the reverse Trendelenburg position to minimize compression of the diaphragm by the abdomen.

Postoperative Period

9. List the potential postoperative complications/ events and frequency that can occur after UPPP.

- Respiratory 1.1–11% (i.e., laryngospasm, post-obstructive pulmonary edema, airway obstruction and oxygen desaturation, emergent tracheotomy, reintubation, and pneumonia)
- Hemorrhage 0.3–14% (biphasic occurrence; immediate postoperatively or several days after surgery)
- Hypertension 2–70%
- Cardiovascular < 0.3% (i.e., arrhythmias, cardiac arrest, angina, MI, cerebrovascular accident, or pulmonary embolism)

Table 5-4   Procedure for Awake Fiberoptic Intubation

1. Discuss need for awake fiberoptic intubation with patient and surgical team.

2. IV access should be obtained as soon as possible and glycopyrrolate 0.2 mg IV (takes up to 20 minutes for peak effect).

3. Difficult airway cart with a fiberoptic bronchoscope (at least 2 mm narrower than the ETT), atomizer, nebulizer, nasal trumpets, viscous lidocaine and lubricant, Ovassapian and Williams airways, sources of oxygen and suction, cotton-tipped applicators, bag valve mask, and additional difficult intubation equipment should be in room.

4. Bronchoscope should be verified for proper functioning and attached to a light source and camera if present. Practice rotating, antiflexing, and retroflexing the scope.

5. Adequate airway topicalization is critical. Techniques include:

   - 4% lidocaine by atomizer or nebulizer

   - 5% lidocaine ointment on top of tongue depressor placed in the back of mouth near posterior pharynx

   - If nasal intubation is needed, the nares should be sprayed with Neo-Synephrine spray, then may use 4% lidocaine in a syringe or atomizer to spray in the nose; 2% lidocaine jelly in a 10-ml syringe can be injected into the nose.

   - Glossopharyngeal and superior laryngeal nerve blocks with 1–2 ml of lidocaine 1–2%. Glossopharyngeal nerve block provides anesthesia to the posterior third of the tongue, anterior epiglottis, posterior and lateral walls of the pharynx, and the tonsillar pillars. The superior laryngeal nerve block abolishes the gag reflex by providing anesthesia of the larynx down to but excluding the vocal cords.

6. If oral intubation is done, a Williams or Ovassapian airway should be used to keep scope midline. The ETT can then be slid close to the cords then pass the fiberoptic scope; alternatively, the scope may be passed first. If nasal intubation, then pass the tube first into the posterior pharynx.

7. Prior to passing the scope through the cords, additional lidocaine can be injected onto the cords via the side port on the scope. Alternatively, a transtracheal injection of local anesthetic can be performed to block the recurrent laryngeal nerve.

8. Suction and oxygen can be attached to the scope and used if needed.

9. If pink tissue is seen, pull the ETT and scope back until the vocal cords can be seen. An assistant may also provide a jaw thrust or cricoid pressure to help open the airway and improve visualization/guidance.

10. Once fiberoptic is passed through the vocal cords advance and avoid touching the carina. Next, slide the ETT over the fiberoptic scope. If resistance is met pull the tube back and rotate the ETT 90 degrees counterclockwise, this turns the tip away from the arytenoids.

11. After placement is confirmed, general anesthesia may be induced.

ETT, endotracheal tube; IV, intravenous.

10. Describe the postoperative management for patients after UPPP with severe OSA.
Anesthetic considerations in the postoperative period include:

- Decreasing postoperative pain
- Ensuring adequate oxygenation
- Observing for airway obstruction
- Positioning the patient in a lateral or semirecumbent position
- Using of CPAP

Patients with severe OSA are at high risk for opioid-induced airway obstruction in the postoperative period and should not be discharged from the recovery room to an unmonitored setting. This is especially important because UPPP surgery is associated with moderate postoperative pain, and patients may require intravenous narcotics and have an increased susceptibility to airway obstruction given the type of surgery. Nonsteroidal anti-inflammatory agents have an opioid-sparing effect and should be considered. Recent research suggests clonidine 2 ug/kg orally in the preoperative period stabilizes intraoperative hemodynamics and reduces intraoperative anesthetics and postoperative opioid requirements. Supplemental oxygen and continuous pulse oximetry should be continued until patients can maintain room air oxygen saturation at baseline or > 90% and not develop airway obstruction when left undisturbed. Patients should be positioned either in the lateral or semirecumbent position, and CPAP should be restarted as soon as it is safe enough in the postoperative period. Finally, patients with severe OSA should be admitted to an intensive care setting for airway observation for up to 24 hours.

REVIEW QUESTIONS

1. Obstructive sleep apnea is associated with periodic, partial, or complete obstruction of the upper airway during sleep and is not associated with:
   a. apnea-hypopnea and frequent arousals.
   b. oxygen desaturation.
   c. daytime hypersomnolence.
   d. hypocarbia.
2. Which classification of OSA is associated with a preoperative apnea–hypopnea index of 25?
   a. None
   b. Mild
   c. Moderate
   d. Severe
3. Which statement is true regarding the pathophysiologic changes associated with obstructive sleep apnea?
   a. Poor upper airway motor control
   b. Increased upper airway motor control
   c. Ventilatory control stability
   d. Increased pharyngeal dilator muscle activity
4. Repeated obstructive and hypoxemic/hypercarbic events do not result in:
   a. sleep fragmentation.
   b. parasympathetic nervous system hyperactivity.
   c. metabolic dysregulation.
   d. systemic inflammation.
5. Postoperative narcotic administration and airway obstruction can increase the risk for life-threatening apnea because of:
   a. stability of the sleep architecture, postoperative pain, and rebound of light REM sleep.
   b. alteration of the sleep architecture alteration, postoperative pain, respiratory depressant effect of opioids, and rebound of deep REM sleep.
   c. alteration of the sleep architecture alteration, decreased postoperative pain, and rebound of deep REM sleep.
   d. inhibition of the airway reflexes, stimulation of the sympathetic nervous system, and increased myocardial oxygen consumption.

REVIEW ANSWERS

1. **Answer: d**
   Obstructive sleep apnea is a syndrome associated with periodic, partial, or complete obstruction of the upper airway during sleep that leads to episodes of apnea-hypopnea, frequent arousals, oxygen desaturation, and daytime hypersomnolence and hypercarbia.
2. **Answer: c**
   Based on the ASA Clinical Practice Guidelines for OSA, an apnea–hypopnea index (AHI) of 25 indicates the patient has moderate OSA. Sources vary, but severe sleep apnea is defined as an AHI > 30 or > 40 per the ASA Practice Guidelines.
3. **Answer: a**
   Patients with OSA display poor upper airway control during sleep, which is associated with

substantial decrements in pharyngeal dilator muscle activity; over time these muscles may develop neural/muscle damage, which further exacerbates the obstruction. OSA is associated with ventilatory control instability that results in increases and decreases in respiratory output to pharyngeal dilator muscles which, when combined with increased fat deposition in the airway and poor upper airway motor control, may further contribute to episodes of obstruction.

4. **Answer: b**

Chronic repeated obstructive events of hypoxemia and hypercarbia cause sleep fragmentation, sympathetic hyperactivity, systemic inflammation with higher C-reactive protein and interleukin-6 levels, endothelial dysfunction, and metabolic dysregulation—all of which can increase the risk for cardiovascular, neuropsychologic, and endocrine disorders and an impaired the quality of life.

5. **Answer: b**

Sleep architecture is altered after surgery with suppression of stage 3 and 4 REM and NREM sleep. Postoperative pain is highest in the first several days after UPPP surgery. Patients with OSA are at greater risk for life-threatening obstructive apnea secondary to respiratory depressive effects of opioids. After the third postoperative day, deep REM sleep rebounds and OSA patients are again at risk for life-threatening deep sleep-induced apnea.

SUGGESTED READINGS

Benumof JL. Obesity, sleep apnea, the airway and anesthesia. *Curr Opin Anaesthesiol* 2004;17(1):21–30.

Chung F, Yegneswaran B, Liao P, et al. Validation of the Berlin questionnaire and American Society of Anesthesiologists checklist as screening tools for obstructive sleep apnea in surgical patients. *Anesthesiology* 2008;108(5):822–830.

Chung SA, Yuan H, Chung F. A systemic review of obstructive sleep apnea and its implications for anesthesiologists. *Anesth Analg* 2008;107(5):1543–1563.

Gross JB, Bachenberg KL, Benumof JL, et al. Practice guidelines for the perioperative management of patients with obstructive sleep apnea: a report by the American society of anesthesiologists task force on perioperative management of patients with obstructive sleep apnea. *Anesthesiology* 2006;104(5):1081–1093; quiz 1117–1118.

Kezirian EJ, Weaver EM, Yueh B, et al. Risk factors for serious complication after uvulopalatopharyngoplasty. *Arch Otolaryngol Head Neck Surg* 2006;132(10):1091–1098.

McNicholas WT, Ryan S. Obstructive sleep apnea syndrome: Translating science to clinical practice. *Respirology* 2006;11(2):136–144.

Moos DD, Prasch M, Cantral DE, et al. Are patients with obstructive sleep apnea syndrome appropriate candidates for the ambulatory surgical center? *AANA J* 2005;73(3):197–205.

Nieto FJ, Young TB, Lind BK, et al. Association of sleep-disordered breathing, sleep apnea, and hypertension in a large community-based study. sleep heart health study. *JAMA* 2000;283(14):1829–1836.

Pawlik MT, Hansen E, Waldhauser D, et al. Clonidine premedication in patients with sleep apnea syndrome: a randomized, double-blind, placebo-controlled study. *Anesth Analg* 2005;101(5):1374–1380.

Somers VK, White DP, Amin R, et al. Sleep apnea and cardiovascular disease: an American Heart Association/American College of cardiology foundation scientific statement from the American heart association council for high blood pressure research professional education committee, council on clinical cardiology, stroke council, and council on cardiovascular nursing. *J Am Coll Cardiol* 2008;52(8):686–717.

General Surgery

II

Exploratory Laparotomy for Bowel Resection

6

Timothy Palmer

KEY POINTS

- Hemodynamic variability is possible and can be attributed to factors such as preoperative dehydration, evaporative fluid loss from the surgical site, sepsis, and blood loss.
- Electrolyte and acid–base abnormalities may occur during the intraoperative management.
- Extensive third space expansion due to extravasation of volume from the intravascular space and from perforated viscera may prohibit abdominal closure at the end of surgery.
- The patient's history and intraoperative course contributes to decisions regarding postoperative management.

CASE SYNOPSIS

A 48-year-old woman is scheduled to have an exploratory laparotomy. She has a 3-day history of increasing episodes of vomiting. A nasogastric tube is inserted and 300 ml of gastric secretions are suctioned. The patient is complaining of feeling bloated and severe abdominal pain.

PREOPERATIVE EVALUATION AND DEMOGRAPHIC DATA

Past Medical/Surgical History

- Hypertension
- Cholecystectomy (open): 2 years ago, no anesthetic complications
- Total abdominal hysterectomy: 12 years ago, no anesthetic complications

List of Medications

- Zestril (lisinopril)
- Nexium (esomeprazole Mg)

Diagnostic Data

- Hemoglobin, 13 g/dl; hematocrit, 39%
- Electrolytes: sodium, 132 mEq/l; potassium, 2.8 mEq/l; chloride, 96 mEq/l; carbon dioxide, 22 mEq/l
- Arterial blood gases: pH, 7.46; $PaCO_2$, 32 mm Hg; HCO_3, 20 mEq/l; base excess, 6

Height/Weight/Vital Signs

- 163 cm, 72 kg
- Blood pressure, 96/62; heart rate, 112 beats per minute; respiratory rate, 28 breaths per minute; room air oxygen saturation, 94%; temperature, 38.5°C
- Electrocardiogram (ECG): Sinus tachycardia, heart rate, 108 beats per minute

PATHOPHYSIOLOGY

There are multiple causes for acute abdominal disease with intestinal obstruction. Obstruction can occur in various portions of the bowel and the etiology of obstruction may be multifactorial; most likely caused by adhesions, strictures, or tumor. Intestinal obstruction may be intraluminal (e.g., due to tumor, sequestration within a hernia, stricture), extraluminal (e.g., cholelithiasis, foreign body), or as part of a process directly involving the bowel tissue (e.g., ulcerative colitis, Crohn disease, ischemic pathology). Pain is the most common initial symptom associated with abdominal disease and is typically present in acute obstructive disease. The etiology of abdominal pain is multifactorial. Pain may initially be localized or nonspecific and referred from one abdominal region to another due to anatomic confluence of common neural pathways from various intraabdominal structures. Abdominal distention may progress dramatically, which strongly suggests the presence of a perforated intraabdominal viscous; a sign that is verified by radiographic findings showing evidence of free air within the abdominal cavity. Associated symptoms include nausea and vomiting, bloating, constipation, and diarrhea.

Other causes of acute obstruction may be attributed to the development of adhesions that occurs as a result of previous abdominal surgery. Incarcerated or strangulated loops of bowel that become trapped within hernias in the abdominal wall may occur. A prior history of abdominal surgery, particularly in the pelvic region, is associated with a greater risk of developing intraabdominal adhesions. Patient's who are sedentary, debilitated, and taking chronic medications (i.e., phenothiazines) are at increased risk of developing hypotonic bowel. Such an area may evolve into a strangulated loop of bowel or into a complete bowel obstruction. Bowel obstruction, strangulation, and perforation results in hypovolemia from causes which include vomiting, diarrhea, extravascular fluid losses, and gastric suctioning. Peritonitis and sepsis, which occur from the bacteria and enterotoxins that are released from the perforated bowel, further magnify fluid loss. These processes can dramatically affect intravascular volume, electrolyte, acid–base balance, and result in sepsis. Multisystem organ dysfunction syndrome is associated with increased mortality, which is initiated via the inflammatory response and may result in acute respiratory distress syndrome.

SURGICAL PROCEDURE

Surgical resection of a diseased portion of intestine is accomplished by creating a midline abdominal incision. This surgery is necessary for a variety of reasons including the presence of a tumor or to remove an ischemic portion of the bowel caused by adhesions, volvulus, or herniation of the intestine. The fascia and the muscle layers are excised and retractors are placed within the abdomen to improve visualization. The peritoneal cavity is inspected. After the disease portion of the bowel is identified and resected, the distal and proximal ends of the bowel are excised as seen in Figure 6-1. An anastomosis is created by inserting a stapling device through a purse string suture that is made at the distal portion. The abdominal incision is closed and dressed.

Diseased part of small
bowel removed

Healthy ends
reattached

Figure 6-1   *Bowel resection performed using open laparotomy.*

ANESTHETIC MANAGEMENT AND CONSIDERATIONS

Preoperative Period

1. Compare and contrast the clinical considerations associated with a large bowel and small bowel obstruction.

Large bowel obstruction typically has a longer prodromal period before acute signs and symptoms occur. It may be associated with fewer acute metabolic derangements because its primary function is storage rather than secretion and absorption. The large bowel is less likely to strangulate than the small bowel but it can become markedly distended under certain conditions, such as toxic megacolon, which may lead to rupture.

Small bowel obstruction generally occurs with a more acute onset. The progression of small bowel obstruction begins with hypotonia (loss of motility with intraluminal stasis), osmotic disequilibrium leading to transudation of fluids into the peritoneum, accumulation of gas, and eventually electrolyte imbalance. Systemic derangements in organ function may be more dramatic and acute in comparison to

large bowel obstruction. A small bowel obstruction is more likely to occur than a large bowel obstruction (75–80%).

The risk of gastric aspiration is increased in patients who have a bowel obstruction due to increased gastric volume resulting in increased gastric pressure. The competency of the lower esophageal sphincter is also compromised and as a result a rapid sequence induction during induction of anesthesia and tracheal intubation is warranted. Tracheal extubation at the end of surgery is undertaken only after the patient demonstrates awareness and control of airway reflexes.

2. Discuss the physiologic concerns associated with toxic megacolon.

Toxic megacolon occurs more frequently in patients that have ulcerative colitis and the condition can occur in critically ill patients undergoing aggressive antibiotic therapy. In this disease process, acute stasis of the large colon permits bacterial overgrowth, promoting a dramatic increase in intraluminal pressure. This results from overproduction of gas within the lumen of the bowel caused by anaerobic metabolism. The result is mucosal inflammation with loss of bowel wall integrity occurs, which facilitates systemic absorption of bacterial endotoxins. Clinical signs include abdominal distention, fever, tachycardia, pain, and the absence of bowel sounds. Anemia, leukocytosis, hypokalemia, and hypoalbuminemia are typically present. Aggressive resuscitation and emergent colectomy is indicated. The mortality rate associated with this condition may be as high as 30%.

3. Describe typical signs and symptoms of bowel obstruction.

The most common signs and symptoms associated with bowel obstruction are included in Table 6-1.

4. Describe the physiologic manifestations associated with bowel perforation.

Bowel perforation results from decreased blood flow, which causes tissue ischemia and a breakdown of the bowel wall resulting from increased intraluminal pressure. Obstruction to blood flow along with impairment in bowel motility leads to sequestration and accumulation of fluid and gas proximal to the level of obstruction. Absorption of intraluminal fluid is impaired because of increased

---

Table 6-1	**Signs and Symptoms Associated with Bowel Obstruction and Perforation**

- Pain
- Abdominal distention
- Bloating
- Constipation
- Nausea and vomiting
- Fever
- Leukocytosis
- Hemodynamic variability
- Intraluminal gas-fluid within the lumen of segments proximal to the obstruction
- Free air present within the peritoneum (suggestive of bowel perforation)

---

intraluminal pressure. Furthermore, hypersecretion of fluid occurs, which is enhanced by the release of prostaglandins. Release of bacteria, endotoxins, and intraluminal contaminants from within the bowel lumen into the peritoneum and into the systemic circulation results in sepsis.

5. Describe the cardiovascular abnormalities associated with bowel obstruction.

Profound alterations in cardiovascular functioning and metabolic homeostasis are possible because of disruption in the integrity of the gastrointestinal tract. Hemodynamic function is particularly susceptible to alterations in fluid, electrolyte, and acid–base balance that occur. Cardiovascular function is affected by decreased preload resulting from an intravascular fluid volume deficit. Compensatory sympathetic responses (tachycardia and vasoconstriction) attempt to restore adequate perfusion to tissues; however, there is a point where the compensatory mechanism will fail. If the bowel is perforated and sepsis occurs, bacterial endotoxins enhance the activity of nitric oxide, inhibits vasopressin or activates ATP sensitive potassium channels in vascular smooth muscle resulting in systemic vasodilation. It is surmised that one or a combination of these mechanisms cause severe hypotension that may or may not be responsive to vasopressor medication during septic shock.

Cardiac conduction abnormalities resulting from hypokalemia during a bowel obstruction can cause ECG abnormalities which include atrial and ventricular dysrhythmias, ST-T wave depression, prominent U wave, prolonged PR interval, and increased P wave amplitude. A rapid progression to shock and systemic organ failure will occur.

6. Define abdominal compartment syndrome and the anesthetic implications.

Abdominal compartment syndrome (ACS) is associated with increased intraabdominal pressure (IAP) which can cause to end-organ dysfunction. Increased IAP decreases cardiac output, glomerular filtration, and mesenteric and hepatic perfusion. Decreased respiratory excursion and functional residual capacity can lead to increased peak airway pressures and hypoxia. Because of pressure on the venous and arterial vasculature within the abdominal cavity, increases in intracranial pressure occur.

Normal IAP approximates atmospheric pressure. Progressive impairment on organ dysfunction occurs as IAP exceeds 25 mm Hg. Abdominal compartment syndrome is associated with abdominal trauma, infarction with necrosis of abdominal viscera, repair of a ruptured abdominal aortic aneurysm, and pancreatitis. Overzealous infusion of colloid and/or crystalloid intravenous solutions during emergent resuscitation can cause ACS. Fulminant ACS is associated with an approximate mortality rate of 50% mortality.

Intraoperative Period

7. Discuss the use of invasive intraoperative monitoring for bowel resection.

The clinical decision to employ invasive monitoring modalities is directed by numerous factors, including the magnitude of the surgical procedure, the length of surgical time anticipated, the degree to which fluid shifts may become problematic, the extent of preoperative preparation of the patient, and the presence of comorbid patient factors.

An arterial line and pressure monitoring allows for beat-to-beat assessment of arterial blood pressure and allows the anesthetist to obtain blood for intraoperative analysis. The use of central venous pressure (CVP) monitoring may be considered. The CVP is used to assess volume status and the cordis can be used to administer fluids, blood, and or vasoactive medications. CVP values have been determined to be unreliable in the presence of both right and left ventricular dysfunction, pulmonary hypertension, valvular dysfunction, and abdominal distention. When utilized, the CVP should be used to monitor trends and responses to fluid boluses used to correct hypovolemia related to hypotension.

Pulmonary artery catheter placement may also be considered for assessment of cardiac output and cardiac index and to measure pulmonary and systemic vascular resistance. There is considerable controversy as to the accuracy of the specificity and sensitivity of data that is obtained during monitoring. Central venous catheterization may increase the risk of infection.

Emerging technologies which are noninvasive and minimally invasive have been studied in clinical trials and allow the anesthetist to assess the arterial waveform contour analysis, stroke volume, and stroke volume variation (SVV) as real-time parameters of cardiac performance and volume status. Data that has been obtained supports these indicators of cardiac performance in comparison with single, point-in-time measurement of cardiac output as obtained by a pulmonary artery catheter.

8. Construct a fluid plan for a patient having a bowel resection.

Implementation of a fluid management strategy is based on assimilated preoperative data and the patient's preexisting comorbidities (e.g. cardiovascular disease, renal insufficiency, pulmonary disease, advanced age). Laboratory values are also pertinent in estimating the magnitude of deficit necessitating replacement as well as in selection of appropriate resuscitative fluid. Fluid losses caused by vomiting and diarrhea are associated with electrolyte losses, which may warrant concurrent replacement in addition to restoration of circulating intravascular volume.

In the presence of bowel obstruction, third space loss occurs into the interstitium within the bowel wall. Fluid may also be sequestered within the lumen of the bowel. Both cases result in bowel dilation leading to failure in barrier function. With the loss of bowel wall integrity, hypoalbuminemia occurs because of loss of protein-rich exudate into the peritoneum. An aberrant osmolar gradient facilitates continued fluid loss into this space.

Patients undergoing elective intraabdominal surgery may undergo a preoperative cathartic bowel cleansing preparation, which is administered orally or via enema. The potential benefits of this intervention include lower wound infection rates and lower rates in peritoneal contamination and anastomotic breakdown. Presently, there is no clinically reliable method available that can accurately account for this fluid loss. The potential magnitude of volume and electrolyte loss can be extreme. Preoperative assessment of volume deficit and electrolyte balance must therefore not only consider losses mediated by diarrhea, vomiting, third space loss, and fasting, but also as secondary to bowel preparation. In patients who are in relatively good health, the effects of bowel preparation are generally well tolerated; however, the physiologic consequences in patients who are malnourished or in medically compromised may result in tachycardia, hypotension, decreased renal blood flow, and possible increased morbidity. An adequate amount or urine output is 0.5–1 ml/kg/hr.

9. Discuss the advantages and contraindications associated with laparoscopic bowel resection as compared to a traditional open approach.

In select procedures with adequate preoperative patient preparation, a laparoscopic or laparoscopic-assisted technique is an option. Laparoscopy has evolved into a standard minimally invasive surgical technique with an ever increasing array of applications and is show in Figure 6-2. The

Table 6-2	Advantages of Laparoscopic Bowel Resection

- Decreased postoperative pain
- Decreased hospitalization time
- Decreased postoperative ileus
- Rapid recovery of pulmonary function
- Improved cosmetic result
- Decreased overall morbidity

benefits associated with laparoscopic surgery for bowel resection are listed in Table 6-2. Surgical trauma necessary for exposure and access is associated with inducing an inflammatory response, which results in a variable degree of systemic manifestations. Due to the minimal invasiveness of laparoscopic bowel resection as compared to the conventional open approach, surgical morbidity is decreased. The contraindications associated with laparoscopic bowel resection are listed in Table 6-3.

10. Describe the anesthetic challenges associated with intraoperative ventilation during pneumoperitoneum.

The creation of a pneumoperitoneum through insufflation of carbon dioxide (CO_2) gas into the abdominal cavity is necessary to perform a laparoscopic bowel resection. Advantages to using CO_2 as an insufflating gas include its nonflammability, its rapidity in movement across lipid membranes, its solubility in the blood, and its rapid removal by the

Figure 6-2 *Laparoscopic bowel resection.*

Table 6-3	Contraindications to Laparoscopic Bowel Resection

- Intestinal obstruction
- Bulky tumors
- Evidence of metastatic tumor growth in adjacent abdominal organs
- Pregnancy

lungs. The effect on the patient's cardiovascular system and pulmonary ventilatory mechanics can be significant.

Absorption of CO_2 that results from the insufflating gas consistently occurs during laparoscopy as increased in end-tidal CO_2 occur. Thus, increased minute ventilation is necessary to achieve normocapnia. Furthermore, insufflation of CO_2 gas under pressure is capable of causing subcutaneous emphysema. If the insufflating trocar is placed inappropriately and/or migrates within the abdominal cavity, then a pathway for CO_2 gas to diffuse into the subcutaneous space.

The use of CO_2 has additional disadvantages and can cause hypercarbia, peritoneal irritation, hypertension, and acidosis. The adverse effects of CO_2 insufflation can be further exacerbated by the effects caused by surgery and anesthesia. The mechanics associated with ventilation during laparoscopy causes increased dead space ventilation, reduction in functional residual capacity, and decreased pulmonary compliance. The lithotomy and Trendelenburg positions further decrease pulmonary compliance causing ventilation perfusion mismatch.

Ventilatory alterations imposed by anesthesia and pneumoperitoneum can be partially offset by administering positive-end expiratory pressure (PEEP) and pressure-control ventilation utilizing a higher ventilatory rate and lower tidal volumes to achieve normocarbia and acceptable peak ventilating pressures. The overall postoperative pulmonary function (forced expiratory volume in 1 second [FEV_1] and forced vital capacity [FVC]) in patients undergoing laparoscopic procedures in comparison with those patients undergoing conventional laparotomy is improved.

of renal venous flow as evidenced by decreased urine output. Reduced cardiac preload with consequent reduction in cardiac output and perfusion pressure may also occur. Systemic blood pressure is usually maintained or increased due to the effect CO_2 exerts in the peritoneum causing increased sympathetic tone and systemic peripheral resistance. Increased cardiac filling pressures may initially occur with insufflation due to increased intrathoracic pressure. Ventricular wall tension and left ventricular function is generally well preserved in healthy patients but pneumoperitoneum may have deleterious consequences in patients with compromised cardiac function. Decreased preload and increased afterload can result in decreased cardiac output and myocardial ischemia in patients with limited cardiac reserve.

A CO_2 gas embolism is a rare event but can result in decreased myocardial and cerebral perfusion. As CO_2 gas is inadvertently entrained into venous circulation, an air lock is created at the level of the inferior vena cava and right atrium. The signs associated with CO_2 air embolism include:

- Hypotension
- Hypoxemia
- Decreased end-tidal CO_2
- Dysrhythmias

The interventions used to treat a venous air embolus include:

- Immediate exsufflation
- Administer 100% oxygen
- Positioning in left lateral decubitus
- Intravenous fluid bolus
- Vasopressors
- Minimizing peak airway pressures
- Aspiration from the central venous pressure line

11. Describe the hemodynamic effects of increased IAP caused by a pneumoperitoneum.

Elevation in IAP can cause obstruct blood flow to the mesentery, liver, and inferior vena cava. Renal function may be compromised due to compression

12. Describe the activation of the neuroendocrine stress response caused by bowel surgery.

Abdominal insufflation as well as intraabdominal exploration induces a stress response as evidenced by increased plasma concentrations of cortisol, renin, vasopressin, epinephrine, norepinephrine, and angiotensin. The plasma levels of these substances can increase mean arterial pressure (MAP), systemic vascular resistance (SVR), and cardiac output. Methods that can be used to attenuate the hemodynamic responses in the susceptible patient include delivery of a balanced, opioid-based anesthetic technique, the use of alpha-2 agonists (dexmedetomidine, clonidine), and beta adrenergic receptor blockade.

13. Discuss the anesthetic options for a laparoscopic bowel resection.

A balanced anesthetic technique utilizing a volatile inhalation anesthetic agent with opioid and muscle relaxation is effective for laparoscopy. Nitrous oxide is best avoided in laparoscopic surgery due to its potential for causing distention of the bowel. Nitrous oxide can also delay resolution of gaseous air embolism and may increase the incidence of postoperative nausea and vomiting (PONV). Laparoscopic surgery is associated with increased PONV, and prophylactic interventions should be used to decrease the incidence.

Extensive intraabdominal procedures requiring significant visceral manipulation and retraction, particularly in the mid and upper abdomen, will dramatically increase the patient's work of breathing. As a result, neuraxial anesthesia is not commonly used as the sole anesthetic technique during bowel resection. However, epidural anesthesia that is combined with general anesthesia is advantageous by decreasing intraoperative medication requirements and providing postoperative analgesia

Postoperative Period

14. Discuss strategies that can be used to decrease postoperative pain after laparotomy.

A number of strategies may be employed for the purpose of providing postoperative analgesia after laparotomy. Epidural analgesia may be used alone or combined with supplemental intravenous or oral medications to control pain. Patient controlled analgesia (PCA) may also be employed effectively as a primary modality or as a supplement to an epidural technique. An epidural infusion may be initiated preoperatively and used as an adjunct in intraoperative anesthetic management and continued to provide for an established level of analgesia for postoperative management. The use of N-methyl-D-aspartase (NMDA) antagonists such as ketamine, administered in low intravenous doses, has been shown to effectively augment the effect of opioids. Nonsteroidal anti-inflammatory drugs (NSAIDS) can be used effectively as single therapy or in combination with opiates. Infiltration of the surgical wound edges with local anesthetic may offer valuable analgesic supplementation.

Pain that occurs in one or both shoulders following a laparoscopic bowel resection commonly occurs and is most effectively treated with ketorolac. It is theorized that shoulder pain that is caused by creation of a pneumoperitoneum is due to subdiaphragmatic peritoneal irritation from either blood, residual carbon dioxide gas or due to stretching of intra-abdominal tissues. Irrigation of the peritoneal cavity and peritoneal instillation of bupivacaine have been shown to decrease the incidence. Ketorolac should not be administered if the patient is coagulopathic or has asthma, renal insufficiency, or gastric ulcers.

REVIEW QUESTIONS

1. Which is not a sign that is associated with an acute bowel obstruction?
   a. Diarrhea
   b. Abdominal distention
   c. Fever
   d. Vomiting
2. Which is an advantage of laparoscopic bowel resection as compared to laparotomy?
   a. Increased postoperative pain
   b. Decreased hospitalization time
   c. Increased postoperative ileus
   d. Delayed recovery of pulmonary function

3. Which is not a contraindication to laparoscopic bowel resection?
   a. Intestinal obstruction
   b. Bulky tumors
   c. Evidence of metastatic tumor growth in adjacent abdominal organs
   d. Obesity
4. Which is a sign of CO_2 gas embolism?
   a. Hypertension
   b. Hypoxemia
   c. Increased end-tidal CO_2
   d. Decreased hemoglobin
5. Pain that is associated with laparoscopic bowel resection is most likely caused by:
   a. release of inflammatory mediators.
   b. Trendelenburg position.
   c. subdiaphragmatic peritoneal irritation.
   d. inflammation of the bowel.

REVIEW ANSWERS

1. **Answer: a**
   Signs that are associated with a bowel obstruction include constipation, abdominal distention, fever, and vomiting.
2. **Answer: b**
   Advantages associate with laparoscopic bowel resection include decreased postoperative pain, decreased hospitalization time, decreased postoperative ileus, and rapid recovery of pulmonary function.
3. **Answer: d**
   Contraindications to laparoscopic bowel resection include intestinal obstruction, bulky tumors, evidence of metastatic tumor growth in adjacent abdominal organs, and pregnancy.

4. **Answer: b**
   Signs that are associated with a CO_2 gas embolus include hypotension, hypoxemia, decreased end-tidal CO_2, and dysrhythmias.
5. **Answer: c**
   Pain that is associated with laparoscopic bowel resection is most likely caused by subdiaphragmatic peritoneal irritation.

SUGGESTED READINGS

Chappell D, Mathias J, Hofmann-Kiefer K, et al. A rational approach to perioperative fluid management. *Anesthesiology* 2008;109:723–740.

Chung D, Evers B. The digestive system. In: O'Leary J, Capote L. eds. *The Pathologic Basis of Surgery*, 3rd ed. Philadelphia: Lippincott Williams & Wilkins, 2002:457–490.

Church J. Laparotomy for acute colorectal conditions in moribund patients: is it worthwhile? *Diseases of the Colon and Rectum* 2005;48:1147–1152.

Crews J. New developments in epidural anesthesia and analgesia. *Anesthesiol Clin N America* 2000;18:251–266.

Hunter J, Damani Z. Intra-abdominal hypertension and the abdominal compartment syndrome. *Anaesthesia* 2004;59:899–907.

Joshi G. New developments in epidural anesthesia and analgesia. *Anesthesiol Clin N America* 2001;19:89–105.

Kehlet H, Dahl J. Anaesthesia, surgery, and challenges in postoperative recovery. *Lancet* 2003;362:1921–1928.

Muravchick S. Preoperative assessment of the elderly patient. *Anesthesiol Clin N America* 2000;18:71–89.

Ng A, Smith G. Gastrointestinal reflux and aspiration of gastric contents in anaesthetic practice. *Anesth Analg* 2001;93:494–513.

Ogunnaike B, Whitten C. Anesthesia and gastrointestinal disorders. In: Barash P, Cullen B, Stoelting R, eds. *Clinical Anesthesia*, 5th ed. Philadelphia: Lippincott Williams & Wilkins, 2006:1053–1060.

Laparoscopic Gastric Bypass

7

Michael Churchin and Paul Aguiar

KEY POINTS

- As the incidence of obesity continues to increase in the United States, the frequency of bariatric surgery is expected to rise.
- Surgical intervention can attenuate and even resolve the pathophysiologic effects of severe systemic disease that are associated with obesity.
- Successful airway management and intraoperative ventilation presents challenges for the anesthetist.
- Patients who present for bariatric surgery frequently have other pathologic conditions that are associated with obesity.

CASE SYNOPSIS

A 56-year-old woman who is morbidly obese has consulted with her physician and consented to have a gastric bypass procedure. The surgeon has chosen a laparoscopic Roux-en-Y procedure for this patient based on her individual needs.

PREOPERATIVE EVALUATION AND DEMOGRAPHIC DATA

Past Medical/Surgical History

- Type II diabetes
- She uses a walker and frequently develops shortness of breath. She is unable to walk up flight of stairs. She is generally inactive.
- Hypertension
- Hypercholesterolemia
- Obstructive sleep apnea
- Gastroesophageal reflux disease
- Smoked 1 pack of cigarettes a day for 25 years, however she stopped 1 year ago
- Appendectomy 20 years ago without associated anesthesia complications

List of Medications

- NPH insulin
- Cimetidine
- Hydrochlorothiazide
- Lisinopril

Diagnostic Data

- Hemoglobin, 12.2 g/dl; hematocrit, 36.6%
- Platelet count, 336/mm^3
- Glucose, 156 mg/dl (took half dose of NPH on morning of surgery), glycosylated hemoglobin, 7.2%
- Blood urea nitrogen (BUN), 19 mg/dl; creatinine, 0.9 mg/dl
- Prothrombin time, 10.2 seconds; activated partial thromboplastin time, 29 seconds; international normalized ratio, 1.0
- Electrolytes: sodium, 134 mEq/l; potassium, 4.3 mEq/l; chloride, 100 mEq/l; carbon dioxide, 24 mEq/l
- Electrocardiogram: normal sinus rhythm with nonspecific ST segment abnormalities
- Liver function: alanine transaminase (ALT), 28 U/I; aspartate transaminase (AST), 31 U/I
- Cardiac echocardiography: left ventricular hypertrophy; normal systolic ventricular function; ejection fraction, 67%
- Chest x-ray within normal limits
- Pulmonary function test: forced expiratory volume in 1 second (FEV$_1$), 70% of predicted

Height/Weight/Vital Signs

- 155 cm, 152 kg; body mass index (BMI) is 63.3kg/m^2, indicating morbid obesity
- Blood pressure,158/92; heart rate, 86 beats per minute; respiratory rate, 22 breaths per minute; room air oxygen saturation, 95%; temperature 36.6°C

PATHOPHYSIOLOGY

When caloric consumption is greater than the bodies physiologic requirements, obesity is likely to occur. However, the cause of obesity is multifactorial, including environmental factors, genetic predisposition, hormonal disorders, behavioral variables, and cultural norms. Obesity has reached epidemic in proportions in the United States and projections suggest that the rate of this disease process will continue to increase in the future.

Approximately two thirds of adults in the United States are overweight (BMI $\geq$ 25 kg/m^2) and one third are considered obese (BMI $\geq$ 30 kg/m^2). The spectrum continues to include people who are morbidly obese ($\geq$ 35 kg/m^2), super obese ($\geq$ 55 kg/m^2), and super-super obese ($\geq$ 60 kg/m^2). Medications, diet, exercise, and behavioral modification techniques all have poor long-term results and are associated with complications and significant cost. Although there are risks associated with bariatric surgery, it is the most successful intervention to achieve long-term weight loss and to improve or resolve the comorbid diseases that are associated with obesity. Patients who are candidates for bariatric surgery generally have a BMI greater than 35 kg/m^2 with one or more comorbid conditions. A comprehensive medical and surgical bariatric program will include a medical evaluation and optimization of all pathologic disease states, psychologic and nutritional counseling, and a weight loss program before surgery will be performed. There are significant risks associated with bariatric surgery and a list of contraindications is highlighted in Table 7-1.

Table 7-1   Contraindications to Bariatric Surgery

- Severe cardiac disease
- Poor myocardial reserve
- Significant chronic obstructive pulmonary disease and or respiratory dysfunction
- Noncompliance with medical treatment
- Psychological disorders prohibiting long-term management
- Significant eating disorders
- Severe hiatal hernia or gastroesophageal reflux disease

SURGICAL PROCEDURE

The goal of bariatric surgery is to reduce the patients' caloric intake by either restricting the amount an individual can consume (restrictive procedure) or by reducing the amount absorbed from the gastrointestinal tract (malabsorptive procedure). It is estimated that between 70 to 80% of excess body weight is frequently lost in patients who undergo gastric bypass. There are a number of gastric bypass procedures that can be performed to treat obesity. The most commonly described technique is the Roux-en-Y gastric bypass procedure that restricts the person's ability to consume a large amount of food by partitioning the stomach and creating a small proximal and distal pouch. After gastric bypass surgery, when the person eats a small amount of food, the proximal pouch rapidly becomes distended and afferent impulses to the brain signal that the person is satiated. A decrease in the absorption of calories and nutrients occurs because the anastamosis of the jejunum is to the proximal pouch of the stomach, which bypasses a significant portion of the small intestine. The Roux-en-Y gastric bypass procedure is one of the most common bariatric techniques performed worldwide. An illustration of the Roux-en-Y procedure is presented in Figure 7-1.

Gastric restrictive procedures such as laparoscopic adjustable gastric banding or vertical banded gastroplasty are less invasive and are associated with a shorter surgical duration, but the long-term results and complications such as dietary restrictions, gastric and intestinal erosion, and migration of the restrictive device are factors that will impact daily life. Adjustable gastric banding may become more popular and effective in the future as new and more effective gastric banding devices and surgical techniques are developed. Roux-en-Y gastric bypass has a greater potential for serious complications as compared with gastric banding. The complications that are associated with a Roux-en-Y procedure are listed in Table 7-2.

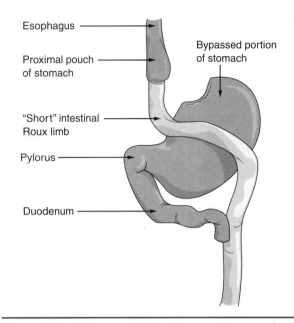

Figure 7-1 *Diagram of the Roux-en-Y procedure.*

ANESTHETIC MANAGEMENT AND CONSIDERATIONS

Preoperative Period

1. Discuss preoperative preparation for a patient having gastric bypass.

Preparation for surgery involves coordination between healthcare disciplines: psychiatry, internal medicine, surgery, and anesthesia. The procedure is described to the patient and the risks, benefits,

Table 7-2 Complications Associated with the Roux-en-Y Procedure
• Hemorrhage
• Respiratory infection
• Deep vein thromboembolism
• Bowel obstruction
• Leakage, stricture, and/or ulcer at the sites of anastomosis
• Infection
• Dumping syndrome
• Nutritional deficiency

and alternatives must be clearly communicated. The patient has also been extensively counseled regarding the typical postoperative course, expectations for weight loss, and dietary limitations. All chronic pathophysiologic conditions need to be medically optimized prior to surgery.

2. Discuss the common coexisting diseases that are associated with patients presenting for bariatric surgery.

Morbid obesity and the associated illness are medically managed in hopes to optimize the patient's level of functioning. Frequently, immobility and joint discomfort become the major motivating factors that drive patients to have of bariatric surgery. Within 1 year after successful bariatric surgery, many of the pathologic disease states such as diabetes, hypertension, and respiratory difficulty improve or resolve. A list of the pathology that is associated with obesity is included in Table 7-3.

3. Outline the positive physiologic effects of weight loss after bariatric surgery.

Obesity is considered by many to occur as a result of behavioral factors and surgery is the final

Table 7-3   Commonly Occurring Pathology Associated with Obesity
• Coronary artery disease
• Atherosclerosis
• Hypertension
• Diabetes mellitus
• Obstructive sleep apnea
• Systemic and pulmonary hypertension
• Gastroesophageal reflux disease
• Non-alcoholic fatty liver disease
• Cholelithiasis
• Deep vein thromboembolic disease
• Degenerative disc disease

intervention. The outcome data associated with bariatric surgery and weight loss demonstrate advantages for both the individual patient and for society by decreasing future expenses that would be incurred as a result of treating multiple chronic disease states. It has been demonstrated that improvement or complete resolution of following pathology occurs:

- 76.8% decrease in type 2 diabetes
- 70% decrease in hypercholesteremia
- 61.7% decrease in hypertension
- 85.7% decrease in obstructive sleep apnea

The survival rate for morbidly obese patients under 40 years who have bariatric surgery is 13.8% as compared to 3.0% for those who did not receive surgical management. The dramatic reduction in body weight is associated with a decreased incidence of cancer, infectious disease, musculoskeletal disorders, respiratory dysfunction, nervous system pathology, psychiatric illness, and reproductive health issues.

4. Discuss the physiologic concerns for patients having bariatric surgery.

Evaluation of the patient presenting for bariatric surgery should focus on optimizing the comorbidities in order to decrease the perioperative risk.

- ***Cardiac function*** should be evaluated via echocardiography, electrocardiogram, exercise, or dobutamine stress testing. The high incidence of hypertension, high cholesterol, and inactivity coupled with the physiologic stress that results from the pneumoperitoneum, surgical procedure and anesthetic management predisposes the patient to untoward perioperative cardiac events. There is a higher incidence of congestive heart failure that occurs in the obese patient population. A cardiomyopathy resulting in cardiomegaly, left ventricular dilation, and myocyte hypertrophy can cause sudden cardiac death. The demand on the heart is further increased as there is an associated increase in total blood volume with obesity. This patient's cardiac ultrasound demonstrated left ventricular hypertrophy, which is consistent with myocardial compensation caused by increased afterload over time. She has normal systolic ventricular function, and adequate ejection fraction of 67%.

- **Pulmonary function** must be scrutinized prior to anesthesia. Due to the excessive adipose tissue present on the chest wall, extrathoracic compliance is decreased causing restrictive lung disease. Oxygen consumption and carbon dioxide production are increased resulting from excessive tissue. Changes in lung volumes that are associated with obesity include decreased vial capacity, decreased total lung capacity, decreased functional residual capacity, and decreased expiratory reserve volume. Closing capacity, the volume at which distal airway closure occurs, is increased—facilitating atelectasis and decreased oxygen transport. This patient has a history of a prolonged period of smoking, which causes obstructive lung disease and the potential for airway hyperreactivity. This patient should have a chest x-ray and pulmonary function testing prior to surgery.

- **Endocrine function** is important to consider since this patient has type 2 diabetes mellitus and requires insulin to maintain normoglycemia. Excessive adipose tissue results in the increased breakdown of free fatty acids that stimulate gluconeogenesis (breakdown of amino acids and the glycerol portion of fat) in the liver to increase blood glucose. Insulin is released to facilitate movement of glucose into cells; however, over a period of time, the cells' responsiveness to the effects of insulin diminishes and insulin resistance occurs. The pancreas compensates by secreting increased amounts of insulin that can result in beta cell dysfunction and decreased insulin production. Her preoperative blood sugar is 156 mg/dl but her hemoglobin A1C, a measure of sustained

glycemic control, is elevated. The increase in blood sugar is frequently a physiologic response to stress. Since she has taken half of her NPH insulin dosage, it would be prudent to check an intraoperative and postoperative blood glucose level.

- **Hepatic function** as assessed using laboratory data may be abnormally elevated in the obese population; however, there is no correlation between routine liver function tests and the liver's capacity to metabolize medications. Drug clearance is usually unimpaired in this patient population. Tests for coagulation are prudent given the potential for hepatic dysfunction, the invasive nature of the surgery, and the administration of low molecular weight heparin for deep vein thrombosis prophylaxis. This patient's liver and coagulation function are within the normal range.

- **Renal function** affects drug excretion, which is often increased in obese patients due to increased renal blood flow and increased glomerular filtration rate. This patient's BUN and creatinine are within normal limits.

- **Gastrointestinal pathology** is believed to exist in patients who are morbidly obese because of increased intragastric pressure and decreased gastric transit time. Additionally, this patient has a history of gastroesophageal reflux disease and is taking cimetidine to control the symptoms. Therefore, aspiration prophylaxis should be instituted in the preoperative period.

- **Venous access** is frequently challenging; however, the need for reliable intravenous access is imperative. Central venous access and arterial line placement is used for those patients who are at high risk with specific conditions that warrant placement.

5. Describe the preinduction preparation for a patient having bariatric surgery.

Anxiety is common for many patients during the preoperative period. The use of midazolam during this time will help to achieve anxiolysis and amnesia as well as decreasing sympathetic nervous system predominance. However, careful titration of all sedative medications administered is vital because significant respiratory depression may lead to rapid and severe hypoxemia.

It is important to know the weight limit for the specific operating table and to secure the patient to the table once they have moved. Airway management is a critical aspect for any patient; however, for morbidly obese patients, due to the potential for redundant airway tissue, large neck, and decreased functional residual capacity, rapid desaturation will occur if the conditions are not optimal. Placement of a ramp under the patient using blankets under their shoulders and then elevating the head will provide optimal "sniffing position" which facilitates the alignment of the oral, pharyngeal, and laryngeal axis. The back of the table can be elevated to help the anesthetist achieve this position and to facilitate improved respiratory excursion during preoxygenation. Figure 7-2 depicts proper positioning for an obese patient prior to the induction of anesthesia.

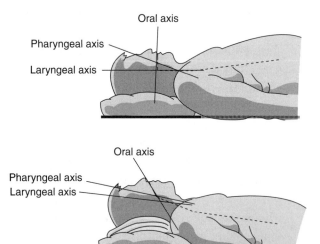

Figure 7-2 *Optimal positioning for airway management.*

Preoxygenation of the patient should occur for as long as possible. Patients must be reminded to take vital capacity breaths prior to induction. Increasing the concentration of oxygen in the blood and also the pulmonary residual volume will increase the time before desaturation occurs after the patient becomes apneic. After induction but before intubation, continuous positive airway pressure (CPAP) can be used to optimize oxygen transfer at the level of the alveoli and help to decrease atelectasis.

A rapid sequence induction is indicated for this patient due to her morbid obesity and history of gastroesophageal reflux. If airway management and intubation prove difficult, then having airway adjuncts available such as a glidescope, Eschmann stylette (elastic gum bougie), and laryngeal mask airway is prudent. The anesthetist should be familiar with and have experience utilizing the American Society of Anesthesiologists' difficult airway algorithm.

The blood pressure cuff should be placed on the patient's upper arm or forearm. Inaccurate blood pressure measurements can occur if the blood pressure cuff is too large or too small. It is necessary to be vigilant regarding positioning and padding of the arms, legs, and pressure points. Continuous assessment of the position and pressure points is imperative because changes in the operating table position or surgical manipulation may cause a shift. Positioning is the responsibility of the entire surgical team and when it is accomplished properly prior to the surgical incision the incidence of a compression injury or nerve palsy can be minimized.

Intraoperative Period

6. Describe the hemodynamic variability and that frequently occur during a laparoscopic Roux-en-Y procedure.

While reverse Trendelenburg positioning is optimal during the induction period and airway management, returning the patient to the supine position facilitates hemodynamic stability and allows the nursing staff to procede with the surgical preparation. The patient is given a bowel preparation solution the day before surgery that facilitates removal of fecal material and water from the gastrointestinal system resulting in dehydration. This process coupled with preoperative fasting and the use of antihypertensive medications can exacerbate hypotension. Depending on the patient's cardiovascular status, an intravenous fluid bolus preinduction will decrease the degree and duration of a hypotensive episode that is caused by the anesthetic induction agents.

The creation of a pneumoperitoneum occurs when the abdominal cavity is insufflated with carbon dioxide gas. If intraabdominal pressures exceed 15 mm Hg, then cardiovascular compromise can occur. Vasopressors can be used to maintain adequate cerebral and coronary perfusion pressure if hypotension exists. However, the degree of hypotension as compared to the patient's preoperative norm, the state of the individual's cardiovascular status, and the degree of surgical stimulation must be taken into account as ephedrine and phenylephrine can both increase myocardial oxygen demand and result in cellular acidosis. A complete list of the cardiovascular and respiratory physiologic changes that are associated with a pneumoperitoneum is included in Tables 7-4 and 7-5.

The anesthetists must be cautious of rapidly developing fluid overload. Attention to the estimated blood loss and urine output is essential.

Table 7-4	Cardiovascular Effects Associated with a Pneumoperitoneum

- Increased neurohumoral response
- Decreased venous return (preload)
- Increased systemic vascular resistance (afterload)
- Increased heart rate
- Increased blood pressure
- Decreased cardiac output

Table 7-5	Respiratory Effects Associated with a Pneumoperitoneum

- Increased carbon dioxide absorption
- Decreased vital capacity
- Increased intrathoracic compliance
- Decreased pulmonary compliance
- Increased peak airway pressure
- Decreased functional residual capacity
- Increased atelectasis
- Increased ventilation/perfusion mismatch

The average blood loss associated with a laparoscopic Roux-en-Y procedure is between 50 and 100 ml; however, as with any laparoscopic surgical intervention, there is always the possibility of inadvertent vascular damage resulting in acute hemorrhage. The signs consistent with fluid volume overload for a patient receiving general anesthesia are included in Table 7-6.

7. Discuss the airway dynamics and ventilation strategy for patients having laparoscopic bariatric surgery.

A reduction in functional residual capacity (FRC) occurs in obese patients and this phenomenon

Table 7-6	Signs of Fluid Overload in an Anesthetized Patient

- Increased peak inspiratory pressures
- Jugular venous distention
- Increased central venous pressure
- Bilateral rales
- Pink frothy secretions in the endotracheal tube
- Hypoxemia/hypercarbia/acidosis
- Dysrhythmias
- Hypotension/hypertension

presents a host of unique challenges during anesthetic management and intraoperative ventilation. Initial tidal volume settings (ventilation based on volume) or pressure settings (ventilation based on pressure to achieve a specific volume) for ventilation should begin at 10–12 ml/kg and positive-end expiratory pressures (PEEP) of 3 to 7 cm H_2O pressure can be used to decrease the development of atelectasis and improve ventilation perfusion mismatch. PEEP can decrease venous return by increasing intrathoracic pressure and contribute to barotrauma. Evidence suggests larger tidal volumes can cause barotrauma even if peak pressures are not excessively high and this maneuver may not improve arterial oxygenation. The tidal volume should be increased or decreased depending on the peak pressure and the oxygen saturation.

Due to the pneumoperitoneum, pressure is exerted on the diaphragm. This fact coupled with the Trendelenburg position that is required during the surgical procedure and morbid obesity dramatically increases peak inspiratory pressures. It is recommended that the initial tidal volume is calculated using the patient's ideal body weight. If peak airway pressures increase significantly greater than 30 mm Hg, then the tidal volume or ventilating pressures can be decreased by 10–30%. The respiratory rate can be increased to maintain the end-tidal carbon dioxide within physiologic parameters.

An attempt should be made to extubate the patient while they are positioned in reverse Trendelenburg to facilitate respiratory excursion. Due to this patient population's compromised respiratory function, rapid desaturation will occur unless adequate spontaneous tidal volume breaths occur postextubation. After the patient moves back to the gurney, they should be placed in a sitting position and supplemental oxygen should be provided for transport. This intervention increases FRC and decreases the incidence of airway obstruction. Atelectasis commonly occurs in obese patients and alveolar recruitment and distention may be addressed by providing CPAP in the immediate postoperative period.

8. Cite the pharmacokinetic implications and dose requirements for patient having bariatric surgery.
Significant increases in the volume of distribution occur due to the high degree of lipid solubility of most of the medications used to provide anesthesia. The literature suggests that the dosages of lipid soluble (fat soluble) medications should be increased by 20% beyond the dose that is calculated for ideal body weight because a portion of the patient's total body weight is lean body mass.

Medications that are lipophilic are sequestered within adipose tissue after intravascular redistribution occurs. If a person has a greater percentage of adipose tissue, then a greater percentage of lipid soluble medications will remain in the body for a prolonged amount of time as compared to lean person. When a drug is bound to adipose tissue, it is not available to undergo hepatic metabolism and or renal excretion. Therefore, inhalation agents with a low blood–gas solubility coefficient (insoluble) will redistribute to adipose tissue to a lesser degree and, when the medication is discontinued, pulmonary elimination will be more rapid. Neuromuscular blocking medications are water soluble and do not redistribute to adipose tissue. The pharmacokinetic profile of this drug class in obese patients is similar to that of patients who have ideal body weight. The amount of nondepolarizing medications that is administered for maintenance of paralysis should be assessed using neuromuscular blocking monitoring.

Although body mass index provides a more accurate determination of patients' ideal body weight because this formula accounts for height calculated in meters squared, the Broca index helps the anesthetist to determine initial drug dosages because the difference is expressed in kilograms. An estimation of ideal body which can be calculated using the following equation.

- Male, Height (cm) − 100 = ideal kilogram weight
- Female, Height (cm) − 105 = ideal kilogram weight

There are many variables that affect drug metabolism and excretion, such as individual variability, liver and renal function, and cytochrome P450 induction or inhibition. The safest method of dosing in light of these factors is to titrate medications as determined by the physiologic response.

9. Identify key aspects of anesthetic maintenance.
- ***Cardiovascular function*** and titration of anesthetic medication, antihypertensive agents, and vasopressors are administered as needed to maintain adequate coronary perfusion. Due to the high incidence of hypertension in this population, these patients may require preoperative level mean arterial pressure. The coronary artery autoregulation curve is shifted to the right in patients with hypertension requiring a higher pressure for adequate myocardial perfusion.
- ***Intraoperative ventilation*** should be titrated to maintain normocarbia, avoid hypoxemia, decrease the development of atelectasis, and minimize peak inspiratory pressures. Awareness of the potential for endotracheal tube migration during changes in the patient position is critical. The immediate result of right mainstem ventilation of a morbidly obese patient in the Trendelenburg position with a pneumoperitoneum is rapidly occurring desaturation.
- ***Neuromuscular blockade*** should be maintained throughout the surgical procedure to decrease the possibility of patient movement, facilitate the creation and maintenance of the pneumoperitoneum, and ensure ideal operating conditions.

- ***Positioning*** a patient that is morbidly obese is difficult and care to ensure that all pressure points are padded and checking throughout the intraoperative period is essential to decrease the possibility of nerve palsy as well as the development of pressure sores.
- ***Maintenance of normothermia*** is imperative for adequate blood coagulation and the metabolism of anesthetic medications. Postoperative hypothermia that results in severe shivering will increase myocardial oxygen consumption by 400 to 600%. The use of a heated air warming blanket, fluid warming system, low fresh gas flow rate, and core temperature monitoring is indicated.
- ***Anesthetic medications*** that are most commonly used for maintenance during this surgical procedure include a combination of narcotics and an inhalation agent. The anesthetic goal throughout the intraoperative period is inhibition of sympathetic nervous system predominance and maintenance of analgesia and unconsciousness. However, the intraoperative titration of these medications will affect the emergence and postoperative period. It is important that morbidly obese patients are able to breathe effectively postoperatively and oversedation should be avoided.
- ***Antibiotic prophylaxis*** using a broad spectrum agent is to be administered within 60 minutes prior to surgical incision to decrease the potential for infection. The antibiotic regimen should be continued during the postoperative period.

10. Describe the anesthetic concerns that are associated with emergence and extubation.
The inhalation agents are lipid soluble medications and are sequestered in adipose tissue. Incremental decreases of the volume percent concentration of the agent prior to complete surgical closure will help to facilitate a more rapid emergence from anesthesia. Reversal of neuromuscular blockade

should be accomplished and guided by the use of a nerve stimulator. Ketorolac can be given prior to emergence to decrease postoperative pain. Relative contraindications to the use of ketorolac include impaired renal function, bleeding, and hyperreactive airway. Narcotics can also be carefully titrated if pain persists in the postoperative area. A combination of medications used as prophylaxis for nausea and vomiting may include antidopaminergics, serotonin receptor antagonists, steroids, and anticholinergics. Once the patient has been moved back to the gurney, the head of the bed should be elevated and supplemental oxygen provided during the transportation to the postoperative area.

Postoperative Period

11. Describe the common complications that are associated with bariatric surgery.

Intestinal leakage at the site of the surgical anastomosis is the most frequent complication associated with bariatric surgery. The development of a deep vein thrombosis that may or may not develop into a pulmonary embolus occurs in approximately 2% of these patients. Low molecular weight heparin is routinely administered during the postoperative period to decrease the potential for deep vein thrombosis. Strictures that develop within the gastrointestinal tract resulting from surgical intervention range from 3 to 8%. The mortality rate for this surgical specialty ranges from 0.1 to 2%. Overall, the postoperative complication rate for laparoscopic Roux-en-Y procedure is 13%; however, incidence of mortality is less than 1%. A complete list of the complications associated with the Roux-en-Y procedure is included in Table 7-2.

REVIEW QUESTIONS

1. A common complication associated with bariatric surgery includes:
   a. cardiovascular collapse.
   b. pitting edema formation.
   c. congestive heart failure.
   d. deep venous thrombosis.

2. Which disease state frequently resolves after significant weight reduction?
   a. Gastroesophageal reflux disease
   b. Osteoarthritis
   c. Diabetes mellitus
   d. Chronic obstructive pulmonary disease

3. Diagnostic abnormalities are expected in the morbidly obese patient for all of the following except:
   a. liver function tests.
   b. creatinine.
   c. cardiac echocardiography.
   d. blood glucose.

4. When calculating the drug dose for lipid soluble drugs administered to a morbidly obese patient, it is suggested to use:
   a. ideal body weight.
   b. ideal body weight and increased lean body mass.
   c. actual weight.
   d. a ratio of ideal body weight to volume of distribution.

5. Which range of abdominal carbon dioxide insufflation pressure is most likely to significantly reduce cardiac output?
   a. 20–30 mm Hg
   b. 1–5 mm Hg
   c. 6–10 mm Hg
   d. 10–20 mm Hg

REVIEW ANSWERS

1. **Answer: d**
   Of the choices that are listed, deep venous thrombosis is the most common complication associated with the laparoscopic Roux-en-Y procedure.

2. **Answer: c**
   Diabetes mellitus is a frequent coexisting disease that can rapidly resolve by successful weight loss postoperatively.

3. **Answer: b**
   Creatinine levels are frequently normal as obesity has limited negative effects on glomerular filtration, renal blood flow, and clearance.

Advanced stages of diabetes can impair renal function, indicating the need for preoperative evaluation of renal function.

4. **Answer: b**

Ideal body weight plus approximately 20% accounts for the increased lean body mass acquired in adaptation to larger overall body mass.

5. **Answer: a**

Abdominal pressures of 20–30 mm Hg can cause cardiovascular compromise as a result of decreased cardiac output, increased systemic vascular resistance, and decreased venous return.

SUGGESTED READINGS

Chand B, Gugliotti D, Schauer P, et al. Perioperative management of the bariatric surgery patient: focus on cardiac and anesthesia considerations. *Cleve Clin J Med* 2006;73(S1):51–56.

Golembiewski J. Considerations in selecting an inhaled anesthetic agent. *Am J Health-System Pharmacy* 2004; 61(20):S10–S17.

Guthrie EW. Bariatric surgery – What all pharmacists need to know. *US Pharmacist* 2007;32(9):27–37.

Hassani A, Kessell G. Neck circumference and difficult intubation. *Anesth Analg* 2008;107(5):1756–1757.

Hutter MH, Randall S, Khuri SF, et al. Laparoscopic versus open gastric bypass for morbid obesity: A multicenter, prospective, risk-adjusted analysis from the national surgical quality improvement program. *Ann Surg* 2006;243(5):657–666.

Lee CW, Kelly JJ, Wassef WY. Complications of bariatric surgery. *Curr Opin Gastroenterol* 2007;23(6):636–643.

Ogunnaike BO, Jones SB, Jones DB, et al. Anesthetic considerations for bariatric surgery. *Anesth Analg* 2002;95:1793–1805.

Pinkney J, Kerrigan K. When should bariatric surgery be used in the treatment of type 2 diabetes? *Br J Diabet Vasc Dis* 2004;4(4):232–237.

Rao SL, Kunselman AR, Schuler HG, et al. Laryngoscopy and tracheal intubation in the head-elevated position in obese patients: a randomized, controlled, equivalence trial. *Anesth Analg* 2008;107:1912–1918.

Open and Laparoscopic Appendectomy

Veronica Davis and Sandra E. Morris

8

KEY POINTS

- The definitive treatment for acute appendicitis is an appendectomy.
- Techniques that are used include laparoscopic appendectomy (LA) or open appendectomy (OA).
- Timely surgery, intravenous (IV) fluids, and antibiotic administration significantly decreases the overall morbidity and mortality associated with acute appendicitis.
- The Trendelenburg position and the creation of a pneumoperitoneum used during laparoscopic appendectomy causes physiologic changes that affect anesthetic management.
- Patients who have experienced a ruptured appendix will develop sepsis. The degree of sepsis encountered by the patient will affect the anesthetic technique and medications that are used.

CASE SYNOPSIS

A 33-year-old woman who is treated in the emergency department complains of a 3-day history of abdominal pain that is localized in the right lower quadrant (RLQ), persistent nausea and vomiting, and a low-grade fever. She has been scheduled for an LA.

PREOPERATIVE EVALUATION AND DEMOGRAPHIC DATA

Past Medical/Surgical History

- Asthma as a child; no current problems with asthma

List of Medications

- Multivitamins
- Birth control pills

Diagnostic Data

- Hemoglobin, 13.5 g/dl; hematocrit, 39.8 g/dl; white blood cells, 15,000 mm^3
- Electrolytes: sodium, 139 mEq/l; potassium, 3.5 mEq/l; chloride, 104 mEq/l; carbon dioxide, 24 mEq/l
- Computed tomography (CT) scan reveals inflammation of a large tubular structure with slight bowel wall thickening; impression, acute appendicitis.

Height/Weight/Vital Signs

- 173 cm, 74 kg
- Blood pressure, 112/68; heart rate, 95 beats per minute; respiratory rate, 18 breaths per minute; room air oxygen saturation, 100%; temporal artery temperature, 100.8°F.

PATHOPHYSIOLOGY

There are more than 250,000 new cases of acute appendicitis in the United States every year, with an overall incidence of 7 to 8% in the US population. Demographically, males between the ages of 10 and 30 years have a higher incidence than females of developing the disease. Appendicitis occurs most often in the second decade of life and the median age is 22 years. Patients with higher fiber intake have a lower incidence of developing appendicitis due to a decreased formation of hard stool, also known as fecalith. Appendicitis can occur at any age, but is rare in infants and octogenarians. Appendectomy is one of the most common surgical procedures performed in the pediatric population.

The appendix is a blind-ended loop of bowel that arises from the cecum 3 to 4 cm below the ileocecal valve. Appendicitis is inflammation of the appendix and it is most commonly caused by a bacterial invasion of an obstructed appendiceal lumen. As the bacteria multiply, the appendix becomes distended, congested, and inflamed. Peritonitis may occur and, if the condition remains untreated, arterial blood flow to this portion of the intestine is compromised and tissue ischemia can develop, which can result in necrosis of the appendiceal wall. A perforation of the appendix can occur, which causes the release fecal contents into the peritoneal cavity. Other less common causes of appendicitis include obstruction resulting from foreign bodies or fecalith, inflammatory strictures, and parasitic infections.

Morbidity and mortality increases significantly if immediate recognition and treatment is not instituted. Once appendicitis has developed, surgery to remove the appendix is necessary, along with IV fluids and antibiotics. Without treatment sepsis occurs and the mortality associated with a ruptured appendix is > 50%. With early surgical intervention, the mortality rate is < 1%.

The appendix has been thought to be a remnant of a digestive organ that has disappeared as a result of evolution in humans. Interestingly enough, the appendix is made of lymph tissue; it may have played a role in immune function. Located at the proximal aspect of the large intestine, the appendix is thought to be a reserve for bacteria. Figure 8-1 depicts the anatomic position of the appendix and the surrounding structures.

The clinical presentation associated with appendicitis includes epigastric or periumbilical pain which migrates to the RLQ. Direct pain and rebound

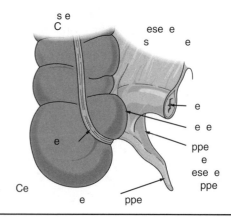

Figure 8-1   *Anatomic position of the appendix and the surrounding structures.*

tenderness may occur at McBurney's point, which is known as McBurney's sign. It is located on the RLQ of the abdomen, two thirds the distance between the umbilicus and the anterior superior iliac spine. Abdominal tenderness in this region does not always occur in patients with acute appendicitis. Other physical signs include Rovsing sign (pain felt in the RLQ when palpating the left lower quadrant [LLQ]), psoas sign (an increase in pain from passive extension of the right hip that stretches the iliopsoas muscle), and a fever of > 38°C. Retractable pain upon palpation of the abdominal wall frequently parallels the severity of the inflammatory process. A leukocyte count > 10,000 cells/ml and an increase in C-reactive protein commonly occurs. A normal white blood cell count should not exclude appendicitis. A contrast-enhanced CT scan is recognized as a useful and accurate method to diagnose appendicitis. A positive CT scan indicating the presence of appendicitis may show a distended appendix, appendiceal or bowel wall thickening, periappendiceal abscess formation, or inflammation of large tubular structure. The CT scan can also assist with the differential diagnosis by revealing other causes of acute abdominal pain such as ovarian cyst, tubal pregnancy, acute salpingitis, mesenteric adenitis, and perforated duodenal ulcer.

SURGICAL PROCEDURE
Open Approach
Through a right paramedian 2- to 4-inch incision in the abdomen, the cecum is exposed and removed through the wound. The appendix is identified, separated from the surrounding tissue, ligated, crushed, and then transected at its base and removed. The surgical site is irrigated, then the layers including the peritoneum, muscle, and fascia are sutured closed. In some instances, when the appendix is perforated and infection has occurred, the wound is maybe left open and a soft Penrose drain is inserted to facilitate drainage out of the surgical site.

Laparoscopic Approach
A laparoscopic appendectomy is performed using 3 to 4 trocar sites, with an initial 10-mm trocar placed at the umbilicus and subsequent trocars placed in lower abdomen according to surgeon's preference. After insufflation of the abdomen or establishing a "pneumoperitoneum," the patient is placed in Trendelenburg position with left tilt to facilitate exposure of the appendix. The base of the cecum is identified, the appendix is mobilized, and the base of the appendix is stapled. After stapling the mesoappendix, the appendix is freed from the intestine, placed in a bag and removed through the 10-mm trocar. Figure 8-2 illustrates the laparoscopic approach for an appendectomy. The umbilical fascia is closed and the skin is approximated.

ANESTHETIC MANAGEMENT AND CONSIDERATIONS
Preoperative Period
1. List the advantages and disadvantages associated with an LA as compared to an OA.
Since the introduction of LA in 1983, the debate continues over the potential advantages and disadvantages comparing LA to the traditional OA. Clear advantages to an LA technique include improved aesthetic result due to smaller incisions, decreased pain, less blood loss and postoperative pulmonary impairment, a reduction in postoperative ileus, shorter hospital stays, faster postoperative recovery, and fewer wound infections. LA has become a standard surgical approach in medical centers; however, the disadvantages associated with LA include longer operative times (related to the surgical experience and skill of surgeon with laparoscopic techniques), increased postoperative nausea and vomiting, and a higher incidence of postoperative intraabdominal abscess and bowel perforation.

As surgeons become more proficient at LA, the advantages of choosing a routine OA over LA are

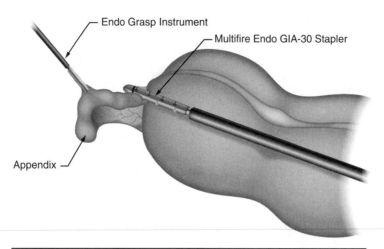

Figure 8-2   *Laparoscopic approach for an appendectomy.*

dwindling. The OA technique was once considered the gold standard for appendectomy and is still an alternative if LA is unsuccessful. A surgeon may consider an open procedure or convert intraoperatively to an OA for patients with a history of complicated perforated appendicitis, previous abdominal surgery with dense scar tissue or adhesions, morbid obesity, inability to gain adequate surgical access to the appendix, or with excessive bleeding during surgery.

2. List the anesthetic options that are available for an OA procedure.

General endotracheal anesthesia (GETA) using a rapid sequence induction is most frequently employed. Patients who have appendicitis generally do not have significant comorbidities. These patients usually have pain and may have recently eaten and therefore it may be prudent to assume that aspiration prophylaxis may be necessary. Administration of metoclopramide (gastrokinetic), cimetidine, ranitidine, or famotidine (H_2 antagonists) and sodium bicitrate (nonparticulate antacid) decreases the risk of aspiration and assists in the control of postoperative nausea and vomiting (PONV). It is worthy to note that if the patient may have a bowel obstruction, metoclopramide should be avoided as the gastrokinetic effects of this drug

can enhance the potential for perforation of the bowel. A combination of air-oxygen with inhalation agents, narcotics, and a muscle relaxant is frequently used during the maintenance period. An orogastric tube can be inserted after induction to drain gastric residual secretions. It has not been conclusively determined that by decompressing the stomach during surgery, the risk of PONV is decreased and antiemetic medications (5-HT3 antagonist) are customarily administered 15 to 30 minutes before the end of surgery.

The administration of regional anesthesia is an option and should be discussed with the patient. Local anesthesia using ilioinguinal, iliohypogastric nerve blocks, and injections at the incision site supplemented with sedation can be accomplished for OA. Neuraxial blockade, subarachnoid, and epidural blocks can be provided if the patient is normovolemic and does not exhibit signs of septicemia. When neuraxial anesthesia and local anesthesia is placed at the surgical incision site, it has been demonstrated to decrease both postoperative pain and the incidence of PONV.

3. List possible complications associated with LA.

The pneumoperitoneum is accomplished by using carbon dioxide gas, which allows the surgeon to perform a laparoscopic procedure. Complications that can arise include:

- The use of pressurized gas increases the possibility of extravasation of CO_2 along the tissue planes, resulting in subcutaneous emphysema, pneumomediastinum, or pneumothorax. Nitrous oxide is highly diffusible and will enter the bowel lumen and possible cause distention and increase the difficulty of the surgical procedure. If nitrous oxide is administered, it should be discontinued and insufflating pressures must be decreased if subcutaneous emphysema occurs.
- The pneumoperitoneum creates a cephalad displacement of the diaphragm which results in decreased functional residual capacity and pulmonary compliance, which promotes the development of atelectasis.
- The celiac reflex can be illicited during the creation and maintenance of the pneumoperitoneum. Pressure in the abdominal cavity causes vagal nerve stimulation that can result mild, moderate, or severe bradycardia. The immediate treatment for severe bradycardia is to have the surgeon immediately release the pneumoperitoneum, administer 100% oxygen, check the blood pressure and consider the use of atropine if severe bradycardia is unrelieved.
- Shoulder tip pain can occur and this phenomena is thought to be caused by diaphragmatic irritation as a result of the CO_2 gas.

4. Identify the challenges during anesthetic management for patients who have experienced a perforated appendix.

When the appendix ruptures, intestinal bacteria infect the peritoneal cavity and cause sepsis. The severity of sepsis will depend on the amount of time that the patient has endured the infection. The signs and symptoms associated with a ruptured appendix are reflective of bacteremia and hypermetabolism and include leukocytosis, fever, vomiting, hypovolemia, tachycardia, pain, and possibly compensated or uncompensated metabolic acidosis. The anesthetist should assess all of these factors and the patient's immediate condition prior to making the decision to use a particular type of anesthetic technique and to administer anesthetic medications. Due to the fever and decreased fluid intake, providing hydration through a large bore no. 18 or no. 16 gauge IV is indicated. Depending on the patient's condition and kilogram weight, a 10–20 ml/kg fluid bolus will help to decrease the tachycardia and hypotension that may occur upon induction of anesthesia.

Administration of antibiotics is required and a third generation cephalosporin given within 1 hour of surgical incision provides maximal coverage. If the appendix has ruptured, a multidose antibiotic regimen is required and the patient is admitted to the hospital.

Intraoperative Period

5. Describe the anesthetic technique that is best suited for LA.

Rapid sequence induction GETA with balanced air–oxygen inhalation, narcotic, and muscle relaxation is the preferred anesthetic choice as this technique minimizes the risk of aspiration from increased intraabdominal pressures during insufflation. Muscle relaxation allows for lower insufflation pressures, provides better visualization, and prevents unexpected patient movement. The duration of the surgical procedure is dependent on the expertise of the surgeon, but this surgical procedure is frequently brief, approximately 30 minutes. Therefore, careful titration of medications is necessary to ensure a timely emergence from anesthesia.

It is possible to provide neuraxial anesthesia during LA; however, because the pneumoperitoneum can illicit visceral discomfort as well as making spontaneous respiration difficult, general anesthesia is most commonly employed.

6. Identify the reasons that CO_2 is used to create a pneumoperitoneum.

Carbon dioxide is the insufflating gas of choice for laparoscopy because it is nonflammable, readily diffuses across membranes, and is rapidly degraded.

7. Describe the physiologic manifestations associated with a CO_2 embolus that can occur during a laparoscopic appendectomy.

A venous CO_2 embolism may also result from unintended insufflation of gas into an open vein. This may lead to hypoxemia, pulmonary hypertension, pulmonary edema, and cardiovascular collapse. A "gas lock" is created at the level of the vena cava and right atrium that disrupts blood flow through the heart. Treatment includes immediate release of the pneumoperitoneum, placing patient on 100% FiO_2, insertion of central venous catheter to aspirate the air, administration of a fluid bolus, administration of a vasopressor, and utilizing Durant's maneuver (patient's head down in a left lateral decubitus position).

8. List the hemodynamic and pulmonary changes that occur with pneumoperitoneum and Trendelenburg position during LA.

The patient will be placed supine and in the Trendelenburg position with both arms tucked at their sides. The patient's body is rotated to the left to increase visualization of the lower abdomen and pelvis. Since gravity promotes blood flow in a cephalad direction, an increase in venous return, central blood volume, and cardiac output occurs. This change increases the myocardial workload and may cause cardiac ischemia or infarction in those patients with cardiovascular disease.

The patient's functional residual capacity and vital capacity decreases secondary to diaphragmatic and abdominal contents displacement, leading to a decrease in pulmonary compliance, increase in ventilation–perfusion mismatch, increase in peak inspiratory pressure (PIP), and increase in $ETCO_2$. In addition to these altered pulmonary dynamics, CO_2 will be absorbed into systemic circulation resulting from the pneumoperitoneum. Lastly, patients who are hypermetabolic have an increased rate of CO_2. Ventilation should be adjusted to normalize $ETCO_2$ ($PaCO_2$) by increasing the minute ventilation. Right mainstem intubation and hypoxemia may occur with this position because the endotracheal tube is secured proximally at the mandible and does not move with the trachea as the diaphragm displaces the lungs and carina cephalad.

Postoperative Period

9. Explain the difference in the length of hospitalization when comparing LA versus OA.

Laparoscopic appendectomy offers advantages over OA by decreasing the postoperative wound infection rate, decreasing the need for postoperative pain medications, shortening the days of hospitalization, decreasing postoperative bowel and pulmonary complications, and decreasing the amount of time before the patient can return to work.

REVIEW QUESTIONS

1. Which is not considered an advantage of a laparoscopic approach for an appendectomy?
   a. Decreased wound infections
   b. Decreased incidence of pulmonary complications
   c. Decreased length of stay in the hospital
   d. Decreased antibiotic administration
2. The intraoperative use of nitrous oxide:
   a. increases the minimum alveolar concentration of the volatile agent used.
   b. decreases the necessity for an oral gastric tube.
   c. increases the degree of bowel distention.
   d. decreases the amount of CO_2 needed for creation of the pneumoperitoneum.

3. During insufflation, the patient's heart rate abruptly decreases to 35 beats per minute. Your initial intervention includes:
   a. call a code, start cardiopulmonary resuscitation, administer atropine.
   b. stop insufflation, deliver 100% oxygen, administer atropine if heart rate does not recover.
   c. obtain a blood pressure, deliver 100% oxygen.
   d. administer atropine before insufflation begins.
4. Physiologic changes that occur during prolonged Trendelenburg positioning include:
   a. metabolic alkalosis.
   b. metabolic acidosis.
   c. respiratory acidosis.
   d. respiratory alkalosis.
5. Durant's procedure is indicated for a:
   a. CO_2 gas embolus.
   b. massive hemorrhage.
   c. pneumothorax.
   d. cardiac tamponade.

REVIEW ANSWERS

1. **Answer: d**
   The perioperative administration of antibiotics is dependent on the individual patient's situation and whether the appendix has ruptured. Therefore, the antibiotic regimen when comparing LA and OA will be the same. Advantages to an LA include improved aesthetic result, smaller incisions, decreased pain, less blood loss, less postoperative pulmonary impairment, a reduction in postoperative ileus, shorter hospital stays, faster postoperative recovery, fewer wound infections, and earlier return to daily functioning.
2. **Answer: c**
   Nitrous oxide is a highly diffusible gas that can cause bowel distention and this effect potentially makes the surgery more difficult to perform.

3. **Answer: b**
   A vagal mediated response initiated as a result of the celiac reflex can result in bronchospasm, bradycardia, and possibly asystole causing cardiovascular collapse. The primary intervention is to have the surgeon evacuate the pneumoperitoneum immediately. Decreasing the amount of peritoneal stimulation can cause the reflex to immediately stop. Other interventions that should be instituted simultaneously includes delivering 100% oxygen, increase fluids, check a blood pressure, and potentially administer atropine 0.5 to 1 mg if the heart rate does not recover.
4. **Answer: c**
   Respiratory acidosis most commonly occurs. The patient's functional residual capacity and vital capacity decreases due to cephalad diaphragmatic and abdominal contents displacement, leading to decreased pulmonary compliance, increased ventilation–perfusion mismatching, increased peak inspiratory pressure, and increased CO_2 that results in respiratory acidosis.
5. **Answer: a**
   Durant's maneuver entails placing the patient's head down below the level of the heart and into the left lateral decubitus position. It is one intervention that can be used to help restore blood flow through the heart during a venous CO_2 embolism.

SUGGESTED READINGS

Corneille MG, Steigelman MB, Myers JG, et al. Laparoscopic appendectomy is superior to open appendectomy in obese patients. *Am J Surg* 2007;194:877–881.

Carbonell AM, Burns JM, Lincourt AE, et al. Outcomes of laparoscopic versus open appendectomy. *Am Surg* 2004;70:759–766.

Friday J. Update on appendicitis: diagnosis and presurgical management. *Curr Opin Pediatr* 2006;18: 234–238.

Jaffe R, Samuels S, eds. *Anesthesiologist's Manual of Surgical Procedures*, 3rd ed. Philadelphia: Lippincott Williams and Wilkins, 2009:509–513.

Kamal M, Qureshi KH. Laparoscopic versus open appendectomy. *Pakistan J Med Res* 2003;42(1):1–7.

Kuwabara K, Imanaka Y, Matsuda S, et al. Cost of open versus laparoscopic appendectomy. *Clin Ter* 2008;159(3):155–163.

Moore DE, Speroff T, Grogan E, et al. Cost perspective of laparoscopic and open appendectomy. *Surg Endosc* 2005;19(3):374–378.

Rybkin AV, Thoeni RF. Current concepts in imaging of appendicitis. *Radiol Clin North Am* 2007;45:411–422.

Schick KS, Hüttl TP, Fertman JM, et al. A critical analysis of laparoscopic appendectomy: how experience with 1,400 appendectomies allowed innovative treatment to become standard in a university hospital. *World J Surg* 2008;32:1406–1413.

Yau KK, Siu WT, Tang CN, et al. Laparoscopic versus open appendectomy for complicated appendicitis. *J Am Coll Surg* 2007;205:60–65.

Cholecystectomy: Open and Laparoscopic Approaches

9

Garrett Peterson

KEY POINTS

- The open technique is utilized in less than 10% of patients having a cholecystectomy.
- It is estimated that less than 5% of these procedures will require conversion to an open technique.
- There are many benefits associated with the laparoscopic surgical technique as compared to the traditional open technique, including: decreased postoperative respiratory dysfunction, decreased postoperative pain, and decreased postoperative analgesic requirements which reduce lethargy, nausea, vomiting, and constipation.
- There are alterations in normal physiologic functioning that occur as a result of the creation of a pneumoperitoneum during laparoscopic cholecystectomy.

CASE SYNOPSIS

A 40-year-old man presents to the emergency room vomiting with severe upper right abdominal pain. The patient is evaluated by a general surgeon with diagnosis of cholecystitis and prepared for emergency cholecystectomy.

PREOPERATIVE EVALUATION AND DEMOGRAPHIC DATA

Past Medical/Surgical History

- Cholelithiasis
- Alcohol abuse
- Left knee anterior cruciate ligament repair; no anesthetic complications

List of Medications

- Thiamin
- Folic acid

Laboratory Tests

- Hemoglobin, 14.8 g/dl; hematocrit, 44%; white blood cells, 7.9/mm^3; platelet count, 270/mm^3
- Blood urea nitrogen (BUN), 20 mg/dl; creatinine, 1.1 mg/dl
- Electrolytes: sodium, 142 mEq/l; potassium, 4.0 mEq/l; chloride, 101 mEq/l; carbon dioxide, 28 mEq/l
- Coagulation: prothrombin time, 10.4 seconds; partial thromboplastin time, 41.1 seconds; international normalized ratio, 1.03
- Liver function: bilirubin, 1.0 mg/dl; aspartate aminotransferase (AST), 28 U/l; alanine aminotransferase (ALT), 30 U/ml; alkaline phosphatase, 1.9 U/ml; and albumin, 3.9 g/dl

Height/Weight/Vital Signs

- 173 cm, 85 kg; body mass index (BMI), 28.4
- Blood pressure, 168/86; heart rate, 95 beats per minute; respiratory rate, 22 breaths per minute; room air–oxygen saturation, 98%; temperature, 37.6°C
- Electrocardiogram: normal sinus rhythm

PATHOPHYSIOLOGY

The gallbladder is a hollow, pear-shaped organ that is located on the underside of the right lobe of the liver. Bile that is produced within the liver is stored in the gallbladder until it is released into the intestine. The cystic duct connects the gallbladder to the common hepatic duct, forming the common bile duct. The gallbladder concentrates and acts as a reservoir for bile. Bile salts, bile pigments, cholesterol, and calcium are component parts that comprise bile. The role of bile is to aid in the intestinal absorption and breakdown of dietary fat.

When the gallbladder becomes full, the sphincter of Oddi will relax, allowing bile to be released into the duodenum. Cholecystokinin, a hormone secreted by the duodenum in response to acid contents, causes contraction of the gallbladder and relaxation of the sphincter of Oddi. Normally, 500 to 1000 ml of bile is secreted per day.

Cholelithiasis results in hard masses formed within the gallbladder. Gallstones are formed from bile, which is composed of bile acids, bile pigments, cholesterol, and calcium. These stones can become lodged in the cystic duct resulting in obstruction. Cholecystitis occurs as a result of infection, inflammation, and from the blockade of bile flow through the cystic duct or common bile duct. This result can cause severe right upper abdominal pain that characteristically radiates to the right shoulder. Patients with cholecystitis typically present with an acute, severe mid-gastric pain that radiates to the right abdominal quadrants. Patient factors that increase the risk for developing cholecystitis include female gender, obesity, parity, and age.

A diagnostic evaluation called Murphy's sign can be used to assess for the presence of cholecystitis. During an abdominal examination, the patient is asked to exhale while the practitioner places their hand over the approximate location of the gallbladder. The patient is instructed to inhale and if the patient stops breathing, this sign may be indicative of abdominal tenderness resulting from gallbladder disease.

The blood test results in patients that have cholecystitis include increased plasma bilirubin, alkaline phosphatase, and amylase. Ileus and localized tenderness may indicate a gallbladder perforation with associated peritonitis. If complete obstruction of the cystic duct occurs, jaundice may occur. Confirmation of cholecystitis is accomplished by cholescintigraph, a contrast study of the gallbladder that is accomplished by ultrasonography.

Patients who have cholecystitis are frequently dehydrated caused by decreased oral intake, vomiting, or nasogastric tube evacuation. Unless other pathophysiologic conditions exist that preclude fluid resuscitation, it is warranted to correct volume depletion. Ileus should be treated with a nasogastric tube. Free air that is determined to be present within the abdomen causes fever, ileus, abdominal rigidity and pain, vomiting, and

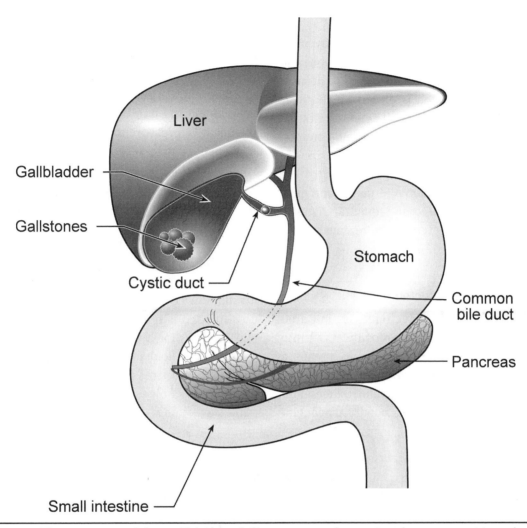

Figure 9-1 *The anatomy of the gallbladder, biliary tree, and associated structures. Note the presence of the gallstones within the gallbladder and cystic duct.*

dehydration. It is estimated that 20% of patients who develop cholecystitis will become symptomatic and develop pain when biliary obstruction occurs. Figure 9-1 shows the anatomy of the gallbladder and biliary tree. Notice the gallstones that are present within the gallbladder and lodged within the cystic duct.

SURGICAL PROCEDURES

A cholecystectomy can be performed as an open procedure or by a laparoscopic approach. Patients who have undergone previous abdominal surgeries, adhesions around the past surgical field can increase the complexity of the surgical procedure. Significant medical problems such as obesity, cardiac and pulmonary pathology, and coagulopathy will complicate the anesthetic management. The open technique is utilized in less than 10% of cholecystectomy procedures performed. It is estimated that less than 5% of laparoscopic cholecystectomy procedures will be converted to the open approach.

Open Cholecystectomy

An open cholecystectomy is performed by making a right subcostal or midline incision into the abdominal wall. Dissection into the peritoneal cavity occurs and traction is placed on the liver and the duodenum until maximum exposure of the gallbladder, cystic duct, cystic artery, and common bile duct are achieved. The gallbladder is excised from the liver bed, followed by isolation of the cystic artery and cystic duct. Alternate techniques include isolation of the cystic duct and cystic artery first, followed by retrograde removal of the gallbladder from the liver bed.

Laparoscopic Cholecystectomy

A laparoscopic cholecystectomy is initiated through insufflation of carbon dioxide (CO_2) into the patient's peritoneum in order to create a pneumoperitoneum. A Veress needle is inserted just below the umbilicus and then introduced into the peritoneal cavity. Correct needle placement is confirmed in several ways. The most common method is for the surgeon to feel and hear a distinct "pop" that occurs when the needle pierces the fascia and peritoneum. A more scientific and safe approach is accomplished by placing a drop of water on the hub of the Veress needle. Due to the negative pressure that is present in the peritoneal cavity, a drop of water will be sucked inward when placed in the hub of the Veress needle, confirming proper placement. An alternative method, the Hasson technique, involves creating a small incision through the abdominal fascia in order to place the trocars in the abdomen. Confirmation of proper location is further demonstrated by percussion of the CO_2 in the abdomen during insufflation. Once correct needle placement is confirmed, it is replaced with a cannula or trocar, which allows for a video laparoscope to visualize the operative field and instruments to be inserted. Figure 9-2 compares the surgical approaches used for an open cholecystectomy and a laparoscopic cholecystectomy.

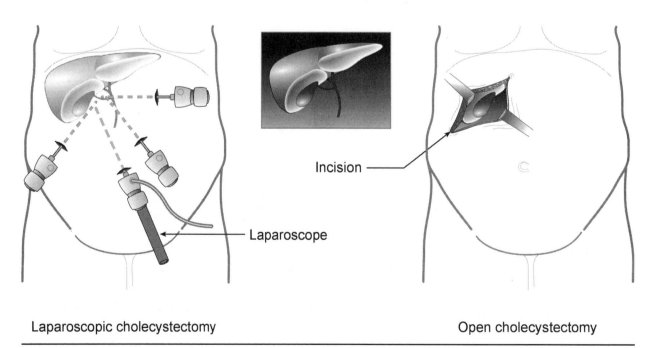

Incision

Laparoscope

Laparoscopic cholecystectomy   Open cholecystectomy

Figure 9-2   *A comparison of the surgical approaches for a laparoscopic cholecystectomy and open cholecystectomy.*

ANESTHETIC MANAGEMENT AND CONSIDERATIONS FOR CHOLECYSTECTOMY

Preoperative Period

1. Identify the associated disease states that commonly occur in patients having a cholecystectomy.

Patients who present for a cholecystectomy often have associated pathologic conditions, including gastrointestinal disorders including paralytic ileus, cirrhosis, hemolytic disorders, choledocholithiasis, and active pancreatitis.

2. Describe the alteration in respiratory dynamics that occur in patients who have cholecystitis.

Patients presenting with symptomatic cholecystitis may exhibit splinting secondary to pain resulting from an acute abdominal process. This may lead to an impaired respiratory function resulting in atelectasis, decreased functional residual capacity, and hypoventilation. The respiratory changes associated with a pneumoperitoneum are discussed later in this chapter. A patient with a history of impaired pulmonary function or chronic pneumonitis may be at increased risk for desaturation and barotrauma during the intraoperative period. Preoperative testing for patients with pulmonary disorders should include a chest x-ray.

3. Describe the potential decreased intravascular volume status and management for patients having a cholecystectomy.

A patient who presents for a cholecystectomy may be dehydrated from vomiting and decreased oral intake. Preoperative evaluation of the patient's hemodynamic status must include blood pressure measurement, heart rate, and the presence of orthostatic hypotension. Fluid resuscitation is recommended for those patients who present with the signs and symptoms of hemodynamic compromise. Preoperative testing for patient with cardiac pathology should include an electrocardiogram (ECG).

4. Describe the benefits of using laparoscopic surgery versus open procedures.

There are many benefits related to the use of a laparoscopic surgical technique as compared to the traditional open technique. Table 9-1 presents the advantages of a laparoscopic approach for surgical procedures.

5. Describe the potential for renal insufficiency for patients having a cholecystectomy.

Occasionally these patients will present with obstructive jaundice that requires the preoperative administration of bile salts, which may cause postoperative renal insufficiency. Preoperative testing should include a urinalysis (UA) and blood urea nitrogen (BUN) and creatinine. These patients' BUN and creatinine are considered to be within the high normal range. The presence of billirubin in the urine is indicative of a bile duct obstruction.

6. Describe the potential for gastrointestinal pathology for patients having a cholecystectomy.

Patients may present with peritonitis, which may result in abdominal distension and paralytic ileus. Preoperative laboratory testing should include bilirubin, aspartate aminotransferase (AST), alanine

Table 9-1	Advantages Associated with a Laparoscopic Approach for Surgical Procedures
•	Faster return to normal activities
•	Decreased time of hospitalization
•	Decreased incidence of ileus and adhesions resulting from less bowel exposure and manipulations
•	Early postoperative ambulation
•	Decreased postoperative pain
•	Decreased postoperative physiologic stress
•	Decreased need for analgesic medication
•	Decreased postoperative respiratory dysfunction
•	Improved cosmetic result

aminotransferase (ALT), alkaline phosphatase (ALP), and albumin. These patients' liver function tests are considered to be within the normal limits. Increased bilirubin, AST, ALT, ALP, and decreased albumin are consistent with hepatic dysfunction.

7. Discuss premedication for the cholecystectomy patient.

Preoperative medications to consider include drugs that will reduce spasm of the sphincter of Oddi. These include anticholinergic medications such as glycopyrrolate or atropine. Vitamin K administration is indicated if the patient has a prolonged prothrombin time. For those patients who are at increased risk of gastric aspiration, a histamine-2 antagonists such as cimetidine, a gastrokinetic such as metoclopramide, and a nonparticulate antacid such as sodium Bicitra should be administered.

Intraoperative Period

8. Describe the anesthetic technique used for laparoscopic cholecystectomy.

The anesthetic technique of choice utilized for cholecystectomy is general anesthesia. Providing general anesthesia and an endotracheal tube used for airway maintenance allows for airway protection and provides the ability to control and manage CO_2 during artificial ventilation. The use of muscle relaxation will help to minimize abdominal insufflation pressures and expedite surgical exposure of the gallbladder. Since cholecystectomy is frequently accomplished as an outpatient procedure, and the degree of postoperative discomfort is rarely extreme, the use of a significant amount of narcotic is not warranted.

9. Which gas is utilized for insufflation during laparoscopic surgical procedures?

Many gasses have been utilized during laparoscopic insufflation including helium, argon, nitrous oxide (N_2O), and CO_2. All of these gasses, with the exception of CO_2, possess properties that can cause untoward physiologic effects. Carbon dioxide is noncombustible and therefore it can be used in conjunction with electrocautery and during laser surgery. Additionally, CO_2 is rapidly and easily eliminated from the lungs by increasing minute ventilation.

Absorption of CO_2 can occur through the intraperitoneal route, which is common as a result of normal laparoscopic insufflation which will result in increased end-tidal CO_2. Inadvertent extraperitoneal insufflation can occur and CO_2 can accumulate in the subcutaneous tissues, between the fascia and the peritoneum and in the pericardium or mediastinum.

End-tidal CO_2 ($ETCO_2$) is an estimate of the $PaCO_2$ levels. In healthy patients, the $PaCO_2$–$ETCO_2$ gradient is typically 3 to 5 mm Hg. However, in patients with severe cardiovascular disease or prolonged laparoscopic surgeries, the $PaCO_2$–$ETCO_2$ gradient will be increased. It is important to attempt to maintain normocapnia through out the procedure since hypercapnia causes coronary and cerebral vascular dilation as well as sympathetic nervous system stimulation.

10. Explain the effect of a pneumoperitoneum during laparoscopic cholecystectomy on the following body systems: cardiovascular, pulmonary, cerebral, renal, and hepatic.

A pneumoperitoneum that is created during insufflation of CO_2 gas results in a variety of physiologic changes and are thought to result from three distinct mechanisms: a direct mechanical effect caused by compression, the presence of a neurohumoral response, and the effects of CO_2 absorption. Insufflation of gas into the peritoneal cavity allows the surgeon to visualize, expose, and manipulate the intraabdominal contents. Other factors that contribute to physiologic changes include anesthetic medication, artificial ventilation, patient positioning, and surgical stimulation.

Cardiovascular A pneumoperitoneum causes several hemodynamic changes during a laparoscopic cholecystectomy. Increases in systemic vascular resistance (SVR) or afterload occurs because of mechanical compression on the arterial system and from sympathetic nervous system stimulation. As a result, mean arterial blood pressure increases. Patients undergoing laparoscopic cholecystectomy have elevated levels of dopamine, vasopressin, epinephrine, norepinephrine, renin, and cortisol levels. Hemodynamic changes occurring in these patients have been most often associated with the release of vasopressin. Catecholamine levels are slightly increased and may be the result of the stress response to the surgical procedure.

Venous return to the heart (preload) is decreased from increased venous resistance, compression of the inferior vena cava, and peripheral pooling of blood in the lower body. This effect is accentuated when intra-abdominal pressure exceeds 20 Torr. The position used during laparoscopic cholecystectomy is reverse Trendelenburg. This position can further result in decreased venous return to the heart.

As SVR increases, a reduction in stroke volume that results in a decrease in cardiac output occurs. A pneumoperitoneum increases cardiac workload and myocardial oxygen requirements, which is the reason laparoscopic procedures are relatively contraindicated for patients who have a severely limited cardiac reserve. Interventions that can be used to minimize the associated reductions in stroke volume include intravenous fluid administration and compression of the patient's lower extremities. Upon discontinuation of the pneumoperitoneum, and return of patient to the supine position, the stroke volume will increase. Table 9-2 summarizes the hemodynamic effects associated with laparoscopic cholecystectomy.

Pulmonary   Patients having laparoscopic surgery have a decrease in postoperative pulmonary complications as compared to an open procedure. However, creation of a pneumoperitoneum causes intraoperative pulmonary dysfunction. The use of CO_2 displaces the diaphragm cephalad resulting in altered pulmonary dynamics, which are listed in

Table 9-3. Insufflation compresses the basilar lobes of the lungs resulting in atelectasis, decreased functional residual capacity (FRC), decreased vital capacity, and increased dead space ventilation. After creation of a pneumoperitoneum, $PaCO_2$ levels will plateau within 40 minutes after insufflation. Inadvertent CO_2 insufflation in extraperitoneal space can result from a misplaced trocar or lack of CO_2 sequestration into the intraperitoneal space. Extraperitoneal CO_2 insufflation results in a rapid increase in $ETCO_2$.

Surgical patients that present with pulmonary dysfunction, such as obstructive lung disease, require careful monitoring of CO_2 levels during laparoscopic surgery. In patients with normal pulmonary physiology, utilization of $ETCO_2$ monitoring provides a proportional relationship between $ETCO_2$ and CO_2. Patients with preexisting

Table 9-2   The Hemodynamic Effects Associated with Laparoscopic Cholecystectomy
1. Neurohumoral response: Activated
2. Venous return (preload): Decreased
3. Systemic vascular resistance (afterload): Increased
4. Heart rate: Increased
5. Blood pressure: Increased
6. Cardiac output: Decreased

Table 9-3   The Respiratory Effects Associated with Laparoscopic Cholecystectomy
1. CO_2 absorption: Increased
2. Vital capacity: Decreased
3. Intrathoracic compliance: Increased
4. Pulmonary compliance: Decreased
5. Peak airway pressure: Increased
6. Functional residual capacity: Decreased
7. Atelectasis: Increased
8. Ventilation–perfusion mismatch: Increased

pulmonary disease may have an inaccurate $ETCO_2$–$PaCO_2$ relationship ultimately underestimating the $PaCO_2$ values. The direct measurement of $PaCO_2$ with blood gas analysis may be necessary in this patient population.

Neurologic Absorption of CO_2 during laparoscopy results in hypercarbia, leading to an increase in cerebral blood flow and intracranial pressure. Pneumoperitoneum itself will also increase intracranial pressure with or without any increase in the $PaCO_2$ levels due to the pressure exerted on the major venous structures within the abdominal cavity. Increased intracranial pressure leads to a decrease in cerebrospinal fluid drainage. Laparoscopic surgery is contraindicated in patients with increased intracranial pressure.

Renal Abdominal insufflation affects the kidneys and causes oliguria as a result of compression of the renal vasculature, compression of the inferior vena cava causing decreased CO_2, and increased antidiuretic hormone secretion. Decreased renal blood flow leads to decreased glomerular filtration rate, urine output, and creatinine clearance sodium excretion; as a result, there is a potential for fluid overload. The anesthetist should avoid extreme hypotension in patients who have preoperative renal impairment. Patient's plasma vasopressin, renin, and aldosterone levels increase during CO_2 insufflation and remain elevated for up to 1 hour after removal of the pneumoperitoneum. The renal effects that are associated with a pneumoperitoneum are listed in Table 9-4.

Table 9-4 The Renal Effects Associated with Laparoscopic Cholecystectomy
1. Renal blood flow: Decreased
2. Glomerular filtration rate: Decreased
3. Renal plasma flow: Decreased
4. Antidiuretic hormone: Increased
5. Urine output: Decreased

Hepatic Decreases in hepatic and splanchnic blood flow are associated with a pneumoperitoneum. Use of low insufflation pressures can help maintain normal hepatic and splanchnic blood flow.

11. Discuss the effects of CO_2 absorption during laparoscopic procedures.
Carbon dioxide can be absorbed during laparoscopic surgeries in various parts of the body and may lead to untoward effects. Direct effects of CO_2 absorption result in decreases in heart rate, contractility, and SVR. The body reacts to these effects with sympathetic nervous system stimulation resulting in increased heart rate, contractility, and SVR. High levels of CO_2 can cause vagal stimulation producing bradycardia and cardiac arrest.

12. Examine the effects of steep reverse Trendelenburg positioning for laparoscopic cholecystectomy.
Patients undergoing a laparoscopic cholecystectomy are placed into the reverse Trendelenburg position and tilted with their left side downward to facilitate visualization of the gallbladder. When the patient is placed into this position, the bowels shift downward away from the liver, which is located in the right upper quadrant. Lung and chest compliance are improved; however, there is the potential for hypotension as gravity pulls blood downward away from the heart. The anesthetist must also be cautious regarding the possibility of endotracheal tube migration or dislodgement.

13. During insufflation of CO_2, the patient's heart rate abruptly decreases from 82 to 36 beats per minute. Identify the cause and treatment of this situation.
Stretching of the abdominal cavity during insufflation can initiate the celiac reflex. The parasympathetic nervous system innervation to the abdominal cavity is via the vagus nerve. The stretching is sensed and transmitted to the brain as an afferent visceral response. The efferent response from the

brain to the heart increases vagal tone resulting in decreased heart rate, decreased contractility, and decreased rate of cardiac impulse conduction.

The treatment for the celiac reflex depends on the severity of bradycardia and the degree of hypotension that ensues. In this particular case, cardiac output is inadequate in most patients whose heart rate decreases to 36 beats per minute. The immediate initial intervention would be to tell the surgeon to rapidly remove the CO_2 gas from the peritoneal cavity. If severe bradycardia persists, an anticholinergic such as atropine should be administered. If the bradycardia is not as dramatic and cardiac output is adequate, then assessing the blood pressure to determine if perfusion is adequate is acceptable. Cardiac arrest can be caused by parasympathetic nervous system predominance as a result of CO_2 insufflation.

14. What are the potential complications associated with open cholecystectomy?
- Injury to the common bile duct
- Hemorrhage
- Infection of the surgical wound
- Injury to intraperitoneal organs, or major abdominal blood vessels
- Postoperative respiratory insufficiency

15. List the potential complications associated with laparoscopic cholecystectomy.
The mortality rate for laparoscopic cholecystectomy is estimated to be 0.1 to 1.0 per 1000 cases.

- Deep vein thrombosis
- Injury to intraperitoneal organs or major abdominal blood vessels
- Hemorrhage
- Increased intracranial pressure
- Increased risk of regurgitation
- Postoperative nausea and vomiting
- Pneumothorax
- Pneumopericardium
- Pneumomediastinum
- Shoulder pain

- Subcutaneous emphysema
- Carbon dioxide venous gas embolism

Subcutaneous Emphysema Subcutaneous emphysema is a known complication of laparoscopic surgery. It is sometimes unavoidable and it is caused by accidental extraperitoneal insufflation. This situation develops as crepitus occurs over the abdominal wall and causes an increase in $ETCO_2$. The CO_2 gas can migrate upward into the head and neck region resulting in airway edema. The crepitus will resolve in time after exsufflation but the patient should be kept intubated until the presence of hypercarbia is resolved. The severity of crepitus is dependent on the amount and the speed of extraperitoneal CO_2 gas extravasation.

Pneumothorax A pneumothorax is a rare but life-threatening complication that can occur during a laparoscopic cholecystectomy. This situation results from CO_2 gas traversing the thorax through a tear in the visceral peritoneum, a disruption of the parietal pleura during dissection, or a congenital defect in the diaphragm. Patients may be asymptomatic or exhibit rapid desaturation, unilateral breath sounds, bronchospasm, increased $ETCO_2$, increased peak airway pressures, and severe hypotension. After removal of the pneumoperitoneum, spontaneous resolution of the pneumothorax may occur within 30 to 60 minutes. If the pneumothorax is large, a thoracocentesis should be performed. Correction of hypoxemia is paramount and ventilation with 100% oxygen is vital while adding positive-end expiratory pressure (PEEP) may be necessary.

Carbon Dioxide Gas Embolism A venous CO_2 gas embolism is a rare but potentially fatal complication associated with laparoscopic surgery. It typically occurs shortly after creation of a pneumoperitoneum, especially in those patients who have had previous abdominal surgery. Carbon dioxide gas enters into the venous system through a disruption created in a vein within the abdominal wall or peritoneum and then it travels into the heart and pulmonary circulation via the inferior vena cava. If a significant amount of gas is entrained over a short period of time, a venous gas embolism can result in significant hemodynamic compromise. An air lock at the level of the right atrium decreasing blood flow through the heart and results in hypotension, decreased cardiac output, tachycardia, pulmonary edema, hypoxemia, hypercarbia, increased peak airway pressure, jugular venous distention, and facial cyanosis.

Treatment of a patient who develops a carbon dioxide gas embolism includes immediate evacuation of the pneumoperitoneum, ventilation with 100% oxygen, administering fluid, and vasopressors. The patient should be placed in the left lateral decubitus position with the head oriented downward to prevent gas bubble entry into the pulmonary and arterial circulation. If a central venous catheter is placed, the gas embolism may be removed by aspiration.

Postoperative Period

16. Identify the key aspects of postoperative anesthetic management for a patient having an open cholecystectomy or laparoscopic cholecystectomy.

Hemodynamic Stability Emergence phenomena can occur during emergence and extubation. However, the hemodynamic effects can persist throughout the initial postoperative phase. The anesthetist should determine if the patient is experiencing pain, which is a potent stimulus of the sympathetic nervous system. Extremes hypertension and tachycardia should be treated with vasodilators, beta blocking, or calcium channel medications. The specific treatment plan should be tailored to the individual patient.

Respiratory Status A rapid assessment of the patient's postoperative respiratory function is imperative. The head of the patient's bed should be elevated to promote respiratory excursion and supplemental oxygen should be administered. Abdominal splinting can occur with pain and results in an inadequate tidal volume and contributes to the development of atelectasis and ventilation perfusion mismatch. Hypoventilation is more often associated with an open cholecystectomy due to the pain caused by the surgical incision. Analgesic medications should be administered to alleviate discomfort and promote adequate respiratory function.

Postoperative Pain The severity of postoperative pain that is experienced is highly variable and is dependent on the individual patient. As stated previously, patients who undergo an open cholecystectomy frequently have more pain as compared to the laparoscopic approach due to the right upper quadrant incision and retraction of the skin and abdominal contents. However, a specific character of pain occurs during a laparoscopic cholecystectomy and it is described as shoulder tip pain. It is believed that this discomfort is caused by diaphragmatic irritation as a result of the CO_2 gas used to create the pneumoperitoneum. A variety of intravenous or oral analgesic medications can be administered. Ketorolac decreases postoperative pain without inhibiting ventilation or causing sedation which is desirable for outpatient surgery.

Nausea and Vomiting The incidence of nausea and vomiting for patients after the administration of anesthesia ranges from 30 to 70%. Multimodal drug therapy has been shown to be more effective in treating this event as compared to monotherapy. Medications that can be used to inhibit nausea and vomiting include propofol, steroids (dexamethasone), serotonin receptor antagonists (ondansetron/dolasetron), and dopamine receptor antagonists (droperidol/metoclopramide). A new medication called *aprepitant* is a neurokinin type 1 receptor antagonist has also been shown to be effective at decreasing nausea and vomiting.

Presently, this medication is being used to treat chemotherapy induced nausea and vomiting.

REVIEW QUESTIONS

1. Which gas is routinely used during laparoscopic surgery to create a pneumoperitoneum?
   a. Argon
   b. Carbon dioxide
   c. Helium
   d. Nitrous oxide
2. Which is not a hemodynamic change associated with a pneumoperitoneum?
   a. Decreased venous return to the heart
   b. Increased abdominal pressures
   c. Increased mean arterial pressure
   d. Increased stroke volume
3. Which respiratory effect occurs during carbon dioxide insufflation for laparoscopic surgery?
   a. Decreased functional residual capacity
   b. Decreased pulmonary compliance
   c. Increased intrathoracic pressure
   d. Increased vital capacity
4. Which renal effect occurs during carbon dioxide insufflation for laparoscopic surgery?
   a. Decreased aldosterone levels
   b. Decreased antidiuretic hormone levels
   c. Decreased urine output
   d. Increased glomerular filtration
5. Which preoperative laboratory test is not indicated for a patient having a cholecystectomy?
   a. Alanine aminotransferase (ALT)
   b. Aspartate aminotransferase (AST)
   c. Bilirubin
   d. Cholesterol

REVIEW ANSWERS

1. **Answer: b**
   All of the following gasses have been utilized during laparoscopic surgery; however, the safety profile of CO_2 allows its use during electrocautery and laser surgery. Carbon dioxide is also easily eliminated from the lungs.

2. **Answer: d**
   Hemodynamic changes that occur with creation of a pneumoperitoneum include decreased venous return to the heart, decreased stroke volume, increased mean arterial pressure, and increased abdominal pressures.
3. **Answer: d**
   Carbon dioxide insufflation during the creation of a pneumoperitoneum affects the pulmonary system by decreasing functional residual capacity, pulmonary compliance, and vital capacity. It will also result in an increased intrathoracic pressure.
4. **Answer: c**
   Carbon dioxide insufflation during the creation of a pneumoperitoneum affects the renal system by increasing aldosterone and antidiuretic hormone secretion, decreasing urine output, and decreasing glomerular filtration rate.
5. **Answer: d**
   Preoperative laboratory tests necessary for patients having a cholecystectomy include ALT, AST, bilirubin, albumin, and alkaline phosphatase.

SUGGESTED READINGS

Bablekos GD, Michaelides SA, Roussou T, et al. Changes in breathing control and mechanics after laparoscopic vs open cholecystectomy. *Arch Surg* 2006;141:16–22.

Cunningham AJ, Brull SJ. Laparoscopic cholecystectomy: anesthetic implications. *Anesth Analg* 1993;76:1120–1133.

Joris JL, Noirot DP, Legrand MJ, et al. Hemodynamic changes during laparoscopic cholecystectomy. *Anesth Analg* 1993;76:1067–1071.

Kaki AM, Abd El-Hakeem EE. Prophylaxis of postoperative nausea and vomiting with ondansetron, metoclopramide, or placebo in total intravenous anesthesia patients undergoing laparoscopic cholecystectomy. *Saudi Med J* 2008;29(10):1408–1412.

Karanicolas PJ, Smith SE, Kanbur B, et al. The impact of prophylactic dexamethasone on nausea and vomiting after laparoscopic cholecystectomy. A systematic review and meta-analysis. *Ann Surg* 2008;248(5):751–762.

Keus F, Ali UA, Noordergraaf GJ, et al. Anesthesiological considerations in small-incision and laparoscopic cholecystectomy in symptomatic cholecystolithiasis: implications for pulmonary function. A randomized clinical trial. *Acta Anaesthesiol Scand* 2007;51:1068–1078.

Keus F, De Vries J, Gooszen H, et al. Laparoscopic versus small-incision cholecystectomy: health status in a blind randomized trial. *Surg Endosc* 2008;22:1649–1659.

Leo J, Filipovic G, Krementsova J, et al. Open cholecystectomy for all patients in the era of laparoscopic surgery – a prospective cohort study. *BMC Surgery* 2006;6:5.

Palmer TJ. Hepatobiliary and gastrointestinal disturbances. In: Nagelhout JJ, Zaglaniczy KL, eds. *Nurse Anesthesia*, 3rd ed. St. Louis, MO: Elsevier Saunders, 2005:678–680.

Ros A, Carlsson P, Rahmqvist M, et al. Non-randomised patients in a cholecystectomy trial: characteristics, procedures and outcomes. *BMC Surgery* 2006;6:17.

Yi NJ, Han HS, Min SK. The safety of a laparoscopic cholecystectomy in acute cholecystitis inhigh-risk patients older than sixty with stratification based on ASA score. *Minim Invasive Ther Allied Tech* 2006;15(3):159–164.

Liver Failure and Nonalcoholic Steatohepatitis

10

Joseph F. Burkard

KEY POINTS

- Hepatic dysfunction is often multifactorial and can be categorized as prehepatic, intrahepatic (hepatocellular), or posthepatic (cholestatic) based on measurement of serum bilirubin, aminotransferases, and alkaline phosphatase.
- Orthotropic liver transplantation (OLT) has emerged as a definitive treatment option for patients with end-stage hepatic disease and this is largely attributable to advances in surgical technique, immunosuppressive therapy, and donor organ procurement.
- Anesthesia-related concerns for patients undergoing OLT are consistent with those for patients undergoing major surgery with severe cirrhosis.
- There is no single anesthetic technique that has been proven superior during anesthetic management of OLT.
- Anesthetic management is strongly influenced by the various hemodynamic manifestations presented during the three major phases of the procedure.

CASE SYNOPSIS

A 38-year-old woman with a history of nonalcoholic steatohepatitis presents with end-stage liver disease and is scheduled for a liver transplant. She was recently hospitalized because of jaundice, fever, confusion, urine incontinence, and progressive abdominal pain and swelling. Two months before admission the patient noted pain and swelling of her elbows. One month later she developed malaise, weakness, and irritability. The patient's clinical status has stabilized with diuretic and albumin therapy, administration of parenteral nutrition, and salt restriction. The patient has been on the liver transplant list for 8 months.

PREOPERATIVE EVALUATION AND DEMOGRAPHIC DATA

Past Medical/Surgical History

- Nonalcoholic steatohepatitis
- Acute renal failure

- Smoked an average of 1 pack a day for 10 years, stopped 1 year ago
- Jaundiced with multiple spider angiomas of the face and trunk
- Abdominal distention due to ascites
- Hematoma present on the anterior wall after a recent paracentesis.

List of Medications

- Accupril, an angiotensin converting enzyme inhibitor (ACEI), interferes with the conversion of angiotensin I to angiotensin II
- Zosyn (2 g piperacillin with 0.25 mg tazobactam) for a staph infection
- Bumex, a loop diuretic

Diagnostic Data

TEST NAME	RESULT		NORMAL RANGE
White blood cell (WBC)	30.2 K/CUMM	(High)	4.8–10.8 K/CUMM
Blood urea nitrogen (BUN)	47.14 mmol/l	(High)	2.9–7.1 mmol/l
Creatinine	411.53 umol/l	(High)	61.9–114.9 umol/l
Bilirubin	110.34 umol/l	(High)	1.7–5.1 umol/l
Aspartate amino-transferase (AST)	260 U/l	(High)	12–38 U/l
Alanine amino-transferase (ALT)	59 U/l	(High)	10–45 U/l
Albumin	17 g/l	(Low)	35–48 g/l
Protein (serum)	70 g/l	(Normal)	60–80 g/l
Protein (urine)	30	(Positive)	Negative trace
Urinalysis (bacteria)	Many	(Positive)	None

Height/Weight/Vital Signs

- 168 cm, 64 kg
- Blood pressure, 150/88 mm Hg; heart rate, 100 beats per minute; respiratory rate, 22 breaths per minute; room air oxygen saturation, 96%; temperature, 38.1°C

PATHOPHYSIOLOGY

When hepatic dysfunction (jaundice) occurs, an analysis of historical data, clinical signs, and symptoms; serial liver function tests; and a search for extrahepatic causes of hepatic dysfunction facilitate development of a differential diagnosis. Table 10-1 lists the causes of hepatic dysfunction and can be categorized as prehepatic, intrahepatic (hepatocellular), or posthepatic (cholestatic) based on measurement of serum bilirubin, aminotransferases, and alkaline phosphatase. Hepatic dysfunction is often multifactorial. Table 10-2 describes factors that can be used to develop a differential diagnosis for hepatic dysfunction.

SURGICAL PROCEDURE

OLT has emerged as a definitive treatment option for patients with end-stage hepatic disease. This is largely attributable to advances in surgical technique, immunosuppressive therapy, and donor organ procurement. Other contributing factors have greatly attenuated the previously formidable morbidity and mortality associated with this procedure, including advances in technologic and perioperative management.

Patients with end-stage hepatic disease who experience progressive life-threatening complications that become increasingly refractory to medical intervention are candidates for OLT. Transplantation may also be considered a therapeutic option in patients with certain viral infections who respond poorly to medical management but are nevertheless deemed physiologically salvageable. In the adult population, postnecrotic (nonalcoholic) cirrhosis constitutes the most common indication for OLT.

Table 10-1 Causes of Hepatic Dysfunction Based on Liver Function Tests

HEPATIC DYSFUNCTION	BILIRUBIN	AMINOTRANSFERASE ENZYMES	ALKALINE PHOSPHATASE	CAUSES
Prehepatic	Increased unconjugated fraction	Normal	Normal	Hemolysis, hematoma, bilirubin overload
Intrahepatic	Increased conjugated fraction	Markedly increased	Normal to slightly increased	Viral, drugs, sepsis, hypoxemia, cirrhosis
Posthepatic	Increased conjugated fraction	Normal to slightly increased	Markedly increased	Biliary tract stones, sepsis

The refinement of immunosuppressive therapy has been instrumental in the increasingly impressive survival rates in patients undergoing OLT. A vital component has been the use of cyclosporine, which interferes with helper T-cell activity and inhibits interleukin (IL)-2 and other proinflammatory cytokines. Cyclosporine is often used concurrently with azathioprine and corticosteroids. Anti-OKT3, a monoclonal antibody directed toward lymphocytes, has also shown efficacy in preventing acute rejection, particularly if it is steroid refractory. Tacrolimus (FK-506) is an effective alternative to cyclosporine. Technical refinements in the procedure and development of more precise support modalities have also contributed to the overall improved outcome in patients undergoing OLT.

Anesthesia-related concerns for patients undergoing OLT are consistent with those for patients undergoing major surgery with severe cirrhosis. The multisystem effects of cirrhosis are underscored. Profound hemodynamic derangements may preexist and are likely to be exacerbated by the numerous stressors imposed during particular phases of the procedure. These include the hemodynamic consequences of clamping and unclamping the portal vein and vena cava, as well as alterations in metabolism. Hyperkalemia and venous air embolism may be encountered with perfusion of the transplanted graft.

Table 10-2 Factors Used to Develop a Differential Diagnosis for Hepatic Dysfunction

1. Review all drugs administered
2. Check for sources of sepsis
3. Evaluate the possibility of an increased exogenous bilirubin load such as a blood transfusion
4. Rule out occult hematoma formation
5. Rule out hemolysis
6. Assess for evidence of hypotension, hypoventilation, and hypovolemia
7. Assess for congestive heart failure and renal insufficiency
8. Consider the possibility of immune-mediated hepatotoxicity

ANESTHETIC MANAGEMENT AND CONSIDERATIONS

Preoperative Period

1. List various causes that result in cirrhosis of the liver.

Cirrhosis can result from a large variety of chronic, progressive liver diseases. Most often cirrhosis is the result of excessive chronic alcohol ingestion or chronic viral hepatitis due to hepatitis B virus (HBV) or hepatitis C virus (HCV) infection. Scarring of the liver results in disruption of normal liver architecture, and regenerating parenchymal nodules are typically seen. A percutaneous liver biopsy establishes the diagnosis of cirrhosis. Computed tomography (CT), magnetic resonance imaging (MRI), and hepatic ultrasonography with Doppler flow studies may reveal findings consistent with cirrhosis (splenomegaly, ascites, irregular liver surfaces). Fatigue and malaise are common with all forms of cirrhosis as well as with almost all forms of acute and chronic liver disease. Characteristic but nondiagnostic physical findings of cirrhosis include palmer erythema, spider angioma, gynecomastia, testicular atrophy, and evidence of portal hypertension (splenomegaly, ascites). A decreased serum albumin concentration and a prolonged prothrombin time are characteristic of cirrhosis. An increase in serum aminotransferase and alkaline phosphate concentration is common. Hepatic and extrahepatic complications of hepatic cirrhosis develop predictably in patients afflicted with progressive liver scarring. Acute hepatic failure is characterized by an increased expression of these complications and includes a list for differential diagnosis found in Table 10-3.

2. Discuss the major features of nonalcoholic steatohepatitis (NASH).

NASH is a common, often "silent" liver disease. This condition resembles findings that are consistent with alcoholic liver disease, but occurs in people who drink little or no alcohol. The major feature in NASH is fat in the liver, along with inflammation and damage.

Table 10-3   Pathologic Consequences Associated with Acute Hepatic Failure
• Portal hypertension
• Esophagogastric varices
• Ascites
• Hyperdynamic circulation
• Anemia
• Coagulopathy
• Arterial hypoxemia
• Hepatorenal syndrome
• Hypoglycemia
• Gallstones
• Hepatic encephalopathy
• Hepatic carcinoma

Most people with NASH feel well and are not aware that they have a liver problem. Nevertheless, NASH can be severe and can lead to cirrhosis, in which the liver is permanently damaged and scarred and no longer is able to function properly. Nonalcoholic steatohepatitis affects 2 to 5% of Americans. An additional 10 to 20% of Americans have fat in their liver, but no inflammation or liver damage, a condition called "fatty liver." NASH is becoming more common, possibly because of the greater number of Americans who are obese. In the past 10 years, the rate of obesity has doubled in adults and tripled in children. Obesity also contributes to diabetes and high blood cholesterol, which can further complicate the health of someone with NASH. NASH is initially suspected in a person who is found to have elevations in liver tests that are included in routine blood test panels, such as alanine aminotransferase or aspartate aminotransferase. When further evaluation shows no apparent reason for liver disease and x-rays or imaging studies of the liver indicate the presence of fat deposition, NASH is suspected. The only confirmatory test for NASH is a liver biopsy which will show fat and inflamed tissues. Nonalcoholic steatohepatitis is usually a silent disease with few or no symptoms.

Patients generally do not develop symptoms in the early stages; however, fatigue, weight loss, and weakness occur once the disease is more advanced or cirrhosis develops. The progression of NASH can take years to develop, and as fibrosis develops and becomes more severe, cirrhosis occurs (Fig. 10-1). The liver becomes scarred, hardened, and, as a result, hepatic function is impaired. Currently, there are no specific therapies used to treat NASH. The most important recommendations given to persons with this disease are to:

1. Reduce their weight
2. Follow a balanced and healthy diet
3. Increase physical activity
4. Avoid alcohol
5. Avoid unnecessary medications

People with NASH often have other medical conditions, such as diabetes, high blood pressure, or elevated cholesterol. Once cirrhosis and liver damage develop, liver transplantation is considered.

Intraoperative Period

3. Identify the anesthetic management and monitoring considerations for liver surgery.
Invasive monitoring modalities are mandatory for OLT. These include intraarterial pressure monitoring and central venous or pulmonary artery catheterization. Owing to the profound fluid shifts and blood loss encountered in these procedures, direct measurement of central filling pressures is vital for guiding volume and blood-product replacement. Large-bore (14- to 16-gauge) intravenous catheters are needed for administration of large volumes using rapid infusion devices. Intravenous fluids should be warmed to prevent hypothermia in order to avoid the untoward effects on coagulation, pharmacokinetics, and other metabolic process. Other measures used to maintain normothermia include forced-air surface warming and possibly increased ambient room temperature. All airway gases should be humidified. Urinary output, as measured via indwelling urinary catheter, should be maintained at a minimum of 0.5 ml/kg/hr.

4. Identify the serial laboratory results that must be assessed during anesthetic management for OLT.
Patients with severe cirrhosis are typically coagulopathic (deficient in coagulation factors and thrombocytopenic). Massive blood loss should be anticipated. Red blood cells, fresh frozen plasma, platelets, and cryoprecipitate should be readily available. Blood-salvaging technology should also be used. Infusion of antifibrinolytics such as aminocaproic acid may also be useful

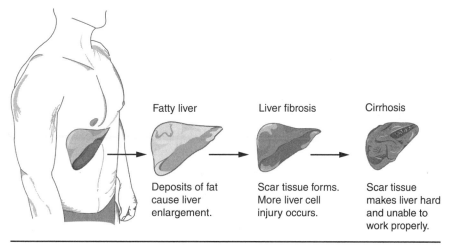

Fatty liver

Liver fibrosis

Cirrhosis

Deposits of fat cause liver enlargement.

Scar tissue forms. More liver cell injury occurs.

Scar tissue makes liver hard and unable to work properly.

Figure 10-1 *Degenerative changes that progress toward cirrhosis.*

perioperatively in efforts to control hemorrhage. Serial laboratory measurements are performed throughout surgery which include arterial blood gases, electrolytes, hemoglobin and hematocrit levels, and metabolic studies assessing ionized calcium and serum glucose. Coagulation parameters are also closely assessed via activated partial thromboplastin time, prothrombin time, fibrinogen, and platelet count.

5. Discuss the anesthetic technique of choice for OLT.

There is no single anesthetic technique that has been proven superior during anesthetic management of OLT. Patients undergoing OLT are considered at increased risk for aspiration of stomach contents because of the likelihood of abdominal distention or history of upper gastrointestinal bleeding. General anesthesia is therefore induced via rapid-sequence technique with cricoid pressure. Premedication may be administered but may be curtailed in the presence of marked encephalopathy. Sodium thiopental, ketamine, propofol, and etomidate are all suitable hypnotic agents, but the requisite doses may be modified based on the patient's preexisting mental and hemodynamic status. Succinylcholine is used for rapid onset of neuromuscular blockade; however, rocuronium may also be used if no difficulty with intubation is anticipated. Maintenance of anesthesia is accomplished through the use of inhalation agent and intravenous opioid by bolus administration or infusion. Patients with severe encephalopathy may have increased intracranial pressure requiring hyperventilation. The minimum alveolar concentration of volatile agent should also be reduced in these patients. The use of nitrous oxide is limited or avoided because of concerns pertaining to its capability to expand air bubbles that may reside in the nonperfused donor liver. Bowel distension is also a consideration with prolonged usage. Patients undergoing OLT typically remain intubated and mechanically ventilated in the intensive care unit postoperatively.

6. Describe the three phases during OLT and the associated anesthetic management.

Intraoperative anesthetic management is strongly influenced by the various hemodynamic manifestations presented during the three major phases of the procedure. During the *preanhepatic* (dissection) phase, a wide subcostal incision is used to provide optimal surgical exposure. Prior abdominal surgeries may have resulted in adhesion formation, thereby potentially increasing blood loss. The liver remains attached to the portal vein, inferior vena cava, biliary tract, and hepatic artery. During the *anhepatic* phase, the vena cava is clamped above and below the liver. The portal vein, common bile duct, and hepatic artery are also ligated. Total excision is then undertaken. Venovenous bypass is generally reserved for patients with pulmonary hypertension or significant cardiovascular disease. Removal of the liver may result in hypocalcemia because of loss of the liver's role in the metabolic removal of citrate from blood products that may have been administered. Citrate is a preservative used in banked blood that binds calcium and the associated hypocalcemia that occurs may also result in cardiac depression. Ionized calcium levels should be regularly assessed and should guide exogenous replacement (200 to 500 mg). Loss of hepatic clearance of acid metabolites from the gastrointestinal tract results in progressive acidosis. Sodium bicarbonate is administered judiciously to prevent hypernatremia, hyperosmolality, and metabolic alkalosis. Should large amounts of sodium bicarbonate be needed, tromethamine should be considered as an alternative. Hyperglycemia may be encountered more commonly than hypoglycemia because of the increased glucose load presented from large amounts of transfused blood products. In general, dextrose-containing intravenous fluids are avoided. Air emboli may result from air entrapped in venous sinusoids and released when the donor liver is reperfused. The incidence of air embolism is reduced by infusing cold crystalloid solution through the venous structures as the graft is being anastomosed. After the portal and suprahepatic caval anastomoses but before infrahepatic caval anastomosis is completed, the liver is flushed by portal blood through the incomplete infrahepatic anastomosis.

Caval clamping is associated with profound hemodynamic changes, particularly decreased cardiac output and hypotension. Renal perfusion may be adversely affected as well. Increased venous back pressure may also increase bleeding and impair splanchnic perfusion. The technique of venovenous bypass consists of cannulation of the inferior vena cava and portal vein and an axillary vein with the intention of diverting blood away from the liver and delivering it directly to the heart. Venovenous bypass is used to minimize hypotension, maintain renal and splanchnic perfusion, and prevent gut edema and ischemia. Heparinization is not necessary because of circuit design technology. Venovenous bypass is associated with an element of risk, however. Venovenous bypass may lengthen operative time and subject the patient to increased risk of air embolic and thromboembolic events. Brachial plexus injury and hypothermia are also recognized side effects. Cannulation of the internal jugular vein rather than the axillary vein as a return circuit also has been used and has been shown to attenuate a number of the side effects of venovenous bypass. Percutaneous methods for establishing venous bypass also have been described. Prophylactic measures for preservation of renal perfusion include the use of mannitol and low-dose dopamine infusion (2–3 mcg/kg/min). Ultimately renal perfusion, as well as overall systemic organ perfusion, is best accomplished by optimizing cardiac output and systemic blood pressure. For this, any of a number of vasoactive and inotropic agents should be available and used as needed.

7. Construct a plan to manage intraoperative electrolyte imbalances.

Hypocalcemia and myocardial depression associated with removal of the liver are managed with periodic administration of calcium chloride, which is guided by assessment of serum ionized calcium concentration. Hyperkalemia may be a consequence of the progressive acidosis frequently encountered during the *anhepatic stage*. Symptomatic hyperkalemia may lead to cardiac dysrhythmias and refractory asystole. Treatment consists of the administration of calcium chloride, sodium bicarbonate, and glucose and insulin and the application of hyperventilation. Maintaining adequate diuresis throughout surgery is crucial to controlling hyperkalemia.

8. Discuss the fluid of choice for perioperative fluid replacement.

Fluid management presents a formidable perioperative challenge because of its unpredictability and variability. This is influenced in large part by the extent and magnitude of portal hypertension, the challenges in dissection, and the coagulation status. Ongoing goals include; maintaining normovolemia, sustaining organ system perfusion, and optimizing oxygen-carrying capacity. Selection of crystalloid is based on these goals and preservation of electrolyte and acid–base balance. Lactated Ringer's solution may increase serum lactate levels and contribute to hyperkalemia. Normal saline may cause hyperchloremic metabolic acidosis. Isotonic solutions with greater compatibility to normal osmolality are therefore preferred. Rapid transfusion devices that allow the infusion of large volumes of warmed fluids and blood products should be used. Correction of acidosis may be accomplished by optimizing systematic perfusion, hyperventilation, and sodium bicarbonate. Excessive sodium bicarbonate may result in hyperosmolality, hypernatremia, central pontine myelinolysis, and metabolic acidosis. Before reperfusion of the grafted donor liver, correction of electrolyte and acid–base abnormalities should be undertaken. Central filling pressures should also be allowed to increase, and hyperventilation should be instituted. Preparation for rapid infusion of warmed blood products, as well as for administration of indicated inotropic and vasoactive agents, allows prompt retrieval of hemodynamic parameters secondary to reperfusion hypotension.

During the *postanhepatic* (revascularization–biliary reconstruction) phase, the venous anastomoses are completed, and circulation to the new liver is accomplished via the anastomosed hepatic artery. A Roux-en-Y choledochojejunostomy connects the bile duct to the recipient gastrointestinal tract. The reperfusion phenomenon can result in acidosis, hypotension, and electrolyte abnormalities—particularly hyperkalemia.

9. Discuss the management of electrocardiographic aberrations during liver transplantation.
Electrocardiographic aberrations may occur and most typically manifest as bradycardia. Management is largely supportive and consists of volume restoration by colloid or crystalloid (as directed by laboratory findings, central filling pressures, and urinary output), calcium chloride, and sodium bicarbonate. Inotropic and vasoactive support may be indicated. This may entail a polypharmacologic approach because of the recipient's possible attenuated response to vasoactive agents. To optimize the activity of these agents, acidosis must be corrected. Postperfusion coagulopathy is commonly encountered after reperfusion. This may be attributable to the release of sequestered heparin in the donor liver or to activity of an endogenous heparinoid.

10. Describe the laboratory technique that is utilized to monitor intraoperative fibrinolysis.
Hyperfibrinolysis is frequently encountered subsequent to increased release of tissue plasminogen activator inhibitor during the anhepatic phase. The use of thromboelastography (TEG) allows for accurate detection of fibrinolysis and abnormalities in platelet activity and is valuable, in addition to laboratory findings, in directing blood and blood-component resuscitation. Platelets and FFP should be available. Cryoprecipitate may also be used for restoration of an adequate fibrinogen level in the presence of fibrinolysis. Desmopressin (DDAVP) may be administered to help improve platelet function. Overtransfusion with blood components and crystalloid should be avoided to prevent pulmonary edema, decreased oxygenation, peripheral edema, and prolonged intubation and ventilation and their attendant risks.

Postoperative Period

11. Identify postoperative complications that are associated with OLT.
Postoperative complications may include:

- Persistent hemorrhage
- Fluid volume overload
- Metabolic and electrolyte abnormalities (hyperglycemia, hyperkalemia, metabolic alkalosis)
- Infection
- Neurologic (encephalopathy, seizures, cyclosporine neurotoxicity, cerebrovascular hemorrhage)

12. Discuss the surgical complications that require surgical reintervention.
Surgical complications that may require surgical reintervention include anastomotic leak or stricture of the biliary reconstruction or dehiscence or thrombosis of the hepatic or portal vessels. Prophylactic antibacterial and antifungal agents are administered in addition to the immunosuppressive agents. The incidence of infection is high. The locus of infection may be an intraabdominal source, an indwelling catheter, the surgical wound, the urinary tract, or an intrapulmonary source. Numerous infective entities may be causative. Commonly encountered are fungi, gram-negative bacteria, viruses, and parasites. Postoperative hepatitis may be caused by herpes virus, Epstein Barr virus, cytomegalovirus, adenovirus, or hepatitis B or C virus. Reactivation of a preexisting viral infection is also a causative possibility. Potential organ rejection is closely monitored and differentially determined by live biopsy. The most common period in which rejection occurs is during weeks 1 to 6 after transplant. Laboratory findings usually reflect a prodromal period before this occurs.

13. Discuss the anesthetic considerations for patients undergoing retransplantation.

Considerations for patients with hepatic failure apply to patients who undergo retransplantation. These patients are immunosuppressed and sensitized to antibodies, which makes blood type and cross-matching more complex. A variable degree of renal insufficiency and hypertension secondary to cyclosporine toxicity may also be present. Patients on immunomodulatory steroids who undergo retransplantation are considered steroid dependent and require steroid supplementation before surgery. Strict aseptic technique is mandatory for all patients who are immunocompromised.

Living donor hepatic transplantation is currently being undertaken in select centers and accounts for approximately 10% of all hepatic transplants. This modality has been made possible through research and experience-based advances in surgical, medical, and perianesthetic techniques and strategies. In living donor hepatic transplantation, the recipient typically receives the healthy right hepatic lobe from the donor. Besides the advantage of a closer graft match and decreased waiting time between donor and recipient, intraoperative ischemic time of the liver graft is significantly minimized. Recipient and donor hepatectomy are performed nearly simultaneously to reduce the time from donation to transplant. Anesthetic concerns for the donor will focus on perioperative management for hepatectomy while attempting to minimize the degree of potentially complicating comorbidities. Posttransplant regeneration of liver tissue within the donor is noted to occur within a year. Return of hepatic function to preoperative levels correlates with the amount of donor liver mass resected. The relative risk for complications in the donor is consistent with the degree of resection (right lobe donor, 32%; left lateral segment, 9%; left lateral lobe, 7.5%). Biliary complications (stricture and leakage), infection, and blood-product transfusion factors are major postoperative donor complications. Reoperation for complications (4.5%) may be necessary.

In cadaveric liver transplantation, the time from retrieval to transplantation is limited to less than 6 hours, even under the most rigorous cooling and preservative protocols. Anesthetic considerations for the recipient of a cadaveric graft are consistent with those of the patient with end-stage liver disease.

REVIEW QUESTIONS

1. Which class of medications is instrumental for survival of patients undergoing OLT?
   a. Antibiotics
   b. Narcotics
   c. Immunosuppressants
   d. Beta adrenergic antagonists
2. Which disease process causes cirrhosis of the liver due to the infiltration of fat?
   a. Hepatitis
   b. Alcohol
   c. Diabetes
   d. Nonalcoholic steatohepatitis (NASH)
3. Which electrolyte imbalance is caused by progressive acidosis resulting from cirrhosis?
   a. Hyperkalemia
   b. Hypercalcemia
   c. Hyponatremia
   d. Hypoglycemia
4. Administration of which of the following substances improves platelet function?
   a. Packed red blood cells (PRBC)
   b. Desmopressin (DDAVP)
   c. Fresh frozen plasma (FFP)
   d. Cryoprecipitate
5. The most common period for rejection of the liver is within:
   a. the first 72 hours.
   b. the first week.
   c. 1 to 6 weeks after the transplant.
   d. 6 months after the transplant.

REVIEW ANSWERS

1. **Answer: c**

   The refinement of immunosuppressant therapy has been instrumental by increasing the survival rates in patients undergoing OLT.

2. **Answer: d**

   The major feature that is associated with NASH is fat deposition within in the liver.

3. **Answer: a**

   Hyperkalemia is a consequence of the progressive acidosis that can lead to cardiac dysrhythmias and asystole that is refractory to treatment.

4. **Answer: b**

   Desmopressin (DDAVP) may be administered to help improve platelet function.

5. **Answer: c**

   The most common period in which rejection occurs is during weeks 1 to 6 after the transplant.

SUGGESTED READINGS

Ahmed A, Keeffe EB. Current indications and contraindications for liver transplantation. *Clin Liv Dis* 2007;11(2):227–247.

Herbert MF, Wacher VJ, Roberts JP, et al. Pharmacokinetics of cyclosporine pre- and post-liver transplantation. *J Clin Pharmacol* 2003;43:38–42.

Huether SE. Alterations of digestive function. In: McCance KL, Heuther SE, eds. *Pathophysiology: The Biological Basis of Disease in Adults & Children,* 5th ed. St. Louis, MO: Mosby, 2006:1414–1427.

Marschall KE. Diseases of the liver and biliary tract. In: Hines RL, Marschall KE, eds. *Anesthesia and Co-Existing Disease,* 5th ed. St. Louis, MO: Saunders, 2008:265–274.

Merritt WT. Living donor surgery: overview of surgical and anesthesia issues. *Anesthesiol Clin North Am* 2004;22(4):633–650.

Murakawa M. Coagulation monitoring and management during liver transplantation. *J Anesth* 2003;17:77–78.

Otte JB. History of pediatric liver transplantation. Where are we coming from? Where do we stand? *Pediatr Transplant* 2002;6:378–387.

Palmer TJ. Hepatobilliary and gastrointestinal disorders and anesthesia. In: Nagelhout JJ, Plaus KL, eds. *Nurse Anesthesia*, 4th ed. St. Louis, MO: Saunders, 2010:762–770.

Webb K, Shephard L, Day E, et al. Transplantation for alcoholic liver disease: report of a consensus meeting. *Liv Transplant* 2006;12(2):301–305.

Zetterman RK. Liver transplantation for alcoholic liver disease. *Clin Liv Dis* 2005;9(1):171–181.

Hepatic Resection

Hamid Mahmood

11

KEY POINTS

- The most common cancers that arise within the liver are due to hepatocellular carcinoma and metastasis from colorectal cancer.
- The majority of hepatic resections are performed for the removal of cancerous tissue.
- Bleeding and hemorrhage are major risks that are associated with hepatic resection.
- Advances in equipment and technology, perioperative management, and surgical techniques have decreased the morbidity and mortality associated with liver resections.
- Epidural analgesia can be used to attenuate the stress response and decrease postoperative pain.

CASE SYNOPSIS

A 65-year-old white man with liver cancer is scheduled for surgery. The planned procedure includes a right hepatic lobectomy for removal of hepatocellular carcinoma.

PREOPERATIVE EVALUATION AND DEMOGRAPHIC DATA

Past Medical/Surgical History

- Colon resection
- Laparoscopic cholecystectomy
- Hernia repair
- Hypertension
- Gastroesophageal reflux disease
- Colon cancer

List of Medications

- Metoprolol
- Lipitor
- Pepcid
- Aspirin

Diagnostic Data

- Hemoglobin, 13.3 g/dl; hematocrit, 39.7%
- Platelet count, 109,000 cells/mm³
- Glucose, 100 mg/dl
- Electrolytes: sodium, 140 mEq/l; potassium, 3.8 mEq/l; chloride, 103 mEq/l; carbon dioxide, 27 mEq/l
- Prothrombin time, 22.5 seconds; partial thromboplastin time, 40 seconds; international normalized ratio, 2.1
- Liver function: aspartate transaminase, 120 U/l; alanine transaminase, 205 U/l; albumin, 2.1 g/dl; bilirubin, 1.2 mg/dl
- Transthoracic echocardiography: ejection fraction of 50%; no evidence of wall motion abnormalities or hypertrophy
- Electrocardiogram: normal sinus rhythm, heart rate 78 beats per minute
- Lungs are clear to auscultation

Height/Weight/Vital Signs

- 175 cm, 84 kg; body mass index (BMI), 27.36
- Blood pressure, 155/89 mm Hg; heart rate, 90 beats per minute; respiratory rate, 15 breaths per minute; room air oxygen saturation, 99%; temperature, 98.9°F

ANATOMY AND PHYSIOLOGY

The liver is a versatile organ weighing about 1.5 kg and is located in the right upper quadrant of the abdominal cavity. It extends from the fifth rib to the lower border of the thoracic cage. It is divided into four anatomic lobes and performs many functions that maintains homeostasis. The basic functional unit of the liver is the liver lobule,

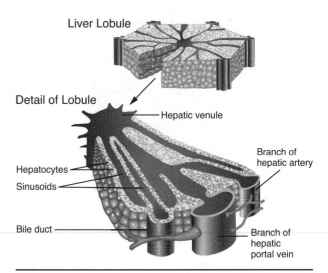

Figure 11-1 *Anatomy of a liver lobule.*

which is composed of hepatocytes, sinusoids, and Kupffer cells in a triangular arrangement around a central vein (Fig. 11-1). Liver lobules are connected together via an intricate network of arteries, veins, and a unique drainage system. In the average adult, normal hepatic blood flow is estimated to be approximately 1500 ml/min or 25 to 30% of cardiac output.

The liver produces and excretes bile into the small intestine where bile is used to emulsify fats. Bile is also stored in the gallbladder and released as needed. Another major function of the liver is the breakdown of carbohydrates, fats, and proteins. Metabolism of carbohydrates includes gluconeo-genesis (synthesis of glucose from amino acids, lactate, and glycerol), glycogenesis (formation of glycogen from glucose), glycogenolysis (break-down of glycogen to glucose), and breakdown of insulin and other hormones. Lipid metabolism includes cholesterol synthesis and lipogenesis or the production of triglycerides (fats). Other meta-bolic functions include drug metabolism via phase 1 (oxidation, reduction, and hydrolysis) and phase 2 (conjugation) reactions.

The liver synthesizes plasma proteins, such as albumin and alpha-1 antitrypsin, that help maintain

Table 11-1	Physiologic Functions Performed by the Liver
Carbohydrate metabolism	
Protein metabolism	
Lipid metabolism	
Drug metabolism	
Breaks down hemoglobin	
Produces and excretes bile	
Converts ammonia to urea	
Produces plasma proteins	
Produces factors for coagulation	

The liver's eight-segment division. Patients undergoing surgery for liver cancer will have a section(s) of their liver removed in which the tumor(s) resides. Following surgery, this section grows back.

Figure 11-2 *Anatomy of the liver and associated vasculature.*

plasma osmotic pressure. Other plasma proteins that are created in the liver include clotting factors I (fibrinogen), II (prothrombin), V, VII, IX, XI, and protein C, S, and antithrombin. The liver functions as a storage site for folate, glycogen, fat soluble vitamins (B12, A, D, E, and K), and minerals such as iron and copper. Hemoglobin from the red blood cells is broken down to bilirubin and is converted to biliverdin by the liver to facilitate excretion. Blood is also filtered for ammonia and the ammonia is subsequently converted to urea. A list of the physiologic functions associated with the liver is included in Table 11-1.

The classic description of the liver is based on the external appearance of four anatomic lobes or segments: right, left, caudate, and quadrate. Right and left lobes are separated by falciform ligament, which is positioned anteriorly. The ligamentum venosum and ligamentum teres divide right and left lobes on the posterior aspect of the liver. The transverse fissure divides the caudate and quadrate lobes. Unfortunately, this classic description does not include internal features such as vessels and biliary duct branching that are vital for hepatic surgery. Therefore, the more common functional anatomic model, Couinaud classification, is used for anatomic liver resections.

Couinaud classification for liver resection divides the liver in eight functionally independent segments with each segment having its own inflow and outflow vasculature, as illustrated in Figure 11-2. The middle hepatic vein divides the liver into the right and left lobes, or hemiliver. The left hepatic vein divides the left hemiliver into a lateral part (corresponding to segments 2, 3) and a median part (corresponding to segment 4 that can be further divided to 4a, superior, and 4b, inferior). The right hepatic vein divides the right hemiliver into an anterior section (corresponding to segments 5, 8) and a posterior section (corresponding to segments 6, 7). Table 11-2 describes the lobes in relation to the segments of the liver.

Table 11-2	Lobes in Relation to the Segments of the Liver
Lobe	**Segment**
Caudate	1
Lateral	2, 3
Medial	4a, 4b
Right	5, 6, 7, 8

PATHOPHYSIOLOGY

Hepatocellular carcinoma (HCC) is the most common primary malignancy affecting the liver. It is also known as primary liver cancer or hepatoma which is primarily caused by chronic hepatitis B or C and cirrhosis due to chronic alcohol abuse. The initial symptoms of HCC are variable with abdominal pain being the most common symptom accompanied with unexplained weight loss. In addition, patients with cirrhosis may develop jaundice, ascites, esophageal varices, and/or portal hypertension.

In those patients who have HCC without evidence of cirrhosis, liver resection is the treatment of choice. However, when cirrhosis is the cause of HCC, liver resectability is limited and may be unsuitable in those patients exhibiting a low platelet count ($< 80,000$ cells/mm^3), a decreased albumin (< 3.5 g/dl), ascites, portal hypertension with esophageal varices, and a prolonged prothrombin time (PT) due to a high risk for postoperative liver failure. Therefore, nonsurgical therapies such as percutaneous ethanol injection and radiofrequency ablation may be an option for treatment. Ultimately, liver resectability is judged by liver function, stage of liver cancer, and overall condition of the patient.

SURGICAL PROCEDURE

Hepatic resection can be performed traditionally via laparotomy or laparoscopically in which one or more complete anatomic segments are removed or a specific nonanatomic division of the liver is resected (wedge resection). The type of resection performed depends on the size, site, and number of tumors and their relation to vascular and biliary structures.

Segmental anatomic surgery involves dissecting the porta hepatis or transverse fissure with mobilization and ligation of the extrahepatic branches of the hepatic artery, portal vein, bile duct, and hepatic vein prior to resecting the liver parenchyma. Nonanatomic division of the liver, or wedge resection, involves ligating and resecting branches of the vessels and hepatic ducts as they are encountered during the resection of the liver parenchyma; only the tumor with a margin of 1 to 2 cm is removed.

ANESTHETIC MANAGEMENT CONSIDERATIONS

Preoperative Period

1. List the components of a thorough preanesthetic evaluation.

- A comprehensive preanesthetic assessment and interview
- Review of pertinent laboratory data: electrolytes, glucose, liver function tests (LFTs), prothrombin time/partial thromboplastin time/international normalized ratio, hemoglobin/hematocrit, and type and cross.
- Review chest x-ray, computed tomography (CT) scan, echocardiogram, and results of an abdominal ultrasound.
- Obtain consent for general anesthesia, central line, and arterial line placement
- Obtain intravenous (IV) access, and placement of an arterial line and a central line
- Attempt to treat/optimize the status of those patient's who have are coagulopathic by administering blood products/antifibrinolytic medication
- Be prepared to administer packed red blood cells and albumin
- A rapid fluid infusing device should be immediately available in the room
- Consider placement of an epidural catheter for intraoperative and postoperative management unless a coagulopathy is present

2. Explain the surgical interventions that are used during hepatic resection.

Three-dimensional (3D) imaging in the surgical planning for hepatic resection is gaining popularity. With the advances in computer scanning technology, a 3D visualization of the tumor is possible. A major advantage of 3D mapping is that it can help determine if a resection is feasible without invasive exploration. Another practice that provides visualization is the intraoperative ultrasound (IOUS), which allows the surgeon to determine the relationship of the tumor and major intrahepatic vessels. Some surgeons use dye injection to stain the segment of choice into the segmental portal vein to aid in the transection of the parenchyma.

Intraoperative blood loss is the most important determinant of survival in the first few days postoperatively. Blood loss can be significant during liver resection and most technologies are focused on reducing blood loss. The introduction of hemostatic stapling has revolutionized hepatic surgery, as well as thoracic and gastrointestinal surgery. During a liver resection, staplers can be used to gain vascular control or to transect parenchyma. Another transection method, ultrasonic dissection using the Cavitron Ultrasonic Surgical Aspirator (CUSA), has become popular.

The clamp crushing technique has traditionally been used for hepatic resection because of its low cost and its effectiveness in controlling blood loss. A clamp is used to "crush" and then divide the parenchyma in small sections. After ligation, the structures that are bleeding or leaking are treated with fine sutures. This makes clamp crushing and ultrasonic dissection the two most popular techniques used to transect the parenchyma in hepatic resection.

3. Describe the use of the Pringle maneuver during liver resection.
The Pringle maneuver is a commonly used technique to prevent intraoperative blood loss that involves occlusion of the main blood vessels that enter the liver. Prolonged application of this procedure can cause significant ischemia and have a detrimental effect on liver function. Most patients can tolerate a repeated 15 to 20 minute clamp time followed by a 5 minute period of reperfusion. Total vascular occlusion is another technique that can be used which involves occlusion of arterial blood flow into the liver and the venous blood flow out of the liver.

4. Identify anesthetic interventions used to treat low central venous pressure (CVP).
Managing CVP appropriately to reduce blood loss is a major goal in the anesthetic management for liver resection. This is typically achieved by fluid restriction, postural changes, vasodilators, and/or diuresis. Maintaining CVP at < 5 mm Hg generally facilitates the goal of achieving a lower blood loss than when CVP is ≥ 6 mm Hg. Intravenous nitroglycerine and furosemide are used as a means to pharmacologically manage CVP, although other vasodilators and diuretics may be employed. Reverse Trendelenburg can also help in decreasing CVP. Oliguria may occur, but the rate of postoperative renal failure does not increase when systolic blood pressure is maintained above 90 mm Hg. At the completion of the liver resection, volume resuscitation is initiated with crystalloid and albumin to normalize the hemodynamic profile and to help the surgeon to discover unrecognized areas of bleeding.

Maintaining a low CVP during anesthesia is vital during liver resection. However by decreasing venous pressure, this intervention increases the risk for developing a venous air embolism. Air embolism is a common occurrence during liver resection although it usually does not result in physiologic compromise. In the event that the patient exhibits signs of a venous air embolism, immediate interventions include:

- Ventilation with 100% oxygen
- Attempt to aspirate the air from the right atrium via the central line
- Trendelenburg and left lateral decubitus position
- Administer intravenous fluids
- Administer vasopressors to help increase the blood pressure

These measures should be utilized in conjunction with advanced cardiac life support (ACLS) resuscitation as appropriate.

5. List the advantages associated with laparoscopic liver resection.

Liver surgeries are commonly performed via an open incision but in selected circumstances a laparoscopic approach can be utilized. Laparoscopic liver resections are performed for cancers that are present on the surface of the liver where the larger blood vessels are not affected. The advantages of laparoscopic surgeries include: absence of a large abdominal incision, decreased postoperative pain, decreased length of stay, and decreased recovery time.

Intraoperative Period

6. Discuss the considerations for anesthetic induction and maintenance for patients having a liver resection.

Considerations for Induction

- Routine monitors: electrocardiogram, invasive and cuff blood pressure monitoring, CVP, temperature, FiO_2, $ETCO_2$, and pulse oximeter
- Consider pharmacologic interventions to reduce gastric volume and increase pH
- Consider performing a rapid sequence induction (RSI) with cricoid pressure
- Consider the patients individual hemodynamic status prior to choosing an induction agent

Consideration for Maintenance Although all muscle relaxants have been used, the most acceptable would be those that do not undergo hepatic or renal metabolism. For example, cisatracurium is degraded by Hoffmann elimination and plasma hydrolysis by nonspecific esterases and its pharmacologic profile is unchanged in patients with hepatic dysfunction. The anesthetist may choose to avoid using nitrous oxide due to the risk of a venous air embolism. Administration of a narcotic

such as fentanyl or sufentanil are both acceptable choices for liver resection and the medications will attenuate intraoperative sympathetic nervous system responsiveness as well as provide for postoperative analgesia.

Glucose levels should be controlled to avoid hypoglycemia and hyperglycemia. Hypothermia inhibits the coagulation cascade and contributes to intraoperative blood loss. The patient's temperature should be maintained within normal limits via a forced air warming blanket and fluid warmer. Coagulation factors should be monitored intraoperatively and platelets, fresh frozen plasma, and cryoprecipitate should be administered as needed. Antifibrinolytics such as aminocaproic acid and tranexamic acid should also be considered perioperatively for procoagulation.

Postoperative Period

7. Discuss the postoperative anesthetic management after liver resection.

The postoperative complications associated with liver resection are included in Table 11-3. Postoperative pain control for the patient that has undergone hepatic resection is challenging. Providing epidural analgesia remains controversial with liver resection mainly due to the associated coagulopathy and epidural hematoma formation. Patient controlled analgesia (PCA) is also an option to treat postoperative pain.

Table 11-3 Postoperative Complications Associated with Liver Resection
• Hemorrhage
• Respiratory complications (atelectasis, effusion, and pneumonia)
• Electrolyte abnormalities
• Hypothermia
• Hypoglycemia
• Disseminated intravascular coagulation

REVIEW QUESTIONS

1. Which intervention can be used to inhibit bleeding caused by decreased coagulation factors?
   a. Administering packed red blood cells
   b. Administering dexamethasone
   c. Administer aminocaproic acid
   d. Administer vitamin K
2. Which is not a physiologic function associated with the liver?
   a. Glycogenesis
   b. Storage of iron and copper
   c. Synthesis of alpha-1 antitrypsin
   d. Corticosteroidogenesis
3. Segments 2, 3, 4a, and 4b constitute the _____ lobe of the liver.
   a. Caudate
   b. Quadrate
   c. Right
   d. Left
4. Which intraoperative factor is associated with increased early postoperative mortality after liver resection?
   a. Severe blood loss
   b. Mean arterial pressure < 70 mm Hg
   c. Urine output less that 1 ml/kg/hr
   d. Presence of metastatic cancer
5. Which is not a postoperative event associated with hepatic resection?
   a. Pneumonia
   b. Hemorrhage
   c. Electrolyte imbalance
   d. Hyperglycemia

REVIEW ANSWERS

1. **Answer: c**
   Of the choices, aminocaproic acid is the only option to decrease acute coagulopathy.
2. **Answer: d**
   Corticosteroidogenesis is not a function that is performed by the liver.
3. **Answer: d**
   Segments 2, 3, 4a, and 4b constitute the left lobe of the liver.
4. **Answer: a**
   The factor that is most closely associated with increased early mortality after liver resection is severe blood loss.
5. **Answer: d**
   Postoperative hypoglycemia is most commonly associated with liver resection.

SUGGESTED READINGS

DeMatteo RP, Fong Y, Jarnagin WR, et al. Recent advances in hepatic resection. *Semin Surg Oncol* 2000;19: 200–207.

Hanazaki K, Kajikawa SS. Survival and recurrence after hepatic resection of 386 consecutive patients with hepatocellular carcinoma. *J Am Coll Surg* 2000;191: 381–388.

Ishizaki Y, Yoshimoto J, Sugo H, et al. Hepatectomy using traditional pean clamp-crushing technique under intermittent pringle maneuver. *Am J Surg* 2008; 196:353–357.

Jaffe RA, Samuels Sl. Hepatic resection. In: *Anesthesiologist's Manual of Surgical Procedures*, 3rd ed. Philadelphia: Lippincott Williams & Wilkins, 2004: 440–444.

Katz SC, Shia J, Liau KH, et al. Operative blood loss independently predicts recurrence and survival after resection of hepatocellular carcinoma. *Ann Surg* 2009; 249(4):617–623.

Longnecker DE. Anesthesia for liver surgery and transplantation. In: *Anesthesiology*. New York: McGraw Hill, 2008:1345.

Poon RTP. Current techniques of liver transection. *HPB* [serial online] 2007;9:166–173.

Redai I, Emond J, Berntjens T. Anethetic considerations during liver surgery. *Surg Clin N Am* 2004;84:401–411.

Saint-Marc O, Cogliandolo A, Piquard A, et al. Early experience with laparoscopic major liver resections: A case-comparison study. *Surg Laparosc Endosc Percutan Tech* 2008;18(6):551–555.

Wang W, Laiang L, Haung X, et al. Low central venous pressure reduces blood loss in hepatectomy. *World J Gastroenterol* 2006;12:935–939.

Endocrine Surgery

III

Anesthesia Case Management for Excision of a Pheochromocytoma

12

Becky Rubin and Michael Rubin

KEY POINTS

- The meaning of pheochromocytoma is dusky colored tumor (*phios* means dusky, *chroma* means color, and *cytoma* means tumor) and the neoplasm is derived from chromaffin cells.
- A pheochromocytoma is most commonly located within the adrenal medulla, but can also be localized within extraadrenal sites.
- Approximately 90% of pheochromocytomas cause a massive amount of norepinephrine to be produced and released into systemic circulation. Epinephrine can also be the predominant catecholamine that is produced.
- The most common triad of symptoms include headache, diaphoresis, and tachycardia.
- Excessive and prolonged alpha 1 receptor stimulation can result in intravascular volume depletion, renal insufficiency, hemorrhagic cerebral infarct, myocardial irritability, ischemia, and infarction. Congestive heart failure and cardiomyopathy can occur if hypertension remains untreated.
- Preoperative management includes adrenergic receptor blockade (alpha receptor blockade followed by beta receptor blockade), intravascular volume replacement, and assessment of end organ damage.
- Intraoperative surges in catecholamine release can occur at the time of laryngoscopy, intubation, and manipulation of the tumor and during ligation of the adrenal vein.
- Postoperative anesthetic concerns include treating pain and stabilizing of blood pressure. Prompt diagnosis and treatment of a pneumothorax, hypoglycemia, and hypoadrenocorticism should also be considered.

CASE SYNOPSIS

A 38-year-old woman presents to the emergency room complaining of severe headaches and palpitations several times a day. She has become increasingly anxious and diaphoretic. Her blood pressure, heart rate, and respiratory rate are elevated. Plasma tests reveal elevated metanephrine levels. An endocrinologist reviews her case and orders further diagnostic testing that includes a computed tomography (CT) scan and a 24-hour urine sample to assess for metanephrines and normetanephrines. The CT scan reveals a right adrenal mass. Medical management of a pheochromocytoma is initiated and she is scheduled for a right sided adrenalectomy in 2 weeks.

PREOPERATIVE EVALUATION AND DEMOGRAPHIC DATA

Past Medical/Surgical History

- Depression
- Cesarean section 2000; no anesthetic complications

List of Medications

- Phenelzine sulfate (Nardil) 15 mg TID

Diagnostic Data

- Hemoglobin, 16.5 g/dl; hematocrit, 49.5%
- Glucose, 170 mg/dl
- Blood urea nitrogen, 33 mg/dl; creatinine, 1.5 mg/dl
- Electrolytes: sodium, 147 mEq/l; potassium, 3.4 mEq/l; chloride, 95 mEq/l; carbon dioxide 24 mEq/l
- Electrocardiogram (ECG): sinus tachycardia, nonspecific T-wave changes, occasional premature ventricular contraction (PVC)
- Echocardiogram (ECHO): mild left ventricular hypertrophy, ejection fraction 55%

Catecholamines and Metabolites

- Urinary vanillylmandelic acid (VMA), 32 mg/24h (normal value 2–7 mg/24 h)
- Urinary metanephrine, 6.8 mg/24 h (normal value < 1.3 mg/24 h)
- Urinary norepinephrine, 458 mcg/24 h (normal value < 100 mcg/24 h)
- Plasma norepinephrine, 1109 pg/ml (normal value 150–450 pg/ml)
- Plasma epinephrine, 37 pg/ml (normal value < 35 pg/ml)

Height/Weight/Vital Signs

- 165 cm, 68 kg
- Blood pressure, 146/80; heart rate, 92 beats per minute; respiratory rate, 24 breaths per minute; room air oxygen saturation, 98%; temperature, 37.3°C

PATHOPHYSIOLOGY

A pheochromocytoma is a catecholamine secreting tumor that originates within the adrenal gland in approximately 90% of cases. These unique tumors can also arise anywhere along the paravertebral sympathetic chain and are known as extraadrenal pheochromocytomas. The tumors are comprised of chromaffin cells that can produce, store, and secrete catecholamines. The majority of extraadrenal pheochromocytomas exist within the abdominal cavity. These tumors most frequently affect a unilateral adrenal gland, and most are benign. Familial pheochromocytomas occur in bilateral adrenal glands in 50% of cases and are usually benign. Pheochromocytomas rarely occur within this population and they are associated with only 0.5% of all patients who have hypertension. This disease affects males and females equally and most frequently manifest between 30–50 years of age. There is an association between pheochromocytoma and multiple-endocrine neoplasia type II A and B, neurofibromatosis, tuberous sclerosis, Sturge-Weber syndrome, and von Hippel-Lindau disease.

Sympathetic nervous system stimulation in patients with pheochromocytoma causes a massive release of catecholamines, predominantly norepinephrine, which stimulates alpha adrenergic receptors. Subsequently, common clinical manifestations associated with a pheochromocytoma include headache, diaphoresis, tachycardia, arrythmias with palpitations, anxiety, pallor, hypertension, hyperglycemia, and paresthesias to the extremities. Orthostatic hypotension and polycythemia occur due to intravascular volume depletion resulting from extreme peripheral vasoconstriction. Cerebral hemorrhage, myocardial infarction, cardiomyopathy, congestive heart failure, and renal insufficiency can occur.

A pheochromocytoma is not directly innervated by the autonomic nervous system and, therefore, is not controlled by neural stimulation. Consequently, stimulation of the tumor resulting in catecholamine release is not completely understood and the precipitating factors are not clearly defined and vary per individual. However, events that are associated with causing tumor activation include hypotension, hypothermia, defecation, physiologic stress, medication, intubation, and surgery.

SURGICAL PROCEDURE

Adrenalectomy for removal of pheochromocytoma is traditionally accomplished by performing an open transperitoneal approach. The patient is placed in supine position and the incision is made in the subcostal or midline regions. The adrenal vein is located and ligated. The adrenal gland is then excised and removed.

Laparoscopic adrenalectomy has become a popular surgical technique for removal of a pheochromocytoma. The patient is placed in the lateral decubitus position for maximal exposure to the surgical site. The close proximity of the inferior vena cava to the adrenal veins increases the potential for rapid and uncontrolled hemorrhage. Because the patient's cardiovascular system may be compromised due to long standing untreated hypertension, the potential for cardiovascular compromise caused by prolonged insufflation should be considered. The adrenal glands are anatomically located on the superior aspect of each kidney, and there is a potential for developing a pneumothorax during the surgical dissection. The advantage of a laparoscopic approach as compared to a tradition open technique is the small incision that results in decreased postoperative pain. The adrenal glands are surrounded by a layer of fat and a thin fibrous capsule which makes the resection complicated and tedious.

ANESTHETIC MANAGEMENT AND CONSIDERATIONS

Preoperative Period

1. Describe the signs and symptoms that are associated with a pheochromocytoma.

A triad of signs and symptoms that is most commonly associated with a pheochromocytoma include headache, diaphoresis, and tachycardia. A list of physiologic signs and symptoms are included in Table 12-1. Hypertension associated with tachycardia is most common; however, the physiologic response is directly proportional to the concentration of catecholamines that are released. It is possible that the patient can develop bradycardia caused by the baroreceptor activation in response to extreme hypertension. Arrythmias, ST-segment changes, nervousness, and anxiety may also be observed.

Table 12-1 Signs and Symptoms Associated with Pheochromocytoma
Headache
Diaphoresis
Tachycardia
Chest pain
Bradycardia
Anxiety
Blurred vision
Seizures

2. Identify various methods that can be used to diagnose pheochromocytoma.

The initial diagnosis of pheochromocytoma is difficult to make because the symptoms are nonspecific, can occur in variety of disease states, vary among individuals and pheochromocytoma is a rare disease. A thorough history and physical is essential and vital in order to correctly diagnose a pheochromocytoma. Further diagnostic tests include plasma free metanephrines, urine catecholamine and metanephrine levels, and a clonidine suppression test.

- **24-hour urine test:** Three urine samples are collected within a 24-hour period and the concentration of metanephrines are analyzed. It is estimated that 95% of patients with pheochromocytomas have increased levels of urinary metanephrines. If urine metanephrine levels are elevated, then three 24-hour urine samples are tested for free catecholamines. If all three samples are within normal limits, the patient is not considered to have a pheochromocytoma.

- **Plasma test:** Elevations in the concentration of norepinephrine in plasma may be indicative of a pheochromocytoma. The plasma test is extremely sensitive to factors such as exercise, stress, and medications—all which may increase catecholamines within the blood.

- **Clonidine suppression test:** Clonidine 0.2 mg is administered by mouth and, within 3 hours, the patient's blood pressure should decrease. Clonidine causes centrally mediated alpha 2 agonism, which decreases catecholamine output from the brain. A patient with a pheochromocytoma will remain hypertensive despite the actions of clonidine because the catecholamine release from the tumor is not centrally controlled.

- **Imaging studies:** A CT scan, positron emission tomography (PET) scan, or magnetic resonance imaging (MRI) is obtained to identify the presence of a tumor and the tumor's size and location.

- **Metaiodobenzylguanidine (MIBG) scintigraphy:** This chemical possesses a high affinity for secretory granules present in chromaffin cells. The chemical structure of MIBG is similar to norepinephrine and, when injected, it concentrates within these granules as a result of reuptake. The sensitivity and specificity of this test for confirming the presence of a pheochromocytoma is 85% and 97%, respectively.

3. Discuss the preoperative pharmacologic preparation for a patient with a pheochromocytoma.

Preoperative pharmacologic management of these patients includes alpha receptor blockade, beta receptor blockade, and volume expansion. Alpha receptor blockade is always instituted prior to beta receptor blockade and is usually accomplished by the administration of phenoxybenzamine, a noncompetitive alpha 1 receptor and alpha 2 receptor antagonist. The patient will take phenoxybenzamine 50 to 400 mg/day for 10 to 14 days preoperatively. Once adequate alpha receptor blockade is established, beta receptor blockade can begin. Initiation of beta receptor blockade prior to alpha receptor blockade can cause a hypertensive crisis and can lead to the development of congestive heart failure. The tachycardia that is either caused by excessive beta receptor activity or vasodilation caused by phenoxybenzamine is managed with beta receptor blockade, most often propranolol. In order to judge the adequacy of volume resuscitation, a decrease of 5% from the baseline hematocrit level is indicative of adequate hydration. Note that this patient is polycythemic prior to adrenergic receptor blockade and fluid resuscitation. Another method that can be used to assess the adequacy of fluid management is to determine if the patient develops orthostatic associated with a decline in the systolic blood pressure greater than or equal to 15%, while maintaining a systolic pressure of at least 80 mm Hg.

Another medication that can be administered preoperatively is metyrosine. This medication has an inhibitory effect on the creation

Figure 12-1 *Biosynthesis of catecholamines.*

of catecholamines, which occurs in adrenergic nerves. This drug decreases the concentration of tyrosine hydroxylase, an enzyme that is necessary during the biosynthesis of catecholamines and this process is shown in Figure 12-1.

This patient has been taking phenelzine sulfate, a nonspecific monoamine oxidase inhibitor. Monoamine oxidase is present within the synaptic cleft of adrenergic nerves and its function is to enzymatically degrade catecholamines. As a result, inhibition of monoamine oxidase increases the concentration of catecholamines within the synaptic junction in adrenergic nerves. Taking phenelzine sulfate in a patient with a pheochromocytoma can result in an uncontrolled hypertensive response. She will have to discontinue taking this medicine 1 to 2 weeks prior to surgery.

4. Explain the optimal preoperative cardiovascular criteria that should be achieved prior to surgery.

The goal of preoperative therapy for a patient with a pheochromocytoma includes control of excessive catecholamine release that causes extreme physiologic aberrations. The following criteria

must be met prior to surgical intervention and anesthesia administration.

- Blood pressure must remain less than 160/90 mm Hg within 48 hours prior to surgery.
- Orthostatic hypotension must occur however the blood pressure must be greater than 80/45 mm Hg.
- The ECG must not have of ST/T wave abnormalities for at least 1 week and have no more than one PVC within 5 minutes.
- Adequate hydration is achieved by a decrease in the hematocrit by approximately 5% from the baseline value.

5. Identify the factors that increase the morbidity and mortality associated with removal of a pheochromocytoma.

Factors that increase the potential for morbidity and mortality include:

- The activity of the pheochromocytoma. A highly active tumor is associated with increased concentrations of catecholamines and a more dramatic physiologic response.

- Inadequate preoperative alpha receptor and then beta receptor blockade.
- Advanced end organ damage.
- Whether the pheochromocytoma is malignant or benign. The 5-year survival rate for a patient with a benign tumor is approximately 90%. However, if the pheochromocytoma is malignant, the survival rate dramatically decreases to 10% due to metastasis resulting from the high amount of blood flow that courses through the adrenal glands.
- The duration of surgery.

Intraoperative Period

6. List the medications that should be avoided during intraoperative management.
Administration of any medications that can cause an increased blood pressure or heart rate or causes the release of histamine should be avoided. Alternative drugs that stimulate the release or inhibit the breakdown of catecholamines should be used. A complete list of anesthetic medications that should be avoided for these patients is included in Table 12-2.

Table 12-2 Anesthetic Medications that Should be Avoided in Patients with a Pheochromocytoma
• Desflurane
• Pancuronium
• Atracurium
• Succinylcholine
• Morphine
• Droperidol
• Metoclopramide
• Phenothiazines
• Ephedrine
• Ketamine
• Atropine
• Naloxone hydrochloride

7. Discuss the anesthetic considerations for a patient with a pheochromocytoma.
General anesthesia and endotracheal intubation is necessary and an epidural placed preoperatively can be used to provide anesthesia during the surgery and analgesia during the postoperative period. The concern when dosing an epidural catheter with local anesthetic medications during the intraoperative period is that after the pheochromocytoma is isolated, the concentration of catecholamines dramatically decreases and hypotension commonly occurs. This fact, along with adrenergic receptor downregulation and alpha receptor blockade, predisposes to severe hypotension. Preganglionic sympathetic B fiber blockade that results in vasodilation from neuraxial anesthesia will augment this effect.

Since rapidly developing hemorrhage is a major concern, two large bore peripheral intravenous lines are indicated. Aside from the American Society of Anesthesiologist basic monitoring modalities, arterial line placement is required for blood pressure monitoring. A central line is indicated to monitor central venous pressure to assess the patient's volume status. The use of a Swan-Ganz catheter should be individually determined and based on the degree of cardiac pathology.

Anesthetic management for a patient with pheochromocytoma begins with preoperative sedation to decrease anxiety and sympathetic nervous system (SNS) activity. An adequate anesthetic depth should be achieved prior to direct laryngoscopy to avoid an exaggerated SNS response. Nitrous oxide should be avoided due to the potential for bowel distention and concerns regarding the development of a pneumothorax. The administration of succinylcholine for muscle paralysis is controversial because the resulting fasciculations cause abdominal rigidity and can increase the release of catecholamines from the pheochromocytoma. The anesthetist should expect blood pressure lability throughout the entire perioperative course.

Hypertension most commonly occurs during intubation, incision, manipulation of tumor, and ligation of the venous drainage of the affected adrenal gland. Hypertension is most effectively managed by:

- Increasing the concentration of inhalation anesthetic agent
- Administering narcotics
- Infusing sodium nitroprusside as an intravenous drip

Hypotension is most common after removal of tumor. Hypotension is most effectively treated by:

- Decreasing the anesthetic depth
- Administering crystalloids, colloids, or packed red blood cells
- Administering a direct acting vasopressor such as phenylephrine

The patient's blood glucose should be assessed preoperatively and incrementally throughout the surgical procedure. Hyperglycemia commonly occurs prior to the tumor removal due to the inhibition of endogenous insulin release due to SNS predominance and glycogenolysis by the liver. Conversely, hypoglycemia can develop rapidly during the postoperative period. If tachycardia occurs and beta receptor blockade is necessary, the advantage for administering esmolol is that the metabolism is extremely rapid and persistent blockade is not a concern.

8. Describe the intraoperative course for a patient having a laparoscopic adrenalectomy for a pheochromocytoma by assessing the hemodynamic variables provided in Figure 12-2.

1. Despite alpha and beta adrenergic blockade, note the degree of hypertension and heart rate variability that occurs during the periods of induction, endotracheal intubation, and placement of an epidural catheter.

2. At 10:00 there is abrupt increase in the blood pressure most probably due to surgical manipulation of the pheochromocytoma. An infusion of nitroprusside is started and titrated to the degree of hypertension that occurs. Notice that the heart rate abruptly decreases to less that 50 beats per minute during the extreme hypertensive response, which was most likely caused by the baroreceptor response or by the administration of labetalol.

3. At approximately 11:00 the venous drainage from the adrenal gland is ligated. High concentrations of catecholamines are present in the venous system, which are forced into systemic circulation prior to ligation. Notice the rapid speed of which the blood pressure decreases as the catecholamines are metabolized. The hypotension is also caused by the administration of anesthesia and the preoperative adrenergic blockade. The blood pressure is supported by decreasing the anesthetic depth and by administering fluids as is reflected by an increase in the central venous pressure.

4. At 11:45 the inhalation anesthetic concentration is decreased and local anesthetic is given in incremental boluses through the epidural catheter.

Postoperative Period

9. Identify potential complications following an adrenalectomy for a pheochromocytoma.

- Hypertension may result from residual pheochromocytoma, pain, hypoglycemia, hypervolemia, and hypoxia
- Hypotension can result from residual alpha adrenergic receptor blockade, hypovolemia, myocardial ischemia or infarction, bleeding, or sepsis.
- Pneumothorax
- Hemorrhage
- Sepsis
- Hypoglycemia
- Hypoadrenocorticism

Figure 12-2 *Intraoperative hemodynamic profile during excision of a pheochromocytoma.*

REVIEW QUESTIONS

1. The classic triad of symptoms associated with pheochromocytoma include:
   a. elevated systolic pressure/swelling/anxiety.
   b. headache/diaphoresis/tachycardia.
   c. elevated diastolic pressure/diaphoresis/tachycardia.
   d. mood swings/increased pulse pressure/arrhythmias.

2. The majority of extraadrenal pheochromocytomas are located in which region of the body?
   a. Thorax
   b. Cranium
   c. Mediastinum
   d. Abdomen

3. Which is true regarding pheochromocytoma excretion of endogenous catecholamines?
   a. Norepinephrine > epinephrine
   b. Norepinephrine < epinephrine
   c. Dopamine > norepinephrine
   d. Epinephrine < dopamine

4. Which of the preoperative vital signs are reflective of adequate for surgery and anesthetic management for a patient scheduled for adrenalectomy for pheochromocytoma?
   a. Heart rate 101, blood pressure 138/66, hematocrit 27
   b. Heart rate 83, blood pressure 149/82, hematocrit 36

c. Heart rate 96, blood pressure 165/66, hematocrit 48

d. Heart rate 62, blood pressure 138/112, hematocrit 51

5. Which sign, symptom, or diagnostic test is most sensitive to diagnose a pheochromocytoma?

   a. T-wave changes on a 12-lead ECG

   b. Idiopathic hypertension

   c. Elevated urinary metanephrine levels on a 24-hour urine collection

   d. Chronic headache

REVIEW ANSWERS

1. **Answer: b**
   All of the following symptoms can occur. However, the classic triad includes headache, diaphoresis, and tachycardia in the presence of hypertension.

2. **Answer: d**
   A pheochromocytoma originates in the adrenal gland 90% of the time. The adrenal gland is located in the abdominal cavity. This tumor can also arise anywhere along the paravertebral sympathetic chain (extraadrenal pheochromocytoma).

3. **Answer: a**
   Catecholamine synthesis occurs within the adrenal medulla. Under normal circumstances, the adrenal medulla secretes 80% epinephrine and 20% norepinephrine. However, pheochromocytomas that are comprised of chromaffin cells secrete norepinephrine at a ratio of 9:1, as compared to epinephrine.

4. **Answer: b**
   The vital signs in choice b are within normal parameters. Proper alpha blockade followed by beta blockade must be accomplished. Hemodilution occurs after vasodilation and intravenous volume loading is established. The blood pressure should be less than 160/90 within 48 hours prior to surgery.

5. **Answer: c**
   Diagnostic tools used to diagnose the presence of a pheochromocytoma include diagnostic imaging, MIBG scanning, 24-hour urine test, plasma test, and a clonidine suppression test. Urine tests include an elevation of metanephrines on three tests in a 24-hour period. Plasma test include elevations in norepinephrine levels.

SUGGESTED READINGS

Adler JT, Meyer-Rochow GY, Chen H, et al. Pheochromocytoma: current approaches and future directions. *Oncologist* 2008;13(7):779–793.

Greco R, Koransky M, Mihm F. Endocrine surgery. In: Jaffe RA, Samuels SI, eds. *Anesthesiologist's Manual of Surgical Procedures*, 4th ed. Philadelphia: Lippincott Williams & Wilkins, 2009:585–587, 675–677.

Higashi, YS. Excess norepinephrine impairs both endothelium dependent and independent vasodilation in patients with pheochromocytoma. *Hypertension* 2002;39(2):513–518.

Humphrey R. Laparoscopic compared with open adrenalectomy for resection of pheochromocytoma: a review of 47 cases. *J Can Chir* 2008;51(4):8–11.

Karlet MC. The endocrine system. In: Nagelhout JJ, Zaglanicy KL, eds. *Nurse Anesthesia*, 3rd ed. St. Louis, MO: Elsevier Saunders, 2005:768–772.

Lodin M. Laparoscopic adrenalectomy: keys to success: correct surgical indications, adequate preoperative preparation, surgical team experience. *Surg Laparosc Endosc Percutan Tech* 2007;17(5): 392–395.

Pacak, K. Preoperative management of the pheochromocytoma patient. *J Clin Endocrinol Metab* 2007;92(11):4069–4079.

Prys-Roberts C. Phaeochromocytoma-Recent progress in management. *Br J Anesth* 2000;85:44–57.

Sesay M. Real time heart rate variability and its correlation with plasma catecholamines during laparoscopic adrenal pheochromocytoma surgery. *Anesth Analg* 2008;106(1):164–170.

Tarant N. Acute Appendicitis in a patient with undiagnosed pheochromocytoma. *Anesth Analg* 2006;102(2): 642–643.

Thyroidectomy

13

Joan Cornachio

KEY POINTS

- Indications for thyroidectomy include increased thyroid function (hyperthyroidism), cancer is present or suspected, decreased thyroid function (hypothyroidism) with a goiter that causes respiratory difficulty, and enlargement of the thyroid gland (idiopathic hypertrophy without increased thyroid hormone synthesis and release).
- Ideally, patients should be rendered euthyroid prior to surgery.
- The systemic effects of hyperthyroidism are manifested as exaggerated sympathetic nervous system responses. Perioperative care should focus on avoiding stimulation of the sympathetic nervous system.
- Hemodynamic stability is essential and should be maintained by providing adequate fluid resuscitation, preoperative administration of antithyroid medications, and avoidance of excessive sympathetic stimulation.
- Thyroid storm is a potentially fatal complication that can occur during the intraoperative and postoperative period.

CASE SYNOPSIS

A 31-year-old African American woman with a history of Graves' disease and toxic multinodular goiter is scheduled by her surgeon to have a total thyroidectomy.

PREOPERATIVE EVALUATION AND DEMOGRAPHIC DATA

Past Medical/Surgical History

- Hyperthyroidism
- No past surgical history

List of Medications

- Propranolol prescribed 10 days preoperatively
- Propylthiouracil prescribed 6 weeks preoperatively
- Sodium iodide prescribed 10 days preoperatively

Diagnostic Data

- Hemoglobin, 13.1 g/dL; hematocrit, 38.2%; white blood cell count, 4,100/mm³; platelet count, 155,000/mm³
- Thyroid studies: total T_4, 11.6 mcg/dl (normal value 5.0–12.0 mcg/dl); free T_3, 176 ng/dl (normal value 70–195 ng/dl); thyroid stimulating hormone, 0.6 mU/L (normal value 0.4–5.0 mU/L)
- Glucose, 125 g/dl
- Electrocardiogram (ECG): sinus tachycardia, heart rate, 86 beats per minute
- Airway evaluation: Mallampati 2, thyromental distance 7 cm, full range of motion of cervical spine and temporomandibular joint. A 3-cm palpable nodule present on the left side of the neck approximating the cricoid cartilage. She denies changes in the quality of her voice or difficulty in breathing while lying flat.

Height/Weight/Vital Signs

- 173 cm, 68 kg
- Blood pressure, 136/82; heart rate, 84 beats per minute; respiratory rate, 14 breaths per minute; room air oxygen saturation, 100%; temperature, 37.2°C

ANATOMY AND PHYSIOLOGY OF THYROID GLAND

The thyroid gland consists of two lobes connected by an isthmus. It is bound to the anterior and lateral aspects of the trachea by the superior border of the isthmus located just below the cricoid cartilage. Two pairs of parathyroid glands which regulate plasma calcium levels are located on the posterior aspect of each lobe, one pair that is superior and one pair that is inferior on each lobe. The posterior aspects of the thyroid gland run alongside the carotid sheath and the esophagus.

The recurrent laryngeal nerve (RLN) and the external superior laryngeal nerve (SLN) are branches of the vagus nerve that innervate the intrinsic muscles of the larynx that serve a variety of functions including adducting and abducting the vocal cords. These nerves exist in proximity to the thyroid gland and they can be damaged during resection of the thyroid gland.

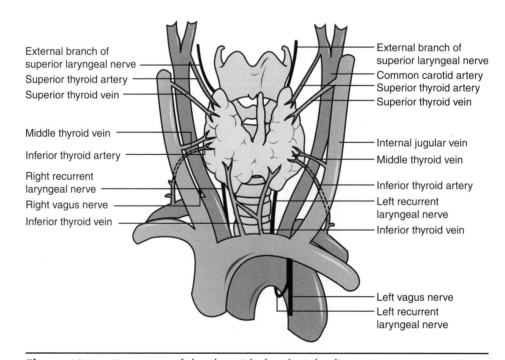

Figure 13-1 *Anatomy of the thyroid gland and adjacent structures.*

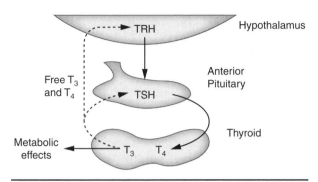

Figure 13-2 *Physiologic control of thyroid hormone secretion.*

Arterial blood is supplied by the superior and inferior thyroid arteries. A venous plexus is formed by the superior, middle, and inferior thyroid veins. In addition, the thyroid gland lies adjacent to the common carotid artery and the anterior jugular vein, which are potential sources of rapid and massive blood loss. Figure 13-1 illustrates the anatomic complexity associated with the thyroid gland and its adjacent structures.

The hypothalamus secretes thyrotropin releasing hormone (TRH) that circulates within the hypophyseal portal system and stimulates the anterior pituitary gland to create thyroid stimulating hormone (TSH). The biosynthesis of thyroid hormone created by the thyroid gland is solely controlled by TSH. The thyroid functions to produce and secrete thyroid hormones T_3 (triiodothyronine) and T_4 (tetraiodothyronine [thyroxine]) in a ratio of 1:10, respectively. When the concentration thyroid hormone is sufficient, T_3 and T_4 have an inhibitory effect on the hypothalamus and anterior pituitary gland creating a negative feedback loop. This process is illustrated in Figure 13-2.

Although T_3 is found in smaller concentrations as compared to T_4, it is approximately four times more potent. Triiodothyronine is found in significantly greater concentration in peripheral tissues as compared to T_4 (90% versus 10%). Table 13-1 compares the physiologic effects of thyroid hormones. In addition to T_3 and T_4, the thyroid gland also produces calcitonin from parafollicular C cells, which in addition to the parathyroid glands also helps to regulate serum calcium levels.

Thyroid hormones regulate the metabolic rate of numerous physiologic processes including tissue growth, oxygen consumption, and the rate at which tissues utilize energy for catabolic processes. The symptomatology associated with thyroid dysfunction is directly related to the increase or decrease in metabolic rate that occurs with hyperthyroid or hypothyroid disease states, respectively. The symptomatology associated with these disease states is presented in Table 13-2.

PATHOPHYSIOLOGY

Hyperthyroidism is a pathologic state in which the thyroid gland secretes an excessive amount of T_3 and T_4 resulting in hypermetabolism. Most cases are a result of Graves disease, toxic multinodular goiter, or toxic adenoma. Common signs and symptoms

Table 13-1 Comparison of the Physiologic Effects of T_3 and T_4		
NAME	**TRIIODOTHYRONINE (T_3)**	**TETRAIODOTHYRONINE (T_4) THYROXINE**
Amount in circulation	5–10%	90–95%
Degree of protein binding	99.80%	99.98%
Potency	4 times greater that T_4	
Onset	6–12 hours	2–3 days
Half life	1–2 days	6–7 days
Activity	80%	20%

Table 13-2   Comparison of Signs and Symptoms of Hyperthyroidism and Hypothyroidism

HYPERTHYROIDISM	HYPOTHYROIDISM
• Heat intolerance	• Cold intolerance
• Weight loss	• Weight gain
• Anorexia	• Depression
• Frequent bowel movements	• Constipation
• Muscle weakness/ fatigue	• Fatigue
• Tremors	• Mood swings
• Tachydysrhythmia (atrial fibrillation)	• Pericardial effusion

that are associated with hyperthyroidism are consistent to hypermetabolism and include:

- weight loss
- exophthalmos
- heat intolerance
- tachycardia
- muscle weakness
- hyperglycemia
- increased deep tendon reflexes
- fatigue

The cardiac manifestations associated with hyperthyroidism include tachycardia, dysrhythmias (atrial fibrillation is most common), and increased cardiac output caused by adrenergic hyperactivity. Ideally, surgical intervention should be postponed until the patient has taken antithyroid medications and is euthyroid, but, if this is not possible, the patient will often receive beta-adrenergic antagonists to maintain hemodynamic stability.

Patients with low levels of T_3 and T_4 are considered to be hypothyroid, which can be caused by an autoimmune disease such as Hashimoto thyroiditis, radioactive iodine, antithyroid medications, or iodine deficiency, among others. The clinical presentation associated with hypothyroidism reflects a decrease in metabolic rate and include:

- weight gain
- lethargy

- decreased deep tendon reflexes
- coronary artery disease
- hypoglycemia
- peripheral vascular disease
- cold intolerance
- constipation
- depression

Decreased cardiac output is caused by a decrease in both heart rate and stroke volume. Although patients who develop hyperthyroidism are at increased risk for perioperative complications, mild hypothyroidism is not considered a contraindication to surgery. Because there is a range of severity associated with thyroid disease, patients with severe hypothyroidism (myxedema coma) may have an increased risk for perioperative complications associated with the physiologic stress of surgery and anesthesia.

SURGICAL PROCEDURE

Removal of the thyroid gland is performed via a transverse neck incision through the platysma and strap muscles, exposing the thyroid gland and its blood supply. Once hemostasis is achieved, resection can begin. Depending of the pathologic condition, a subtotal thyroidectomy or lobectomy (one lobe of the thyroid gland is removed) can be accomplished. The amount of thyroid gland tissue that is removed depends on the severity of thyroid disease, and the intraoperative findings. The muscle and fascia layers are sutured closed using dissolvable material and the wound edges are approximated and then sutured or stapled.

ANESTHETIC MANAGEMENT AND CONSIDERATIONS

Preoperative Period

1. Discuss the key findings that should be evaluated preoperatively in a patient presenting for thyroidectomy.

All elective cases should be postponed until antithyroid medications can allow the patient to achieve a euthyroid state. Serum thyroid levels

Table 13-3	Normal Lab Values for Thyroid Function Tests
TSH	0.4–5.0 mU/l
Total T$_4$	5.0–12.0 mcg/dl
Free T$_4$ (F T$_4$)	0.9–2.4 ng/dl
Free T$_3$ (F T$_3$)	70–195 ng/dl
Free thyroxine index (F T$_4$ index)	1.2–4.9 ng/dl
T$_3$ resin uptake (R T$_3$U)	24–39%

should be within normal limits as these values are shown in Table 13-3. The patient should be evaluated for signs and symptoms such as tachycardia, fever, dysrhythmias, or agitation. Airway assessment and management may be complicated in patients having a thyroidectomy. The anesthetist must be aware that a potentially difficult intubation may occur in a patient with an enlarged thyroid gland. A nodule or goiter may displace the larynx and distort the normal airway anatomy, thus obscuring the view during laryngoscopy. Additionally, one should note the quality of the patient's voice and if changes have occurred, as hoarseness may indicate recurrent laryngeal nerve palsy caused by compression from the enlarged thyroid gland.

2. Describe the mechanism of action and indications for medications used to achieve a euthyroid state for patients who are hyperthyroid.

- **Thioamides**: Propylthiouracil (PTU) and methimazole (Tapazole) are thioamide medications that decrease the formation of thyroid hormone by inhibiting thyroid peroxidase, which catalyzes the conversion of iodide to iodine in the thyroid follicle cell. Additionally, these medications inhibit the organification process by decreasing the iodination of iodine onto tyrosine decreasing diiodotyrosine and monoiodotyrosine. Methimazole is 10 times more potent as compared to PTU. The patient will be prescribed one of these medications.

- **Iodides**: Sodium iodide or potassium iodide inhibits the organification process, the production and release of thyroid hormone, and the size and vascularity or the thyroid gland if hyperplasia exists. Because 60% of T$_3$ and T$_4$ is composed of iodine, it would seem counterintuitive to administer iodide. However, the Wolff-Chaikoff effect is an autoregulatory process that inhibits thyroid activity for several days to weeks if excessive quantities of iodide are present.

- **Radioactive iodine**: The isotope I[131] is administered orally, collects within the follicle, and emits radiation that destroys the thyroid cells. Patients can achieve a euthyroid state within several weeks after treatment.

- **Beta adrenergic blockade**: Beta-blocking medications that do not possess intrinsic sympathomimetic activity inhibit the peripheral conversion of T$_4$ to T$_3$ and decreases the cardiac manifestations consistent with enhanced sympathetic nervous system activity.

- **Corticosteroids**: Steroids have an inhibitory effect on TSH. These medications can be used in conjunction with others to achieve a euthyroid state.

3. Identify anesthetic induction agents that can be administered for patient having a thyroidectomy.

Thiopental, propofol, and if indicated etomidate are acceptable medications to use for induction. It has been determined that thiopental possesses antithyroid activity; however, the degree of inhibition is dependent on the dose given. In order for thiopental to affect thyroid function in this way it has been postulated that very large doses, those greater than that given to a human, would need to be administered. The choice of the specific drug and dose to be administered should be based on the individual patient's status. Ketamine is not a reasonable choice for an induction agent due to the potential sympathetic stimulation.

Intraoperative Period

4. Describe patient positioning for thyroidectomy and associated anesthetic considerations.

Patients are placed supine with the head elevated 30 degrees and the neck extended. The eyes should be carefully taped, especially for patient's who have developed exopthalmos, in order to avoid corneal abrasions. The anesthetist should be aware that there is a possibility of endotracheal tube migration during neck extension and flexion. The surgeon may request a shoulder roll and extend the patient's head to achieve the ideal position for maximal surgical exposure. It is important to support the occiput in order to avoid postoperative neck discomfort or brachial plexus injury.

5. Discuss the effect of hyperthyroidism on the maintenance of adequate anesthetic depth.

Maintenance of anesthesia should focus on attenuating sympathetic nervous system stimulation. This can be achieved by obtaining adequate depth of anesthesia to prevent an exaggerated response to surgical stimulation and avoidance of drugs that excite the sympathetic nervous system. Isoflurane, sevoflurane, and desflurane are all acceptable choices for inhalational anesthetic and may be used in combination with nitrous oxide. Some anesthetists avoid the use of desflurane because of the potential for sympathetic nervous system activation.

Although hyperthyroidism increases metabolic requirements, clinical evidence does not support an increase in minimum alveolar concentration (MAC) requirements for these patients. MAC requirements may be increased in the presence of hyperthermia; on average, a 4–5% increase in MAC occurs with every degree that the temperature increases above 37°C. For this reason, continuous temperature monitoring is essential.

6. Identify measures that can be taken to maintain hemodynamic stability.

Hemodynamic stability should be closely monitored and appropriately managed to maintain stability and prevent onset of a thyrotoxic crisis. The ECG may reveal atrial fibrillation, a common tachydysrhythmia seen with hyperthyroidism. The onset of tachycardia that is unresponsive to fluid replacement may indicate the need for additional beta adrenergic receptor blockade. Hypotension that is unresponsive to fluid resuscitation is best treated with a direct acting vasoconstrictor such as phenylephrine. Ephedrine, an indirect agonist for catecholamine release, is best avoided because patients with hyperthyroidism may have an exaggerated sympathetic nervous system response to catecholamines.

7. Explain the rationale for the use of a nerve integrity monitoring (NIM) endotracheal tube during a thyroidectomy.

The NIM endotracheal tube uses electromyelographic (EMG) information to determine the real time integrity of the right and left RLNs. The electrodes that are present on the proximal end of the tube are inserted into a monitor that interprets the signals and allows the surgeon to determine if RLN function remains intact throughout surgery. Neuromuscular blockade and laryngeal tracheal lidocaine have an inhibitory effect on EMG and their use is contraindicated if this endotracheal tube is used. If the patient must remain intubated for a prolonged period, the NIM endotracheal tube should be replaced with a standard endotracheal tube because of the potential for kinking and rupturing. Presently, there is no conclusive objective evidence to show that the use of the NIM endotracheal tube decreases RLN injury during thyroidectomy.

8. Discuss the signs, symptoms, differential diagnosis, and treatment of thyroid storm.

Early detection and prevention of thyrotoxic crisis (i.e., thyroid storm) is essential and resuscitative measures should be instituted as soon as possible to prevent circulatory collapse or decompensation of one or more organ systems.

Patients who develop thyroid storm are hypermetabolic due to an abrupt increase of circulating thyroid hormone. In most cases, diagnosis of thyroid storm is based on clinical findings alone, as onset is abrupt and treatment precludes diagnosis with laboratory tests or other screening measures. The signs and symptoms that are most often associated with thyroid storm include hyperthermia, tachycardia and tachydysrhythmia, central nervous system symptoms such as psychosis or altered mental state, and can also include rhabdomyolysis. Although thyrotoxic crisis can occur intraoperatively, the onset more frequently occurs 6 to 18 hours postoperatively. Precipitating factors include infection, surgery, diabetic ketoacidosis, congestive heart failure, pregnancy, and extreme physiologic stress. Without treatment, thyroid storm can be fatal and mortality ranges from 10 to 75%.

Thyroid storm can be mistaken for hypermetabolic states caused by different pathologic processes such as malignant hyperthermia or hypertensive crisis resulting from a pheochromocytoma. A comparison of the signs and symptoms associated with various hypermetabolic states is included in Table 13-4. Thyroid storm is most commonly occurs in patients who are not euthyroid preoperatively, and is most strongly linked to patients with Graves disease.

Treatment of thyroid storm involves pharmacologic treatment to decrease circulating thyroid hormone, as well as providing supportive interventions which include:

- Increasing the fraction of inspired oxygen concentration because the increased metabolic rate will lead to increased O_2 consumption.
- Fluid resuscitation with cooled intravenous (IV) fluids in the presence of hyperthermia
- Serial electrolyte and arterial blood gas analysis
- Propylthiouracil or methimazole can be administered to further inhibit the synthesis of thyroid hormone. Most authorities recommend the use of methimazole for thyroid storm because it acts more rapidly and is associated with fewer side effects than propylthiouracil.
- Sodium iodide is given to block release of hormone from the thyroid gland.
- Acetaminophen is the antipyretic of choice, as aspirin can displace thyroid hormone from proteins thereby increasing circulating free hormone.
- Beta-adrenergic antagonists should be administered to control the cardiovascular effects associated with sympathetic nervous system predominance. Propranolol or a continuous infusion of esmolol can be administered.
- Steroid administration such as dexamethasone or hydrocortisone may also be considered.
- Other treatment options include attempts to increase the clearance of circulating thyroid

Table 13-4 Differentiation Between Thyroid Storm, Malignant Hyperthermia, and Pheochromocytoma

THYROID STORM	MALIGNANT HYPERTHERMIA	PHEOCHROMOCYTOMA
Hyperthermia	Hyperthermia	Paroxysmal hypertension
Tachycardia and tachydysrhythmia	Tachycardia	Tachycardia
Hypertension	Hypertension	Headaches
Altered mental status	Hypercarbia	
	Elevated ETCO$_2$	
	Masseter spasm	

hormone, whether by hemodialysis, plasmapheresis, or administration of cholestyramine, to clear hormone via the gastrointestinal tract.

Postoperative Period

9. Identify postoperative complications associated with thyroidectomy and discuss prevention and/or treatment.

- **Recurrent laryngeal nerve damage** can be either unilateral or bilateral. Unilateral damage will manifest as hoarseness, whereas bilateral nerve palsy may result in aphonia, stridor, or respiratory distress. The incidence of permanent vocal cord paralysis is rare (0.5–2.4%, with incidence of temporary paralysis being 2.6–5.9%) and can be avoided by surgically identifying the location of the recurrent laryngeal nerve intraoperatively prior to resection of the thyroid gland. Vocal cord function can be assessed either via direct laryngoscopy following deep extubation or by having the patient phonate 'e' postoperatively. Recurrent laryngeal nerve dysfunction, whether unilateral or bilateral, may require reintubation and reexploration of the surgical site for possible nerve compression.

- **Hematoma formation** can cause further compression or collapse of the airway secondary to tracheomalacia (a weakening of the walls of the trachea). The incidence is rare (approximately 1%), and typically occurs within 6–24 hours postoperatively. Inadequate surgical hemostasis, coagulopathy, acute hypertension, and straining from postoperative nausea and vomiting can increase the potential for postoperative bleeding. The definitive treatment involves immediate evacuation of the hematoma and reexploration of the surgical site.

- **A pneumothorax** is a rare complication associated with a thyroidectomy. Because the apices of the lungs extend above the level of the clavicles very close to the surgical site, there is the potential for air to enter the thoracic cavity.

- **Acute hypocalcemia** resulting from inadvertent removal of the parathyroid glands. The incidence of postoperative hypocalcemia ranges from 10–50% and, for this reason, the anesthetist may be asked to obtain serum calcium levels intraoperatively or immediately postoperatively to help predict the potential for hypoparathyroidism. Hypocalcemia is most likely to occur 24 to 48 hours after surgery is complete. Parathyroid dysfunction is typically transient, and normal function may return in 4 weeks postoperatively. Inadvertent parathyroid resection will result in permanent dysfunction and both situations are treated with oral calcium and vitamin.

- **Thyroid storm**, as discussed previously.

REVIEW QUESTIONS

1. Which is the preoperative goal of pharmacologic prophylaxis for patients with hyperthyroidism?
   a. To maintain a hyperthyroid state via administration of exogenous thyroid hormone
   b. To blunt the sympathetic nervous system by obtaining an adequate depth of anesthetic and avoiding drugs that cause sympathetic stimulation
   c. To stimulate the sympathetic nervous system via administration of cardiac stimulants
   d. To observe complete muscle paralysis via administration of a nondepolarizing neuromuscular blocker

2. Which sign is not commonly observed during thyroid storm?
   a. Hypertension
   b. Hyperthermia
   c. Tachycardia
   d. Hypercarbia

3. Which best describes the physiologic sequence that leads to the biosynthesis of thyroid hormone?
   a. Thyroid stimulating hormone stimulates the thyroid gland to produce T_3 and T_4

b. Thyrotropin releasing hormone stimulates the thyroid gland to produce thyroid hormone

c. T_3 and T_4 directly stimulate the thyroid gland to produce thyroid hormone

d. T_3 and T_4 directly stimulate the hypothalamus to produce thyroid stimulating hormone

4. Which best describes the relationship between the minimum alveolar concentration (MAC) of an inhalational, hyperthyroidism and a temperature of 38.1°C?

a. Increased MAC of inhalational agents

b. Decreased MAC of inhalational agents

c. MAC of inhalational agents remains unaffected

d. Increased MAC can precipitate hyperthyroidism

5. Due to its close proximity to the thyroid gland, accidental removal of the parathyroid gland may result in:

a. hypokalemia.

b. hypomagnesemia.

c. hypermagnesemia.

d. hypocalcemia.

REVIEW ANSWERS

1. **Answer: b**

   The goal of anesthetic maintenance is to attenuate the sympathetic nervous system by maintaining an adequate depth of anesthesia and avoiding drugs that cause sympathetic stimulation.

2. **Answer: d**

   Hypercarbia is not commonly associated with hyperthyroidism.

3. **Answer: a**

   Thyrotropin releasing hormone (TRH) is secreted by the hypothalamus, which stimulates the anterior pituitary gland to produce thyroid stimulating hormone (TSH) which causes the thyroid gland to synthesize T_3 and T_4.

4. **Answer: a**

   Although hyperthyroidism does increase metabolic requirements, studies have not indicated that hyperthyroidism causes an increase in MAC of inhalational agents. However, hyperthermia does increase MAC values.

5. **Answer: d**

   Accidental removal of the parathyroid glands results in hypocalcemia.

SUGGESTED READINGS

Amathieu R. Difficult intubation in thyroid surgery: myth or reality? *Anesth Analg* 2006;103(4):965–968.

Asari R, Passier C, Kaczirek K, et al. Hypoparathyroidism after total thyroidectomy: a prospective study. *Arch Surg* 2008;143(2):132–137.

Glinoer D, Andry G, Chantrain G, et al. Clinical aspect of early and late hypocalcaemia after thyroid surgery. *Eur J Surg Oncol* 2000;26(6):571–577.

Grimes CM. Intraoperative thyroid storm: a case report. *AANA J* 2004;72(1):53–55.

Leyre P, Desurmont T, Lacoste L, et al. Does the risk of compressive hematoma after thyroidectomy authorize 1-day surgery? *Langenbeck's Arch Surg* 2008;393(5):733–737.

Minogue SC, Ralph J, Lampa MJ. Laryngotracheal topicalization with lidocaine before intubation decreases the incidence of coughing on emergence from general anesthesia. *Anesth Analg* 2004;99(4):1253–1257.

Morrison MP, Schroeder A. Intraoperative identification and management of thyroid storm in children. *Otolaryngol Head Neck Surg* 2007;136(1):132–133.

Myssiorek D. Recurrent laryngeal nerve paralysis: anatomy and etiology. *Otolaryngol Clin North Am* 2004;37(1):25–44.

Shindo M. Incidence of vocal cord paralysis with and without recurrent laryngeal nerve monitoring during thyroidectomy. *Arch Otolaryngol* 2007;133(5):481–485.

Young WF. Adrenal causes of hypertension: pheochromocytoma and primary aldosteronism. *Rev Endocr Metabol Dis* 2007;8(4):309–320.

Trauma Surgery

IV

Emergency Airway Management for the Trauma Patient

14

Matthew D'Angelo

KEY POINTS

- A traumatic airway injury necessitates rapid assessment and emergency management in critically ill patients.
- Properly executing a rapid sequence induction (RSI) is a vital and fundamental skill. Anesthesia providers must be proficient at performing an RSI during rapid airway maintenance.
- Patients who have sustained a potential or actual cervical spine injury must be intubated using in-line manual axial stabilization.

CASE SYNOPSIS

A 38-year-old man who has been assaulted arrives via ambulance to a trauma center. He has sustained multiple stab wounds to the face, neck, and torso. Blood is streaming out of his mouth and he is combative.

PREOPERATIVE EVALUATION AND DEMOGRAPHIC DATA

Past Medical/Surgical History

- Unknown. Medical alert bracelet on right wrist reads, "Diabetic."

List of Medications

- Unknown

Diagnostic Data

- None

Height/Weight/Vital Signs

- 193 cm, 87 kg
- Blood pressure, 88/39; heart rate, 126 beats per minute; respiratory rate, 32 breaths per minute; room air oxygen saturation, 88%; temperature, 36.8°C

Physical Exam

The primary trauma assessment is rapidly completed upon arrival. The findings include: a patient who is a well-developed male with obvious deep tissue lacerations along his face and neck with multiple 2- to 3-cm punctures along his chest wall, primarily situated around the right 4th rib at the midclavicular line. He arrived with a cervical collar in place and on a backboard. His initial airway examination indicates the following signs: respiratory stridor, hemoptysis, broken teeth, facial lacerations, and a large hematoma on the right side of his neck near the 6th cervical vertebrae. You are immediately consulted by the trauma team and asked to secure the patient's airway. During laryngoscopy and direct visualization of the oropharyngeal region of the airway, you notice the presence of supraglottic edema and left-sided tracheal deviation.

TRAUMATIC AIRWAY OVERVIEW

Endotracheal intubation is a mainstay of anesthesia practice. Despite its routine use during general anesthesia, intubation and airway management can be challenging when caring for an acutely injured patient. Difficult tracheal intubation is the third most common respiratory-related event that leads to brain damage and death. Although many patients who endure a traumatic injury will not have an airway that is difficult to manage, the anesthetist frequently will not have the opportunity to perform an airway examination. Therefore, it is vitally important for the anesthetist to have a contingency plan if a difficult airway is encountered.

RSI is the preferred method that should be used for traumatic airway management. One of the greatest differences between performing a routine anesthetic induction and an RSI is the timing of administration of a muscle relaxant. In an RSI, the patient is paralyzed without the anesthetist knowing if the patient can be mask ventilated. The use of muscle relaxants in this situation increases the risk of a "can't intubate/can't ventilate" scenario. Muscle relaxation is associated with the highest overall rate of successful airway management and provides the greatest possibility for rapidly securing the airway.

Emergency intubation for the trauma patient should adhere to the American Society of Anesthesiologists (ASA) difficult airway algorithm. In addition to requiring a secured airway, trauma patients are assumed to have delayed gastric emptying and are at increased risk for aspiration. The anesthesia provider must be skilled in utilizing a variety of airway adjuncts including the laryngeal mask airway (LMA).

Cervical Spine Injuries

Patients who have sustained a blunt or penetrating injury to the neck and face must be considered to have cervical spine instability. Direct laryngoscopy with the use of manual in-line manual axial stabilization of the cervical spine has been shown to be safe and effective in patients with potential or actual cervical spine injuries. Cricoid pressure (Sellick maneuver) assists the anesthetist by displacing the larynx posteriorly and providing an improved view of the vocal cords. This procedure may also help to prevent both gastric insufflation during bag-valve-mask ventilation and passive reflux of gastric contents during laryngoscopy. A disadvantage of providing cricoid pressure to a patient with a cervical spine injury is that pressure is exerted on the cervical vertebrae that could possible result in spinal cord and vascular injury.

Rapid Sequence Induction

Patients with traumatic injury present in varying degrees of injury and may not require emergent airway management. The most common indications for endotracheal intubation include: inadequate oxygenation/ventilation; loss of airway reflexes; decreased level of consciousness; and, in some cases, the need to secure the airway in order to provide deep sedation during painful procedures. Once it is deemed that the patient must be intubated, it should be accomplished by using an RSI. An RSI is conducted to rapidly control a patient's airway, while reducing the likelihood of gastric aspiration. The procedure consists of five primary components: (1) preoxygenation, (2) cricoid pressure, (3) induction/muscle relaxation, (4) apneic ventilation, and (5) direct laryngoscopy. Each of these steps is discussed in the following text.

Preoxygenation

Thorough preoxygenation of the patient is imperative prior to the induction of anesthesia for RSI. Preoxygenation provides an increased time period after the patient stops breathing before hypoxemia ensues which occurs by increasing the concentration of oxygen contained within the functional residual capacity. The procedure is accomplished by administering 100% high-flow (10–15 l) oxygen via a nonrebreathing face mask or bag-valve-face mask. It is estimated that four to eight tidal volume breaths provides an adequate degree of preoxygenation.

Adequate preoxygenation is challenging for patients who are unable to deep breathe or follow commands. In these circumstances, it is appropriate to provide *controlled* positive pressure bag-valve-mask ventilation throughout the induction period.

Cricoid Pressure

Cricoid pressure was first described by Sellick in 1961. The goal of this maneuver is to reduce the risk of pulmonary aspiration of gastric contents by compressing the esophagus against the cricoid cartilage and the cervical vertebrae. Cricoid pressure is maintained throughout the RSI and is not released until endotracheal tube (ETT) placement has been confirmed to be bilaterally equal. Aspiration of gastric contents can occur if the ETT cuff is placed too deeply and migrates into the right mainstem bronchus.

Induction Agents

The anesthetic induction that is used for RSI can be achieved by using a variety of agents, but care should be taken when selecting an initial dose. Any induction agent has the potential for causing a dramatic decrease in blood pressure especially in

the presence of hypovolemia. This effect can occur due to the inhibition of high circulating catecholamine levels and because of an increased sensitivity of the brain during shock. The precise dose of induction agent that should be used in a trauma patient is variable and highly individualized. Induction agents should be titrated to response, realizing that sympathetic nervous system (SNS) inhibition can have dramatic cardiovascular effect in patients who have hypovolemic shock. Although there is no induction agent that is contraindicated for this patient, the dose should be reduced to minimize the potential for hemodynamic decompensation.

The choice to administer succinylcholine or a nondepolarizing muscle relaxant for paralysis may be complex because there are advantages and disadvantages to using these medications. A discussion of inducing paralysis and the type of neuromuscular blocking medication that should be used will occur later in this chapter.

Apneic Ventilation

Apneic ventilation is the concept of providing pulmonary ventilation using high-flow oxygen. The purpose of this procedure is to reduce the risk of gastric distension and pulmonary aspiration from positive pressure ventilation while preventing hypoxemia. The principle of apneic ventilation is based on Boyle's law in which gas leaves the face mask, fills the lungs, and exchanges within the lungs based on the concentration gradient of gases in the alveoli. Unfortunately, optimal gas exchange may not occur, resulting in hypoxemia.

Apneic ventilation used for RSI for the trauma patient is intended to reduce the risk of aspiration for a potential full stomach, yet many trauma patients are unable to inhale deeply and take tidal volume breaths prior to induction, resulting in a reduced functional residual capacity and reduced pulmonary reserve. Avoiding the potential for hypoxemia is important and clinical modifications have been made to RSI that include bag-valve-mask ventilation through cricoid pressure. To date, there does not appear to be any increase in aspiration by bag-valve-mask ventilation while cricoid pressure is achieved.

Direct Laryngoscopy

There is no evidence to show that there is an optimal laryngoscope blade or size for laryngoscopy to accomplish RSI. The anesthetist should use the equipment with which they are most comfortable. Successful ETT placement is immediately confirmed by the presence of carbon dioxide, bilateral equal and clear breath sounds, the absence of sounds over the stomach, and chest rise and fall. If the initial attempt at laryngoscopy is unsuccessful, a second attempt should incorporate a change in the technique (operator, laryngoscope blade, patient position). Experiences gained at shock trauma centers have demonstrated that the intubating stylet is a valuable tool for trauma airway management. This simple and inexpensive device is of enormous benefit in trauma patients because it is readily available and specifically designed to facilitate blind or limited view intubation in the nonsniffing position during in-line manual axial stabilization. Many anesthetists are familiar with placing an LMA and this device is used in emergency situations and in the operating room. However, the gold standard for securing the airway is an ETT. Supporting oxygenation throughout the intubation process is of paramount importance. An understanding of airway management adjuncts and the ability to be proficient with these techniques is critical to provide safe patient care. The process of performing an RSI for a trauma patient with a suspected airway and cervical spine injury is shown in Figure 14-1.

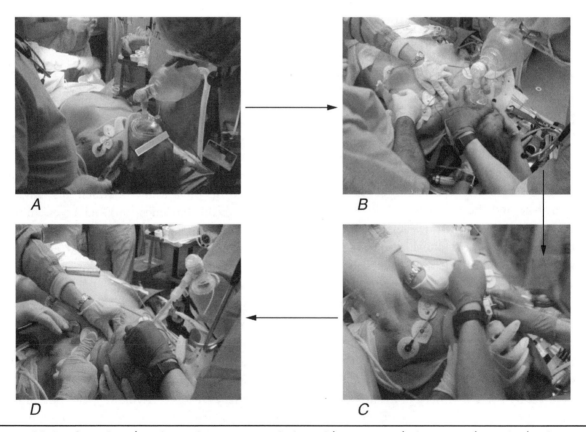

Figure 14-1 *Securing the airway in a trauma victim with suspected airway and cervical spine injuries using a rapid sequence induction with in-line manual axial stabilization. (See Color Plate.)*

ANESTHETIC MANAGEMENT AND CONSIDERATIONS

1. Describe the immediate concerns regarding airway management for a patient who has sustained a traumatic injury.

This patient is exhibiting signs of significant respiratory distress as determined by the following.

- ***Respiratory compensation***: Respiratory rate is 32 breaths per minute, audible stridor, and oxygen delivered by nonrebreathing oxygen face mask. The patient's oxygen saturation is 88%.

An increased respiratory rate can occur for a variety of reasons; however, in this scenario, the patient's physiologic compensatory mechanism for hypoxia includes increasing minute ventilation. Despite a supraphysiologic concentration of inhaled oxygen that is being delivered, the patient's SpO_2 remains 88%. The most accurate method of assessing the degree of hypoxemia is by obtaining an arterial blood gas. According to the values present on the oxyhemoglobin dissociation curve, an SpO_2 of 90% is consistent with a PaO_2 of approximately 60 mm Hg indicating the presence of arterial hypoxemia.

This patient is exhibiting signs of compensated hypovolemic shock as determined by the following:

- ***A potential for vascular injury***: Blood pressure, 88/39; heart rate, 126 beats per minute; evidence of a hematoma and edema on the right side of his neck; the presence of hemoptysis; blood is streaming out of his mouth.

The SNS response associated with hypoxia and hypovolemic shock is powerful and involves the release of major neurovascular mediators such as epinephrine, norepinephrine, and cortisol. By increasing cardiac output and systemic vascular resistance, the physiologic compensatory response should result in increasing blood pressure and thus systemic perfusion, which results in oxygen and substrate delivery and carbon dioxide removal to body tissues. However, this patient's blood pressure

Figure 14-2 *Supraglottic edema and displacement of trachea. (See Color Plate.)*

remains low suggesting the possibility of moderate to severe hypovolemic shock.

The loss of blood from his mouth indicates the possibility of intraoral or pharyngeal laceration. This fact, along with his broken teeth and hematoma on his neck, will complicate direct laryngoscopy by obscuring the anesthetist vision and distorting the structures that comprise the airway anatomy as seen in Figure 14-2. It is also necessary to determine if the patient has sustained a pulmonary contusion that is actively bleeding. In this case, lung isolation using a double lumen ETT or a bronchial blocker is indicated. Hemoptysis and respiratory distress make it unlikely that this patient will cooperate and be able to take tidal volume breaths for adequate preoxygenation. It is imperative to perform a secondary assessment for this patient because there is the possibility that he has sustained other injuries that may be contributing to his state of shock.

This patient should be allowed to sit upright and be permitted to suction his oral pharynx as tolerated. Gravity will likely facilitate movement of fluids from his airway. At the same time, high flow oxygen should be supplied via a nonrebreathing face mask, face tent, or blow-by oxygen to optimize pulmonary reserve prior to induction. An arterial blood gas, hemoglobin and hematocrit values, and a type and cross should be rapidly obtained. A surgeon should evaluate the type and extent of his vascular injures and a plan for surgical intervention is necessary. The anesthetist should expect hypotension to occur after induction and vasopressor medication should be prepared. Preparation for immediate surgical airway intervention is warranted.

2. Identify the most safe and efficient method for acute airway management for this patient.

Airway management for this patient should include an RSI and in-line manual axial stabilization. Performing an awake fiberoptic intubation should not be considered because the patient is hypoxic and not likely to cooperate. This patient presents with several unique problems for the anesthetist. Despite the presence of penetrating injuries and the potential for cervical spine injury, he will likely not tolerate lying supine. In this instance, it may be necessary to begin induction in the high-Fowler's position. Supplemental oxygen via bag-valve-mask should be placed over the patient's face. Induction should begin when all participants are prepared to provide cricoid pressure, administer induction agents, lower the head of the bed, and hold in-line manual axial stabilization. It would be prudent to have a surgeon or another provider skilled in cricothyrotomy in the event that airway management is unsuccessful. After airway control has been established, in-line manual axial stabilization with use of a cervical spine collar should be maintained.

3. Discuss the advantages and disadvantages of using succinylcholine or rocuronium to facilitate intubation during RSI.

Succinylcholine (1.5 mg/kg) provides the most rapid onset of muscle relaxation to facilitate intubation, and is the preferred agent in any patient

Table 14-1	Contraindications for the Use of Succinylcholine

- Malignant hyperthermia
- Hyperkalemia
- Spinal cord injury (chronic injury—is safe for acute airway management)
- Crush injury (massive trauma)
- Stroke
- Guillain-Barré syndrome
- Burn injury (> 24 hrs)
- Muscular dystrophy
- Motor neuron disease
- Mitochondrial myopathies
- Hyperkalemic periodic paralysis
- Pseudocholinesterase deficiency

without a specific contraindication to its use. Table 14-1 lists contraindications for the use of succinylcholine. Life threatening hyperkalemia following the administration of succinylcholine is a risk for patients with neurologic deficits that are caused by spinal cord injuries. Nicotinic cholinergic receptor upregulation occurs within after 24–48 hours postinjury and it is after this period that the administration of succinylcholine is absolutely contraindicated. High dose rocuronium (1.2 mg/kg) can also be used for RSI and adequate intubating conditions are present within 1 minute. The prolonged duration of paralysis produced by rocuronium will necessitate ongoing sedation, and will make any subsequent neurologic assessment more difficult.

4. Describe an appropriate management strategy for a failed attempted direct laryngoscopy.

The anesthetist must approach every airway management opportunity with several alternative plans in the event of a failed intubation. The ASA difficult airway algorithm helps the anesthetists to organize a plan in the event of an airway emergency. However, the algorithm was not designed with the intent for airway management of a trauma patient. As such, alternative airway management strategies may be required. The literature demonstrates a place for the gum elastic bougie (intubating stylet) for traumatic airway management. The gum elastic bougie facilitates nearly blind passage of the ETT. Regardless of any plan, prolonged apnea may necessitate the need for bag-valve-mask ventilation while cricoid pressure is maintained and, in approximately 1% of situations, the creation of a surgical airway is necessary.

5. Discuss the physiologic implications that occur resulting from a prolonged period of apnea due to failed intubation.

The failure to secure a patent airway for the trauma patient will rapidly result in physiologic decompensation. Thus, airway management for the trauma patient often occurs during an acute, unstable period requiring immediate and life-saving intervention.

Apnea and hypoventilation cause a variety of pathologic responses related to increases in $PaCO_2$ and decreases in PaO_2. These changes are exacerbated in the trauma patient due to increased metabolic demands. The peripheral chemoreceptors that are located within the aortic and carotid bodies produce an excitatory response caused by decreased PaO_2, increased $PaCO_2$ and decreased pH which stimulates an increase in SNS outflow. The SNS stimulates increased cardiac excitation and vasoconstriction.

In this patient scenario, a rightward shift of the oxyhemoglobin dissociation curve occurs due to hypercarbia, hypoxemia, and increased 2,3 diphosphoglycerate (DPG). The creation of 2,3 DPG occurs in red blood cells and is a byproduct that is associated with metabolism. Increased 2,3 DPG is associated with anaerobic metabolism. This results in a conformational change in the hemoglobin molecule that creates a decreased affinity between oxygen and hemoglobin which favors the release of oxygen to the tissues.

The rate and increase of arterial carbon dioxide accumulation during apnea is predictable. The average $PaCO_2$ accumulation is 6 mm Hg for the first minute and 3–4 mm Hg for each additional minute. Additionally, the metabolic tissue demand for the average adult is approximately 3 ml/kg/min. Assuming that the pulse oximeter reading in this patient scenario is accurate, his PaO_2 of 88% SaO_2 would be less than 60 mm Hg. This equates to rapid desaturation and worsening hypoxemia.

Severe hypoxia will rapidly progress to cardiovascular collapse as a result of anaerobic respiration, cellular energy depletion, hydrogen ion and lactate accumulation, and acidosis. If hypoxia continues, the patient will exhibit decompensation as the cardiac rhythm will progress from tachydysrhythmias or bradydysrhythmias to asystole.

6. Identify the concerns related to emergency airway management for a patient with a suspected cervical spine injury.

Cervical spine injuries remain a significant concern during airway management of the trauma patient. The incidence of cervical spine injury after trauma is approximately 3–6% of all trauma patient and approximately 10% for patients who have experienced a traumatic brain injury. It is prudent for the anesthetist to assume that the patient has a cervical spine injury until it can be definitively determined by physical examination and radiography or computed tomography (CT) scan that the spinal cord and cervical vertebrae are intact. Immobilization of the neck is essential and in-line manual axial stabilization allows for the removal of the front of the cervical collar, allowing jaw and mouth movement necessary to insert the laryngoscope blade, while limiting the risk for further injury.

The management and intubation of patients with suspected cervical spine injuries remains an area of controversy. There is presently no scientific evidence to support that a fiberoptic intubation results in a superior patient outcomes as compared with direct laryngoscopy and in-line manual axial stabilization.

7. Discuss the appropriate anesthetic management for severe hypotension that occurs following positive pressure ventilation after successful endotracheal intubation.

A tension pneumothorax occurs as a result of air becoming trapped in the thorax due to a defect or rupture in the lung tissue. The pathology related to a tension pneumothorax is unique in that it allows gas to escape from the lung into the pleural cavity during inspiration. However, gas is trapped in the thoracic cage due to a flap in the tissue that acts as a one-way valve and decreases the volume of gas that is exhaled. As pressure continues to increase within the thoracic cavity, pressure is exerted on the mediastinum which impinges on the heart and major vasculature, and results in diminished cardiac filling, reduced cardiac output, and, if left untreated, pulseless electrical activity. Typically, a tension pneumothorax will occur shortly after the implementation of positive pressure ventilation. The anesthetist should be aware of the signs associated with a tension pneumothorax and these are listed in Table 14-2.

Release of the thoracic tension via chest tube thoracoscopy or needle decompression is required to manage this complication. Needle decompression is accomplished by placing a 2- to 3-in angiocatheter into the second intercostal space at the midclavicular line on the affected side of the chest. If cardiac function does not immediately improve, the other side of the patient's chest should be decompressed and the advanced cardiac life support protocol initiated. Once needle decompression occurs, the angiocatheter must remain until

Table 14-2   Signs Associated with a Tension Pneumothorax
Pulmonary Manifestations
• Hypoxemia
• Hypercarbia
• Increase peak inspiratory pressures
• Decreased pulmonary compliance
• Absence of breath sound on the affected side
• Tracheal deviation in the opposite direction of the pneumothorax
Cardiac Manifestations
• Hypotension
• Tachycardia
• Mediastinal shift in the opposite direction of the pneumothorax
• Distended neck veins

a chest tube is placed to avoid the reaccumulation of air.

REVIEW QUESTIONS

1. Which patient should receive in-line manual axial stabilization for a rapid sequence induction and emergency airway management?
   a. Sustained blunt airway injury
   b. Sustained an acute head injury
   c. Involved in a high speed car accident
   d. All of these patients should receive a rapid sequence induction

2. The administration of succinylcholine during a rapid sequence induction is appropriate for a patient with:
   a. hypokalemia.
   b. a spinal cord transection that occurred 2 weeks ago.
   c. a history of malignant hyperthermia.
   d. a crush injury to the left thigh.

3. A patient has a $PaCO_2$ of 47 mm Hg prior to induction. It takes 4 minutes to successfully intubate the patient. The anesthetist should expect the patients $PaCO_2$ to increase by:
   a. 7 mm Hg.
   b. 18 mm Hg.
   c. 52 mm Hg.
   d. 65 mm Hg.

4. The _____ reflex activates the sympathetic nervous system when hypoxemia or hypercarbia occurs.
   a. baroreceptor
   b. chemoreceptor
   c. oculocardiac
   d. atrial stretch

5. Which best describes correct placement of an angiocatheter for a patient that has a tension pneumothorax?
   a. At the level of the sternal notch
   b. Above the 5th rib at the midaxillary line
   c. In the 2nd intercostal space at the midclavicular line
   d. On the side opposite of the direction of the tracheal deviation

REVIEW ANSWERS

1. **Answer: d**
   In all of these scenarios, the patient should be suspected of having an acute cervical spine injury until the possibility is definitively excluded by physical exam and radiologic evidence.

2. **Answer: a**
   Succinylcholine can cause hyperkalemia due acetylcholine receptor upregulation in a patient with a spinal cord injury after the first 24–48 hours and a patient with a crush injury. Succinylcholine is also a known triggering agent for malignant hyperthermia. Patients who have sustained a crush injury associated with muscle trauma and at risk of developing hyperkalemia.

3. **Answer: d**
   It is estimated that carbon dioxide (CO_2) increases 6 mm Hg during the first minute and 3–4 mm Hg/minute while an adult patient is apneic. In this scenario, the CO_2 increases 6 mm Hg for the first minute and 4 mm Hg for every minute thereafter (3 minutes). The total increase for the time that the patient is apneic is 18 mm Hg which, when added to the existing $PaCO_2$ of 47 mm Hg (47 + 18), is 65 mm Hg.

4. **Answer: b**
   The chemoreceptor reflex is initiated via the carotid and aortic bodies (peripheral chemoreceptors) in response to decreased PaO_2, increased $PaCO_2$ and increased hydrogen ion concentration. The result is sympathetic nervous system activation.

5. **Answer: c**
   The correct placement for needle decompression of a tension pneumothorax is opposite of the direction of the tracheal deviation in the 2nd intercostal space at the midclavicular line.

SUGGESTED READINGS

Cheney FW. The American Society of Anesthesiologists Closed Claims Project: what have we learned, how has it affected practice, and how will it affect practice in the future? *Anesthesiology* 1999;91:552–556.

Dutton RP. Airway trauma. In: Yao FF, ed. *Anesthesiology Problem Oriented Patient Management*, 6th ed. Philadelphia: Lippincott Williams & Wilkins, 2007: 993–1006.

Dutton RP, McCunn M. Anesthesia for trauma. In: Miller RD, ed. *Miller's Anesthesia*, 6th ed. Philadelphia: Churchill Livingston, 2005:2451–2495.

Frass M. *Airway Management: Principles and Practice*. St. Louis: Mosby, 1996:444–451.

Ghafoor AU, Martin TW, Gopalakrishnan S, et al. Caring for the patients with cervical spine injuries: what have we learned? *J Clin Anesth* 2005;17(8):640–649.

Gronert GA, Theye RA. Pathophysiology of hyperkalemia induced by succinylcholine. *Anesthesiol* 1975;43(1): 89–99.

Heier T, Feiner JR, Lin J, et al. Hemoglobin desaturation after succinylcholine-induced apnea: a study of the recovery of spontaneous ventilation in healthy volunteers. *Anesthesiol* 2001;94(5):754–759.

Johnson KB, Egan TD, Kern SE, et al. The influence of hemorrhagic shock on propofol: a pharmacokinetic and pharmacodynamic analysis. *Anesthesiology* 2004;101:647–659.

Patel M, Fernando R. Preoxygenation in women: effect of posture. *Anesth Analg* 1993;77(5):1081–1082.

Suderman VS, Crosby ET, Lui A. Elective oral-tracheal intubation in cervical spine injured adults. *Can J Anaesth* 1992;39(5 Pt 1):516–517.

Craniotomy for Acute Head Injury

15

Greta Bray

KEY POINTS

- It is estimated that 1.5 million acute head injuries (AHI) occur every year in the United States, most often caused by motor vehicle accidents, sports injuries, and falls.
- Pupillary abnormalities such as size, light reflex, and symmetry occur in 20–30% of patients presenting for craniotomy for AHI.
- The primary objective for induction and maintenance of anesthesia is to decrease elevated intracranial pressure (ICP) if present, optimize cerebral perfusion and oxygenation, and avoid secondary injury from hypoxia and hypotension.
- Hypotension with systolic blood pressure < 90 mm Hg is a major contributor to poor outcome after acute brain injury.

CASE SYNOPSIS

A 21-year-old man has developed an epidural hematoma after falling off of his skateboard and hitting his head on the ground. He is scheduled by his neurosurgeon to have an emergent craniotomy for evacuation of an epidural hematoma.

PREOPERATIVE EVALUATION AND DEMOGRAPHIC DATA

Past Medical/Surgical History

- Tonsillectomy at age 10; no anesthetic complications
- No known allergies

List of Medications

None

Diagnostic Data

- Hemoglobin, 14.0 g/dl; hematocrit, 40.0%
- Glucose, 98 mg/dl

- Prothrombin time, 12 seconds; partial thromboplastin time, 34 seconds; platelets, 350,000/ml
- Electrolytes: sodium, 136 mEq/l; potassium, 4.2 mEq/l; chloride, 107 mEq/l; carbon dioxide, 26 mEq/l
- Blood urea nitrogen, 14 mg/dl; creatinine, 0.9 mg/dl
- Computed tomography (CT) scan of head without contrast demonstrates a large epidural hematoma to the right temporal region. His cervical spine was not injured.

Height/Weight/Vital Signs

- 183 cm, 90 kg
- Blood pressure, 170/85; heart rate, 110 beats per minute; respiration rate, 26 breaths per minute; room air saturation, 97%; temperature, 37.2°C

PATHOPHYSIOLOGY

An epidural hematoma is considered a focal brain injury in that the damage produced by a direct mechanical impact and the acceleration–deceleration stress onto the skull and brain tissue results in skull fractures and intracranial lesions. Epidural hematoma is often caused by skull fracture and laceration of the middle meningeal artery or anterior cerebral artery allowing bleeding to occur between the skull and dura. Epidural hematomas are most commonly located in the temporoparietal and temporal regions of the brain.

A multitude of physiologic compensatory mechanisms are initiated in order to increase cerebral perfusion. The cardiovascular responses that are typically observed in the compensatory stage AHI include tachycardia, hypertension, and increased cardiac output. Hypotension and decreased cardiac output are associated with substantial blood loss and/or progressive or irreversible stage of injury. The respiratory responses that occur as a result of AHI include apnea and abnormal respiratory patterns. Respiratory insufficiency and hyperventilation frequently occur. Cerebral blood flow (CBF) and the cerebral metabolic rate of oxygen consumption ($CMRO_2$) are decreased in the core area of injury. If ICP increases, then a diffuse and more profound hypoperfusion and hypometabolism of the brain will ensue. Acute brain swelling and cerebral edema develop concomitantly after acute brain injury which further decreases CBF resulting in cerebral ischemia. Cerebrovascular autoregulation is also impaired. The decision to perform a craniotomy for AHI is typically based on the patient's Glasgow coma score (GCS), pupillary exam, associated comorbidities, CT scan findings, and ICP values.

SURGICAL PROCEDURE

Evacuation of an epidural hematoma will depend on the location of the injury. A frontotemporal craniotomy is performed for most AHIs that require surgical intervention, as shown in Figure 15-1. Most likely the entire surface of the head is shaved free of hair and the head is placed in a headrest of pins, suction cups, or horseshoe, based on the surgeon's preference. The scalp incision begins anterior to the tragus and continue superiorly in a question mark shape to the frontal area. The scalp is then peeled back and the skull bone is exposed. The skull is punctured using a cranial drill at the temporal site. Additional burr holes are made in the skull, avoiding injury to the major venous structures, with the anterior burr hole being placed above the frontal sinus. A formal bone flap is then removed, allowing access to the dura, and bleeding is controlled. The dura may also be lacerated and in this instance the opening is repaired.

Depending on the degree of cerebral edema, the bone flap may or may not be reapplied at the time of surgical closure. A drain may be placed and extend through a separate incision near the surgical site. An intracranial pressure monitor may be placed at the end of surgery to monitor postoperative ICP.

LEFT FRONTOTEMPORAL CRANIOTOMY

Figure 15-1 *Frontotemporal craniotomy performed to treat a cerebral epidural hematoma.*

ANESTHETIC MANAGEMENT AND CONSIDERATIONS

Preoperative Period

1. Describe the importance of establishing a patent airway and providing ventilation for a patient with an AHI presenting for craniotomy.
Many patients with AHI exhibit partial or complete airway obstruction caused by the tongue blocking the posterior pharyngeal space. Additionally, patients with an AHI who require a craniotomy often have a full stomach, decreased intravascular volume, and potentially a cervical spine injury. Immediate oxygenation and securing of the airway with an endotracheal tube (ETT) may be necessary during the brief and rapid preoperative assessment. If the patient is found to be hemodynamically stable, then rapid sequence induction with inline neck manual axial stabilization is appropriate; however, intubation may produce an elevation in blood pressure and ICP. In hemodynamically unstable patients, the induction drug dosages are decreased or omitted. Once the airway is secured, a nondepolarizing muscle relaxant should be given and mechanical ventilation initiated to achieve low normocarbia, partial arterial pressure carbon dioxide ($PaCO_2$) of approximately 35 mm Hg. Prolonged and aggressive hyperventilation of $PaCO_2 < 30$ mm Hg is to be avoided because hypocarbia causes cerebral vasculature constriction which decreases CBF. CBF decreases by 1 ml/100 g brain tissue/minute for each 1 torr decrease in $PaCO_2$. Hypoxia, if present, should be corrected immediately as decreased cerebral oxygenation is associated with poor neurologic outcomes.

2. Discuss the importance of an initial preoperative neurologic evaluation.

With diagnosis of epidural hematoma caused by an AHI, 22 to 56% of patients are comatose immediately before surgery. A lucid interval, where there is wakefulness and rapid neurologic deterioration, may also be observed. A quick neurologic assessment must be performed with special attention to the level of consciousness, presence or absence of increased ICP, and extent of focal deficits.

The GCS is a valid and reliable method for assessing neurologic status and is shown in Table 15-1. Pupillary abnormalities such as size,

Table 15-1 Adult Glasgow Coma Scale	
RESPONSE	**SCORE**
Eye Opening (E)	
Spontaneous, open and blinking	4
To speech	3
To pain	2
None	1
Verbal Response (V)	
Oriented	5
Answers but confused	4
Inappropriate but recognizable words	3
Incomprehensible sounds	2
None	1
Best Motor Response (M)	
Obeys to verbal commands	6
Localizes painful stimuli	5
Withdraws from painful stimuli	4
Decorticate posturing (upper extremity flexion)	3
Decerebrate posturing (upper extremity extension)	2
No movement	1

GCS ≤ 8, deep coma, severe head trauma, poor outcome; GCS 9–12, conscious patient with moderate injury; GCS > 12, mild injury.

Table 15-2   Signs Associated with Increased ICP
• Cushing's Triad
1. widening pulse pressure (increased systolic blood pressure, decreased diastolic pressure)
2. bradycardia
3. irregular respirations
• Headache
• Nausea
• Papilledema
• Unilateral pupillary dilation
• Nystagmus
• Abducens and oculomotor palsies
• Altered level of consciousness
• Seizures

light reflex, and symmetry occur in 20–30% of patients presenting for craniotomy for AHI. Other presenting symptoms may include hemiparesis, decerebration, and seizures. Signs of increased ICP are included in Table 15-2. The importance of the preoperative assessment is for initial understanding of the patient's baseline neurologic status and urgency for craniotomy; however, equally important is the evaluation used for comparison of the postoperative neurologic assessment once the craniotomy is completed.

3. Examine the initial cardiovascular changes in a patient with an AHI.

The most common early cardiac manifestations associated with AHI include cardiac dysrhythmias, systemic hypertension, and tachycardia, possibly leading to bradycardia. Most patients with AHI initially exhibit hypertension and tachycardia, which is the central nervous system's response to brain ischemia. After AHI, blood flow to the vasomotor center in the brain may be decreased causing cerebral ischemia. With this decrease in blood flow, the vasoconstrictor and cardioaccelerator neurons in the vasomotor center reacts to the ischemia by becoming excited. The result of this excitation is an increase in systemic arterial pressure and heart rate. Cushing's triad, which includes widening pulse pressure (increased systolic blood pressure and decreased diastolic blood pressure), irregular respirations, and bradycardia, is indicative of severely elevated ICP, profound cerebral ischemia, and possible cerebral herniation. If the AHI is accompanied with significant blood loss, additional multiple systemic injuries, or late stage recognition of injury, hypotension and decreased cardiac output may be noted during initial cardiovascular exam. A systolic blood pressure of less than < 90 mm Hg is associated with poor neurologic outcomes.

Intraoperative Period

4. Discuss the choice of anesthetic used for induction and maintenance of anesthesia for patients presenting for craniotomy resulting from AHI.

The primary objective for induction and maintenance of anesthesia is to decrease elevated ICP if present, optimize cerebral perfusion and oxygenation, and avoid secondary injury from hypoxia and hypotension. Laryngoscopy with ETT placement, if not already performed preoperatively, is best achieved using medications that blunt response to stimulation of laryngoscopy and decrease ICP, all while maintaining systolic blood pressure > 90 mm Hg.

- Hypnotic agents decrease ICP, $CMRO_2$, CBF, and brain metabolism. Both propofol and thiopental are good choices for induction of anesthesia in the AHI patient, provided the blood pressure at time of induction is adequate or easily supported with fluids and vasopressors. If hemodynamic instability is present with induction, preservation of the existing blood pressure may best be achieved by administering etomidate or

dexmedetomidine, a potent selective alpha 2 adrenoreceptor agonist.

- Due to the sympathomimetic action, the administration of ketamine is contraindicated as it will increase CBF and ICP.

- Inhalation agents are appropriate to administer for maintaining anesthesia during craniotomy. Dissimilarities between isoflurane, desflurane, and sevoflurane in regard to metabolic suppression and CBF are minor but all have an advantageous effect of decreasing $CMRO_2$. The negative effects of the inhalation agents is that they cause cerebrovascular dilation and increase CBF which may further increase ICP. However, this effect is dependent on the dose administered and with concentrations < 1 MAC, ICP can be maintained. The use of nitrous oxide (N_2O) is contraindicated. N_2O is a modest cerebrovascular dilator and can increase ICP and CBF. N_2O does not provide cerebral protection and may lessen the protective effects of propofol, thiopental, or other inhalation agents. N_2O may also contribute to expansion of a venous air embolism or pneumocephalus should these complications occur.

- Opioids are a useful part of a balanced anesthesia in craniotomy; all have negligible effects on CBF and a dose dependent effect on cerebral metabolism. Once laryngoscopy is achieved, opioids for craniotomy due to AHI should be used conservatively, so that respiratory depression causing hypercarbia resulting in increased ICP is avoided upon emergence. Morphine and hydromorphone will be eliminated more slowly based on their fat soluble properties and have potential to cause respiratory depression and delay neurologic assessment due to sedation once the craniotomy is completed. Short-acting synthetic opioids, such as a remifentanil infusion used during the craniotomy, may be advocated due to the short duration of action and rapid metabolism resulting in a shortened period of respiratory depression and allows the anesthetist to perform a more accurate neurologic assessment at the end of the case.

• Muscle relaxants administered during craniotomy can aid in mechanical ventilation and reduce ICP that can be caused by bucking or straining. The use of a succinylcholine in this patient population is controversial because the fasciculations caused by total body depolarization will increase ICP. If succinylcholine is necessary for emergent control of the airway, a defasciculating dose of a nondepolarizing muscle relaxant should be administered first. If muscle relaxation is required throughout the maintenance period, all muscle relaxant medications with the exception of pancuronium are suitable for administration and have nominal effects on ICP, blood pressure, or heart rate. Pancuronium is not recommended due to its vagolytic effect, possibly leading to increased ICP caused by hypertension and tachycardia.

5. Discuss methods used to decrease elevated ICP during craniotomy for AHI.

Located within the cranium are three major components that comprise the intracerebral volume: the brain including neurons and glia, the cerebrospinal fluid (CSF) and extracellular fluid, and blood that perfuses the brain. Initially, intracranial volume can rise without causing an appreciable increase in ICP. However, there is a point (critical volume) when the cerebral volume within the cranium has reached maximum size and small increases in intracranial volume produce extreme increases in ICP that must be managed rapidly to avoid reductions CBF and cerebral herniation. Figure 15-2 depicts the relationship comparing intracranial volume and ICP.

Cerebral perfusion pressure (CPP) is directly related to both mean arterial pressure (MAP) and ICP as shown in Equation 15-1. If ICP is increased and becomes greater than MAP, CPP is reduced, resulting in reduced CBF. Normal ICP is equal to or

Figure 15-2 *Relationship comparing intracranial pressure and intracranial volume.*

less than 10 mm Hg and normal CPP varies between 80–100 mm Hg. Therefore, the major determinant of CBF is MAP. Management of increased ICP during craniotomy is performed using several different techniques.

• Hyperventilation to a $PaCO_2$ of 25 to 30 mm Hg can be instituted as a rapid and effective method to manage severely increased ICP by decreasing CBF and the blood volume within the brain. However, prolonged hypocarbia is associated with poor neurologic outcome. CBF becomes less sensitive to the effects of hyperventilation within 24 to 48 hours.

• Diuretic therapy using mannitol, an osmotic diuretic, can provide effective ICP reduction intraoperatively. Mannitol administered as a bolus 1 g/kg over 10 minutes or slow infusion 0.25 to 1 g/kg over 20 minutes, and may improve CBF and oxygen delivery by reducing blood viscosity. Hypotension and

Equation 15-1
CPP = MAP − ICP or CVP
CPP, cerebral perfusion pressure; CVP, central venous pressure; ICP, intracranial pressure; MAP, mean arterial pressure.

hypovolemia are possible side effects with mannitol administration and serum osmolarity must be monitored frequently if multiple doses are administered. Serum osmolarity should not exceed 320 mOsm/L. Furosemide, a loop diuretic, provides a synergistic effect with mannitol and may be administered for persistently increased ICP.

- Increasing the level of the patient's head from 10 to 30 degrees increases cerebral venous and CSF drainage, therefore lowering ICP. This position should be maintained throughout the perioperative period. Severe flexing or turning of the head may obstruct cerebral venous drainage and increased ICP may result.
- Barbiturates, such as pentobarbital, decrease ICP during instances of refractory elevation. Barbiturates provide cerebral protection by decreasing $CMRO_2$ and ICP.

6. Discuss fluid requirements and circulatory management for a patient having a craniotomy.
Hypotension with systolic blood pressure < 90 mm Hg is a major contributor to a poor neurologic outcome after acute brain injury. Fluid resuscitation and circulatory management should begin immediately and inotropic and vasopressor medications should be considered to stabilize blood pressure if hypotension ensues. Administration of dopamine or phenylephrine infusions are recommended to maintain CPP 60–110 mm Hg. A bolus dose of a vasopressor must be used cautiously, as a sudden increase in blood pressure can elevate ICP. Hypertension may be caused by Cushing reflex, which causes sympathetic nervous system hyperactivity in response to increased ICP. This event is associated with profound bradycardia caused by baroreceptor activation. Prior to treating the hypertension, heart rate along with adequate oxygenation and anesthetic depth should be considered.

Fluid resuscitation should be guided by assessing blood pressure, urinary output, and central venous pressure (CVP) readings if available. Rapid administration of crystalloid and colloid solutions to restore intravascular volume should be monitored to achieve a CPP > 60 mm Hg, while trying to avoid additional brain swelling.

Glucose containing solutions, such as Ringer's lactate, should be avoided in acute brain injured patients undergoing craniotomy because hyperglycemia is associated with poor neurological outcomes caused by further intracellular acidosis. Ringer's lactate solution, which is slightly hypotonic and contains glucose, promotes swelling in uninjured portions of the brain. Therefore, the crystalloid of choice to be given via rapid infusion is isotonic normal saline.

Colloid solutions, such as hydroxyethyl solutions, and human plasma products can also be given to sustain intravascular volume up to 20 ml/kg. Monitoring the coagulation status should be performed because patients with an AHI are at higher risk for developing coagulopathies. Blood transfusions may be necessary and, although there is not one absolute hemoglobin or hematocrit value that mandates transfusion, patients with an hematocrit below 30%, may need a transfusion to promote oxygen delivery to the brain. Careful fluid resuscitation using crystalloid solutions and blood products must be assessed to minimize cerebral swelling. Blood pressure, urine output, and CVP readings may become crucial to assess the need for blood product or fluid based on the intravascular volume status.

7. Describe methods used for cerebral protection during craniotomy for AHI.
Cerebral protection can be achieved using various methods. One method includes the use of intraoperative hypothermia which reduces core body temperature to between 33 and 35°C. Hypothermia is believed to reduce metabolic demand, suppress excitatory neurotransmitters, diminish free radical formation, and reduce edema of the brain.

A decrease of each degree Celsius decreases $CMRO_2$ by 7%. Hypothermia is achieved by cooling intravenous fluids, decreasing ambient temperature, applying a cooling blanket beneath the patient on the operating room table, and applying ice bags to pulse points on the body. The benefits of controlled hypothermia for cerebral protection remain controversial. The potential side effects associated with induced hypothermia include hypotension, cardiac arrhythmias, pneumonia, and coagulopathies. However, hyperthermia is definitively associated with poor neurologic outcome. Hyperthermia depletes ATP stores and increases calcium influx into cells. Often, AHI patients' thermoregulatory processes are disrupted and hyperthermia persists, which can be detrimental to recovery. Cerebral protection via hypothermia is still being investigated.

8. Identify intraoperative monitoring modalities used during craniotomy for AHI.

Standard American Society of Anesthesiologists (ASA) monitors are essential for the intraoperative monitoring. Additionally, intraarterial blood pressure measurement, central venous pressure monitoring, and urine output are used.

Intraarterial line measurement is necessary for management of CPP and to assess the correlation between arterial blood gases measurements, especially $PaCO_2$ with the $ETCO_2$ display via capnography. The intraarterial transducer should be placed at the level of the tragus of the ear at the external auditory canal to improve accuracy. Arterial blood pressure monitoring also allows for measurement of hematocrit, electrolytes, glucose, and serum osmolarity.

A CVP catheter is often inserted intraoperatively for a craniotomy for AHI. These patients are at risk for fluid volume deficits and CVP monitoring allows for intraoperative fluid volume management. The CVP catheter can be placed in an antecubital vein, subclavian vein, or internal jugular vein. Placement depends on the risk of venous air embolism (VAE) during surgery, and whether the patient can tolerate their head being placed in a dependent position during the insertion process. If the patient has a possible risk for VAE, the location of choice for the CVP catheter placement is subclavian, with the tip of the CVP catheter located 3 cm below the right atrium–superior vena cava junction in the heart. This is the optimal location to withdraw air from the CVP catheter if a VAE occurs during opening of the venous sinuses of the brain.

Doppler ultrasound is frequently used to monitor for VAE during craniotomy. The Doppler is placed between the third and sixth intercostal space on the right sternal border and auditory classic mill wheel murmur is monitored throughout surgery. During craniotomy for AHI, air can potentially enter the circulation through defects in the skull such as burr holes or pin holes from the head holder, and when the head is positioned 10 cm above the mid-thorax. Doppler ultrasound is a sensitive, noninvasive method for detecting a VAE.

Postoperative Period

The total operative time of the surgical craniotomy for evacuation of epidural hematoma following AHI was 240 minutes. In the operating room, the patient demonstrated the following evaluation: delayed awakening, irregular respiratory pattern, blood pressure of 108/62, respiratory rate of 1 per minute, inadequately low tidal volume respirations, heart rate of 65 beats per minute, room air saturation of 98%, and temperature of 35.5°C.

9. List potential postoperative complications and diagnostic criteria following craniotomy for AHI.

Potential postoperative complications after craniotomy include:

- **Delayed awakening**: consider preoperative neurologic baseline, residual anesthetic effects allowing at least 2 hours for residual anesthesia to metabolize, fully reverse muscle paralysis, consider the amount of opioid use intraoperatively and need for naloxone.

- *Hypothermia*: slow active rewarming with forced air warming device.
- *Seizures*: treat with a loading dose of phenytoin 1 g intravenously slowly to avoid developing hypotension.
- *Postoperative cerebral edema*: continued administration of mannitol or furosemide postoperatively, limit fluids, monitor CVP readings, position patient with head up 10 to 30 degrees, patients demonstrating hydro-cephalus may require a shunt procedure to decrease the volume of CSF within the cere-bral ventricles.
- *Metabolic or electrolyte disturbances*: obtain postoperative electrolytes and carefully correct imbalances such as glucose, sodium and potassium especially after mannitol and furosemide administration.
- *Hematoma*: evaluate with CT scan of head, obtain coagulation studies, administer fresh frozen plasma and platelets if necessary to cor-rect coagulopathy.
- *Irregular respiratory pattern and inability to extubate*: consider brain stem ischemia; evaluation of this complication includes a CT scan of the head.

Treatment for this patient postoperatively would include continuous ventilatory support in the inten-sive care unit, hourly neurologic evaluations, active rewarming to achieve normothermia, a CT scan of the head, fluid volume management, and circula-tory support to maintain CPP 60–110 mm Hg.

REVIEW QUESTIONS

1. Which is the initial intervention used to manage severely increased ICP?
   a. Administration of mannitol
   b. Hyperventilation
   c. Head up 10 to 30 degrees
   d. Administration of barbiturates

2. Cerebral perfusion pressure is determined by which two factors?
   a. MAP and urine output
   b. CVP measurement
   c. MAP and ICP
   d. ICP only

3. A systolic value of ____ mm Hg is a major contributor to poor neurologic outcome after craniotomy for AHI.
   a. > 100 mm Hg
   b. < 120 mm Hg
   c. < 80 mm Hg
   d. < 90 mm Hg

4. Which crystalloid solution should be avoided in acute head injured patients presenting for craniotomy?
   a. Normal saline
   b. Albumin
   c. Ringer's lactate
   d. Packed red blood cells

5. Headache, nausea, papilledema, unilat-eral pupillary dilation, abducens, and occulomotor palsies are symptoms that are associated with:
   a. increased ICP.
   b. decreased cerebral perfusion.
   c. cervical spine injury.
   d. hypovolemia.

REVIEW ANSWERS

1. **Answer: b**
   Hyperventilation can be used as the initial intervention used to decrease severely elevated ICP because hypocarbia rapidly decreases ICP.

2. **Answer: c**
   Cerebral perfusion pressure is determined by MAP and ICP.

3. **Answer: d**
   A systolic blood pressure < 90 mm Hg is associated with poor neurologic outcome in patients who have sustained an AHI.

4. **Answer: c**

   Ringer's lactate should be avoided in patients presenting for craniotomy following AHI because it can increase brain swelling and it contains glucose. Due to worsening intracellular acidosis, hyperglycemia is associated with poor neurologic outcomes.

5. **Answer: a**

   Headache, nausea, papilledema, unilateral pupillary dilation, abducens, and occulomotor palsies are all symptoms associated with increased ICP.

SUGGESTED READINGS

Bendo A, Kass IS, Hartung J, et al. Anesthesia for neurosurgery. In: Barash PG, Cullen BF, Stoelting RK, eds. *Clinical Anesthesia*, 5th ed. Philadelphia: Lippincott Williams and Wilkins, 2006:746–772.

Bullock RM, Chestnut RM, Clifton Gl, et al. Guidelines for the management of severe traumatic brain injury. *J Neurotrauma* 2000;17:451–553.

Capan LM, Miller SM. Trauma and burns. In: Barash PG, Cullen BF, Stoelting RK, eds. *Clinical Anesthesia*, 5th ed. Philadelphia: Lippincott Williams and Wilkins, 2006:1269–1272.

Elf K, Nilsson P, Ronne-Engstrom E, et al. Temperature disturbances in traumatic brain injury: relationship to secondary insults, barbiturate treatment and outcomes. *Neurolog Res* 2008;30(10):1097–1105.

Guyton AC, Hall JE. *Textbook of medical physiology*. Philadelphia: Elsevier Saunders, 2006.

Janik D. Anesthesia for craniotomy. In: Duke J, ed. *Anesthesia Secrets*, 3rd ed. Philadelphia: Elsevier Mosby, 2006:488–492.

Sakabe T, Bendo AA. Anesthesia management of head trauma. In: Newfield P, Cottrell JE, eds. *Handbook of Neuroanesthesia*, 4th ed. Philadelphia: Lippincott Williams and Wilkins, 2007:91–109.

Sakamoto GT, Shuer LM, Chang SD. Craniotomy for trauma. In: Jaffe RA, Samuels SI, eds. *Anesthesiologist's Manual of Surgical Procedures*, 3rd ed. Philadelphia: Lippincott Williams and Wilkins, 2004:32–37.

Seppelt I. Intracranial hypertension after traumatic brain injury. *Indian J Crit Care Med* 2004;8:120–126.

Penetrating Traumatic Injuries

16

Jeremy S. Heiner

KEY POINTS

- The severity of injuries that are produced by penetrating trauma vary from minor to life threatening.
- Penetrating injuries can occur from a variety of objects including gun shot wounds (GSWs), stab wounds, or projectiles from a shotgun blast.
- Control of the airway and resuscitative interventions are the anesthetist's primary objectives when caring for a patient with a penetrating traumatic injury.

CASE SYNOPSIS

A 22–year-old man with a GSW to the abdomen is being treated in the emergency department. The entrance wound is observed in the left lower quadrant as a small hole with mild bleeding. The exit wound is present in the right upper flank on the back with moderate bleeding. He is scheduled for a diagnostic laparotomy. He is alert, talking, and states that he is having severe abdominal pain.

PREOPERATIVE EVALUATION AND DEMOGRAPHIC DATA

Past Medical/Surgical History

- Denies

List of Medications

- Admits to smoking marijuana yesterday

Diagnostic Data

- Hemoglobin, 10.1 g/dl; hematocrit, 30.5%
- Platelets, 235,000 per microliter
- Electrolytes: sodium, 141 mEq/l; potassium, 3.9 mEq/l; chloride, 107 mEq/l; carbon dioxide, 25 mEq/l
- Blood glucose, 97 mg/dl
- Computed tomography (CT) scan reveals blood in the peritoneum

Height/Weight/Vital Signs

- 173 cm, 73 kg
- Blood pressure, 136/91; heart rate, 121 beats per minute; respiratory rate, 20 breaths per minute; room air oxygen saturation, 100% on face mask O_2 at 15 liter/min flow; temperature, 36°C

PATHOPHYSIOLOGY

Penetrating trauma caused by a GSW has the potential to cause a tremendous amount of tissue destruction. The resulting damage is dependent on the type of instrument or projectile (e.g., knife, bullet, or fragment), the velocity of the projectile at the time of impact, and the characteristics of the tissue through which the projectile passes (e.g., fat, muscle, nervous tissue, bone, blood vessels, or organs). The amount of damage caused is a result of the amount of energy transferred to the body tissue. This phenomenon is explained by Newton's law of kinetic energy as shown in Equation 16-1. Whereas doubling the projectile's mass will double the energy, doubling the projectile's velocity will *quadruple* the energy.

When a high-velocity projectile enters body tissue, it creates a permanent and a temporary cavity as illustrated in Figure 16-1. High-velocity projectiles are classified as those traveling greater than 750 m/s. The permanent cavity is created by direct contact with the projectile. This is the area that experiences the greatest amount of tissue damage. Projectiles usually follow a tumbling motion, known as yaw, within the tissue which can increase tissue destruction. The temporary cavity is created by the transfer of kinetic energy from the projectile to surrounding tissues (like an energy shock wave). The higher the velocity of the projectile, the more kinetic energy trans-ferred and the greater the production of energy which causes tissues to stretch and tear beyond the radius of the projectile, as shown in Figure 16-1. This effect is very brief, lasting only a few milliseconds.

Projectiles may fragment and ricochet within the body damaging other structures. Solid and dense organs tend to shatter, and they are disrupted to a greater degree by high-velocity projectiles and the temporary cavity created by the transfer of kinetic energy. Elastic tissue can be directly injured or stretched and damaged by the temporary cavity. The risk of infection and sepsis is high if certain organs, such as the bowel, are ruptured or perforated. The wound can become contaminated from dirt, debris, or clothing which is due to a vacuum effect caused by the velocity of the penetrating object. Finally, bleeding from damaged blood vessels or organs into the abdominal cavity is potentially life threatening.

SURGICAL PROCEDURE

Exploratory or diagnostic laparotomy is used to visualize and examine the structures inside of the abdominal cavity to determine the extent of injury or source of pain and to perform repairs if needed. A GSW to the abdomen is an indication for an exploratory laparotomy. Sometimes a single incision extending from the xiphoid process to pubic symphysis is used, especially during trauma surgery. An upper midline incision extends from the xiphoid process to the umbilicus and a lower midline incision is limited by the umbilicus superiorly and by the pubic symphysis inferiorly. The midline incision allows wide access to most of the abdominal cavity. The objectives of a laparotomy are to locate and control hemorrhage, identify bowel injuries and manage fecal contamination within the peritoneum, locate and manage injuries to organs or supporting structures, and, finally, to determine whether definitive repair is needed.

Equation 16-1 Newton's Law of Kinetic Energy
Kinetic energy $= \frac{1}{2}$(Mass $\times$ Velocity^2)

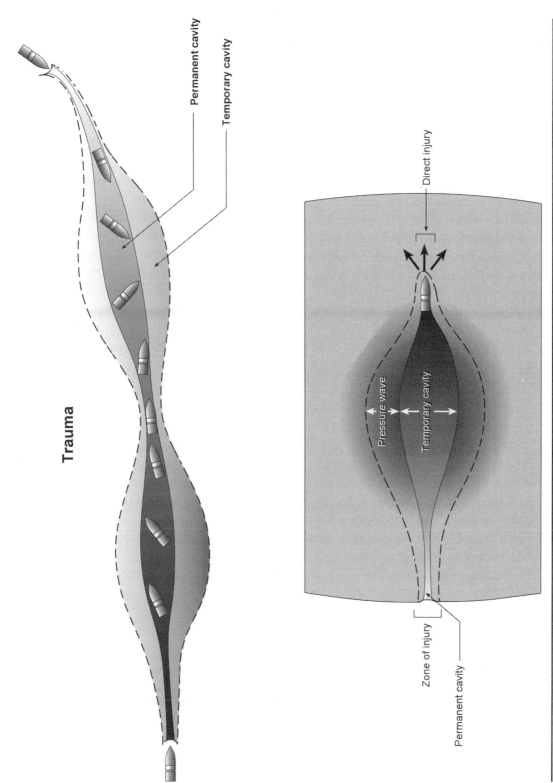

Figure 16-1 *The cavities produced as a penetrating missile passes through tissue.*

ANESTHETIC MANAGEMENT AND CONSIDERATIONS

Preoperative Period

1. Discuss the importance of a head-to-toe physical exam for this patient.

The head-to-toe physical exam allows the anesthetist to identify deficiencies in airway, breathing, or circulation, as well as to assess the possibility of tissues and/or organs damaged. Each part of the body should be inspected and palpated for pain, tenderness, crepitus, or injury, including the posterior when patients are supine. In critically ill trauma patients, assessment and treatment of traumatic injuries occurs concomitantly by a trauma team.

2. Identify the rationale for administering antibiotics during the preoperative period.

Traumatic injuries can introduce pathogens into the body. Pathogens may enter the body via the penetrating object, the skin, the victim's clothing, any foreign material that enters or gets sucked into the wound, or by the perforation and spillage of stomach or colon contents into the peritoneum. A broad-spectrum antibiotic, which covers gram-positive and gram-negative bacteria, such as a third- or fourth-generation cephalosporin agents combined with metronidazole (Flagyl) is recommended by the American College of Surgeons to treat wound contamination and infection.

3. Describe the types of monitoring that are required during exploratory laparotomy for a gun shot wound.

Electrocardiograph (ECG), noninvasive blood pressure, and pulse oximetry are often initiated in prehospital treatment and continued throughout emergency treatment and the perioperative period. End tidal carbon dioxide should be monitored once the airway is controlled and because the patient can rapidly loose heat core temperature monitoring should be initiated. Depending on the severity of the injury and the intraoperative course,

additional monitoring may include invasive blood pressure monitoring via an arterial catheter, central line placement with central venous pressure monitoring, placement of a Swan-Ganz catheter to monitor pulmonary artery and wedge pressures, and/or intracranial pressure monitoring via an intraventricular catheter or a subarachnoid bolt.

4. Discuss the need for intravenous (IV) access that is required for this injury.

At least two large-bore IV (14–18 gauge) should be placed during initial assessment in the upper extremities. Additional large-bore IV catheters should be placed if multiple fluid and blood product administration is anticipated. The external or internal jugular, femoral, or subclavian veins can be considered for central venous catheter placement. A level I transfusion infuser should be available for rapid administration of fluid and blood products.

5. Discuss which laboratory values should be monitored.

Serial laboratory evaluation should include hemoglobin, hematocrit, and platelets; serum chemical constituents including sodium, potassium, magnesium, carbon dioxide, blood urea nitrogen, creatinine, and calcium; and serum coagulation studies consisting of prothrombin time, international normalized ratio (INR), and partial thromboplastin time. If major hemorrhaging occurs, large blood transfusions are instituted, or if the patient's medication regimen dictates, these values should be repeated as long as clinically relevant. Additionally, blood glucose and arterial blood gas values should be continuously evaluated.

If a significant amount of banked blood is transfused, the patient may develop acute hypocalcemia. The preservative that is used to store blood is citrate, phosphate, dextrose, and adenine (CPDA). Citrate chelates or binds free ionized calcium decreasing its availability for physiologic functioning. The symptoms associated with acute hypocalcemia are listed

Table 16-1　Symptoms Associated with Acute Hypocalcemia

Perioral tingling (early symptom of hypocalcemia)

Paresthesia (early symptom of hypocalcemia)

Tetany

Muscle spasms

Weakness

Hyperactive tendon reflexes

Laryngospasm

Bronchospasm

Hypotension

Cardiac dysrhythmias

ECG changes (prolonged QT interval, widened QRS complex, and/or flattened T wave)

in Table 16-1. The treatment for acute hypocalcemia is to administer intravenous calcium chloride. Administration of calcium should be guided by serial blood calcium values.

6. Compare and contrast the injuries that are caused by a high-velocity missile (HVM) and a low-velocity missile (LVM) wounds.

LVMs travel at lower velocities, between 100 and 300 m/s, and exert a relatively low amount of energy, between 10 and 300 joules. LVMs crush and lacerate the surrounding tissues and structures that are in their path to form a drill hole wound, known as the permanent cavity. This cavity approximates the same diameter as the bullet. They produce a small temporary cavity and these types of missiles may fragment or ricochet within the body damaging other structures.

HVMs travel at greater than 750 m/s, and exert a greater amount of energy, between 2000 and 3000 joules. The amount of energy transferred to surrounding tissues can create a temporary cavity 10–20 times the size of the permanent cavity during an HVM injury. An illustration of an HVM wound is shown in Figure 16-1. The temporary cavity expands

and collapses in a very short period of time causing tissues to stretch and tear. Additionally, debris can be sucked into the wound consequently leading to wound infection.

7. Describe how tetrahydrocannabinol (THC) affects anesthesia during both acute and chronic use.

The main substance that causes the drug effect in marijuana is THC. THC is extremely lipid soluble with a half-life of up to 59 hours. Acute marijuana use decreases the anesthetic requirement (decreasing minimum alveolar concentration [MAC]) due to its central nervous system depressant effects. Chronic use (this patient denies currently using) increases the anesthetic requirement (increasing MAC) due to liver enzyme induction. Similar to smoking cigarettes, chronic marijuana smoke can increase secretion production and airway hyperactivity, result in alveolar destruction, and decrease lung compliance consistent with chronic obstructive pulmonary disease.

8. Describe how acute alcohol intoxication and chronic abuse affects anesthesia.

Acute ingestion of alcohol decreases the anesthetic requirements (decreasing MAC) due to its depressant effects. Additionally, alcohol has an inhibitory effect on the release of antidiuretic hormone. Therefore, patients who have consumed a large amount of alcohol can develop hypovolemia. This fact coupled with the vasodilation and myocardial depression associated with inhaled anesthetic agents can result in severe hypotension, especially if the situation is complicated due to hemorrhage. There is the potential for withdrawal, resulting in tremors or seizures during the postoperative course. Long-acting benzodiazepines, such as diazepam (Valium) and chlordiazepoxide (Librium), have been shown to be a safe and effective treatment for alcohol withdrawal. Chronic ingestion of alcohol increases the anesthetic requirement (increasing MAC) due to enzyme induction. Long-term abuse can result in hepatocellular degeneration and decreased production of coagulation factors.

9. Describe how acute and chronic use of stimulants such as amphetamines or cocaine affects anesthesia.

Acute ingestion of stimulants, such as cocaine or amphetamines, increases the anesthetic requirement (increasing MAC) due to stimulation of the sympathetic nervous system. These chemical substances are thought to increase the release or decrease the reuptake of catecholamines from postsynaptic adrenergic nerve terminals. Intense vasoconstriction occurs as a result of continuous catecholamine stimulation. When anesthesia is administered, there is a potential for severe hypotension due to vasodilation especially in the presence of hypovolemia.

Chronic use decreases or has no effect on the anesthetic requirement due to continual sympathetic nervous system stimulation and the possible depletion of catecholamines. For patients who are acutely intoxicated or chronically abusing stimulants, it is recommended that use of a direct-acting vasopressor, such as phenylephrine, be administered. A summation of the physiologic effects and their influence on anesthetic management is present in Table 16-2.

Intraoperative Period

10. Describe the physiologic changes that are associated with induction of anesthesia in a hypovolemic patient.

Anesthesia induction agents (with the exception of ketamine and to a lesser degree etomidate) cause direct myocardial depression and decrease systemic vascular resistance in a dose-dependent manner. Even mild decreases in systemic vascular resistance in the presence of significant hypovolemia can lead to severe hypotension. The anesthetic management for severe hypotension should be individualized to the specific patient; however, decreasing the anesthetic depth, infusing fluids or blood products, and considering administering a vasopressor should be considered.

11. Discuss the physiologic consequences of aspiration in the trauma patient.

Trauma patients are at risk for aspiration as a result of the possibility of a full stomach and the potential for decreased airway reflexes. Aspiration of gastric contents can lead to pulmonary aspiration, aspiration pneumonitis, airway obstruction, and hypoxemia.

12. Construct a plan as it relates to induction of anesthesia for this patient.

Initiating a fluid bolus of 500–1000 ml prior to induction in order to decrease the severity of hypotension is prudent. A hemodynamic goal should include maintenance of systolic blood pressure greater than 90 mm Hg. Oxygen (O_2) administration at 100% should be given at least 5 minutes prior to induction of anesthesia to increase the hemoglobin O_2 saturation during the period of apnea following induction. The goal of preoxygenation is to achieve an SpO_2 value of greater than 90%.

Suction should be readily available. A rapid sequence induction using cricoid pressure is the standard of care in all trauma patients. Succinylcholine or rocuronium may be used for neuromuscular blockade. Etomidate may be used for induction of anesthesia due to their relatively stable hemodynamic profile. Propofol, in small doses, may be used if blood pressure is stable. Hypnotics, such as midazolam, may be administered to prevent recall or to provide sedation for patients who are anxious. Narcotics are frequently used because traumatic injuries can cause severe pain.

13. Discuss the intraoperative anesthetic maintenance for this patient.

Administration of sedative and amnesic medications should be titrated according to the patient's blood pressure. A high percentage of oxygen

Table 16-2 Physiologic Effects and Anesthetic Considerations Associated with Acute Substance Abuse		
STIMULANTS	**SUBSTANCE PHYSIOLOGIC EFFECTS**	**ANESTHETIC CONSIDERATIONS**
Cocaine and amphetamines	Tachycardia, hypertension, dys-rhythmias, mydriasis, hyperreflexia, euphoria, hyperpyrexia, sweating	May require increased doses of anesthetic agents; amphetamine users may have loose or rotting teeth
Phencyclidine (PCP) and lysergic acid diethylamide (LSD)	Tachycardia, hypertension, hallu-cinations, weak analgesic effects, psychosis in high doses	May require increased doses of anesthetic agents; PCP produces dissociative anesthesia with increased doses
DEPRESSANTS		
Cannabis	Tachycardia, labile blood pressure, euphoria, dysphoria, hunger	May require decreased doses of anesthetic agents; may exhibit hyperactive airway and increased secretions
Opioids	Respiratory depression, hypotension, bradycardia, constipation, euphoria, miosis	May require decreased doses of anesthetic agents; IV access may be difficult in heroin users

should be administered throughout the periop-erative course due to the possibility of decreased tissue perfusion. Nondepolarizing muscle relax-ation should be provided to facilitate abdom-inal exposure during exploratory laparotomy. Anesthetic maintenance can be achieved using inhalational agents, or in combination with IV medications such as propofol and opioids, and these medications should be titrated to the hemo-dynamic response. If the trauma patient can-not sustain an adequate blood pressure while anesthetic agents are being administered, these medications should be abandoned in favor of hemodynamic support while maintaining ade-quate neuromuscular blockade.

The patient with a major traumatic injury has a 10–43% chance of intraoperative recall. Scopolamine 0.2–0.4 mg administered intramuscularly (IM) or IV can help prevent recall if other hypnotic medications cannot be administered because of the patient's critical hemodynamic profile. Scopolamine crosses the blood-brain barrier and can cause amnesia within 10 minutes of administration for up to 2 hours.

14. Explain the risks associated with administering nitrous oxide (N_2O) for the trauma patient.
The use of nitrous oxide can be problematic because of it is highly diffusible and has a propensity to accumulate in closed air spaces. If administered, it can worsen gas-containing conditions such as pneumothorax, pneumocephalus, air embolism, or obstructed bowel. These conditions may not occur, but over time the effects of nitrous oxide may become clinically relevant. For these reasons nitrous oxide is best avoided in the trauma patient.

15. Examine the use of various IV fluids and blood products for a trauma patient.
Crystalloid solutions such as lactated ringers and sodium chloride are used as initial volume expand-ers while awaiting blood for transfusion. The intravascular half life of crystalloids is 20–30 min-utes. Large volumes of crystalloid administration should be calculated and based on the patient's kilogram weight. Overzealous IV hydration can cause acute pulmonary edema. Colloid solutions such as hextend, hetastarch, and albumin are

administered for intravascular fluid deficits prior to the arrival of blood for transfusion or for conditions associated with large protein losses (i.e., burn injuries). Blood products such as packed red blood cells (PRBC), fresh frozen plasma (FFP), platelets, and cryoprecipitate are used to replace blood and clotting factors which can become deficient in the trauma patient. The patient's specific blood type should be evaluated and requested from the blood bank for administration. If life-threatening hypovolemia ensues, O-negative blood can be used for immediate transfusion.

The anesthetist should be aware that when administering large volumes of PRBCs (greater than 5 units), FFP and platelets should be added to avoid or treat coagulation abnormalities. The most common cause of continuous bleeding after extreme volume resuscitation is dilutional thrombocytopenia. Patients with decreasing platelet values of less than 100,000 µl should receive a platelet transfusion. The anesthetist should consider infusing 2–4 units of FFP and 4–6 units of platelets after infusion of 8–10 units of PRBCs (1 blood volume in a 70-kg person). Cryoprecipitate, which contains factor VIII, von Willebrand factor, and fibrinogen, can be used to treat thrombocytopenia and/or hypofibrinogenemia.

16. List the signs and symptoms of intraoperative hemorrhage.

The signs and symptoms associated with acute hemorrhage include:

- Hypotension
- Tachycardia
- Decreased urine output
- Decreased central venous pressure/pulmonary capillary wedge pressure
- Diminishing hematocrit values

Repeated surgical suctioning, use of multiple saturated lap-sponge pads, blood in the surgical field, and/or blood around the surgical field (i.e., on the floor) are further evidence of large amounts of blood loss. Some trauma patients can have a severe decrease in blood pressure caused by additional hemorrhage after incision because of the release of a blood clot that has been causing a tamponade effect within the abdominal vasculature.

17. Discuss the potential adverse effects of a massive blood transfusion.

Coagulopathies can develop from dilution of coagulation factors from massive IV fluid and blood product administration. Hypothermia can occur due to cold IV fluid and/or blood administration. A blood transfusion reaction can result if there is an incompatibility to the blood products that are administered. Anaphylaxis can develop due to antibody/antigen reactions. Hypocalcemia can arise from large amounts of banked blood being infused. Calcium is needed during myocardial contractile excitation coupling, and hypocalcemia can cause further hypotension by decreasing myocardial contractility. Hyperkalemia may occur, though it is rare, from the high-potassium concentration contained in the banked blood preservative and from cellular breakdown. Infectious disease transmission is a potential complication. A summary of the characteristic of PRBCs is included in Table 16-3.

18. Compare and contrast the types of vasopressor medications used to maintain blood pressure in a hypovolemic, hypotensive trauma patient.

Ephedrine is a direct–indirect-acting vasopressive agent. It may not be as efficacious as a direct-acting vasopressor due to the trauma patient's potential depletion of sympathetic neurotransmitters (catecholamines), especially for those patients using stimulants. Phenylephrine is a direct-acting vasopressive agent which can directly stimulate sympathetic receptors and cause increases in systemic vascular resistance. Inotropic agents such as dopamine and small intermittent boluses of epinephrine can be used to positively stimulate

Table 16-3 Characteristics of Stored Packed Red Blood Cells	
Sodium citrate	Can lead to decreased levels of ionized calcium due to chelation of the serum ionized calcium; initially acidic, sodium citrate is converted to sodium bicarbonate in the liver and can lead to metabolic alkalosis
Deficient in platelets and clotting factors	Can lead to dilutional coagulopathy
Decreased levels of 2,3 DPG	Large replacements of 2,3 DPG-depleted blood may cause hemoglobin to have increased affinity for oxygen, leading to decreased cellular oxygenation
Increased levels of potassium	Can lead to hyperkalemia in rapid, massive blood transfusion
Microaggregates	Can cause obstruction in small capillaries (i.e., pulmonary vasculature)
Stored at 4°C	Hypothermia

sympathetic alpha and beta receptors on the heart and blood vessels resulting in increases in blood pressure and heart rate. Additionally, epinephrine in ACLS doses is used in emergency situations for resuscitative efforts.

19. List the potential complications associated with a GSW to the abdomen.
- Soft tissue injury
- Severe hemorrhage from vascular injury
- Solid organ injury
- Hollow organ injury
- Diaphragm injury
- Musculoskeletal injury
- Infection and sepsis
- Hypovolemia
- Spinal cord injury
- Death

20. List the organs that can be injured caused by a GSW to the abdomen.
- Liver
- Spleen
- Small bowel
- Large bowel
- Stomach
- Bladder

21. List the organs that can be injured by a projectile in the retroperitoneal regions.
- Kidneys
- Pancreas
- Aorta and/or vena cava

22. Discuss the surgical goals during a laparotomy for a penetrating abdominal injury.
The primary goal of a laparotomy for a penetrating abdominal injury is to stop hemorrhage. This is accomplished by initially locating injuries such as vascular damage, organ damage and/or structural injuries, and controlling hemorrhage. Other goals include controlling fecal contamination from damaged organs, and determining whether temporary repair (damage control surgery) or definitive repair of an injury should occur.

23. Explain the concept of damage control surgery (DCS).
The decision to provide DCS is made due to life-threatening injuries which necessitate a rapid decision to move the patient to the operating room for emergency surgery. The philosophy of DCS consists of controlling hemorrhage, preventing contamination, limiting sepsis, and protection from further injury. DCS is a rapid initial intervention to control

life-threatening injuries and to prevent further injury. It provides time to improve the physiologic state of the trauma patient until a more definitive surgical repair can be accomplished.

24. Explain the difference between penetrating injuries that occur to solid organs as compared to hollow organs.

Solid organs such as the liver and spleen are more vascular, dense, and are more rigid as compared to hollow organs such as the stomach and intestines. A penetrating injury to a solid organ causes shattering or fracturing which can lead to severe hemorrhage. A penetrating injury to a hollow organ leads to a perforation and spillage of contents into the peritoneum that can cause severe infections which may lead to sepsis.

25. Explain how a patient with a penetrating abdominal injury would be a risk for developing sepsis.

Intestinal perforation causes spillage of fecal matter and bacteria into the peritoneum. Sepsis can develop in as little as 2–4 hours after colon injury. The peritoneum may also be contaminated by bacteria from the penetrating object and/or foreign material from the skin. Thus, removal of the contaminating substance, irrigation of the peritoneal cavity, and serial antibiotic administration is essential.

26. Discuss the potential complications associated with a GSW in thoracic region.
- Soft tissue damage
- Pneumothorax
- Hemothorax
- Tension pneumothorax or hemothorax
- Lung contusion
- Cardiac tamponade
- Cardiac contusion
- Direct cardiac injury from projectile
- Aorta and/or vena cava laceration or transaction
- Tracheobronchial laceration or transaction

- Esophageal laceration or transaction
- Diaphragmatic injury
- Rib fracture
- Spinal cord injury
- Death

27. Describe the physiological alterations in ventilation in a patient with a penetrating abdominal injury.

Sympathetic nervous system stimulation in response to trauma causes the patient's heart rate and blood pressure to increase causing an increase in myocardial oxygen demand. The compensatory mechanism includes increasing minute ventilation. A rapid shallow pattern of breathing is not uncommon as a result of pain in the abdominal region or because of a direct lung injury. Additionally, abdominal organ injuries can lead to severe hypovolemia resulting in hypotension which can cause loss of consciousness and apnea.

28. Describe the physiologic alterations in ventilation in a patient with a penetrating thoracic injury.

Pneumothorax, hemothorax, or tension pneumothorax/hemothorax can lead to hypoventilation, hypoxia, and ventilation perfusion mismatches. Open chest injuries can lead to sucking chest wounds when air enters the thoracic cavity but is unable to leave, therefore worsening lung compression and hypoxia. Lung contusions, rib fractures, or diaphragmatic injuries can cause hypoventilation and hypoxia. Tracheobronchial disruption can cause life-threatening hypoxia and/or subcutaneous emphysema.

29. Describe the physiologic alterations in ventilation during and after an exploratory laparotomy with a large midline incision.

Manipulation of abdominal organs during open laparotomy, use of general anesthesia, and administration of neuromuscular blockade can cause pressure on the diaphragm and lungs decreasing volumes, functional residual capacity, and increasing inspiratory pressures. Edema from tissue damage may lead to abdominal compartment syndrome preventing laparotomy closure and creating pressure on the diaphragm and lungs. The increased diaphragmatic pressure increases inspiratory pressures and decreases functional residual capacity promoting atelectasis and hypoventilation. Excessive narcotic administration can lead to bradypnea or apnea. The physiologic consequences of hypoventilation can lead to hypercarbia, decreased tissue oxygenation, acidosis, and death.

30. Discuss the physiologic implications of hypothermia during exploratory laparotomy.

The trauma patient is at risk of developing hypothermia due to exposure to the environment and/or the administration of cold IV fluids. Conductive heat loss can be caused by cold beds and gurneys. Clothing is removed in order to fully assess the extent of injuries which results in radiative heat loss. The patient is exposed to convective heat loss from cold emergency and operating rooms. Physiologic alterations caused by hypothermia include:

- Impaired cardiorespiratory function
- Impaired coagulation
- Impaired hepatorenal function
- Decreased drug clearance
- Impaired immune response
- Impaired wound healing

Additionally, the oxyhemoglobin disassociation curve is shifted to the left during periods of hypothermia. The result is a greater affinity or a tighter bond between oxygen and hemoglobin that decreases oxygen delivery to the tissues.

31. Develop a plan to minimize heat loss and prevent hypothermia in a trauma patient.

Preexisting hypothermia is common in the trauma patient and is attributable to environmental exposure prior to entering the hospital, during resuscitative efforts in the emergency department, and

during the operative procedure. Interventions used to treat or minimize hypothermia include:

- Removing wet clothing
- Warming the operating room
- Using forced air warmers
- Warming intravenous fluids
- Warming/humidifying airway gases
- Heating peritoneal or pleural lavage fluids
- Extracorporeal rewarming (i.e., hemodialysis or cardiopulmonary bypass)

Postoperative Period

32. Describe the risks associated with extubation after open laparotomy and repair of a penetrating injury.

Complications from penetrating trauma and massive blood transfusions can cause acid–base disturbances, coagulopathies, and hypothermia, which may render the patient unable to maintain adequate oxygenation and ventilation without assistance. In addition, large amounts of fluid volume and/or blood replacement may lead to third spacing and pulmonary edema; this may cause a decrease in pulmonary compliance and functional residual capacity rendering the patient susceptible to oxygen desaturation. Finally, a large midline incision has the potential to cause intense postoperative pain which can lead to hypoventilation, atelectasis, hypercarbia, and acidosis. The decision to extubate the patient should be individualized to each specific situation and is best guided by factors such as arterial blood gas values, the extent of the injury and surgical intervention, other associated traumatic injuries, current hemodynamic status, and the amount of volume resuscitation.

33. Explain the concerns for postoperative pain management after penetrating abdominal injury.

Narcotic requirements may be considerable as a result of surgical trauma to the rectus abdominis muscles and the extent of the tissue damage and surgical intervention. Pain can be managed by using patient-controlled analgesia and/or parenteral narcotics. Epidural anesthesia using narcotics or low-dose local anesthetics may be considered if there is no evidence of coagulopathy. Epidural anesthesia has been shown to be beneficial for those patients with rib fractures.

34. Discuss the postoperative laboratory values which would be relevant after an open laparotomy with a massive blood transfusion.

The anesthetist should continue to monitor blood hemogram, coagulation, and chemical constituents. The following is suggested:

- Hemoglobin and hematocrit
- Platelet count
- Prothrombin time, partial thromboplastin time, INR
- Serum sodium, potassium, calcium, chloride, blood urea nitrogen, creatinine
- Blood glucose level
- Arterial blood gas values
- If disseminated intravascular coagulation is suspected or if there is evidence of unexplained bleeding, fibrin split products and a fibrinogen level should be evaluated

REVIEW QUESTIONS

1. Which is the correct method to induce and intubate a trauma patient?
   a. Rapid sequence induction (RSI) followed by airway adjunct of choice
   b. Standard induction maintaining in-line cervical stabilization
   c. Emergency cricothyrotomy
   d. Blind nasal intubation

2. Which anesthetic agent should be avoided in the acute anesthetic management of a patient with a penetrating abdominal injury?
   a. Ketamine
   b. Succinylcholine
   c. Propofol
   d. Nitrous oxide

3. Which statement regarding substance abuse is correct?
   a. Acute ingestion of alcohol increases the anesthetic requirement.
   b. Acute ingestion of marijuana decreases the anesthetic requirement.
   c. Acute ingestion of cocaine decreases the anesthetic requirement.
   d. Acute ingestion of a narcotic has no effect on the anesthetic requirement.

4. Venous air embolism can occur following trauma to which anatomic structure?
   a. Stomach
   b. Small bowel
   c. Liver
   d. Bladder

5. Which is a characteristic of a low-velocity missile wound?
   a. Produces a large temporary cavity
   b. Occurs with guns that have a high muzzle velocity
   c. Tissues are stretched and torn as a result of a large temporary cavity and a high energy shock wave.
   d. Tissue destruction can be extensive.

REVIEW ANSWERS

1. **Answer: a**
   RSI with cricoid pressure is the most correct method to induce and intubate a trauma patient due to increased possibility of aspiration. All trauma patients should be considered to have a full stomach.

2. **Answer: d**
   Nitrous oxide is highly diffusible and accumulates in closed air spaces. The use of nitrous oxide could potentially increase the size of a pneumothorax, pneumocephalus, and cause bowel distention.

3. **Answer: b**
   Acute ingestion of depressant substances decreases the anesthetic requirement. Depressants, such as alcohol, marijuana, and

narcotics, have a synergistic depressant effect when combined with anesthetic agents and, when combined, can lead to marked hypotension and bradycardia.

4. **Answer: c**

The liver is extremely vascular and large vessels, such as the portal vein hepatic artery and hepatic vein, can be damaged. Injury to the liver or associated vasculature can result in the entrainment of air within the venous system leading to a venous air embolism.

5. **Answer: d**

Low-velocity missiles have the potential to fragment and ricochet within the body, which, depending on the tissue or structures damaged, can lead to extensive tissue destruction.

SUGGESTED READINGS

Barton CR. Trauma anesthesia. In: Nagelhout JJ, Zaglaniczny KL, eds. *Nurse Anesthesia*. St. Louis, MO: Elsevier Saunders, 2005:810–827.

Capan LM, Miller SM. Trauma and burns. In: Barash PG, Cullen BF, Stoelting RK, eds. *Clinical Anesthesia*. Philadelphia: Lippincott Williams & Wilkins, 2006:1262–1297.

Cherry RA, Eachempati SR, Hydo L, et al. The role of laparoscopy in penetrating abdominal stab wounds. *Surg Laparosc Endosc Percutan Tech* 2005; 15(1):14–17.

Holcomb JB, Wade CE, Michalek JE, et al. Increased plasma and platelet to red blood cell ratios improves outcome in 466 massively transfused civilian trauma patients. *Ann Surg* 2008;248(3):447–458.

Massive transfusion and control of hemorrhage in the trauma patient. International Trauma Anesthesia and Critical Care Society. Available online at http://www.itaccs.com. Accessed June 18, 2008.

Johnson JW, Gracias VH, Schwab CW, et al. Evolution in damage control for exsanguinating penetrating abdominal injury. *J Trauma* 2001;51(2):261–271.

Kirkpatrick AW, Ball CG, D'Amours SK, et al. Acute resuscitation of the unstable adult trauma patient: bedside diagnosis and therapy. *Can J Surg* 2008;51(1):57–69.

Riskin DJ, Spain DA, Hill CC, et al. Trauma surgery. In: Jaffe RA, Samuels SI, eds. *Anesthesiologists Manual of Surgical Procedures*. Philadelphia: Lippincott Williams & Wilkins, 2009:713–740.

Wilson WC. Anesthesia considerations for abdominal trauma. In: Smith CE, ed. *Trauma Anesthesia*. New York: Cambridge University Press, 2008:155–171.

Yoganandan N, Pintar FA, Kumaresan S, et al. Dynamic analysis of penetrating trauma. *J Trauma* 1997; 42(2):266–272.

Blunt Thoracic Injuries

17

Matthew D'Angelo

KEY POINTS

- Blunt trauma to the chest is the third leading cause of traumatic injury.
- Lung injury is the most common problem resulting from thoracic trauma.
- A pneumothorax occurs in as many as 40% of all blunt thoracic injuries.
- Signs of cardiac tamponade are associated with Beck's triad, which includes jugular venous distention, muffled heart sounds, and hypotension.

CASE SYNOPSIS

A 65-year-old woman arrives in the emergency department after sustaining injuries in a motor vehicle accident (MVA). She was the driver of a sport utility vehicle who was struck by another vehicle at approximately 60 mph. She was wearing her seatbelt and the airbags deployed.

The patient arrives to the trauma center wearing a cervical collar and on a backboard. She is presently complaining of mild shortness of breath. The emergency medical technician reports that the patient has sustained an open left femur fracture. Her electrocardiogram (ECG) tracing shows normal sinus rhythm with occasional premature ventricular contractions.

PREOPERATIVE EVALUATION AND DEMOGRAPHIC DATA

Past Medical/Surgical History

- Osteoporosis
- Hyperlipidemia.
- Caesarian section 35 years ago, spinal anesthesia administered, no problems noted

List of Medications

- Fosamax
- Lipitor

Diagnostic Data

- Initial chest x-ray was significant for multiple rib fractures to the left side of her chest
- Open left femur fracture

Height/Weight/Vital Signs

- 160 cm, 73 kg
- Blood pressure, 132/68; heart rate, 122 beats per minute; respiratory rate, 16 breaths per minute; room air oxygen saturation, 93% on 6 liters of oxygen administered by nasal cannula

Physical Exam

The primary trauma assessment is rapidly completed upon arrival. The patient presents with an obvious orthopedic injury and complains of significant shoulder and left chest pain. She has a cervical neck collar in place and is secured to a backboard. Her breath sounds are diminished bilaterally.

PATHOPHYSIOLOGY

Blunt trauma to the chest is the third leading cause of traumatic injury; closely following traumatic brain injury and extremity trauma. In developed nations, thoracic trauma is most often associated with motor vehicle collisions. Blunt thoracic trauma patients present a unique series of concerns for the trauma team. These patients are frequently severely injured and multisystem involvement commonly occurs. Blunt injuries account for nearly 25–50% of all traumatic deaths.

Pulmonary Injuries

The most commonly reported thoracic injuries are associated with the lungs and include pulmonary contusion, pneumothorax, and hemothorax. These injuries are most consistent with high-velocity trauma and are associated with abrupt deceleration. A pulmonary contusion represents the most common lung injury. It is reported that as many as 70% of patients who sustain blunt thoracic traumatic injuries have some degree of pulmonary contusion. The pathologic mechanism of a pulmonary contusion

includes injuries to the alveoli without disruption of the distal air sacks. The result is a *bruise* to the lung tissue resulting in the disruption of the alveolar capillary membrane which allows protein-rich fluid to exit the pulmonary capillaries and collect within the alveolar capillary interstitium and alveoli. Due to the widening of the pulmonary capillary membrane, pulmonary contusions result in varying degrees of reduced gas diffusion. The degree of hypoxia and hypercarbia that is induced may or may not be clinically relevant.

Pneumothoraces occur in as many as 40% of all blunt thoracic injuries. The size and location of the pneumothorax may vary throughout the lung field. It is estimated that as many as 50% of pneumothoraces are not initially detected by radiographic analysis. This presents a number of intraoperative management issues and may alter an anesthetic plan. Like a pneumothorax, acute identification of a hemothorax is unreliable with conventional radiology. The use of early computed tomography (CT) has increased early detection, with nonoperative management via tube thoracoscopy. Despite the possibility of minimal intervention, the anesthetist needs to monitor blood loss from the chest tube and anticipate acute decomposition and massive hemorrhage (> 1500 ml).

This patient has sustained multiple rib fractures to the left aspect of her chest. Rib fractures are associated with a pneumothorax, hemothorax, and/or thoracic vascular injury. Since nitrous oxide is highly diffusible and decreases the total fraction of inspired concentration, its use during this patient's anesthetic course is contraindicated.

Chest Wall Injuries

Injuries to the chest wall are a common finding in blunt chest trauma, resulting in nearly 50% of trauma admissions. Injuries can vary from individual rib fractures to a flail chest. The most common chest wall injury is a rib fracture. While often clinically insignificant, this finding may serve as sign of underlying pathology and pulmonary injury. Fractures to the first three ribs is associated with significant underlying injury. The scapulae and thoracic musculature protects the upper thorax and fractures that occur to the first three ribs are reflective of a high-energy trauma. This injury is associated with brachial plexus and subclavian vascular injuries. An injury that involves the lower three ribs is associated with kidney, liver, and splenic injuries.

A flail chest is defined as a series of three or more contiguous ribs that are fractured at two or more places. These fractures typically occur on the anterior or anterior lateral surface of the chest. A flail chest produces paradoxical chest wall movement during spontaneous breathing. In addition to causing respiratory compromise and extreme pain, flail chest is indicative of significant thoracic injury. It is estimated that more than 50% of patients who endure a flail chest will require surgical intervention in order to repair additional thoracic injuries.

Cardiac Injuries

The incidence of blunt cardiac trauma is between 5% and 50% depending on the definition and the clinical criteria used to evaluate cardiac injuries. Blunt cardiac trauma, similar to pulmonary injuries, result from occult injury to the thorax, deceleration injuries, and compression of the heart against bony structures such as the sternum. Blunt cardiac trauma are categorized into those that are low- and high-energy events.

Low-energy blunt cardiac injuries are typically a result of a sudden strike to the precordium. While the mechanism can vary widely, these injuries can be caused by objects such as a baseball or fist. The effect of this injury can result in ventricular fibrillation or cardiac arrest depending on the severity of the impact time the trauma is sustained and its relation to the cardiac cycle. Advanced cardiac life support procedures will begin prior to hospital admission and the anesthetist will assist with cardiopulmonary resuscitation. High-energy blunt cardiac injuries are a result of tremendous force that is transferred to the cardiac tissue resulting in significant injury. Sequelae can range from lethal arrhythmias to myocardial septal rupture and massive hemorrhage. Perioperative management is variable and depends

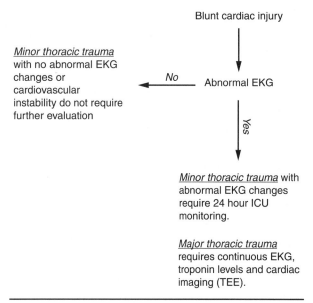

Figure 17-1 *Management of blunt cardiac injuries.*

on the extent of the injury. Clinical management can range from cardiac monitoring and assessing a cardiac enzyme profile to emergency thoracotomy and cardiac repair. Figure 17-1 describes various treatment strategies that depicts a treatment algorithm that is dependent on the severity of the blunt cardiac injury that is sustained.

Thoracic Vascular Injuries

Injuries sustained to the thoracic aorta injuries are caused by rapid deceleration resulting in intimal tears of the thoracic aorta and often occur near the left subclavian artery. If untreated, thoracic aortal injuries can result in vascular rupture and death. In the United States, the majority of injuries to the thoracic aorta result from motor vehicle collisions, which accounts for 10–15% of motor vehicle fatalities.

Surgical management of thoracic aortic injuries has evolved from open vascular repair to endovascular stent grafting (EVSG). This advance in management has demonstrated a significant reduction in morbidity and mortality for these patients. Initial management for thoracic aortic injuries should focus on deliberate blood pressure control and blood replacement. Perioperative goals should include meticulous blood pressure control to reduce sheer wall stress and the risk of aortic rupture. The exact "range" of blood pressure measurements that should be achieved for patients with cardiac tamponade remains unclear. Maintenance of the systolic blood pressure less than or equal to 100 mm Hg is reasonable. Pharmacologic adjuncts such as beta-blockers (esmolol) and nitrates can be used to acutely control hypertension.

Airway Injuries

Airway injuries represent a potentially lethal consequence associated with blunt thoracic trauma. The relative infrequency of airway injuries that are treatable in a trauma center (0.2–8.0%) is likely due to high incidence of rapid mortality that occurs at the site of the accident and is associated with this injury. Recognition of the presence of airway injuries is often challenging. Patients with associated airway trauma that are treated at a trauma center are often unrecognized during the primary assessment despite airway management, direct laryngoscopy, and endotracheal tube (ETT) placement. This is because the majority of thoracic airway injuries occur below the level of the carina and definitive diagnosis is only possible during direct visual inspection by bronchoscopy or CT examination. Nevertheless, the management of a patient with a recognized or unrecognized airway injury is the same; if hypoxia, acidosis, and respiratory distress are evident, airway management and ETT intubation is mandatory.

ANESTHETIC MANAGEMENT AND CONSIDERATIONS

1. Describe the immediate concerns regarding airway management for a patient who has sustained a high-energy blunt thoracic injury from an MVA.
Blunt thoracic trauma that is associated with a high-energy mechanism poses significant issues for both the surgical and anesthesia teams. Following advanced trauma life support (ATLS) protocol, airway assessment is the first priority of management for this patient. Acute respiratory distress or impending respiratory failure will require immediate

airway intervention. A delay in airway management can result in severe hypoxemia and acidosis which will result in cardiopulmonary decompensation. Chapter 14 describes the appropriate procedure for performing a rapid sequence induction (RSI) technique for this patient.

There is a high probability of pulmonary injury as a result of high-energy blunt thoracic injuries and the anesthetist should be prepared to manage a variety of potential complications. The anesthetist should anticipate rapid desaturation upon induction. While all thoracic injuries are concerning, reductions in functional residual capacity (FRC) from injury or a pneumothorax may exacerbate arterial hypoxemia. Rapid desaturation should be anticipated. Simple techniques, such as prolonged and thorough preoxygenation, will be beneficial. During cricoid pressure, the anesthetist should consider bag-valve-mask ventilation using minimal peak pressures to maintain oxygenation and avoid sustained periods of desaturation. The risk of gastric aspiration exists; however, severe hypoxemia that occurs over the course of several minutes will have a negative effect on the patient's postoperative neurologic condition.

Once the ETT is in place and the location is confirmed, the patient should be closely monitored for signs of an unrecognized pneumothorax and/or tension pneumothorax. It should be remembered, that the absence of a pneumothorax on radiograph does not guarantee that there is not an injury to the lung. Additionally, a tension pneumothorax is a clinical diagnosis made on the basis of cardiovascular collapse after positive pressure ventilation ensues. Needle decompression on the affected side at the second intercostal space at the midclavicular line or chest tube thoracoscopy should be performed immediately if decompensation occurs.

2. Describe acute respiratory distress syndrome (ARDS) and the clinical criteria to recognize this condition.
ARDS occurs acutely within the first 24–48 hours after traumatic injury and can occur as a result

of direct pulmonary injury (aspiration, blunt thoracic trauma) or extrapulmonary injury such as sepsis or multiple organ dysfunction syndrome. The diagnosis is based on several factors which include a PaO_2/FiO_2 ratio of < 200 mm Hg, acute onset, the presence of hypoxia, and specific cause such as thoracic trauma. The pathologic progression occurs over a 21- to 28-day span. The acute phase of ARDS occurs over the first 7 days of injury. Tissue trauma causes activation of inflammatory mediators which causes leakage of protein-rich fluid from the capillaries that accumulates into the alveolar capillary membrane and alveoli and causes diffuse alveolar disruption and fibrosis. As a result, atelectasis occurs due to the dilution of surfactant and injury to type II pneumocytes. The thickening of the alveolar septum caused by the formation of edema leads to a reduction in gas diffusion, increased ventilation perfusion mismatching, hypoxemia, and hypercarbia. In severe cases, arterial hypoxemia results in hypoxic pulmonary vasoconstriction and can potentially lead to acute congestive heart failure which is a common cause of rapidly increasing pulmonary pressure. While ARDS is a progressive disorder, the primary challenge for the anesthetist is to maintain a normal PaO_2 to provide adequate ventilation and to avoid barotrauma. Decreased pulmonary compliance commonly results in increased peak airway pressures.

3. Describe an appropriate ventilation strategy for a patient who has sustained a pulmonary contusion caused by blunt trauma. The patient's intraoperative situation during mechanical ventilation includes SpO_2, 91%; arterial hypoxemia (PaO_2 is 97 mm Hg with an FiO_2 of 0.5); and increased ventilating pressures are required to achieve an adequate tidal volume (Tv).

Unlike elective surgery, canceling or postponing surgery for patients who have sustained major traumatic injuries is not possible and delaying the operative procedure may result in increased morbidity and mortality. While complex, managing

pulmonary injuries is a common challenge that faces the anesthetist. Providing adequate oxygenation while minimizing excessive peak airway pressures and dead space ventilation are the ventilatory goals.

A variety of ventilation strategies have been described to best manage intraoperative ventilation for patient with an acute lung injury (ALI). Techniques vary from conventional strategies to inverse ratio ventilation (IRV). Unfortunately, a definitive protocol that outlines the "best practice" for managing ALI during the perioperative period does not currently exist. The findings of the ARDSnet study randomized patients with ALI to a low Tv (6 ml/kg) group or a high tidal volume (10–15 ml/kg) group. The amount of tidal that was used was based on ideal body weights and plateau and peak airway pressure were monitored over a 28-day period. A significant reduction in mortality and the number of days that patients were ventilator dependent occurred in the group that received low tidal volumes.

Intraoperative management for this patient should be focused on maximizing oxygenation and ventilation without causing further pulmonary injury and compromise. Nitrous oxide should be avoided to due to the potential expansion of an unrecognized pneumothorax. Oxygen should be diluted with air and titrated to the lowest inspired oxygen concentration to maintain an arterial oxygen saturation greater than 60 mm Hg. Inhalational anesthetics will reduce hypoxic pulmonary vasoconstriction (HPV) in a dose-dependent fashion. While changes to HPV have been demonstrated in the laboratory, the clinical relevance has not been demonstrated.

As previously discussed, ALI/ARDS can cause noncardiogenic pulmonary edema that results in atelectasis and reduced gas diffusion, which often requires higher pressures to adequately facilitate positive pressure ventilation. Increasing the pressure during mechanical ventilation likely increases ventilation/perfusion mismatching and high-pressure alveolar trauma.

Management of these patients should focus on treating the cause of hypoxemia (i.e., atelectasis). An appropriate ventilation strategy for this patient would begin with a low Tv approximately 6–8 ml/kg, a respiratory rate of 12–14 breaths per minute and positive-end expiratory pressure (PEEP). It is recommended that plateau pressures be maintained less than 30 cm H_2O in order to reduce ventilator-associated barotrauma. The plateau phase of mechanical ventilation represents the longest period of alveolar stretch during the ventilation cycle. Peak airway pressures should be closely monitored; however, plateau pressures are more accurate in predicting high-pressure barotrauma. Figure 17-2 represents the zone for optimal ventilation.

The primary role of PEEP during mechanical ventilation is to maintain alveolar patency during exhalation, avoiding derecruitment or collapse. In addition, PEEP can increase the overall mean airway pressure during positive pressure ventilation, facilitating gas diffusion across the alveolar membrane. This is essential for the patient with ALI/ARDS. While there is no consistent recommendation for the amount of PEEP that should be administered to patients with ALI/ARDS because lung compliance and opening pressures vary, many anesthetists initiate PEEP at 8–10 cm H_2O. Table 17-1 summarizes the strategies that can be used to help manage patients who have developed ALI/ARDS.

Table 17-1	Perioperative Strategies Used to Manage Patients with ARDS

- Maintain tidal volume at 6–8 mL/kg
- Minimize peak inspiratory pressure < 30 cm H_2O
- PEEP
- Pressure ventilation mode
- Inverse ratio ventilation
- High frequency jet ventilation
- Avoid aggressive fluid therapy if possible

4. Discuss the pathophysiology, symptomatology, and treatment for cardiac tamponade.

Cardiac tamponade is an accumulation of blood that pools within the pericardium from an intramyocardial perforation or coronary artery laceration. This type of injury is consistent with a high-speed MVA and associated rib fractures. The fibrous pericardium is extremely durable and as little as 50 to 100 ml of acute blood accumulation in this area can cause death. If untreated, intrapericardial pressure progressively increases, which impinges on the heart and decreases cardiac performance. The pathogenesis associated with cardiac compressive shock includes decreased diastolic filling which decreases left ventricular volume and cardiac output. A cycle resulting from systemic hypoperfusion leads to systemic acidosis, myocardial ischemia, and worsening hypotension.

The symptomatology that can be used for diagnosis of cardiac tamponade is included in Table 17-2. Objective factors that are definitively associated with this process are described by Beck's triad which includes elevated central venous pressure resulting in jugular venous distention, muffled heart sounds, and hypotension. Since the pressure exerted on the heart is equivalently distributed on each region, left- and right-sided heart pressures will become similar. Evaluation with cardiac echocardiography is a definitive method for determining the presence of blood within the pericardium.

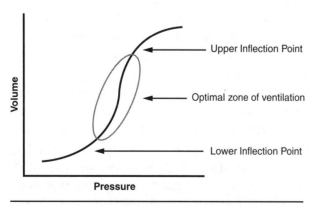

Figure 17-2   *Optimal zone of ventilation.*

Table 17-2	Signs Associated with Cardiac Tamponade

- Tachycardia
- Hypoxemia
- Hypercarbia
- Myocardial ischemia
- Dysrhythmias
- Pulsus paradoxus
- Widened mediastinum
- Decreased cardiac output
- Equivalent left- and right-sided heart pressures
- Beck's triad

The treatment that is used to treat cardiac tamponade is for the surgeon to create an opening in the pericardium, pericardial window, or to perform a pericardiocentesis. The goals of anesthetic management are to maintain preload and to minimize myocardial depression. Bradycardia will cause acute decompensation as the increased heart rate is the primary determinant of stroke volume in this situation. Due to its sympathomimetic effects, ketamine can be used for the induction of anesthesia. The use of etomidate is also acceptable.

REVIEW QUESTIONS

1. The most common injury as a result of blunt thoracic trauma is:
   a. cardiac contusion.
   b. pneumothorax.
   c. pulmonary contusion.
   d. tracheal injuries below the carina.
2. Using the recommendations of the ARDSnet, which is an appropriate range of tidal volume for a male patient who is 84 kg and 72 in tall?
   a. 350 to 500 ml
   b. 450 to 550 ml
   c. 500 to 650 ml
   d. 600 to 750 ml

3. Which factor is most predictive of the potential for barotrauma during mechanical ventilation?
   a. Plateau pressure
   b. Peak airway pressure
   c. Mean airway pressure
   d. Positive-end expiratory pressure
4. Which statement regarding blunt thoracic trauma is false?
   a. A flail chest is a continuous section of three or more rib fractures in two or more locations.
   b. ARDS is defined as a PaO_2/FiO_2 ratio less than 200 mm Hg.
   c. A chest radiograph is insensitive for detecting a pneumothorax following a blunt thoracic injury.
   d. Management of a thoracic aneurysm requires blood pressure control to decrease the heart rate and hemorrhaging.
5. Which best describes the pathologic changes that are consistent with ARDS?
   a. Ventilation perfusion mismatching is decreased.
   b. Hypercarbia occurs due to alveolar capillary membrane fibrosis.
   c. Right ventricular pressure is decreased.
   d. Atelectasis formation cause by increased surfactant.

REVIEW ANSWERS

1. **Answer: c**
   Pulmonary contusions are present in 70% of blunt thoracic injuries. The most definitive method for identification is a CT scan.
2. **Answer: c**
   Lung volumes do not increase with body weight. Appropriate Tv ventilation should be based on the patient's ideal body weight. While various methods can be used to determine ideal body weight, the formula $2.54 \times$ height in inches $- 100 =$ IBW. For the scenario described in question 2, the

patient's ideal weight is near 84 kg (calculated at 82 kg). Based on this, tidal volumes should be between 6 and 8 ml/kg as determined by the ARDSnet.

3. **Answer: a**
The plateau pressure is the longest period of alveolar distension. The ARDSnet demonstrated that plateau pressure (period of stretch) was most indicative of volu-trauma.

4. **Answer: d**
Management of an aortic aneurysm requires blood pressure control to reduce transmural pressure on the lining of the blood vessels. Increased pressure can result in further dissection of the injured vasculature leading to rupture. Blood pressure control can occur via reductions in systemic vascular resistance (SVR) or cardiac output by reducing heart rate.

5. **Answer: b**
Hypercarbia and hypoxemia occur in patients with ARDS due to alveolar capillary edema and fibrosis, increased ventilation perfusion mismatching, and atelectasis and decreased surfactant. Pulmonary hypertension occurs due to chronic hypoxia which increases right ventricular pressure.

SUGGESTED READINGS

Buchman TG, Hall BL, Bowling WM, et al. In: Tintinalli JE, Kelen GD, Stapczymski JS, eds. *Emergency Medicine A Comprehensive Study Guide*, 6th ed. New York: McGraw-Hill, 2003:1595.

Kaewlai R, Avery LL, Asrani AV, et al. Multidetector CT of blunt thoracic trauma. *Radiographics* 2008;28(6):1555–1570.

Lebl DR, Dicker RA, Spain DA, et al. Dramatic shift in the primary management of traumatic thoracic aortic rupture. *Arch Surg* 2006;141:177–180.

Lin PH, Bush RL, Zhou W, et al. Endovascular treatment of traumatic thoracic aortic injury: should this be the new standard of treatment? *J Vasc Surg* 2006;43:22A–29A.

Mattox KL, Flint LM, Carrico CJ, et al. Blunt cardiac injury (formerly termed "myocardial contusion"). *J Trauma* 1992;33:649–650.

Miller PR, Croce MA, Kilgo PD, et al. Acute respiratory distress syndrome in blunt trauma: identification of independent risk factors. *Am Surg* 2002;68(10):845–850.

Moloney JT, Fowler SJ, Chang W. Anesthetic management of thoracic trauma. *Curr Opin Anaesthesiol* 2008;21(1):41–46.

Orliaguet G, Ferjani M, Riou B. The heart in blunt trauma. *Anesthesiology* 2001;95:544–548.

Stafford RE, Linn J, Washington L. Incidence and management of occult hemothoraces. *Am J Surg* 2006;192(6):722–726.

Tomashefski J. Pulmonary pathology of acute respiratory distress syndrome. *Clin Chest Med* 2005;21(3):435–466.

Thoracic Surgery

V

Pneumonectomy

18

Mark Gabot

KEY POINTS

- Lung cancer is the second most common cancer, and the most common cause of cancer-related death in both men and women in the United States. The majority of pulmonary resection procedures are performed for the removal of lung cancer.
- The term pulmonary resection refers to a variety of procedures including: (1) segmentectomy (i.e., wedge resection), (2) lobectomy, (3) pneumonectomy (e.g., intrapericardial and extrapericardial), (4) completion pneumonectomy, (5) radical pneumonectomy, and (6) carinal pneumonectomy. Each procedure differs in terms of indication, technique, and extent of pulmonary resection.
- The anesthetist should thoroughly evaluate the degree and severity of pulmonary disease, cardiovascular disease, and comorbidities during the preoperative assessment.
- Findings from basic physical examination and preoperative testing dictate: (1) the histologic type and stage of lung cancer, (2) the need for preoperative optimization, (3) the necessity for advanced intraoperative monitoring, (4) optimal one-lung ventilation (OLV) methods, (5) perioperative risk stratification based on the patient's ability to tolerate the proposed resection, and (6) the perioperative anesthetic plan.
- OLV allows for lung separation and provides optimal surgical visualization. It can be achieved through various methods including: (1) dual-lumen endobronchial tube (ETT), (2) bronchial blocker, or (3) endobronchial intubation with a single-lumen ETT.
- Complications of pneumonectomy include: (1) cardiac herniation, (2) hemorrhage, (3) bronchial disruption, (4) arrhythmias, (5) respiratory failure, (6) right heart failure, and (7) neural injury.

CASE SYNOPSIS

A 70-year-old man is admitted to the hospital for right-sided, non–small cell lung carcinoma. He is scheduled by his thoracic surgeon to have a right extrapericardial pneumonectomy.

PREOPERATIVE EVALUATION AND DEMOGRAPHIC DATA

Past Medical/Surgical History

- Hypertension, chronic obstructive pulmonary disease, insulin-dependent diabetes mellitus, and gastroesophageal reflux disease
- Cigarette smoking: 50 pack years of cigarette smoking, stopped 1 month ago
- Computed tomography (CT) guided fine-needle biopsy: pathologic examination reveals right-sided, non–small cell lung adenocarcinoma
- Mediastinoscopy with lymph node biopsy: pathologic examination reveals no mediastinal metastases, no mediastinal lymph node involvement
- Bronchoscopy: gross visual examination reveals right bronchial involvement, without carinal extension, no tracheobronchial compression

List of Medications

- Atenolol (Tenormin)
- Albuterol (ProAir)
- Regular insulin (Novolin R)
- Omeprazole (Prilosec)

Diagnostic Data

- Hemoglobin, 15.3 g/dl; hematocrit, 45.9%; platelets 300,000 mm^3
- Electrolytes: sodium, 147 mEq/l; potassium, 4.1 mEq/l; chloride, 107 mEq/l; carbon dioxide, 30 mEq/l
- Glucose, 135 mg/dl
- Blood urea nitrogen, 12 mg/dl; creatinine 1.2 mg/dl
- Chest radiograph (anterior, posterior, and lateral): Bilateral hyperinflation with increased vascular markings. Right lung: centrally located opacity of pulmonary parenchyma, approximately 10 cm in diameter. Cardiac hypertrophy noted. No gross tracheal or bronchial deviation.
- Chest CT: Right lung, 10 cm centrally located pulmonary mass. No cardiac or tracheobronchial compression. Vascular involvement as indicated by contrast-enhanced CT.
- Chest magnetic resonance imaging (MRI): Right lung, 10 cm centrally located, high-intensity pulmonary mass. No cardiac and tracheobronchial compression.
- Pulmonary function test (pre- and postbronchodilator therapy): FVC, 3 l; FEV_1, 2 l; $FEV_1/FVC = 67\%$
- Arterial blood gas (21% oxygen): pH, 7.37; $PaCO_2$, 44 mm Hg; HCO_3, 25 mEq/l; PaO_2, 70 mm Hg
- Electrocardiogram (ECG), normal sinus rhythm, heart rate 67 beats per minute

Height/Weight/Vital Signs

- 170 cm, 83 kg
- Blood pressure, 135/86; heart rate, 65 beats per minute; respiratory rate, 25 breaths per minute; room air oxygen saturation, 95%; temperature, 36.9°C

PATHOPHYSIOLOGY

Pulmonary resection procedures have been performed for a variety of etiologies such as: (1) pulmonary masses, (2) malignant mesothelioma, (3) bronchiectasis, (4) tuberculosis, (5) and thoracic trauma. Pulmonary masses may present as benign or malignant pathology. Benign pulmonary masses include: carcinoid tumors, hemangiomas, bronchopulmonary sequestrations, and infection. The majority of pulmonary resection procedures are performed for the removal of malignant tissue (e.g., bronchogenic carcinoma).

Lung cancer is the second most common cancer (15%) and the most common cause of cancer-related deaths (29%), in both men and women in the United States. The majority of patients have an extensive history of smoking and less than 10% of patients presenting with lung cancer are nonsmokers. In these cases, lung cancer can often be attributed to environmental exposure (i.e., passive smoking) or industrial exposure (i.e., asbestos or heavy metals).

Lung cancer is traditionally divided into two categories: small cell lung carcinoma (SCLC) and non–small cell lung carcinoma (NSCLC). SCLC (e.g., oat-cell carcinoma) accounts for 25% of all lung cancer. Treatment for SCLC rarely involves surgery because patients typically present with advanced staging and metastases have frequently occurred upon initial evaluation. Endocrinopathies and paraneoplastic neurologic syndromes are common in patients with SCLC. NSCLC accounts for the remaining 75% of all lung cancer. Less than 20% of NSCLC patients present at a stage that is amendable by surgical intervention. Depending on the type and stage of lung cancer, treatment options include a combination of surgery, radiation, chemotherapy, and targeted biological therapy.

SURGICAL PROCEDURE

Extrapericardial pneumonectomy involves making a posterolateral or lateral thoracotomy incision through the fifth intercostal space allowing exposure of the pulmonary hilum and lateral mediastinum. Partial or total rib resection may be necessary to facilitate surgical visualization. Surgical evaluation of the thoracic cavity, mediastinum, pulmonary parenchyma, and all pleural surfaces are assessed. Instances of metastases, multistation lymph node involvement, and/or invasion of the major vascular and mediastinal structures preclude complete resection. Based on the patient's presenting pathology, the surgeon determines if a pneumonectomy is indicated or if a less dramatic pulmonary resection procedure can be performed.

Once the need for pneumonectomy is established and resectability is deemed favorable, the surgeon performs a methodical biopsy of the thoracic lymph nodes. Attention is then directed to the pulmonary hilum. The surgical ligation of the hilar structures includes the: (1) pulmonary artery, (2) pulmonary veins, and (3) bronchus ipsilateral to the thoracic pathology. Meticulous surgical resection is undertaken to prevent unwarranted

damage to major vascular and mediastinal structures. Surgical ligation is performed through the use of traditional sutures and/or vascular staples.

Following surgical resection and hemostasis, the affected lung is extracted though the thoracotomy incision and will be examined by a pathologist. If the surgeon desires, the in vivo bronchial stump may be reinforced with synthetic material or autografted tissue/muscle. An appropriately sized chest tube is inserted and the thoracic cavity is closed in traditional surgical fashion.

ANESTHETIC MANAGEMENT AND CONSIDERATIONS

Preoperative Period

1. Describe the anatomy of the pulmonary hilum and lungs and its bearing on pneumonectomy.

The pulmonary hilum refers to the site of contact between the lung parenchyma and the mediastinum. Figure 18-1 depicts the anatomy of the left and right pulmonary hila. The left and right pulmonary hila have four common structures: (1) the pulmonary artery; (2) superior and inferior pulmonary veins; (3) main bronchus; and (4) hilar lymph nodes. The pulmonary hila lie in intimate proximity to major vascular and mediastinal structures including the (1) heart, (2) aorta, (3) main pulmonary artery, (4) trachea, (5) esophagus, (6) vena cava, and (7) nerves (i.e., phrenic, vagus, and recurrent laryngeal nerves). Vigilance must always be exercised by the anesthetist, since surgical damage to major vascular and mediastinal structures is a constant risk.

The major function of the lungs is for gas exchange (i.e., oxygenation and ventilation), which is dependent on the quantity and quality of functional lung tissue. The right lung represents up to 60% of the total lung volume, while the left lung represents the remaining 40%. Following right-sided pneumonectomy, total lung are decreased to a greater degree than with a left-sided pneumonectomy. A right-sided pneumonectomy is therefore more physiologically taxing and is associated with a significantly higher mortality rate.

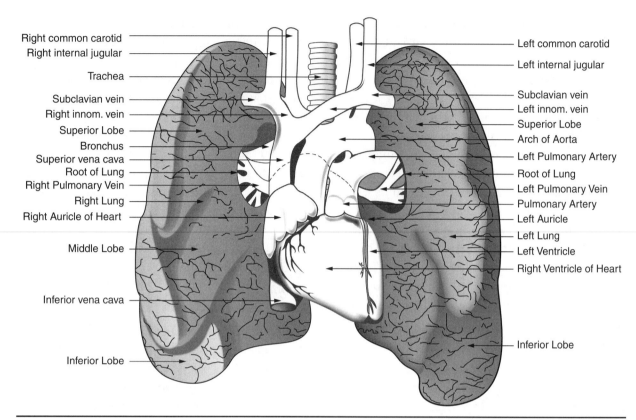

Right common carotid
Right internal jugular
Trachea
Subclavian vein
Right innom. vein
Superior Lobe
Bronchus
Superior vena cava
Root of Lung
Right Pulmonary Vein
Right Lung
Right Auricle of Heart
Middle Lobe
Inferior vena cava
Inferior Lobe

Left common carotid
Left internal jugular
Subclavian vein
Left innom. vein
Superior Lobe
Arch of Aorta
Left Pulmonary Artery
Root of Lung
Left Pulmonary Vein
Pulmonary Artery
Left Auricle
Left Lung
Left Ventricle
Right Ventricle of Heart
Inferior Lobe

Figure 18-1 *Anatomy of the left and right pulmonary hila. The left and right pulmonary hila have four common structures: (1) the pulmonary artery; (2) superior and inferior pulmonary veins; (3) main bronchus; and (4) hilar lymph nodes.*

2. Discuss an appropriate preoperative assessment for patients presenting for scheduled pneumonectomy.

As with any disease process, the optimal anesthetic plan is based on a thorough clinical evaluation and preoperative testing that should be tailored to each patient's presenting condition and symptomatology. Preoperative symptoms exhibited by patients with bronchogenic carcinoma are listed in Table 18-1. Findings from basic physical examination and preoperative testing dictate: (1) the histologic type and stage of lung cancer, (2) the need for preoperative optimization, (3) the necessity for advanced intraoperative monitoring, (4) optimal OLV methods, (5) perioperative risk stratification based on the patient's ability to tolerate the proposed resection, and (6) the perioperative anesthetic plan.

The chest radiograph is the most common preoperative test used to evaluate intrathoracic pathology. When the patient develops symptoms consistent with bronchogenic carcinoma, a chest radiograph is frequently ordered. Anterior, posterior, and lateral chest radiographs provide information regarding tumor: (1) size, (2) location, (3) density, and (4) cardiopulmonary abnormalities.

CT, MRI, and positron emission tomography (PET) studies provide more accurate information regarding tumor: (1) size, (2) location, (3) density, (4) and metabolic activity. Information from these studies is used to determine the presence, type, and stage of lung cancer. Instances of metastases to distal sites or invasion of the major vascular and mediastinal structures preclude complete resection.

Table 18-1	Preoperative Symptoms Exhibited by Patients Presenting with Bronchogenic Carcinoma	
SYMPTOM CATEGORY	**ANATOMY INVOLVED**	**SYMPTOM**
Bronchopulmonary symptoms	• Bronchial irritation	• Cough or wheezing
	• Obstruction	• Dyspnea
	• Infection	• Chest pain, rales, rhonchi, or pneumonia
	• Ulceration	• Hemoptysis
Extrapulmonary intrathoracic symptoms	• Pleura	• Pleural effusion
	• Chest wall	• Chest pain
	• Esophagus	• Dysphagia
	• Superior vena cava	• Superior vena cava syndrome
	• Pericardium	• Pericardial effusion or pericarditis
	• Brachial plexus	• Arm pain
	• Recurrent laryngeal nerves (unilateral or bilateral)	• Hoarseness or stridor
	• Spinal cord	• Parathesia or paralysis
	• Cervical sympathetic nerves	• Horner syndrome
Extrathoracic metastatic symptoms	Multiple sites throughout body	• Dependent on site and tumor involvement.
Extrathoracic nonmetastatic symptoms	• Endocrinologic syndromes	• Syndrome of inappropriate antidiuretic hormone hypersecretion (SIADH)
	• Paraneoplastic syndromes	• Cushing syndrome
		• Eaton-Lambert syndrome
Nonspecific	Variant	• Weight loss
		• Nocturnal diaphoresis
		• Anemia
		• Weakness
		• Anorexia
		• Lethargy
		• Malaise

Preoperative bronchoscopic and mediastinoscopic examination is imperative in patients presenting with bronchogenic carcinoma. Examination allows evaluation of the patient's airway and the opportunity to obtain biopsies from tracheobronchial pathology. Gross findings and pathological examination provide insight regarding: (1) histologic typing, (2) stage of lung cancer, and (3) optimal OLV methods based on abnormalities in airway anatomy.

Pulmonary function tests provide invaluable diagnostic information regarding a patient's ability to tolerate the proposed pulmonary resection (e.g., perioperative risk stratification). Pulmonary function testing should commence in a tiered approach, with each tier increasing in sensitivity,

Table 18-2 Three Tiers of Preoperative Pulmonary Function Testing and Indicators of Increased Perioperative Risk

TIER 1 WHOLE LUNG FUNCTION TESTING	TIER 2 SPLIT-LUNG FUNCTION TESTING	TIER 3 POSTOPERATIVE FUNCTIONAL CAPACITY TESTING
Arterial blood gas on room air $PaCO_2$: > 45 mm Hg **Spirometry** • FEV_1: < 2 liters • FEV_1/FVC: < 50% predicted • Maximum breathing capacity: < 50% predicted **Lung volume** RV/TLC: > 50% **Diffusing capacity CO_2** $DLCO_2$: < 60% predicted	Split-lung spirometry with DLT or regional lung radiospirometry (i.e., V/Q scan) • Predicted postoperative FEV_1: < 0.85 l or < 40% predicted • Blood flow to affected lung: > 70%	Temporary unilateral occlusion of the right or left pulmonary artery or bronchus. • Mean PA pressure: > 40 mm Hg • $PaCO_2$: > 60 mm Hg • PaO_2: < 45 mm Hg (with supplemental oxygen) • Signs of respiratory failure

specificity, and invasiveness. Table 18-2 describes the three tiers of preoperative function testing.

The pulmonary and cardiovascular systems are physiologically intertwined. Therefore, a thorough preoperative evaluation of right- and left-sided cardiac function is crucial in determining a patient's ability to tolerate pneumonectomy. Right and/or left ventricular dysfunctions (i.e., as indicated by decreased exercise capacity), indicate the need for preoperative optimization (e.g., medical management, angioplasty, or coronary artery bypass graft [CABG]) prior to surgery.

3. Describe preoperative interventions that can be used to optimize high risk patients for pneumonectomy.

The purpose of preoperative optimization is to treat or manage conditions that predispose the patient to perioperative complications (i.e., atelectasis and pneumonia), ideally decreasing morbidity and mortality in the process. Pulmonary optimization procedures include: (1) cessation of smoking, (2) bronchodilation therapy, (3) decreasing viscosity of secretions, (4) secretion mobilization, and

(5) adjunct care (e.g., pharmacologic and psychologic). As discussed previously, cardiac optimization to maximize ventricular function must be instituted prior to surgery.

Patients that present with lung cancer typically have multiple risk factors. Preoperative interventions should be implemented with consideration of "the four Ms": (1) mass effects (e.g., bronchopulmonary and extrapulmonary intrathoracic symptoms), (2) metabolic effects (e.g., endocrinopathies and paraneoplastic neurological syndromes), (3) metastases, and (4) medications (i.e., bleomycin and other chemotherapy drugs).

4. Describe contraindications to performing pneumonectomy.

The contraindications for having a pneumonectomy are due to distal metastases and/or a patient's inability to tolerate the physiological stresses of surgery. Physical examination, preoperative testing, and preoperative optimization are aimed at determining which patients are optimal surgical candidates. Table 18-3 describes contraindications to a pneumonectomy procedure.

Table 18-3	Contraindications for a Pneumonectomy Procedure

- Metastases and/or multistation lymph node involvement
- Invasion of the major vascular and/or mediastinal structures
- Inadequate pulmonary function as indicated by pulmonary function tests
- Hemodynamic instability with clamping of pulmonary artery (1 to 5 min) prior to ligation

5. Describe the significance of SCLC in a patient for pneumonectomy.

Endocrinologic abnormalities and paraneoplastic neurologic syndromes are common in patients with SCLC. Table 18-4 describes common syndromes and anesthetic considerations in patients with SCLC. SCLC cells are derived from neuroendocrine tissue and commonly produce physiologically active factors. These factors clinically manifest as paraneoplastic endocrine syndromes including syndrome of inappropriate antidiuretic hormone (SIADH) and Cushing syndrome. SIADH is present in up to 40% of patients with SCLC.

Myasthenic syndrome (e.g., Eaton-Lambert syndrome) may also be present in patients with SCLC. An autoimmune reaction between tumor-related (immunoglobulin G) antibodies and presynaptic calcium channels causes a decreased presynaptic release of acetylcholine. Clinical manifestations of myasthenic syndrome frequently precede cancer identification and should be considered in patients undergoing diagnostic procedures.

Table 18-4   Common Syndromes and Anesthetic Considerations in Patients with SCLC

	SIADH	CUSHING SYNDROME	MYASTHENIC SYNDROME
Signs and symptoms	• Increased urine osmolarity • Increased sodium concentration with serum hyponatremia • Decreased serum osmolarity	• Systemic hypertension • Hypokalemia • Hyperglycemia • Skeletal muscle weakness • Osteoporosis • Obesity • Poor wound healing	• Limb weakness (proximal, legs greater than arms) • Strength improved with exercise • Muscle pain common • Reflexes decreased or absent
Treatment	• Fluid restriction • Diuretics • Electrolyte replacement therapy	• Fluid and electrolyte therapy • Surgical treatment of primary cause	• Steroids • 3,4 diaminopyridine • Plasma exchange • Intravenous immunoglobulin
Anesthetic considerations	• Hyponatremia associated with altered consciousness • Diuretics may cause hypovolemia and hypotension with induction	• Blood pressure, electrolyte, and blood glucose management • Decreased doses of muscle relaxants • Need for postoperative ventilation possible	• Sensitive to succinylcholine • Sensitive to nondepolarizing muscle relaxants • Need for postoperative ventilation possible

Intraoperative Period

6. Describe the different classifications of pneumonectomy.

Pneumonectomy for lung carcinoma is typically performed for large and centrally located pulmonary masses untreatable by segmentectomy (e.g., wedge resection) or lobectomy. Several types of pneumonectomy exist. Selection of the type of pneumonectomy is dependent on the type, stage, and location of lung carcinoma. A standard pneumonectomy involves the sole removal of the affected lung. Intrapericardial and extrapericardial pneumonectomy refers to a standard pneumonectomy with the extent of surgical resection in relation to the cardiac pericardium. Completion pneumonectomy involves removing the affected lung, following previous lung resection, which has experienced a recurrence of carcinoma. Radical pneumonectomy (e.g., extrapleural pneumonectomy) is commonly performed as treatment for malignant mesothelioma and involves removal of the entire lung, ipsilateral pleura, hemopericardium, and hemidiaphragm. Carinal pneumonectomy is the removal of the entire lung, ipsilateral mainstem bronchus, and carina. This procedure requires surgical anastomosis of the remaining mainstem bronchus and distal trachea.

7. Describe indications for lung separation and OLV.

OLV allows for lung separation and provides optimal surgical visualization during thoracic procedures. It can be accomplished through various methods including: (1) dual-lumen endobronchial tube (DLT), (2) bronchial blocker, or (3) endobronchial intubation with a single-lumen endotracheal tube. Absolute and relative indications for lung separation techniques and OLV are given in Table 18-5.

8. Describe unique features of DLTs, bronchial blockers, and endobronchial intubation.

A DLT consists of two separate channels for independent ventilation of the distal bronchus and the

Table 18-5   Absolute and Relative Indications for OLV and/or Lung Separation Techniques

NEED	INDICATION	EXAMPLES
Absolute	Unilateral lung isolation	Infection and massive hemorrhage
	Unilateral ventilation control	Fistula (i.e., bronchopleural or bronchopleural cutaneous fistula), tracheobronchial surgery or disruption, large lung parenchymal mass (i.e., cyst or bulla), and unilateral lung disease causing life-threatening hypoxemia
	Unilateral pulmonary lavage	Treatment for alveolar proteinosis
Relative	Surgical exposure (high priority)	Thoracoscopy, mediastinal exposure, thoracic aortic aneurysm surgery, pneumonectomy and upper lobectomy
	Surgical exposure (low priority)	Segmentectomy, middle and lower lobectomy, esophageal surgery, minimal invasive cardiac surgery, transmyocardial revascularization, and thoracic spine surgery
	Status postcardiopulmonary bypass	Following removal of unilateral pulmonary emboli
	Unilateral lung disease	Severe hypoxemia related to lung pathology

Table 18-6	Advantages, Disadvantages, Complications, Relative Contraindications, and Types of DLTs
	DUAL-LUMEN ENDOBRONCHIAL TUBE
Advantages	• Effective suction for secretions and lung deflation
	• Application of CPAP to nonventilated lung
	• Easy conversion between OLV and two-lung ventilation
Disadvantages	• Difficult or impossible placement with abnormal anatomy
	• If postoperative ventilation is required, removal may pose risk to patient
Complications	• Tracheobronchial trauma
	• Laryngeal trauma
	• Accidental suturing to mediastinal structures
Relative contraindications	• Full stomach
	• Difficult airway
	• Ventilator dependent, critically ill
Types	• Robertshaw
	• Carlens
	• White

trachea. DLTs are designed to accommodate the left or right mainstem bronchus. The choice of a left-versus right-sided DLT is dependent on the type and side of operation. Most surgical procedures can be performed with a left-sided DLT. However, choice of a left- versus right-sided tube is not absolute. Stenosis, disruption, obstruction, or absence of a mainstem bronchus warrants placement of a DLT on the opposite side. During surgical procedures involving the mainstem bronchus (e.g., pneumonectomy), the choice of left- versus right-sided DLT must be carefully considered to avoid interference of the bronchial lumen during resection. Table 18-6 describes advantages, disadvantages, complications, relative contraindications, and types of DLTs.

When compared to the left mainstem bronchus, the right mainstem bronchus is shorter in length with variable location of the right upper lobe orifice. Right-sided DLTs have a separate opening, embedded in the endobronchial cuff, to ventilate the right upper lobe. Inadvertent obstruction of the ventilation slot has occurred. Therefore, proper DLT placement

should be ensured to avoid inadequate ventilation of the right upper lobe. An anomalous right upper lobe orifice that emerges above the tracheal carina is a contraindication for a right-sided DLT.

Choosing the correct size of DLT may be based on gender, height, weight, tracheal width, and/or bronchial diameter. It is important to remain cognizant that the patient's height more accurately correlates to the appropriate DLT size as compared to the patient's weight. The ideal DLT size is one that: (1) can safely traverse the glottis; (2) minimizes tracheobronchial trauma; (3) minimizes airway resistance; (4) allows the passage of the fiberoptic bronchoscope and suction catheter; and (5) requires no greater than 1–2 ml of air to create an adequate endobronchial cuff seal. Size recommendations, placement techniques, and confirmation of placement recommendations for DLTs are given in Table 18-7.

There are three methods of confirming DLT placement: (1) chest radiograph, (2) clinical signs, and (3) fiberoptic bronchoscopy. Table 18-8 describes

Table 18-7	Sizing Recommendations, Placement Techniques, and Confirmation of Placement Recommendations for DLT
	DUAL-LUMEN ENDOBRONCHIAL TUBE
Sizing recommendations	*Height:* 4'6" to 5'5": 35 or 37 French 5'6" to 5'10": 37 or 39 French 5'11" to 6'4": 39 or 41 French Pediatrics (> 8 years): 26 or 28 (only available as left-sided DLT) *Gender:* Adult female: 35 or 37 French Adult male: 39 or 41 French
Placement technique (i.e., blind technique)	• Direct laryngoscopy with appropriate laryngoscope blade to maximize visualization (i.e., Macintosh recommended) • DLT passes with distal curvature concave anteriorly • After the tip passes the larynx, the DLT is rotated 90 degrees into appropriate mainstem bronchus • Advanced to proper depth (Fig. 18-2)
Confirmation of placement	• Chest x-ray • Clinical signs • Fiberoptic bronchoscopy

Table 18-8	Proper Sequence of Determining DLT Placement by Clinical Signs		
BRONCHIAL SIDE VENTILATED	**TRACHEAL SIDE VENTILATED**	**SITUATION**	**ACTION**
Unilateral breath sounds on correct side	Unilateral breath sounds on correct side	DLT placed in the correct position	None required
Unilateral breath sounds	Unilateral breath sounds or no breath sounds	DLT advanced too far, tracheal lumen in mainstem bronchus	Retract DLT until properly positioned
Bilateral breath sounds	No breath sounds	DLT advanced not far enough, bronchial lumen in trachea	Advance DLT to proper positioning
Unilateral breath sounds on wrong side	No breath sounds or breath sounds on wrong side	DLT advanced into wrong mainstem bronchus	Retract DLT into trachea and rotate into appropriate mainstem bronchus
No breath sounds	No breath sounds	DLT not in trachea (e.g., esophageal placement)	Remove DLT and reattempt placement

Figure 18-2 *Placement of left-sided DLT (i.e., blind technique) and confirmation of placement via fiberoptic bronchoscopy. A DLT passes with distal curvature concave anteriorly.*

the proper sequence of assessing DLT placement using clinical signs. Fiberoptic bronchoscopy has revealed malpositioning of the DLT in 78 to 83% of cases despite proper positioning as confirmed by relying on clinical signs. It is recommended that an appropriately sized fiberoptic bronchoscope be used in conjunction with clinical signs to confirm placement. Proper positioning of the DLT should be confirmed following: (1) initial placement, (2) changes in position, and (3) instances of hypoxemia. Figure 18-2 depicts proper placement

of a left-sided DLT and confirmation of placement via fiberoptic bronchoscopy. Table 18-9 describes two methods to assist in difficult placement of a DLT.

Bronchial blockers can be placed: (1) in conjunction with a preexisting endotracheal tube (i.e., Fogarty catheter), (2) via a specially designed large caliber endotracheal tube with a small integrated channel for a built-in bronchial blocker (i.e., Univent tube), (3) wire-guided endobronchial blocker (i.e., WEB blocker), or (4) with the aide of

Table 18-9   Two Methods to Assist in Difficult DLT Placement

Step 1	• DLT is positioned with both the bronchial and tracheal lumens within the trachea, the tracheal cuff is inflated
Step 2	• Bilateral lungs are ventilated and the position is confirmed such as with a single-lumen endotracheal tube

METHOD 1	METHOD 2
Step 3	*Step 3*
Appropriately sized fiberoptic bronchoscope is inserted into the bronchial lumen and the carina is visualized	Appropriately sized fiberoptic bronchoscope is inserted into the tracheal lumen and the carina is visualized
Step 4	*Step 4*
Under direct visualization the fiberoptic bronchoscope is passed into the appropriate mainstem bronchus	The tracheal cuff is deflated, and under direct visualization the right- or left-sided bronchial lumen is passed into the appropriate mainstem bronchus
Step 5	*Step 5*
The tracheal cuff is subsequently deflated and the right- or left-sided DLT may then be passed over the fiberoptic bronchoscope using it as a conduit for proper placement	Assess proper depth of insertion
Step 6	
The fiberoptic bronchoscope can then be inserted into the tracheal lumen to assess proper depth of insertion.	

a looped suture that can be attached to a fiberoptic bronchoscope (i.e., Arndt blocker). Advantages, disadvantages, confirmation of placement recommendations for bronchial blockers, and endobronchial intubation are given in Table 18-10.

9. Describe hypoxic pulmonary vasoconstriction and methods to optimize oxygenation during pneumonectomy.

Hypoxic pulmonary vasoconstriction (HPV) is a normal physiologic response during instances of: (1) primary hypoxia (i.e., low FiO_2), (2) hypoventilation, and/or (3) atelectasis to maximize oxygenation. During HPV, blood vessels perfusing nonventilated, poorly oxygenated alveoli constrict causing a regional increase in pulmonary vascular resistance. Blood flow from these alveoli is diverted to the ventilated, well-oxygenated alveoli. This physiologic response to hypoxia decreases intrapulmonary shunt, while maintaining oxygenation in the process. Persistent alveolar hypoxia and pulmonary vasoconstriction may manifest as pulmonary hypertension, pulmonary vascular remodeling, and may progress to cor pulmonale. The mechanism of HPV involves the activation of reduction–oxidation mitochondrial units within pulmonary artery smooth muscle cells, which regulate calcium influx and vascular tone.

In an effort to maintain patient oxygenation during instances of permissive atelectasis (e.g., OLV), it is imperative to avoid factors that inhibit HPV. Pharmacologic agents utilized in anesthesia have been implicated in HPV inhibition (i.e., inhalation anesthetics, calcium channel blockers, isoproter-

Table 18-10 Advantages, Disadvantages, Confirmation of Placement Recommendations, and Types of Bronchial Blockers and Endobronchial Intubation

	BRONCHIAL BLOCKER	ENDOBRONCHIAL INTUBATION
Advantages	• In situ endotracheal tube may be used for postoperative ventilation • May be used for pediatric patients when DLT is not possible • May be used in prone position • May be easier to place in difficult airway situations • Selective partial lung collapse possible (i.e., lobular) • Application of CPAP possible	• May be placed acutely in instances of thoracic hemorrhage or hemoptysis when visualization with a fiberoptic bronchoscope is inadequate
Disadvantages	• Small lumen of bronchial blocker may provide ineffective suction for secretions • Prolonged lung deflation and reinflation • Lumen of bronchial blocker easily occluded by secretions and blood • Bronchial blocker cuff prone to intraoperative leak or mucosal damage (e.g., improper inflation and prolonged use) • Lumen of bronchial blocker increases diameter of endotracheal tube • Malpositioning causes ineffective lung separation and impaired ventilation	• Limited in function • Allows only OLV • Inability to suction nonventilated lung • Inability to apply CPAP to nonventilated lung increases intrapulmonary shunt • Variant placement in right lung can cause ineffective ventilation of right upper lobe
Confirmation of placement	• Placed in conjunction with a self-sealing diaphragm and fiberoptic bronchoscope	• Placed blindly into mainstem bronchus in emergent situation • Self-sealing diaphragm and fiberoptic bronchoscope
Types	• Fogarty catheter • Univent • WEB blockers • Arndt blocker	• Standard endotracheal tube

enol, nitrous oxide, and vasodilators). Inhibition of HPV does not preclude the use of these medications during anesthetic management. However, the degree of HPV inhibition is dependent on the amount of drug that is administered.

As with any surgical procedure, it is vital to maintain adequate patient oxygenation. Various maneuvers can be instituted during the intraoperative period such as:

• **High FiO$_2$**
   Utilization of a high fraction of inspired oxygen (up to 100%) maximizes arterial oxygenation. Utilization of 100% oxygen has been associated

with absorption atelectasis and oxygen toxicity. However, the benefit of increasing PaO_2 in patients with marginal respiratory reserve exceeds the risks associated hypoxia.

- *Continuous positive airway pressure (CPAP) and positive-end expiratory pressure (PEEP)*
  The application of 5–10 cm H_2O of CPAP to the nonventilated lung is effective in minimizing alveolar hypoventilation, decreasing intrapulmonary shunt, and maintaining oxygenation during OLV. Furthermore, the application of PEEP to the ventilated lung has also been shown to be effective in maintaining oxygenation during OLV by preventing alveolar collapse and increasing functional residual capacity. The amount of PEEP should be maintained at less than 5 mm Hg if possible to avoid increasing pulmonary vascular resistance and barotrauma.

- *Tidal volume and respiratory rate*
  During OLV, a tidal volume set to approximately 8 to 10 ml/kg should be used to prevent atelectasis, increases in airway pressure, and increases in pulmonary vascular resistance. Despite the ventilation and perfusion mismatch that occurs during OLV, a 20 to 30% increase in respiratory rate is frequently adequate to maintain normal minute ventilation and physiologic $PaCO_2$.

10. Describe physiologic differences in ventilation and perfusion comparing: (1) the upright versus lateral decubitus position, (2) the awake versus anesthetized patient, (3) spontaneously breathing versus controlled ventilation patient, and (4) the closed versus open chest.

Distribution of perfusion to the pulmonary parenchyma is affected by gravitational forces. In the upright lung, gravity causes a proportionally larger blood flow to the inferior areas when compared with the superior areas. In the lateral decubitus position, pulmonary blood flow to the dependent lung functions much like the inferior areas of the upright lung. The increased perfusion of these areas is consistent through the physiological states described in Table 18-11. Figure 18-3 depicts the zones of the lung proposed by West. Note the distribution of blood flow between the upright and lateral decubitus positions.

Table 18-11   Summary of the Physiology of Positioning, Anesthesia, Ventilation, and Chest Opening

STATE	PHYSIOLOGY	VENTILATION: PERFUSION (V/Q) RATIO
Upright, awake, spontaneous respiration, closed chest	• Ventilation: ↑ inferior lung regions • Perfusion: ↑ inferior lung regions	Relatively matched
Lateral, awake, spontaneous respiration, closed chest	• Ventilation: ↑ dependent lung • Perfusion: ↑ dependent lung	Relatively matched
Lateral, anesthetized, spontaneous respiration, closed chest	• Ventilation: ↑ nondependent lung • Perfusion: ↑ dependent lung	Mismatch
Lateral, anesthetized, controlled respiration, closed chest	• Ventilation: ↑ nondependent lung • Perfusion: ↑ dependent lung	Mismatch
Lateral, anesthetized, controlled respiration, open chest	• Ventilation: ↑ nondependent lung • Perfusion: ↑ dependent lung	Mismatch
Lateral, spontaneous respiration, and open chest	• Mediastinal shift • Paradoxical respiration	Mismatch

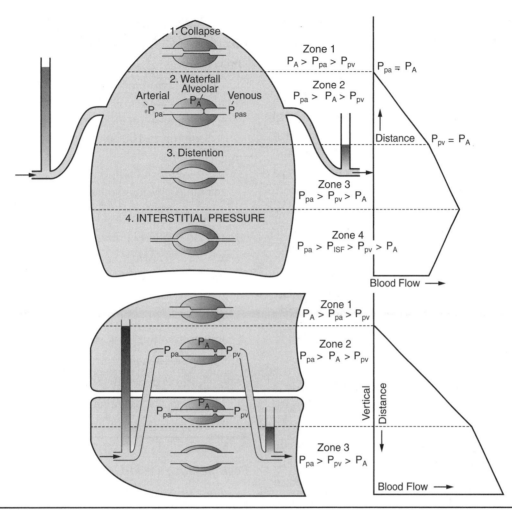

Figure 18-3 *The zones of the lung proposed by West. Note the distribution of blood flow in the upright and lateral decubitus positions.*

Pulmonary compliance refers to the stiffness or mechanical compliance of lung tissue. It is defined as the change in volume for a given change in pressure. Equation 18-1 can be used to calculate pulmonary compliance (C). Regional differences in pleural pressure causes inferior areas of the upright lung to be more compliant when compared to the superior portions. For a given and equal change in transpleural pressure, the inferior areas of the lung receive a larger portion of the tidal volume (e.g., increased ventilation). In the lateral decubitus position, the dependent lung functions much like the inferior regions of the upright lung.

During spontaneous respiration, the increased ventilation of the inferior or dependent areas of the lung is relatively matched to the increased perfusion in these same areas. However, with the institution of: (1) anesthesia, (2) controlled ventilation, and (3) thoracotomy (e.g., open chest), the dependent lung in the lateral decubitus position

---

Equation 18-1

C (liters/cm H_2O) $= \Delta V$ (change in volume) / ΔP (change in pressure)

undergoes a decrease in pulmonary compliance, while the nondependent lung undergoes a relative increase in ventilation. Due to the fact that perfusion does not change to the dependent area of the lung, a mismatch of ventilation and perfusion ensues. Table 18-11 summarizes the physiology of positioning, anesthesia, ventilation, and chest opening. Regional differences in ventilation and perfusion affect anesthetic management in regard to: (1) maintaining oxygenation and ventilation; (2) alterations in pulmonary resistance and compliance; and (3) interpretation of data from invasive monitoring (i.e., pulmonary artery catheter).

Scenario: After 20 minutes of surgical resection, the following scenario occurs: blood pressure, 70/30; heart rate, 120; room air oxygen saturation, 75%; respiratory rate, 10; tidal volume, 20 ml; peak inspiratory pressure, 45 cm H$_2$O.

11. List potential intraoperative complications that could cause this clinical scenario and the appropriate initial anesthetic interventions.

Treatment for this patient would include immediately informing the surgeon, ventilating with 100% oxygen, and diagnosing the etiology of this scenario prior to instituting further treatment. A treatment plan for severe hypoxemia is given in Table 18-12. Potential intraoperative complications that can occur during pneumonectomy include:

- Pneumothorax: Treatment, emergent needle decompression, subsequent chest tube placement
- Venous air embolism: Treatment, flooding the surgical field with normal saline solution; Durant position, aspiration of the air embolus via central venous catheter, supportive measures as needed
- Hemorrhage: Treatment, surgical hemostasis, administration of crystalloids, colloids, and blood products
- Airway obstruction: Treatment, ensure airway device (e.g., lung separation and OLV method) is not occluded or surgically attached to bronchus

---

Table 18-12 Treatment Plan for Severe Hypoxemia

Prevention:

1. Maintain two-lung ventilation until parietal pleura is exposed to atmosphere
2. Utilization of a high fraction of inspired oxygen (up to 100%)
3. OLV: Tv 8–10 ml/kg and adjust respiratory rate to maintain physiologic PaCO$_2$

Treatment:

1. Check position of lung isolation/OLV method
2. Assess and correct hemodynamic status (e.g., mechanical or pharmacologic therapy)
3. Nondependent lung CPAP
4. Dependent lung PEEP
5. Intermittent two-lung ventilation
6. Clamp pulmonary artery (i.e., pneumonectomy)

Alternative oxygenation methods:

1. High-frequency ventilation
2. Low-flow apneic ventilation (apneic insufflation)

Postoperative Period

12. Describe serious postoperative complications specifically related to pneumonectomy.

A variety of postoperative complications have been reported after pneumonectomy including: (1) cardiac herniation, (2) hemorrhage, (3) bronchial disruption, (4) arrhythmias, (5) respiratory failure, (6) right heart failure, and (7) neural injury. Constant vigilance is necessary during the postoperative period.

Cardiac Herniation An intrapericardial approach for pneumonectomy may result in a large pericardial defect if it is unable to be closed. Herniation of the heart through this defect into the empty hemithorax causes severe impairment of cardiac function with a mortality rate of 50%. Immediate surgical exploration of the thoracic cavity is necessary.

Hemorrhage Systemic arterial bleeding, diffuse bleeding from thoracic parenchyma, failure of staples/sutures, and tracheobronchial trauma resulting from management of the airway have been reported. Uncontrolled postoperative bleeding and hypovolemia necessitate emergency thoracotomy.

Bronchial Disruption The severity of a bronchopleural fistula is dependent on the size of the bronchial disruption, the accumulation of fluid within the pleural space, and the presence of a chest drain. The development of tension pneumothorax necessitates prompt resuscitation. The in vivo bronchial stump should be assessed for air leaks prior to closure of the thoracic cavity.

Arrhythmias Approximately 25% of patients undergoing thoracic surgery experience postoperative atrial dysrhythmias, of which atrial flutter and fibrillation are the most common. Trauma from cardiac manipulation, vagal stimulation, cardiopulmonary disease, and right atrial enlargement from increased pulmonary vascular resistance can precipitate cardiac dysrhythmias.

Respiratory Failure Acute respiratory insufficiency is the most common and serious complication following pulmonary resection of bronchial carcinoma. Preexisting pulmonary pathology, pulmonary trauma, unilateral reexpansion pulmonary edema, and/or postoperative pain can precipitate inadequate respiratory effort.

Right Heart Failure The decrease in functional pulmonary vasculature after pulmonary resection causes an increase in pulmonary vascular resistance. The resultant increase in right ventricular afterload can precipitate acute right heart failure (e.g., cor pulmonale) and right-to-left intracardiac shunting across a patent foramen ovale.

Neural Injury During dissection the phrenic, vagus, and recurrent laryngeal nerves may be inadvertently injured or deliberately sacrificed. Damage to the spinal branches of the intercostal arteries by dissection or diathermy may cause spinal cord ischemia. Fistula formation between the pleura and epidural space can cause spinal cord compression and ischemia from hematoma formation.

13. Describe available pain management modalities for patients presenting for pneumonectomy.

Intercostal nerve damage plays a significant role in the development of pain following thoracic surgery. Nerve dysfunction and muscle damage following incision, retraction, and suture placement is common. Analgesic therapies used to treat postoperative pain after pneumonectomy is included in Table 18-13. Although effective analgesic therapy reduces the prevalence and intensity of pain after thoracic surgery, up to 21% of patients still develop chronic pain. Since there are multiple pathways of nociceptive input to the central nervous system, a multimodal approach to pain management may also include a combination of nonsteroidal anti-inflammatory drugs, use of patient-controlled analgesia, and narcotics.

Treating pain after pneumonectomy is important for the following reasons: (1) patient comfort and satisfaction; (2) allowing optimal respiratory effort, and (3) minimizing pulmonary complications (i.e., atelectasis and pneumonia). Lung volume may be greatly reduced after thoracic surgery and effective analgesic therapy has been shown to improve pulmonary function.

Thoracic epidural analgesia is the current gold standard for postthoracotomy pain and has gained increasing acceptance in providing subjectively better analgesia than any other method

Table 18-13 Effective Analgesic Therapies Used to Treat Postoperative Pain After Pneumonectomy

- Epidural analgesia (i.e., thoracic or upper lumbar)
- Interpleural regional anesthesia
- Cryoanalgesia
- Intercostal nerve block
- Paravertebral block
- Local anesthetic infiltration
- Systemic analgesia (i.e., patient-controlled analgesia)

in thoracic surgery. Epidural anesthesia has been utilized in thoracic surgery performed in the awake patient, a testament to its versatility as an analgesic therapy. In the absence of contraindications, patients undergoing major open thoracic surgical procedures should have a thoracic epidural catheter placed preoperatively. Typically a thoracic epidural catheter is placed in the T6–T8 interspace. This is to be done in patients who are awake in order to assess proper placement and the presence of postprocedural complications. A clear plan must be created for the intraoperative utilization and management of a thoracic epidural catheter such as the type and volume of local anesthetic to be injected for the initial bolus and maintenance doses. The benefit of intraoperative analgesia should be weighed against the potential for sympathectomy resulting in hypotension for patients with marginal hemodynamic reserve. Postoperatively, the epidural solution used for infusion typically combines a low concentration of a long-acting local anesthetic such as bupivacaine or ropivacaine and a lipophilic opioid which includes fentanyl or hydromorphone.

Scenario: Following right-sided extrapericardial pneumonectomy, the following scenario occurs: blood pressure,160/89; heart rate, 98; room air oxygen saturation, 88%; respiratory rate, 45; tidal volume, 150 ml; spontaneous respirations, FiO$_2$ 100%.

14. Describe the standard tracheal extubation criteria for patients presenting with pulmonary resections and available methods for DLT exchange.

In patients presenting for pulmonary resection procedures, the plan for tracheal extubation should be

---

Table 18-14   Standard Extubation Criteria for Patients Presenting for Pulmonary Resection Procedures

Global criteria:

1. Acceptable hemodynamic status

2. Normothermia

3. Ability to maintain patent airway
   - Return of laryngeal and cough reflexes
   - Appropriate level of consciousness

4. Adequate muscular strength
   - Reversal of neuromuscular blockade as indicated by: train-of-four ratio > 0.9, tetanic response to 100 hz for 5 seconds, and double-burst stimulation without fade
   - Head lift > 5 s and strong, constant hand grip

5. Acceptable metabolic function indicators
   - Electrolytes
   - Acid–base balance

6. Acceptable hematologic function indicators
   - Hemoglobin level consistent with adequate oxygen delivery

7. Adequate analgesia for optimal respiratory effort

Respiratory criteria:

1. Adequate respiratory mechanics
   - Vital capacity > 15 ml/kg
   - Maximal negative inspiratory force > −20 cmH$_2$O

2. Ability to maintain adequate oxygenation (with FiO$_2$ < 50%)
   - SpO$_2$ > 90%
   - PaO$_2$ > 60 mm Hg

3. Ability to maintain adequate alveolar ventilation
   - PaCO$_2$ < 50 mm Hg
   - Spontaneous respiratory rate (breaths/min) to tidal volume (l) ratio (e.g., rapid shallow breathing index) < 100 breaths/min/l

considered within the early postoperative period to decrease the risk of pulmonary barotrauma and infection. Patients with marginal cardiopulmonary reserve may require postoperative mechanical respiratory support and should remain intubated until standard extubation criteria are met. Standard extubation criteria for patients presenting for pulmonary resection procedures are given in Table 18-14. Oftentimes it is impossible and impractical to fulfill the criteria in its entirety. However, the anesthetist should exercise sound judgment in determining which patients are suitable for postoperative tracheal extubation.

If the decision to continue postoperative mechanical respiratory support is made and a DLT has been utilized for OLV, it should be replaced at the end of surgery with a single-lumen endotracheal tube. The DLT tube may be replaced under direct laryngoscopy or with the assistance of an airway exchange catheter depending on the preoperative history (i.e., difficult intubation). During this procedure care should be exercised by the anesthetist to minimize airway trauma, maintain adequate oxygenation, and prevent barotrauma if ventilation through the airway exchange catheter is possible.

Physical examination, preoperative testing, and preoperative optimization are aimed at determining which patients are optimal surgical candidates. Pulmonary function tests provide invaluable diagnostic information regarding a patient's ability to tolerate the proposed pulmonary resection. Pulmonary function testing should commence in a tiered approach, with each tier increasing in sensitivity, specificity, and invasiveness. Table 18-2 describes the three tiers of preoperative function testing. Postoperative predicted (pop) FEV_1 is a method of estimating postoperative ventilatory function after pulmonary resection. It is based on the amount of functional lung tissue remaining after resection and can be calculated from ventilation and perfusion scanning of each individual lung by radioisotope. Equation 18-2 can be used to calculate the $popFEV_1$. A $popFEV_1$ of less than 0.85 l or less than 40% of predicted is associated with increased morbidity and mortality rates.

Equation 18-2

$$popFEV_1 = preop\ FEV_1 - (\%\ contribution\ of\ diseased\ lung \times preop\ FEV_1)$$

REVIEW QUESTIONS

1. The majority of pulmonary resection procedures are performed for the removal of:
   a. malignant tissue.
   b. mesothelioma.
   c. bronchopulmonary sequestrations.
   d. thoracic trauma.

2. Which endocrinopathy is present in up to 40% of patients with SCLC?
   a. SIADH
   b. Cushing syndrome
   c. Myasthenic syndrome
   d. Carcinoid syndrome

3. Which accurately describes the correct placement and depth of insertion of a left-sided dual lumen tube following fiberoptic bronchoscopy?
   a. Bronchial cuff in the right mainstem bronchus, visible just below the carina
   b. Bronchial cuff in the left mainstem bronchus, not visible below the carina
   c. Bronchial cuff in the left mainstem bronchus, herniating above the level of the carina
   d. Bronchial cuff in the left mainstem bronchus, visible just below the carina

4. During which physiologic states are ventilation and perfusion most closely matched?
   a. Lateral, awake, spontaneous respiration, closed chest
   b. Lateral, anesthetized, spontaneous respiration, closed chest
   c. Lateral, anesthetized, controlled respiration, closed chest
   d. Lateral, anesthetized, controlled respiration, open chest

5. During a pneumonectomy, what surgical maneuver can be performed to decrease intrapulmonary shunt and prevent hypoxemia?
   a. Clamping of the mainstem bronchus
   b. Clamping of the superior pulmonary vein
   c. Clamping of the pulmonary artery
   d. Clamping of the inferior pulmonary vein

REVIEW ANSWERS

1. **Answer: a**
   Pulmonary resection procedures have been performed for a variety of etiologies including: (1) pulmonary masses, (2) malignant mesothelioma, (3) bronchiectasis, (4) tuberculosis, (5) and thoracic trauma. Pulmonary masses may present as benign or malignant pathology. Benign pathology includes carcinoid tumors, hemangiomas, bronchopulmonary sequestrations, and infection. The majority of pulmonary resection procedures are performed for the removal of malignant tissue (e.g., bronchogenic carcinoma).

2. **Answer: a**
   Endocrinologic abnormalities and paraneoplastic neurological syndromes are common in patients with SCLC. These syndromes include: (1) SIADH, (2) Cushing syndrome, and (3) Myasthenic syndrome (e.g., Eaton-Lambert syndrome). SIADH is present in up to 40% of patients with SCLC.

3. **Answer: d**
   Following fiberoptic bronchoscopy, correct placement and depth of insertion of a left-sided dual lumen tube should reveal that the blue, bronchial cuff is situated in the left mainstem bronchus and is visible just below the level of the carina without herniation.

4. **Answer: a**
   During spontaneous respiration, the increase ventilation of the inferior/dependent areas of the lung is relatively matched to the increase perfusion in these same areas. However, with the institution of: (1) anesthesia, (2) controlled ventilation, and (3) thoracotomy (e.g., open chest), the dependent lung in the lateral decubitus position undergoes a decrease in pulmonary compliance, while the nondependent lung undergoes a relative increase in ventilation. Due to the fact that perfusion does not change to the dependent area of the lung, a mismatch of ventilation and perfusion ensues.

5. **Answer: c**
   Surgical clamping of the pulmonary artery inhibits arterial blood flow to the nonventilated lung. By eliminating intrapulmonary shunt from the nonventilated lung, physiologic shunt is decreased and hypoxemia is decreased in the process. Hemodynamic instability (e.g., due to the increase in right ventricular afterload and decrease in left ventricular preload) with clamping of pulmonary artery prior to ligation is a contraindication to continuing with the pneumonectomy procedure.

SUGGESTED READINGS

American Cancer Society. *Cancer Facts & Figures 2008*. Available online at http://www.cancer.org/downloads/STT/2008CAFFfinalsecured.pdf. Accessed February 10, 2009.

Campos JH. Current techniques for perioperative lung isolation in adults. *Anesthesiology* 2002;97(5):1295–1301.

Cohen E, Neustein SM, Eisenkraft JB. Anesthesia for thoracic surgery. In: Barash PG, Cullen BF, Stoelting RK, eds. *Clinical Anesthesia*, 5th ed. Philadelphia: Lippincott Williams & Wilkins, 2006:813–855.

Datta D, Lahiri B. Preoperative evaluation of patients undergoing lung resection surgery. *Chest* 2003;123(6):2096–2103.

Gottschalk A, Cohen SP, Yang S, et al. Preventing and treating pain after thoracic surgery. *Anesthesiology* 2006;104(3):594–600.

Grichnik KP, Clark JA. Pathophysiology of one-lung ventilation. *Thorac Surg Clin* 2005;15(1):85–103.

Kirby TJ, Fell SC. Pneumonectomy and its modifications. In: Shields TW, Locicero J, Ponn RB, Rusch VW, eds. *General Thoracic Surgery*, 6th ed. Philadelphia, Lippincott Williams & Wilkins, 2004:470–485.

Mineo TC. Epidural anesthesia in awake thoracic surgery. *Eur J Cardiothorac Surg* 2007;32(1):13–19.

Nagelhout JJ. Respiratory anatomy: thoracic surgery. In: Nagelhout JJ, Zaglaniczy KL, eds. *Nurse Anesthesia*, 3rd ed. St. Louis, MO: Elsevier Saunders, 2005:574–590.

Wilson WC, Benumof JL. Anesthesia for thoracic surgery. In: Miller RD, ed. *Miller's Anesthesia*, 6th ed. New York: Churchill Livingstone, 2005:1847–1939.

Mediastinoscopy

19

Mary C. Karlet

KEY POINTS

- Mediastinoscopy is a diagnostic procedure used for biopsy of mediastinal masses and staging of lung cancer.
- Compression of vital respiratory structures by a large mediastinal mass can create airway collapse or edema with severe respiratory compromise. An asymptomatic patient can develop severe respiratory compromise with anesthesia and any change in position.
- Mediastinal tumors can produce cardiac dysfunction secondary to compression of the heart and great vessels. The compression of vascular structures in the mediastinum can produce serious hemodynamic problems, including a condition called superior vena cava (SVC) syndrome. Effects of SVC obstruction may worsen in the supine position and with the onset of general anesthesia.
- Mediastinal and thoracic tumors can produce abnormal hormone production, autocoids, or autoantibodies that have systemic effects and can potentially affect anesthesia management.
- Major complications of mediastinoscopy include: hemorrhage, pneumothorax, compression of major blood vessels, esophageal perforation, tracheal or bronchial trauma, and recurrent laryngeal nerve injury.

CASE SYNOPSIS

A 57-year-old woman reports to her physician that she has had a recent history of respiratory distress. A chest radiograph reveals the presence of a large mediastinal mass and the patient is subsequently scheduled for a mediastinoscopy for histological biopsy and possible staging of tumor.

PREOPERATIVE EVALUATION AND DEMOGRAPHIC DATA

Past Medical/Surgical History

- Right-sided mastectomy with axillary node dissection for breast carcinoma 5 years ago

- During the past month, the patient reports increasing dyspnea, orthopnea, and a feeling of fullness in her neck.
- Smoking ½ pack per day for 35 years

List of Medications

- None

Diagnostic Data

- Hemoglobin, 13.2 g/dl; hematocrit, 39.4%; glucose, 139 mg/dl; blood urea nitrogen (BUN), 15 mg/dl; creatinine, 1.1 mg/dl
- Electrolytes: sodium, 139 mEq/l; potassium, 3.9 mEq/l; chloride, 104 mEq/l; carbon dioxide, 24 mEq/l
- Chest x-ray and magnetic resonance imaging (MRI) reveal a widened mediastinum due to the suspected metastatic tumor

Height/Weight/Vital Signs

- 160 cm, 58 kg
- Blood pressure, 152/84; heart rate, 78 beats per minute; respiratory rate, 24 breaths per minute; room air oxygen saturation, 97%; temperature, 36.8°C
- Electrocardiogram (ECG): normal sinus rhythm; heart rate, 86; ejection fraction, 60%
- Mallampati class III airway, midline trachea, clear breath sounds bilaterally

PATHOPHYSIOLOGY

The mediastinum is the region between the two pleural cavities, containing the heart, great vessels, thymus gland, esophagus, and tracheobronchial tree. The borders of the mediastinum are anterior—the sternum, posterior—the thoracic vertebrae, lateral—the pleural sacs and thoracic inlets, and inferior—the diaphragm. Evaluation of the mediastinum and its contents is often performed by mediastinoscopy, a diagnostic procedure that was first described by Carlens in 1959. The procedure is used to obtain tissue for histological diagnosis and to help identify treatment options for various thoracic diseases.

Table 19-1	Predisposing Factors Associated with Mediastinal Masses
Tumors	Thymus gland tumors
	Thyroid and parathyroid tumors
	Lymphoma
	Esophageal cancer
	Neurogenic tumors
Benign conditions	Esophageal and bronchogenic cysts
	Tuberculosis lymphadenopathy
	Sarcoidosis lymphadenopathy
	Aortic aneurysms

Mediastinoscopy is an important tool for staging bronchogenic cancer to determine resectability and prognosis. Lymph fluid from the lungs drains directly into mediastinal lymph nodes, and node biopsy helps determine the extent of disease metastasis. Diseases presenting with mediastinal lymphadenopathy (e.g., sarcoidosis, lymphoma, infectious granulomatous diseases) may be diagnosed and staged with mediastinal tissue biopsy. When performed for cancerous lung tumor staging, the procedures sensitivity is greater than 80% and specificity of 100%. Table 19-1 lists conditions that are associated with mediastinal masses.

Despite the availability of newer and less invasive imaging and diagnostic techniques (e.g., MRI, positron emission tomography [PET]), mediastinoscopy is still widely used and remains the diagnostic standard used to identify the histology of various mediastinal masses.

SURGICAL PROCEDURE

Most mediastinoscopy procedures are performed under general anesthesia by way of the cervical approach, through a small incision in the suprasternal notch. A tunnel created by blunt dissection through fascial layers, anterior and lateral to the trachea, allows the mediastinoscope to gain access to the subcarinal area (paratracheal,

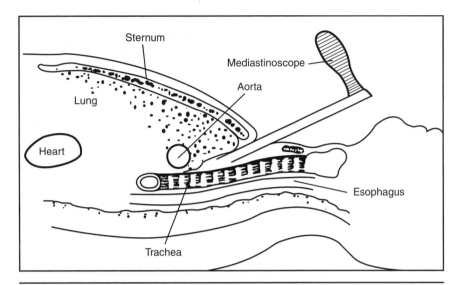

Figure 19-1 *A tunnel created by blunt dissection through fascial layers, anterior and lateral to the trachea, allows the mediastinoscope to gain access to the subcarinal area (paratracheal, subaortic, and bronchial lymph nodes).*

subaortic, and bronchial lymph nodes) as shown in Figure 19-1. An alternate anterior or transthoracic approach (Chamberlain procedure) is used less frequently to inspect the lower and anterior mediastinum. The anterior approach involves entry through the second, third, or fourth left intercostal space lateral to the sternal border.

Table 19-2	Relative and Absolute Contraindication to Mediastinoscopy
RELATIVE CONTRAINDICATIONS	**ABSOLUTE CONTRAINDICATIONS**
Previous mediastinoscopy	Superior vena cava obstruction
Severe tracheal deviation	Thoracic aortic aneurysm
Cerebrovascular disease	Coagulopathy
Severe cervical spine disease that limits neck extension	
Previous chest radiotherapy	

The relative contraindications for cervical mediastinoscopy include factors that may distort the anatomy or interfere with the facial plane for mediastinal dissection (scarring from a previous mediastinoscopy, radiation to the chest). Absolute contraindications to mediastinoscopy include coagulopathy, SVC obstruction, and thoracic aneurysm. Table 19-2 lists relative and absolute contraindications associated with mediastinoscopy.

ANESTHESIA MANAGEMENT CONSIDERATIONS

Preoperative Period

1. Describe comorbidities often present in patients having a mediastinoscopy procedure.
Patients scheduled for mediastinoscopy often have significant cardiac and respiratory problems, such as coronary artery disease, peripheral vascular disease, and chronic obstructive pulmonary disease. Many of these patients are smokers, and the associated comorbidities require a thorough preoperative evaluation.

2. Discuss preoperative evaluation of the patient scheduled for a mediastinoscopy.

Anesthetic management is complicated by the presence of a large mediastinal masses or enlarged mediastinal lymph nodes that compress nearby vital structures, such as the superior or inferior vena cava or the tracheobronchial tree. Preoperative evaluation should include an ECG, chest radiograph, and CT/MRI scan to determine the size and location of the mass and any compression on adjacent vital structures. Echocardiography in the upright and supine positions may be indicated for the patient with cardiac symptoms.

Patients with tracheobronchial compression may exhibit wheezing, cyanosis, orthopnea, coughing, dyspnea, and stridor. A thorough preoperative assessment of the airway is imperative to detect distortion or obstruction. Patients should be questioned about the effect of position changes on their ventilation. Pulmonary function tests and flow-volume loops (in the upright and supine positions) provide useful information regarding effects of the tumor on pulmonary function and airway dynamics. The inspiratory limb of the flow-volume loop is blunted by extrathoracic obstruction; the expiratory limb is dampened by intrathoracic obstruction. Preoperative sedation must be avoided if clinical manifestations or laboratory tests reveal suspected or demonstrated airway obstruction.

Table 19-3 lists factors that predict an increased risk of perioperative respiratory problems in patients with a mediastinal mass. It is noteworthy that some surgical patients who do not present with symptoms may exhibit severe respiratory and cardiovascular compromise during or after anesthesia and surgery.

3. Explore the paraneoplastic syndromes that may be associated with lung and mediastinal tumors.

Paraneoplastic syndromes are diseases or symptoms that occur as a consequence of cytokines or hormones produced by, or in response to, a cancerous tumor. Hormones or hormone-like substances secreted from lung and mediastinal tumors can produce paraneoplastic syndromes. Disorders that may result from the liberation of abnormal humoral factors include hyperparathyroidism (parathyroid hormone secreted), Cushing syndrome (adrenal corticotropic hormone secreted), syndrome of inappropriate antidiuretic hormone (ADH secreted), and carcinoid syndrome (serotonin secreted).

Some mediastinal tumors produce humoral factors that affect muscle function. The preoperative history should include an assessment of the patient's muscle strength, as muscle weakness can be associated with thymomas or oat-cell (small cell) tumors of the lung.

Oat-cell tumors may be associated with Eaton-Lambert syndrome (myasthenic syndrome). These tumors can produce autoantibodies that inhibit calcium-dependent acetylcholine release at the presynaptic neuromuscular junction, which causes profound proximal muscle weakness results. The muscle weakness associated with Eaton-Lambert syndrome typically improves with repeated movement, in contrast to the muscle weakness of myasthenia gravis which worsens with repeated activity.

Tumors of the thymus gland (thymomas) are associated with myasthenia gravis, an autoimmune disease caused by antibodies that destroys nicotinic acetylcholine receptors on the postsynaptic neuromuscular junction. The resulting muscle weakness may be temporarily reversed by rest and anticholinesterase medications.

Table 19-3	Predictors of Perioperative Respiratory Insufficiency	
Preoperative cardiopulmonary clinical manifestations	Peak expiratory flow rate < 40% of predicted
Both obstructive and restrictive respiratory impairment	Tracheal diameter < 50% of predicted on CT scan

Surgical patients with Eaton-Lambert syndrome or myasthenia gravis may be at risk for aspiration and perioperative respiratory failure and they are extremely sensitive to nondepolarizing muscle relaxants.

4. Define the anesthetic implications associated with SVC syndrome.

SVC compression by a mediastinal mass occurs in approximately 6–7% of patients with lung cancer. Masses that produce SVC compression are usually malignant and often consist of oat cell carcinoma or non-Hodgkin lymphoma. Obstruction of the SVC by a mediastinal tumor can result in blocked venous drainage from the head, neck, and upper extremities. Depending on the severity, patients may present with dyspnea, dilated veins across the upper chest and neck, fullness in the face, or rubor of the upper body. Symptoms of SVC obstruction may be exaggerated in the supine position, and may be relieved by head elevation. Steroids or diuretics are used to help control SVC congestion.

Tongue swelling and upper airway edema associated with SVC obstruction can make intubation difficult or impossible, and minor trauma during intubation can result in bleeding. SVC obstruction is considered to be a contraindication to mediastinoscopy. The surgeon may schedule radiation or chemotherapy to reduce the size of the tumor prior to mediastinoscopy. As compared to patients undergoing mediastinoscopy without SVC obstruction, patients with SVC syndrome have a significantly higher incidence of morbidity.

Intraoperative Period

5. Describe the necessary equipment and monitoring modalities required for safe anesthetic management of a mediastinoscopy.

Standard intraoperative monitors are used for most mediastinoscopy procedures. Assiduous neuromuscular blockade monitoring is particularly important for patients with mediastinal or thoracic tumors. An arterial line is optional, based on the anticipated hemodynamic stability of the patient. Preparation, a plan, and equipment for emergency thoracotomy should always be in place.

Intraoperative blood loss is usually minimal with a mediastinoscopy, but blood should be type and crossmatched because of the surgery's proximity to great vessels. The most serious complication associated with mediastinoscopy is massive hemorrhage. At least one large-bore intravenous catheter should be placed prior to induction of anesthesia. Should major blood loss occur through lacerated vasculature in the mediastinum, fluid and blood replacement through upper extremity cannulation sites may flow directly into the mediastinum. Under these conditions, and for the patient with SVC syndrome, fluids should be administered through lower extremity intravenous sites.

During the procedure, the rigid mediastinoscope can cause compression of major blood vessels, especially the innominate (brachiocephalic) artery (Fig. 19-2). Decreasing innominate blood flow, which perfuses the right common carotid and right subclavian arteries, increases the risk of cerebral ischemia or loss of the right radial pulse. Continuous monitoring of arterial flow in the right arm is necessary to alert the surgeon should repositioning or removal of the mediastinoscope be necessary. Intra-arterial monitoring of the *right radial artery pressure or obtaining a right pulse oximetry* reading from a right finger probe may be used to monitor blood flow. If noninvasive blood pressure monitoring is used, the blood pressure cuff should be placed on the patient's left arm and the pulse oximeter on the right finger.

Close monitoring of breath sounds and ventilation pressures during the procedure is important to help detect the development of a pneumothorax or compression of the tracheobronchial tree by the mediastinoscope. The surgeon should be alerted immediately if any acute increase in airway pressure or change in breath sounds occurs.

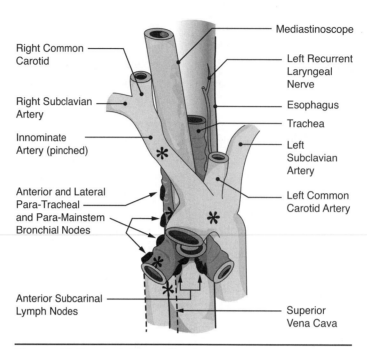

Right Common Carotid

Right Subclavian Artery

Innominate Artery (pinched)

Anterior and Lateral Para-Tracheal and Para-Mainstem Bronchial Nodes

Anterior Subcarinal Lymph Nodes

Mediastinoscope

Left Recurrent Laryngeal Nerve

Esophagus

Trachea

Left Subclavian Artery

Left Common Carotid Artery

Superior Vena Cava

Figure 19-2 *A rigid mediastinoscope can cause compression of major blood vessels, especially the innominate (brachiocephalic) artery.*

6. Describe the positioning considerations for a mediastinoscopy.

Typically, the surgical patient is positioned supine with the shoulders elevated on a shoulder roll and the head extended and supported on a head cushion. A slight head-up position may be employed to help reduce congestion in the great veins and reduce compression on the airway. A head-up position will increase the risk of venous air embolism, especially if the patient breathes spontaneously. Changes in the patient's respiratory or cardiovascular state can occur suddenly, and plans should be in place to rapidly turn the patient if needed.

7. Explain the key considerations for safe anesthetic management of the patient undergoing a mediastinoscopy.

General anesthesia with mechanical ventilation is the preferred anesthetic management technique for mediastinoscopy. The ideal general anesthetic

should produce profound depression of airway reflexes during instrumentation followed by rapid emergence. Due to the risk of pneumothorax with this procedure, nitrous oxide should be avoided. Cardiovascular changes during mediastinoscopy can occur suddenly, and administering vasoactive medications may be necessary for hemodynamic support. The nodes and tissue biopsies will be sent to pathology for interpretation prior to wound closure. The absence of surgical stimulation during this period may predispose the patient to developing profound hypotension. Titration of the inhalation agent is important and the individual's hemodynamic response should dictate the concentration that is administered.

The patient's preoperative respiratory status is an important determinant of the type of anesthesia induction. A slow controlled induction in the sitting position is often the prudent choice for the patient with SVC syndrome. Suspected or documented obstruction of the tracheobronchial tree may necessitate an awake fiberoptic-guided intubation under local anesthesia. Case reports of cardiovascular collapse or an inability to ventilate with anesthesia induction reflect decreased thoracic muscle tone and loss of transmural distending pressure associated with the onset of anesthesia and muscle paralysis. Changing the patient's position (prone, lateral, sitting) may dramatically reverse cardiorespiratory distress by moving a mediastinal mass off of vital structures.

Equipment for emergency airway management (fiberoptic or rigid ventilating bronchoscope) should be available. A single-lumen reinforced endotracheal tube may be used to minimize the risk of kinking during the procedure.

High intrathoracic pressures associated with positive-pressure ventilation and a large tidal volume decrease venous return. In a patient with venous congestion, controlled ventilation must be adjusted to provide the lowest ventilating pressure compatible with oxygenation and normal end-tidal carbon dioxide levels.

Muscle paralysis is important to prevent movement and coughing. Spontaneous ventilation with generation of negative intrathoracic pressure can increase the risk of air embolism through open venous structures. The patient should exhibit full return of reflexes and recovery of neuromuscular function prior to extubation.

The complication rate for mediastinoscopy is 1.5–3%. Table 19-4 outlines major complications associated with this procedure.

Table 19-4 Complications that are Associated with Mediastinoscopy	
HEMORRHAGE	**PNEUMOTHORAX**
Esophageal perforation	Recurrent laryngeal nerve injury
Pulmonary artery injury	Tracheal or bronchial trauma
Compression of major blood vessels	Air embolism
Dysrhythmias	

Postoperative Period

8. Review the important postoperative considerations for the patient who is recovering from a mediastinoscopy.

Routine postoperative monitoring is usually sufficient for an uncomplicated mediastinoscopy. The head of the bed should be elevated to improve respiratory function and decrease airway and surgical site edema. An uncomplicated cervical mediastinoscopy in an asymptomatic patient may be performed on an outpatient basis and the patient can return home the same day. A transthoracic mediastinoscopy generally requires at least one night of observation in the hospital prior to discharge.

Respiratory distress in the recovery room may be the result of inadequate reversal of muscle relaxant, airway edema, damage to the recurrent laryngeal nerve, paratracheal hematoma, compression of the tracheobronchial tree by tumor, or pneumothorax. The patient with unilateral recurrent laryngeal nerve damage will be hoarse and require close observation. Bilateral recurrent laryngeal nerve damage requires immediate reintubation. Tracheomalacia that has developed as a result of long-standing tracheal compression can cause an unexpected airway obstruction during the recovery period. A chest x-ray obtained in the postanesthesia care unit is necessary to rule out the possibility of a pneumothorax.

9. Describe future trends and developments for diagnosing and managing lung and mediastinal tumors.

Newer, less invasive staging techniques are being developed that may redefine the need for surgical mediastinoscopy in patients with lung cancer. Video mediastinoscopy is increasingly used in selected cases and is associated with fewer complications. Endobronchial or transesophageal endoscopic ultrasound-guided fine-needle aspirations are promising, accurate, safe, and minimally invasive tools for mediastinal staging.

REVIEW QUESTIONS

1. Eaton-Lambert syndrome (myasthenic syndrome) is associated with:
   a. antibody-mediated depression of postsynaptic acetylcholine receptor synthesis.
   b. oat cell carcinoma of the lung.
   c. profound skeletal muscle weakness that improves with rest.
   d. derangements in calcium release from skeletal muscle sarcoplasmic reticulum.

2. Myasthenia gravis is associated with which type of mediastinal tumor?
   a. Thymoma
   b. Oat cell carcinoma
   c. Lymphoma
   d. Adenoma

3. Which is classified as an absolute contraindication to a mediastinoscopy?
   a. Coagulopathy
   b. Myasthenic syndrome
   c. Distortion of the airway
   d. Previous chest radiotherapy

4. Anesthetists should monitor flow in the right radial artery during a mediastinoscopy to detect instrument compression on the

   _____.
   a. superior vena cava
   b. common carotid
   c. innominate artery
   d. right atrium

5. Near the end of a mediastinoscopy procedure, the patient becomes hypotensive and the peak inspiratory pressure increases. The trachea is noted to be deviated to the left. Which is the most likely cause of this situation?
   a. Pneumothorax
   b. Recurrent laryngeal injury
   c. Incomplete muscle relaxant reversal
   d. Bronchospasm

REVIEW ANSWERS

1. **Answer: b**
   Eaton-Lambert syndrome is most often associated with oat cell carcinoma, which is also known as small cell carcinoma of the lung.

2. **Answer: a**
   Thymomas (tumors of the thymus gland) are commonly observed in patients with myasthenia gravis. These tumors play a role in the formation of antibodies that attack nicotinic acetylcholine receptors at the postsynaptic neuromuscular junction.

3. **Answer: a**
   Mediastinoscopy would pose a severe risk for bleeding in the patient who has a coagulopathy, and therefore, this surgical procedure is contraindicated.

4. **Answer: c**
   The innominate artery is a branch of the thoracic aortic arch, and gives rise to the right common carotid artery and the right subclavian artery. Compression of the innominate artery will decrease blood flow to the right arm by decreasing blood flow into the right subclavian artery.

5. **Answer: a**
   A pneumothorax may result from inadvertent puncture of the pleura during a mediastinoscopy. Positive-pressure ventilation can cause the rapid accumulation of air within the pleural space creating a tension pneumothorax which results in cardiac and respiratory compromise.

SUGGESTED READINGS

Ahmed-Nusrath A, Swanevelder J. Anaesthesia for mediastinoscopy. *Cont Educ Anaesth Crit Care Pain* 2007; 7:6–9.

Dosios T, Theakos N, Chatziantoniou C. Cervical mediastinoscopy and anterior mediastinoscopy in superior vena cava obstruction. *Chest* 2005;128:1551–1556.

Lemaire A, Nikolic I, Petersen T, et al. Nine-year single center experience with cervical mediastinoscopy:

complications and false negative rate. *Ann Thorac Surg* 2006;82:1185–1189.

Leschber G, Sperling D, Klem W, et al. Does video-mediastinsocopy improve the results of conventional mediastinoscopy? *Eur J Cardiothorac Surg* 2008;33: 289–293.

Leyn PD, Lerut, T. Conventional mediastinoscopy. *Eur Ass Cardio-Thoracic Surg* 2005:1–10.

Tournoy KG, DeRyck F, Vanwalleghem LR, et al. Endoscopic ultrasound reduces surgical mediastinal staging in lung cancer: a randomized trial. *Am J Respir Crit Care Med* 2008;177:531–535.

Vander Els NJ. Abnormal flow volume loops in patients with intrathoracic Hodgkin's disease. *Chest* 2000; 117(5):1256–1261.

Vueghs PJ, Schurink GA, Vaes L, et al. Anesthesia in repeat mediastinoscopy: a retrospective study of 101 patients. *J Cardiothorac Vasc Anesth* 1992;6: 193–195.

Wallace MB, Pascual JM, Raimondo M, et al. Minimally invasive endoscopic staging of suspected lung cancer. *JAMA* 2008;299:540–546.

Wilson LD. Superior vena cava syndrome with malignant causes. *N Engl J Med* 2007;356:1862–1869.

Video-Assisted Thoracoscopic Surgery for Mediastinal Mass

20

Mark Gabot

KEY POINTS

- Improvements in video technology, endoscopic instruments, and surgical techniques have permitted a variety of diagnostic and therapeutic procedures to be performed using video-assisted thoracoscopic surgery (VATS).

- The advantages of VATS as compared to open thoracotomy include decreased postoperative pain, reduced incidence of postoperative respiratory dysfunction, shorter postoperative course, and rapid recovery resulting in reduced duration of hospitalization and decreased cost.

- Open thoracotomy remains the gold standard surgical approach for thoracic surgery. A VATS procedure may be emergently converted to an open thoracotomy and this possibility must be considered during the creation of an anesthetic care plan.

- The presence of a mediastinal mass may be associated with cardiac and respiratory derangements which include: direct cardiac and great vessel compression; superior vena cava syndrome; and tracheobronchial obstruction. Complete airway obstruction can develop perioperatively in patients regardless of the presence of clinical symptoms associated with airway compression.

- Preoperative optimization of a patient with a mediastinal mass may include: (1) a comprehensive preoperative assessment; (2) selective radiation and chemotherapy in sensitive groups, and (3) a biopsy of the mass under local anesthesia.

- Anesthetic management of high-risk patients includes: (1) administration of general anesthesia without the use of muscle relaxants; (2) maintenance of spontaneous respirations; (3) remaining cognizant that cardiopulmonary bypass may be required for distal airway obstructions and hypoxemia; and (4) airway obstruction has been relieved by placing the patient in a lateral, prone, or semirecumbent position.

CASE SYNOPSIS

A 26-year-old man is admitted to the hospital for a 3-cm right infrabronchial mass. He is scheduled by his thoracic surgeon to have a VATS for an excision of the mediastinal mass.

PREOPERATIVE EVALUATION AND DEMOGRAPHIC DATA

Past Medical/Surgical History

• The patient has had a persistent nonproductive cough for 6 months which has been unresponsive to conventional medical treatment.

List of Medications

• Guaifenesin (Robitussin)

Diagnostic Data

• Hemoglobin, 14.1 g/dl; hematocrit, 42.3%; platelets 250,000 mm^3
• Electrolytes: sodium, 135 mEq/l; potassium, 4.1 mEq/l; chloride, 107 mEq/l; carbon dioxide, 26 mEq/l,
• Blood urea nitrogen (BUN), 10 mg/dl; creatinine, 1 mg/dl
• Chest radiograph (anterior, posterior, and lateral): 3-cm right infrabronchial opacity; normal cardiac silhouette and pulmonary parenchyma; no tracheal or bronchial deviation
• Chest computed tomography (CT) scan: 3-cm right infrabronchial mass; homogeneous in nature; no cardiac and tracheobronchial compression; minimal vascular involvement as indicated by contrast-enhanced CT scan
• Magnetic resonance imaging (MRI): 3-cm right infrabronchial, high-intensity mass; no cardiac, great vessel, and tracheobronchial compression
• Pulmonary function tests (upright and supine): FVC, 4 l; FEV$_1$, 3 l; FEV$_1$/FVC = 75%

Height/Weight/Vital Signs

• 170 cm, 68 kg
• Blood pressure,120/86; heart rate, 90 beats per minute; respiratory rate, 25 breaths per minute; room air oxygen saturation, 98%; temperature 36.9°C

PATHOPHYSIOLOGY

Mass lesions in the mediastinum encompass a variety of pathologic etiologies and are classified as anterior, middle, or posterior based on their relationship to the heart, which occupies the middle mediastinum as shown in Figure 20-1. Due to the tenuous proximity to thoracic structures within a confined space, mediastinal masses may be associated with cardiac and respiratory derangements including: (1) direct cardiac and great vessel compression; (2) superior vena cava syndrome; and (3) tracheobronchial obstruction.

The incidence of mediastinal masses vary according to the age of the patient and location of the lesion. In adults, most mediastinal tumors occur in the anterior mediastinum. The two most common neoplasms of the anterior mediastinum are thymomas and lymphomas which account for 30% of the pathology. In children, most mediastinal tumors occur in the posterior mediastinum. Tumors of the posterior mediastinum are typically

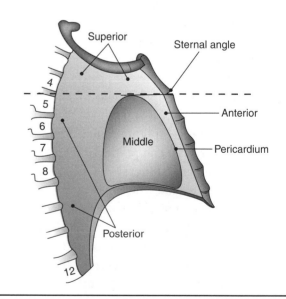

Figure 20-1 *Anatomic representation of the mediastinum with associated mediastinal pathological abnormalities.*

neurogenic in nature and comprise 12 to 21% of all mediastinal masses.

SURGICAL PROCEDURE

Improvements in video technology, endoscopic instruments, and surgical techniques have permitted surgeons to perform a variety of diagnostic and therapeutic procedures using the VATS technique. The indications for VATS procedures are listed in Table 20-1. VATS involves making three or more small incisions through which access ports are inserted into the chest wall. This allows the introduction of a high-resolution video camera and endoscopic surgical instruments into the thoracic cavity for surgical resection.

Typically the sixth or seventh intercostal space in the midaxillary line is ideal for initial access to the pleural cavity. This allows for the introduction of a high-resolution video camera and a clear view of the mediastinum, all pleural surfaces, and the pulmonary parenchyma. Under direct thoracoscopic vision additional intercostal access ports are created allowing the introduction of various surgical instruments into the thoracic cavity. The positioning of the

Table 20-1 Indications for Diagnostic and Therapeutic VATS	
Pulmonary disease	• Biopsy and staging of cancer
	• Identification of disease (i.e., tuberculosis, mesothelioma, pulmonary interstitial fibrosis, and solitary nodules)
	• Lung resection or lobectomy
	• Lung volume reduction surgery
	• Drainage and treatment of pleural effusions (e.g., pleurodesis by talc, thermal, chemical, or mechanical means)
	• Traumatic thoracic injury evaluation
	• Diaphragmatic disease
	• Tissue resection (i.e., decortication, empyemectomy, bullae, blebs, and granulomas)
Esophageal disease	• Biopsy and staging of cancer
	• Tissue resection (i.e., vagotomy, Heller myotomy, Zenker diverticulum, and esophagectomy)
	• Gastroesophageal reflux treatment (e.g., Nissen fundoplication)
Mediastinal disease	• Biopsy and staging of cancer
	• Surgical resection of tumors of the anterior, middle, and posterior mediastinum
Cardiac and vascular procedures	• Patent ductus arteriosus ligation
	• Internal mammary artery dissection
	• Pericardial window and stripping
	• Minimally invasive direct coronary artery bypass
Miscellaneous	• Sympathectomy (i.e., treatment of hyperhydrosis or chronic reflex pain syndrome)
	• Thoracic anterior vertebral surgery
	• Removal of intrathoracic foreign bodies (i.e., sheared catheters)

patient, operating team, video monitor, camera, and surgical access ports are determined by the location within the thoracic cavity of the area of surgical concern. Positioning varies and it is dependent on the individual surgeon's needs, but the principle of triangulation used for laparoscopic surgery is applicable to the thoracic cavity for VATS as shown in Figure 20-2. The thoracoscopic camera and endoscopic instruments should be oriented to face the target pathology from the same direction and triangulate the lesion.

Following meticulous surgical resection of the mediastinal mass and hemostasis, a retrieval device is used for extraction of the mass. The tissue that is removed will be examined by a pathologist to determine if the specimen is cancerous. The

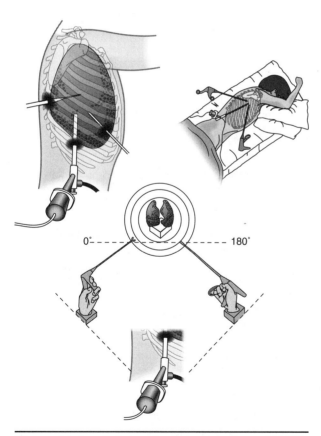

Figure 20-2 *Schematic representation of VATS. Note the triangular fashion in which the high-resolution video camera and surgical instruments are placed to promote adequate surgical visualization and resection.*

adequacy of pulmonary reexpansion is observed under direct visualization. An appropriately sized chest tube is then inserted and the thoracic cavity is closed in traditional surgical fashion.

ANESTHETIC MANAGEMENT AND CONSIDERATIONS

Preoperative Period

1. Describe the anatomy of the mediastinum and its bearing on mediastinal masses.

The mediastinum extends superiorly to the thoracic inlet, inferiorly to the diaphragm, and is bound laterally by the mediastinal parietal pleura. The mediastinum is separated into the superior and inferior mediastinum by an imaginary plane that extends from the sternal angle to the lower body of the fourth thoracic vertebra. The inferior mediastinum is further separated into the anterior, middle, and posterior mediastinum based on their relationship to the heart, which occupies the middle mediastinum.

At the convergence of the superior, anterior, and middle mediastinum are: (1) the middle portion of the superior vena cava, (2) the tracheal bifurcation, (3) the main pulmonary artery, (4) the aortic arch, and (5) the cephalad surface of the heart. Mediastinal masses are associated with direct cardiac and great vessel compression, superior vena cava syndrome, and tracheobronchial obstruction. Each of these complications is potentially life threatening, resulting in acute cardiac and respiratory deterioration and death during anesthesia if not appropriately managed.

2. Discuss an appropriate preoperative assessment for patients presenting with mediastinal masses.

As with any disease process, the optimal anesthetic plan is based on a thorough clinical evaluation and preoperative testing that should be tailored to each patient's presenting condition and symptomatology. Preoperative symptoms exhibited by patients presenting with mediastinal masses are listed in Table 20-2. This is of utmost importance in patients with mediastinal masses

Table 20-2   Preoperative Symptoms Exhibited by Patients Presenting with Mediastinal Masses

SYMPTOM CATEGORY	ANATOMY INVOLVED	SYMPTOM
Bronchopulmonary symptoms	• Bronchial irritation • Obstruction • Infection • Ulceration	• Cough or wheezing • Dyspnea • Chest pain, rales, rhonchi, or pneumonia • Hemoptysis
Extrapulmonary intrathoracic symptoms	• Pleura • Chest wall • Esophagus • Superior vena cava • Pericardium • Brachial plexus • Recurrent laryngeal nerves (unilateral or bilateral) • Spinal cord • Cervical sympathetic nerves	• Pleural effusion • Chest pain • Dysphagia • Superior vena cava syndrome • Pericardial effusion or pericarditis • Arm pain • Hoarseness or stridor • Paresthesia or paralysis • Horner syndrome
Extrathoracic metastatic symptoms	• Brain • Skeleton • Liver • Kidneys • Adrenal glands • Gastrointestinal tract • Pancreas	• Dependent on site and tumor involvement • Detection of metastases precludes curative surgery
Extrathoracic nonmetastatic symptoms	• Endocrinologic syndromes • Paraneoplastic syndromes	• Myasthenia gravis • Syndrome of inappropriate secretions of antidiuretic hormone (SIADH) • Cushing syndrome • Carcinoid syndrome • Eaton-Lambert syndrome • Pheochromocytoma
Nonspecific	• Variant	• Weight loss • Nocturnal diaphoresis • Anemia • Weakness • Anorexia • Lethargy • Malaise

due to the possibility of cardiac, great vessel, and tracheobronchial compression. Findings from basic physical examination and preoperative testing dictate: (1) the severity of the mediastinal mass, (2) the necessity for advanced intraoperative monitoring, and (3) the perioperative anesthetic plan.

The chest radiograph is the most common preoperative test used to evaluate intrathoracic pathology. When the patient develops symptoms consistent with a mediastinal mass, the chest radiograph is frequently ordered. Anterior, posterior, and lateral chest radiographs provide information regarding mediastinal mass: (1) size, (2) location, (3) density, and (4) cardiopulmonary compression.

CT with contrast-enhancement and MRI studies provide more accurate information regarding the location and density (i.e., solid, cystic, soft-tissue, or vascular) of a mediastinal mass. The degree of cardiac and airway compression, which is not always obvious on chest radiograph, can be quantified. Perioperative risk of airway obstruction increases in patients with tracheal compression greater than 50% of predicted cross-sectional area. Table 20-3 lists indicators of patients who are at high risk for perioperative complications from a mediastinal mass.

Pulmonary function tests performed in the upright and supine positions can be useful in differentiating between obstructive versus restrictive mediastinal pathology. In addition, variable intrathoracic, variable extrathoracic, and fixed airway obstructions can be determined. This makes it a valuable diagnostic tool for evaluating the dynamic nature of the mediastinal mass and its compression of tracheobronchial structures throughout the respiratory cycle.

When constructing the anesthetic plan additional tests may be advantageous for staging, planning operative therapy, and deciding on the method for one-lung ventilation. These tests should only be performed when the condition and age of the patient allows. These preoperative tests include: (1) transthoracic echocardiography, (2) ultrasonography, (3) venography, (4) angiography, (5) radionucleotide scan, (6) biochemical marker testing, and (7) awake fiberoptic bronchoscopy.

3. Evaluate the significance of superior vena cava syndrome.

Mediastinal masses may cause compression of the superior vena cava or major tributaries, causing obstruction to venous drainage from the upper thorax. The two most common causes of superior vena cava obstruction are bronchial carcinoma and malignant lymphoma. The inherent low pressure of the venous circulatory system, including the pulmonary artery, predisposes it to extrinsic compression. The resultant increase in central venous pressure causes a myriad of symptoms which can create physiologic instability. Patients who present with superior vena syndrome are at high risk for developing perioperative cardiopulmonary collapse. Table 20-4 lists the signs, symptoms, and anesthetic considerations for patients who present with superior vena cava syndrome.

4. Describe the preoperative interventions that can be used to optimize high-risk patients with a mediastinal mass.

The mediastinal mass is a foreign structure within the small confines of the thoracic cavity and

Table 20-3	Indicators of Patients Who Are at High Risk of Perioperative Complications

- Cardiopulmonary signs and symptoms at presentation (i.e., dyspnea or orthopnea)
- Combined obstructive and restrictive pattern on pulmonary function tests
- Tracheal compression greater than 50% of predicted cross-sectional area
- Pericardial effusion at presentation

Table 20-4	Signs, Symptoms, and Anesthetic Considerations Associated with Superior Vena Cava Syndrome

Signs and symptoms

- Dilation of jugular veins and collateral veins of the neck and upper thorax
- Edema of the face, neck, and upper thorax
- Cyanosis
- Papilledema or edema of the conjunctiva
- Central nervous system symptoms (i.e., headache, visual disturbances, or altered mental status)

Anesthetic considerations

- Placement of central or peripheral venous catheter below the level of obstruction (i.e., femoral vein or lower extremity)
- Drug distributions from upper extremity intravenous injections are unpredictable and are therefore less desirable
- The presence of facial and neck edema correlates with edema of the mouth, oropharynx, and hypopharynx; a careful airway assessment is imperative
- Increase in venous bleeding is possible due to high venous pressures (e.g., as high as 40 mm Hg)
- Increase in arterial bleeding is possible due to vessel compression and/or difficult mass dissection

further compression occurs when the patient lies in a supine position. Therefore, mediastinal masses pose a dilemma for the anesthetist due to the possibility of cardiac, great vessel, and tracheobronchial compression. These situations can result in hypotension, hypoxia, and cardiac arrest. Procedures such as tumor debulking, cystic aspiration, and tracheobronchial stenting have been cited in literature and have successfully alleviated extrinsic compression.

Most anterior mediastinal masses that cause airway obstruction are lymphomatous in origin and are usually responsive to radiation and chemotherapy. Preoperative radiotherapy and chemotherapy have been used to reduce mediastinal mass size and compression. Significant diminution in mediastinal mass size and an improvement in symptoms after a single dose of chemotherapy have been reported.

Determination of a mediastinal mass' sensitivity to radiation and chemotherapy can be determined only after biopsy. However, the induction of

general anesthesia in symptomatic patients with mediastinal masses is associated with increased perioperative risk. Therefore, it is prudent to perform diagnostic procedures such as fine needle or cervical node biopsy by administering local anesthesia and minimal sedation in cooperative and age-appropriate patients.

5. Describe contraindications to performing VATS.
The contraindications for having a VATS procedure are often due to a tenuous patient condition and/or inadequate surgical exposure. The specific contraindications for VATS are listed in Table 20-5. An open thoracotomy remains the gold standard approach to thoracic procedures. Conversion of a VATS procedure to an open thoracotomy always exists and should be considered when formulating the anesthetic plan. Conversion to a limited thoracotomy or a standard open thoracotomy is justified if the patient's diagnostic and therapeutic condition is severely compromised.

Table 20-5   Contraindications for VATS
• Hemodynamic instability and indication(s) for emergent open thoracotomy
• Bleeding diathesis (i.e., coagulopathy or grossly abnormal coagulation studies)
• Visceral and parietal pleural adhesions secondary to empyema, granulomatous infection, pleurodesis, or previous thoracotomy
• Inability to tolerate OLV or lateral decubitus position as manifested by acute or chronic respiratory insufficiency and/or dependency on mechanical ventilation
• Pulmonary resection due to inaccessible location or size

Intraoperative Period

6. Describe the effects of general anesthesia on airway compression in a patient with a mediastinal mass.

Surgery and general anesthesia are associated with a variety of physiologic changes which can precipitate acute airway compression in a patient with a mediastinal mass. These physiologic effects include:

- Placement of the patient in the supine position causes a decrease in the anterior–posterior diameter of the chest wall and cephalic displacement of the diaphragm. These actions increase the risk of airway compression by reducing the anatomic dimensions of the thoracic cavity and total lung capacity.
- Placement of the patient in the supine position causes an increase in central blood volume. In highly vascular mediastinal masses, this phenomenon can cause an increase in tumor blood volume and size which exacerbates external compression of the tracheobronchial tree.
- Induction of anesthesia and institution of inhalation anesthetics cause a decrease in tracheobronchial smooth muscle tone. This increases the extrinsic compressibility of the trachea and bronchi.

- Institution of positive-pressure ventilation eliminates the normal transpleural pressure gradient. This decreases airway diameter and increases the risk of extrinsic compression.
- Even in the absence of extrinsic tracheal compression, the presence of tracheomalacia and weakening of tracheal structures can cause complete tracheal collapse.

7. Describe the effects of muscle relaxants and positive pressure ventilation on airway compression in a patient with a mediastinal mass.

Under normal circumstances, inspiratory muscle contraction during spontaneous ventilation causes caudal movement of the diaphragm and an increase in the anterior–posterior diameter of the chest wall. The opposing interaction between the expanding chest wall and the elastic recoil of the lungs creates a negative intrathoracic pressure (-3 to -5 cm H_2O). In addition, a transpleural pressure gradient develops within the thoracic cavity. These distending forces that result from spontaneous respiration increase airway diameter and minimize airway compression.

The use of muscle relaxants and/or the institution of positive-pressure ventilation inhibit spontaneous respiration and effectively eliminate the normal transpleural pressure gradient. The resulting decrease in the caliber of the airways increases the risk of partial or complete airway obstruction.

8. Describe three methods of induction of general anesthesia that preserve spontaneous respiration.

Preanesthetic optimization is imperative to minimizing risks associated with induction of general anesthesia. Prior to induction of anesthesia, patients who exhibit signs and symptoms of respiratory difficulty should be placed in the semirecumbent position to relieve preexisting airway obstruction. In high-risk patients, cannulation of the femoral vein and arteries, in anticipation of the need for cardiopulmonary bypass, has been suggested. Cardiopulmonary bypass may be required for distal airway obstructions and hypoxemia that is untreatable by conventional emergency airway methods. Emergency tracheotomy or placement of a rigid ventilating bronchoscope may prove futile if the airway compression occurs in the distal trachea or bronchial segments.

The following methods preserve spontaneous respiration and are used to minimize the risks associated with induction of general anesthesia:

- Awake intubation, followed by a gradual intravenous or inhalation induction.
- Inhalation induction with a volatile anesthetic, followed by intubation.
- Intravenous induction with ketamine, followed by intubation.

9. Describe methods to optimize visualization and maintain oxygenation during VATS.

As with any surgical procedure, it is of utmost importance to provide adequate surgical visualization and maintain adequate patient oxygenation. Various maneuvers can be instituted during the intraoperative period such as:

Visualization
- **Position**

  The positioning of the patient (i.e., supine, prone, or lateral decubitus) is determined by the location of the mass within the thoracic cavity. The lateral decubitus position allows for intercostal surgical access and visualization of mediastinal structures. The affected side is typically placed in a nondependent position. The operating room table can then be rotated and manipulated (i.e., Trendelenburg, reverse Trendelenburg, or flexed positioned) utilizing gravity to increase surgical visualization.
- **One-lung ventilation (OLV)**

  A dual-lumen endobronchial tube (DLT), bronchial blocker, or endobronchial intubation with a single-lumen endotracheal tube allows:

(1) ventilatory control, (2) selective lung separation, (3) deflation of the lung ipsilateral to the area of surgical concern, and (4) improved surgical exposure. Suction that is applied to the DLT can facilitate rapid lung deflation. Due to the relatively small diameter of the bronchial blocker, it may take up to 30 minutes for complete lung collapse to occur. Allowing adequate time for lung deflation is imperative in order to provide adequate surgical exposure.
- **Carbon dioxide insufflation**

  In rare circumstances, carbon dioxide can be insufflated into the pleural cavity to facilitate visualization. It may be used at the beginning of the procedure to facilitate expedious and complete ipsilateral lung collapse. Insufflation pressure should be maintained as low as possible (less than 5 mm Hg) and the CO_2 inflow rate kept less than 2 l/min. Higher pressures and/or a rapid insufflation rate can cause mediastinal shift and hemodynamic compromise as occurs in a tension pneumothorax.

Oxygenation
- **High FiO$_2$**

  Utilization of a high fraction of inspired oxygen (up to 100%) maximizes arterial oxygenation. It is important to note that the utilization of 100% oxygen has been associated with absorption atelectasis and oxygen toxicity. However, the benefits of increasing PaO_2 in patients with marginal respiratory reserve exceed the risks.
- **Continuous positive airway pressure (CPAP) and positive-end expiratory pressure (PEEP)**

  By minimizing intrapulmonary shunt, the application of 5–10 cm H_2O of CPAP to the nonventilated lung is effective in maximizing oxygenation during OLV. Furthermore, the application of PEEP to the ventilated lung has also been shown to be effective in maintaining oxygenation during OLV by preventing alveolar collapse and increasing functional residual capacity. PEEP should be maintained at less than 5 mm Hg to avoid adversely increasing pulmonary vascular resistance.

- **Tidal volume and respiratory rate**
During OLV, a tidal volume set to approximately 8 to 10 ml/kg should be used to prevent: (1) atelectasis, (2) increases in airway pressure, and (3) increases in pulmonary vascular resistance. Despite the ventilation and perfusion mismatch that occurs during OLV, a 20 to 30% increase in respiratory rate is frequently adequate to maintain normal minute ventilation and physiologic $PaCO_2$.

Scenario: After 20 minutes of surgical resection, the following scenario occurs: blood pressure, 70/30; heart rate, 110; room air oxygen saturation, 87%; respiratory rate, 10; tidal volume, 20 ml; peak inspiratory pressure, 40 cm H_2O.

10. List potential intraoperative complications and appropriate initial interventions during VATS for mediastinal mass that could cause this clinical scenario.
Treatment for this patient would include immediately informing the surgeon, ventilating with 100% oxygen, and diagnosing the etiology of this scenario prior to instituting further treatment. Potential intraoperative complications that can occur during VATS for mediastinal mass include:

- Pneumothorax: Treatment, emergent needle decompression, subsequent chest tube placement.
- Embolism: Treatment, left lateral decubitus positioning (Durant's position), aspiration of embolus via central venous catheter, supportive measures as needed.
- Hemorrhage: Treatment, surgical hemostasis, administration of crystalloids, colloids, and blood products.
- Cardiac, great vessel, and tracheobronchial compression: A treatment plan is included in Table 20-6.

Postoperative Period

11. Describe serious postoperative complications specifically related to VATS.
A variety of postoperative complications have been reported after VATS and constant vigilance is necessary during the postoperative period.

- **Airway obstruction**
Despite adequate surgical resection of a mediastinal mass, the presence of tracheomalacia

Table 20-6   Treatment Plan for Cardiac, Great Vessel, and Tracheobronchial Compression
• Stop surgery
• Minimize or reverse the deleterious effects of: (1) general anesthesia, (2) muscle relaxants, and (3) positive-pressure ventilation
• Change patient position to lateral, prone, or semirecumbent to decrease compression
• Place rigid ventilating bronchoscope to apply tension to weakened tracheobronchial tree
• Place rigid ventilating bronchoscope to bypass distal obstructions
• Helium-oxygen mixture to reduce the resistance to airflow through compressed airway
• Emergency thoracotomy, median sternotomy, and tumor debulking to decrease extrinsic compression
• Utilize advanced cardiac life-support protocol as needed
• Cardiopulmonary bypass to restore oxygenation

and inadequate cartilaginous tracheal support can cause tracheal collapse and necessitate postoperative intubation and ventilatory support.

- **Hemorrhage**
  Systemic arterial bleeding, diffuse bleeding from thoracic parenchyma, failure of endoscopic staples/sutures, and tracheal lacerations resulting from management of the airway have been reported. Uncontrolled postoperative bleeding and hypovolemia necessitate emergency thoracotomy.

- **Arrhythmias**
  Trauma from cardiac manipulation, vagal stimulation, and cardiopulmonary disease can precipitate cardiac dysrythmias. Approximately 25% of patients undergoing thoracic surgery experience postoperative atrial dysrythmias, of which atrial flutter and fibrillation are the most common.

- **Respiratory insufficiency**
  Acute respiratory insufficiency is the most common and serious complication following pulmonary resection which occurs in nearly 5% of patients after resection of bronchial carcinoma. Preexisting pulmonary pathology, pulmonary transudate, pulmonary trauma, and/or postoperative pain can precipitate inadequate respiratory effort.

- **Neural injury**
  During dissection of mediastinal masses, the phrenic, vagus, and recurrent laryngeal nerves may be inadvertently injured or deliberately sacrificed. Damage to the spinal branches of the intercostal arteries by dissection or diathermy may cause spinal cord ischemia. In addition, following dissection in the posterior mediastinum a fistula can form between the pleura and epidural space in which blood can enter and cause spinal cord compression and ischemia.

12. Describe available pain management modalities for patients presenting for VATS.
The advantages of VATS over open thoracotomy include: decreased postoperative pain, reduction

Table 20-7	Effective Analgesic Therapies Used to Treat Postoperative Pain After VATS
• Epidural analgesia (i.e., thoracic or upper lumbar)	
• Interpleural regional anesthesia	
• Cryoanalgesia	
• Intercostal nerve block	
• Paravertebral block	
• Local anesthetic infiltration	
• Systemic analgesia (i.e., patient-controlled analgesia)	

in the incidence of postoperative respiratory dysfunction, shorter postoperative course, and the promotion of a rapid recovery. These benefits result in a reduced length of hospital stay and decreased costs. Analgesic interventions that are used to treat postoperative pain after VATS are included in Table 20-7.

Despite this minimally invasive approach to thoracic surgery, there is an incidence of 22 to 26% of chronic pain in patients following VATS. Intercostal nerve damage resulting from chest wall trauma and muscle damage from instrumentation can result in intercostal neuritis, postoperative neuralgia, and chronic pain.

Treating pain after VATS is important for the following reasons: (1) patient comfort and satisfaction; (2) allowing optimal respiratory effort, and (3) minimizing pulmonary complications (i.e., retention of secretions, airway closure, and atelectasis). Thoracic epidural analgesia is the current gold standard for postthoracotomy pain and has gained increasing acceptance in providing subjectively better analgesia than any other method in VATS.

Typically a thoracic epidural catheter is placed preoperatively in the T6-T8 interspace. This is to be done for patients who are awake in order to assess proper placement and the presence of postprocedural complications. A clear plan must be created for the intraoperative utilization and management of a thoracic epidural catheter such as the type and volume of local anesthetic to be injected for the initial bolus and maintenance doses. The benefit of intraoperative analgesia should be weighed against the potential for sympathectomy resulting in hypotension for patients with marginal hemodynamic reserve. Postoperatively, the epidural solution used for infusion typically combines a low concentration of a long-acting local anesthetic, such as bupivicaine or ropivacaine, and an opioid which includes fentanyl or hydromorphone.

Since there are multiple pathways of nociceptive input to the central nervous system, a multimodal approach to pain management may also include a combination of nonsteroidal anti-inflammatory drugs, use of patient-controlled analgesia, and narcotics.

REVIEW QUESTIONS

1. The two most common neoplasms present in the anterior mediastinum are:
   a. thymoma and lymphoma.
   b. lymphoma and teratoma.
   c. teratoma and bronchogenic cyst.
   d. bronchogenic cyst and neurogenic tumor.
2. Which is not associated with a mediastinal mass?
   a. Cardiac compression
   b. Aortic and pulmonary artery dilation
   b. Superior vena cava syndrome
   c. Tracheobronchial obstruction
3. Which can precipitate tracheobronchial compression?
   a. Maintaining spontaneous ventilation
   b. Local anesthesia and minimal sedation
   c. Tracheomalacia
   d. Intravenous induction with ketamine

4. Which statement is false regarding VATS?
   a. Diagnostic and therapeutic procedures can be performed using VATS.
   b. Principle of surgical triangulation is applicable to VATS.
   c. VATS is associated with more pain than an open thoracotomy.
   d. Conversion from a VATS procedure to open thoracotomy may be necessary.
5. Which is the most common postoperative complication following VATS for bronchial carcinoma?
   A. Respiratory insufficiency
   B. Airway obstruction
   C. Neural injury
   D. Hemorrhage

REVIEW ANSWERS

1. **Answer: a**
   The incidence of mediastinal masses vary according to the age of the patient and location of the lesion. In adults, most mediastinal tumors occur in the anterior mediastinum. The two most common neoplasms of the anterior mediastinum are thymomas and lymphomas which account for 30% of the pathology.
2. **Answer: b**
   At the convergence of the superior, anterior, and middle mediastinum is: (1) the middle portion of the superior vena cava, (2) the tracheal bifurcation, (3) the main pulmonary artery, (4) the aortic arch, and (5) the cephalad surface of the heart. Mediastinal masses are associated with direct cardiac and great vessel (i.e., aorta and main pulmonary artery) compression; superior vena cava syndrome; and tracheobronchial obstruction. Each of these complications is potentially life threatening and can result in death during surgery and anesthesia.

3. **Answer: c**

   Despite adequate surgical resection of a mediastinal mass, the presence of tracheomalacia and inadequate cartilaginous tracheal support can cause tracheal collapse and necessitate postoperative intubation and ventilatory support.

4. **Answer: c**

   The advantages associated with VATS as compared to an open thoracotomy include: decreased postoperative pain, reduction in the incidence of postoperative respiratory dysfunction, shorter postoperative course, and the promotion of a rapid recovery resulting in reduced length of hospital stay and cost.

5. **Answer: a**

   Acute respiratory insufficiency is the most common and serious complication following pulmonary resection which occurs in nearly 5% of patients after resection of bronchial carcinoma. Preexisting pulmonary pathology, pulmonary transudate, pulmonary trauma, and/or postoperative pain can precipitate inadequate respiratory effort.

SUGGESTED READINGS

Béchard P, Létourneau L, Lacasse Y, et al. Perioperative cardiopulmonary complications in adults with mediastinal mass. *Anesthesiology* 2004;100(4):826–834.

Cirino LM, Campos JR, Fernandez A, et al. Diagnosis and treatment of mediastinal mass by thoracoscopy. *Chest* 2000;117(6):1787–1792.

Cohen E, Neustein SM, Eisenkraft JB. Anesthesia for thoracic surgery. In: Barash PG, Cullen BF, Stoelting RK, eds. *Clinical Anesthesia*, 5th ed. Philadelphia: Lippincott Williams & Wilkins, 2006:813–855.

Duwe BV, Sterman DH, Musani AI. Tumors of the mediastinum. *Chest* 2005;128(4):2893–2909.

Gottschalk A, Cohen SP, Yang S, et al. Preventing and treating pain after thoracic surgery. *Anesthesiology* 2006;104(3):594–600.

Massone PBG, Lequaglie C, Magnani B, et al. The real impact and usefulness of video-assisted thoracoscopic surgery in the diagnosis and therapy of clinical lymphadenopathies of the mediastinum. *Ann Surg Oncol* 2003;10(10):1197–1202.

Nagelhout JJ. Respiratory anatomy: thoracic surgery. In: Nagelhout JJ, Zaglaniczy KL, eds. *Nurse Anesthesia*, 3rd ed. St. Louis, MO: Elsevier Saunders, 2005:574–590.

Wilson WC, Benumof JL. Anesthesia for thoracic surgery. In: Miller RD, ed. *Miller's Anesthesia*, 6th ed. New York: Churchill Livingstone, 2005:1847–1939.

Anesthesia Management for Thymectomy

21

Bernadette T. Higgins Roche

KEY POINTS

- The thymus is responsible for the production of T lymphocytes that are involved in cell-mediated immunity.
- Thymomas are frequently associated with paraneoplastic syndromes which include hypogammaglobulinemia, pure red cell aplasia, Cushing syndrome, Graves disease, pernicious anemia, and several autoimmune diseases, especially myasthenia gravis (MG).
- Symptoms that are associated with a thymoma are primarily due to the impingement of mediastinal structures or they are related to MG.
- MG and Lambert-Eaton myasthenic syndrome (LEMS) are two different physiologic disease processes that are associated with implications for anesthetic management.
- Anticholinesterase medications are the primary treatment for symptoms associated with MG.

CASE SYNOPSIS

A 52-year-old woman with a history of Class III MG and a stage III thymoma is admitted for a thymectomy. Prior to admission, she received a 3-month course of chemotherapy with doxorubicin, cisplatin, vincristine, and cyclophospha-mide. She is scheduled for a postoperative course of mediastinal radiation.

PREOPERATIVE EVALUATION AND DEMOGRAPHIC DATA

Past Medical/Surgical History

- MG Class III for 14 years
- Stage III thymoma
- Thyroidectomy for Graves disease 4 years ago
- Laparoscopic cholecystectomy 10 years ago

List of Medications

- Pyridostigmine 600 mg daily
- Prednisolone 100 mg every second day
- Synthroid 0.15 mg daily

Diagnostic Data

- Hemoglobin, 11.9 mg/dl; hematocrit, 35%
- Glucose, 88 mg/dl
- Electrolytes: sodium, 139 mEq/l; potassium, 3.8 mEq/l; chloride, 106 mEq/l; carbon dioxide, 22 mEq/l
- Electrocardiogram (ECG): Normal sinus rhythm, heart rate 88

Height/Weight/Vital Signs

- 163 cm, 63 kg
- Blood pressure, 1300/84; heart rate, 80 beats per minute; respiratory rate, 16 breaths per minute; temperature, 37°C; room air oxygen saturation, 98%

PATHOPHYSIOLOGY

Named for its resemblance to the bud of the thyme herb, the thymus is embryonically derived from the third, and occasionally the fourth, pair of pharyngeal pouches. As seen in Figure 21-1, it is composed of two fused different-sized lobes, enclosed by a dense capsule. The thymus is located in the upper thorax, at the level of the fourth costal cartilage, right beneath the sternum. It can extend upward into the neck as high as the lower border of the thyroid gland. Each thymic lobe is made up of numerous lobules of varying size. The cortical portion of the lobules is mainly composed of lymphoid cells and the medulla is primarily epithelial cells. Blood supply to the thymus is derived from the internal mammary and superior and inferior thyroid arteries. Venous blood drains into the innominate veins and the thyroid sinus. The organ receives both sympathetic and parasympathetic innervation (vagus). The thymus gland weighs 10–30 mg at birth. It increases in size throughout childhood until puberty, at which time it starts to atrophy in response to increased levels of sex hormones; over time it is gradually replaced by adipose tissue.

There are two main types of immune system cells, B lymphocyte (B-cells) and T lymphocytes (T-cells). B-cells are produced by bone marrow stem cells

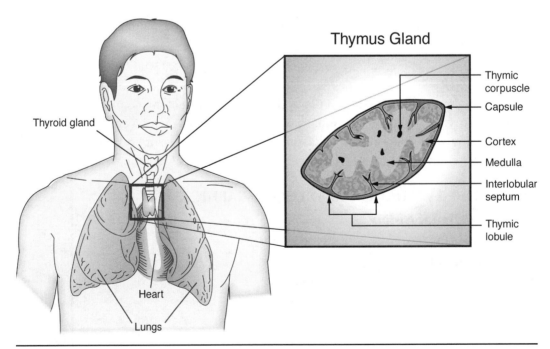

Figure 21-1 *Anatomy of the thymus gland.*

and are responsible for humoral immunity that is mediated by antibody production and complement activation. T-cells, bone marrow stem cells that mature in the thymus, are involved in cell mediated immunity and include helper T-cells (effector T-cells or T_h-cells), cytotoxic T-cells, (T_C cells), memory T-cells, (regulatory T-cells, T_{reg} cells, formerly known as suppressor T-cells), natural killer T-cells, (NKT), and gamma/delta T-cells ($\gamma\delta$ T cells). In addition to their role in fighting infection and cancer, T-cells are responsible for rejection of transplanted organs, autoimmune diseases, and allergies.

The main function of the thymus is the development of immunocompetent T-cells. Bone marrow stem cells migrate to the thymus and enter the cortex of the thymic lobules, where they mature into T-cells, in response to the thymic hormones, thymopoietin and thymosin. Each stem cell has T-cell receptor (TCR) genes, which undergo genetic rearrangement during thymocyte maturation. The resultant T-cells have a unique TCR that can recognize specific cell-bound antigens in lymphoid organs. T-cells account for approximately 65% of blood lymphocytes; they are also found in lymphoid organs.

SURGICAL PROCEDURE

There are three cell types that cause thymic cancers. Epithelial cells give rise to thymic carcinoma and thymomas; lymphocytes are associated with Hodgkin disease or non-Hodgkin lymphomas; Kulchitsky cells (neuroendocrine cells) give rise to thymic carcinoid tumors. Thymolipoma is composed of thymic tissue and fatty tissue. Thymomas are the most common type of thymic tumor. Although the overall incidence is low, 0.15 cases per 100,000 and < 0.5% of all cancers, they account for 20% of all mediastinal tumors and 50% of anterior mediastinal tumors. Surgery is the mainstay of treatment; despite their indolent nature, thymomas have the potential for local spread, especially into the pleural space. Chemotherapy may be instituted preoperatively to shrink large, malignant tumors; postoperative chemotherapy and radiation may

be indicated for large invasive tumors. Thymomas are frequently associated with several autoimmune diseases, especially MG which is found in 30–65% of patients with a thymoma. Approximately 10–15% of patients with MG have a thymoma, and myasthenic patients are routinely screened for thymic tumors.

Surgical thymectomy is also indicated for patients with generalized MG to induce remission or sufficiently reduce symptoms to allow a reduction in immunosuppressive medication. Due to the role of the thymus in development of the immune system, it is preferable to delay thymectomy until puberty. After the age of 60, there is a questionable amount of viable thymic tissue which reduces the probability of a positive response to thymectomy in older patients who have MG. Of the paraneoplastic syndromes associated with thymomas, only MG, pure red cell aplasia, and hypogammaglobulinemia have a positive response to thymectomy.

ANESTHETIC MANAGEMENT AND CONSIDERATIONS

Preoperative Period

1. Describe the symptoms that are commonly associated with thymomas.

Thymomas are capable of local invasion and the majority of symptoms are due to impingement of mediastinal structures or associated myasthenic symptoms. Patients may present with a chronic cough from phrenic nerve encroachment, superior vena cava syndrome, dysphagia, and shortness of breath (SOB) as a result of a paralyzed hemidiaphragm, hoarseness, chest pain, hemoptysis, and pleural effusion. However, 30–50% of patients have no symptoms and the mass is discovered incidentally during chest x-ray (CXR) or computed tomography (CT) scan for an unrelated problem. Thymomas are rare in children and adults older than 40 years; they affect females and males equally.

In addition to MG, thymomas are also associated with other paraneoplastic syndromes. These rare disorders are due to an immune system response to a neoplasm. The symptoms occur remotely from the tumor and can affect multiple systems, including the endocrine, neuromuscular or musculoskeletal, cardiovascular, cutaneous, hematologic, renal, or gastrointestinal systems. Symptoms of a paraneoplastic syndrome are due to humoral factors emanating from the tumor or an immune response to the tumor; they are frequently present before the neoplasm is actually recognized. Paraneoplastic syndromes that are associated with thymomas and thymic carcinoma include pure red cell aplasia, Graves disease, acquired hypogammaglobulinemia, Cushing syndrome, and pernicious anemia.

2. Compare the impact of thymic dysfunction in adults and children.

After puberty, the thymus gradually decreases in size and thymic tissue is replaced by adipose tissue. The majority of T-cells are produced early in life and thymic dysfunction or a thymectomy has no significant impact on immune function in the adult. In contrast, congenital athymia or loss of thymus gland function in childhood is associated with a lack of functional T-cells, resulting in severe immunodeficiency and increased susceptibility to infection. DiGeorge syndrome, a congenital disorder due to deletion of genes from chromosome 22, causes developmental abnormalities in the third and fourth pharyngeal pouches. Characteristics of DiGeorge syndrome includes facial abnormality; congenital heart defects; absence or hypoplasia of the thymus; hypoparathyroidism; conotruncal abnormalities; cognitive, behavioral, and psychiatric problems; and increased susceptibility to infections. Immune deficiency is seen with partial DiGeorge syndrome but improves over time. Patients with athymia are categorized as having complete DiGeorge syndrome, have few detectable peripheral T-cells, and usually die within the first 2 years of life unless they undergo thymus transplantation.

3. Discuss the relationship between the thymus gland and MG.

MG is an antibody-mediated autoimmune disease of the neuromuscular junction (NMJ), specifically the postsynaptic membrane. Immunoglobulin G antibodies (IgG) to the alpha-subunit of the postsynaptic nicotinic acetylcholine receptor (nAChR) are present in approximately 80% of patients with the disease. The antibodies mechanically block the acetylcholine (ACh) binding sites on the nAChR and ultimately destroy them. Over time, the architecture of the postsynaptic membrane changes and takes on a simplified appearance with a decreased number of nAChR and junctional folds on the postsynaptic membrane; the resultant widening of the postsynaptic cleft increases the chance of ACh escaping before it can reach the postsynaptic membrane. Symptoms of MG are present when the number of functional nAChRs is < 30% normal. The thymus contains myeloid (musclelike) cells which expose the T-cells to the nAChR; this may help to explain the relationship between MG and the thymus. The nicotinic cholinergic receptors of the autonomic nervous system (ANS) and the central nervous system (CNS) have a different antigenicity, accounting for the lack of ANS and CNS symptoms in MG patients. Thymectomy improves the symptoms of MG but does not cure the disease, supporting the theory that nAChR antibodies are also produced in organs other than the thymus.

4. Review the diagnosis and treatment for MG.

Muscle weakness is a common symptom associated with many neuromuscular disorders and it is not uncommon for a delayed diagnosis in the myasthenic patient. Weakness of the skeletal muscles is characteristic but symptoms can vary in type and severity. Muscular weakness increases with activity and improves after periods of rest, frequently affecting muscles that control eye and eyelid movements, facial expression, chewing, talking, and swallowing. In some patients, muscle weakness is limited to the eye muscles (ocular

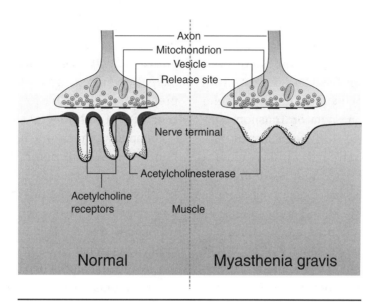

Figure 21-2 *Differences in postsynaptic acetylcholine receptor functioning comparing normal neuromuscular transmission and myasthenia gravis.*

myasthenia). In 20% of patients, MG will initially affect the bulbar muscles but the majority of patients present with generalized weakness involving the limbs. Respiratory involvement occurs late in the disease and is associated with numerous other symptoms. Common symptoms of generalized MG include ptosis, diplopia, facial muscle weakness, dysphagia, dysarthria, dysphonia, limb weakness, and shortness of breath. The highest incidence of MG is found in females < 40 years and males > 60 years. Classifications of MG are listed in Table 21-1.

Standard electromyography (EMG), single-fiber electromyography (SFEMG), and repetitive

Table 21-1 Osserman Classification System for Myasthenia Gravis
Class I: Eye muscle weakness (Ocular myasthenia)
Class II: Eye muscle weakness, mild weakness of other muscles
Class IIa: Predominantly limb or axial muscle weakness
Class IIb: Predominantly bulbar and/or respiratory muscle weakness
Class III: Eye muscle weakness, moderate weakness of other muscles
Class IIIa: Predominantly limb or axial muscle weakness
Class IIIb: Predominantly bulbar and/or respiratory muscle weakness
Class IV: Eye muscle weakness, severe weakness of other muscles
Class IVa: Predominantly limb or axial muscle weakness
Class IVb: Predominantly bulbar and/or respiratory muscle weakness
Class V: Myasthenic crisis

nerve stimulation (RNS) are used for diagnosis of the disease. Diagnostic specificity for MG is close to 100% when nAChR antibodies are present: they are detected in > 80% of patients with MG but may be absent in patients with ocular myasthenia. The edrophonium or Tensilon challenge test is also used for diagnosis of MG; improvement in muscle strength within 5 minutes after administration of edrophonium 10 mg IV is confirmatory for the disease. A positive response is not completely specific for MG and can be seen with other conditions such as amyotrophic lateral sclerosis (ALS). The sensitivity of both RNS and the edrophonium challenge is dependent on the type and severity of symptoms. SFEMG is the most sensitive test for ocular and generalized muscle involvement. CT can identify an abnormal thymus gland or thymoma.

Pregnancy can cause exacerbation or remission of the disease; it is also associated with a transient neonatal myasthenia in response to placental transfer of maternal antibodies. Normally, alpha-fetoprotein inhibits binding of maternal nAChR antibodies to fetal ACh receptors and < 20% of neonates born to myasthenic mothers have transient myasthenia. Alpha-fetoprotein may also contribute to the remission that often occurs during the second and third trimesters of pregnancy. Signs of neonatal myasthenia are usually present at birth and include difficulty in sucking, swallowing, and breathing; ptosis; and facial weakness. In severe cases, the infant is treated with oral neostigmine. Maternal antibodies are present in breastmilk and may accentuate neonatal myasthenia. Spontaneous remission of symptoms usually occurs within 2–4 weeks with no risk of relapse.

Treatment of MG includes administration of anticholinesterase medication, immune suppression, and thymectomy. Anticholinesterase agents are the first line of treatment and pyridostigmine (Mestinon) is the most widely used anticholinesterase. It has a half-life of 4 hours and effects are seen within 30 minutes. Dosage is patient depen-

dent; the average dose is 600 mg daily, spaced to provide maximum effects during periods of intense muscle activity. Higher doses are associated with increased muscle weakness. A sustained-release preparation is available for night administration for treatment of nighttime or early morning weakness.

Immunosuppression can attenuate the destruction of the nACh receptor. High-dose steroid treatment includes prednisolone (Prednisone) 100 mg per day for 2–4 weeks and then 100 mg every other day; improvement of symptoms is typically seen within 2–3 weeks. High-dose steroids are associated with a transient deterioration of NMJ function during the first weeks of treatment. For less severe cases, prednisolone 10–20 mg/day is initiated and increased by 5 mg every 3–5 days. The target daily dose of 100 mg is reached within 6–8 weeks, at which time the patient is switched to alternate-day dosing. This approach minimizes the negative effects on the NMJ but the onset of improvement will be significantly prolonged.

Administration of the antimetabolite, azathioprine (Imuran), is associated with inhibition of T-cells and decreased plasma levels of nAChR antibodies. It is beneficial for patients who relapse on prednisolone or as a steroid-sparing precaution in patients with a history of long-time steroid use. The response to azathioprine is much slower than steroids and can take 3–12 months; consequently, a combination of corticosteroids and azathioprine may be used for the initial treatment of myasthenic patients. Another immunosuppressant, cyclosporine (Sandimmune, Neoral), is also used for management of myasthenic symptoms. It inhibits helper T-cells, facilitates suppressor T-cells, and blocks the production and secretion of interleukin-2. Long-term use of both azathioprine and cyclosporine is associated with an increased risk for malignancy. With similar efficacy and significantly reduced toxicity, mycophenolate mofetil (MyM, CellCept), an immunosuppressive agent used in organ transplantation, is an effective alternative to azathioprine and cyclosporine.

Plasmapheresis involves exchanges of 3–5 liters of plasma; 4–6 exchanges effectively remove nAChR antibodies from the circulation and allow recovery of the nAChR. Improvement of symptoms is seen within days and can last for several weeks. Plasmapheresis is especially effective for treatment of myasthenic crisis, and it is frequently used to improve muscle strength prior to thymectomy. Chronic, intermittent plasmapheresis may be indicated for patients refractory to other treatment modalities. Approximately 65% of myasthenic patients show improvement within days to weeks after receiving intravenous immunoglobulin (IVIg). Its exact mechanism of action is unknown and IVIg has no consistent effect on plasma nAChR antibody levels. The incidence of side effects is low and IVIg is used for treatment of MG patients who are refractory to other immunosuppressive agents. Cost of the drug is a significant limitation to its use. Thymectomy, with or without the presence of thymoma, is an effective treatment for MG, especially if performed within 1 year of the onset of symptoms. The remission response to thymectomy is not immediate and only 25% achieve remission within the first year.

5. Contrast MG and the Lambert-Eaton myasthenic syndrome.

In contrast to MG, which is associated with postsynaptic nAChR antibodies, the LEMS is associated with autoantibodies that antagonize the function of the presynaptic ACh voltage-gated Ca^{2+} channels. The antibodies interfere with the opening of the calcium channels and restrict the release of ACh. Decreased ACh release, characteristic of LEMS, is associated with muscle weakness in the proximal limbs, depressed tendon reflexes, posttetanic potentiation, and ANS abnormalities including gastroparesis, orthostatic hypotension, and urinary retention. Presynaptic ACh stores and the postsynaptic response to ACh remain intact; consequently, rapid repetitive stimulation

or voluntary activation will increase ACh release and improve muscle strength. Symptoms of LEMS include progressive muscle weakness but it does not usually involve the facial or respiratory muscles. Muscle weakness is worse in the morning and improves with exercise or nerve stimulation. Autonomic symptoms are frequently present. The presence of calcium-channel antibodies and improved muscle strength with RNS is confirmatory for the disease. Guanidine hydrochloride enhances the release of ACh and is used to improve muscle strength; 3,4-diaminopyridine increases the action potential duration by blocking the potassium channel efflux. This allows the Ca^{2+} channels to remain open and release a larger amount of ACh. Patients with LEMS may also be treated with steroids. Plasmapheresis and IVIg are associated with transient improvement in muscle strength; anticholinesterases have little effect. Similar to other paraneoplastic syndromes, the majority of patients with LEMS have an identifiable cancer, most notably small cell which is also known as oat cell carcinoma of the lung.

6. Design a preoperative assessment plan of patient with MG.

Optimizing the patient's preoperative condition can markedly improve the surgical outcome for myasthenic patients. Onset, duration, and severity of the disease should be determined and close attention should be paid to a history of related autoimmune diseases. Preoperative evaluation must include assessment of voluntary muscle strength. The ability to cough, clear secretions, and maintain a patent airway should be assessed, especially in patients with bulbar involvement. Pulmonary function testing (PFT) is mandatory in patients with generalized MG; serial forced vital capacity (FVC) measurements are a good indicator of respiratory reserve and can help identify the patients who may need postoperative mechanical ventilation. Pulmonary flow-volume loops in the supine and sitting position can identify fixed or dynamic respiratory impairments in patients with a thymoma. Patients who have a dynamic impairment are at risk for an intrathoracic airway obstruction during induction of general anesthesia. All myasthenic patients should be informed of the possibility of postoperative intubation and mechanical ventilation. Patients undergoing thymectomy for a thymoma may present with undiagnosed MG; complaints of generalized weakness and reduced exercise tolerance that improves with rest should alert the anesthetist to the possibility of the disease. It may be prudent to order preoperative PFT on these individuals.

Patients with advanced stages of MG should receive their full morning dose of pyridostigmine; patients with mild disease may take half or skip their morning dose. Prior to induction, hydrocortisone 100 mg IV should be administered to patients on steroid therapy; the dose can be repeated twice within 24 hours. To allow time for restoration of coagulation factors, plasma cholinesterase levels, and immunoglobulins, plasmapheresis should not be performed within 24 hours of surgery. Careful attention should be paid to the drug history of the myasthenic patient as many medications may provoke acute exacerbations. A list of these drugs is provided in Table 21-2. Premedication is best avoided, especially in patients with limited respiratory reserve and bulbar symptoms. Aspiration prophylaxis is mandatory in patients with bulbar symptoms.

Table 21-2   Medications Associated with Acute Exacerbations of Myasthenia Gravis

Antibiotics: macrolides, fluoroquinolones, aminoglycosides, tetracycline, and chloroquine

Antidysrhythmics: beta-blockers, calcium channel blockers, quinidine, lidocaine, procainamide

Miscellaneous: diphenylhydantoin, lithium, chlorpromazine, muscle relaxants, levothyroxine, adrenocorticotropic hormone (ACTH), trimethaphan, and, paradoxically, corticosteroids

Intraoperative Period

7. Differentiate between a myasthenic crisis and a cholinergic crisis.

Myasthenic crisis is an acute exacerbation of symptoms associated with MG that requires immediate intubation and mechanical ventilation. Increasing generalized weakness may precede the crisis. Failure of the respiratory muscle to maintain adequate ventilation will trigger acute hypoxemia, hypercarbia, and acidosis; and inability to clear bronchial secretions can result in pneumonia. Severe bulbar weakness is associated with a poor or absent gag reflex and an increased risk for aspiration. Myasthenic crisis can be precipitated by fever, infection, stress, menstruation, radiographic contrast dyes, certain mediations, and insufficient treatment with anticholinesterase and/or immunosuppressant medications.

Cholinergic crisis is due to a large amount of ACh at the NMJ, the consequence of overadministration of an anticholinesterase medication. The excess ACh causes increased stimulation of striated muscle, producing a flaccid muscle paralysis that is clinically indistinguishable from the weakness seen during a myasthenic crisis. However, deep tendon reflexes are preserved during a cholinergic crisis. Bradycardia, bronchospasm, miosis, increased lacrimation and salivation, urinary incontinence, and diarrhea are usually present.

There are no laboratory tests to differentiate between a myasthenic crisis and cholinergic crisis but the presence of muscarinic symptoms support the suspicion of a cholinergic crisis. The edrophonium challenge test is useful for distinguishing between the two occurrences. Following tracheal intubation and initiation of mechanical ventilation, an initial intravenous test dose of edrophonium 1 mg is administered, followed by varying increments to a maximum of 10 mg. During myasthenic crisis, the patient will demonstrate an immediate and dramatic improvement in muscle strength, respiratory function, and facial expression. If cholinergic crisis is the problem, the patient will respond to edrophonium with increased salivation and bronchopulmonary secretions, diaphoresis caused by further increases in ACh, but improvement in muscle strength will not occur.

Although the half-life of edrophonium is short, approximately 10 minutes, the patient must be monitored carefully during the test because serious side effects, including significant bradycardia, heart block, and asystole can occur. Patients with myasthenic crisis will require additional doses of an anticholinesterase; pyridostigmine 1 mg IM or IV is equivalent to 30 mg orally. Other treatments of myasthenic crisis include plasmapheresis and IVIg administration. Steroids should be used cautiously as they may worsen the degree of muscle weakness. Management of cholinergic crisis includes discontinuation of all cholinergic medications and intravenous administration of atropine sulfate 1–2 mg, followed by 1–2 mg IM every 2–4 hours until symptoms abate. Continued intubation and mechanical ventilation may also be necessary in these patients.

8. Discuss the surgical resection of a thymoma or the thymus.

Surgical resection is the preferred treatment of patients with a thymoma. To rule out a lymphoma, which is not treated surgically, an initial biopsy is indicated for large masses with indistinct margins. The World Health Organization (WHO) uses a histologic classification system to classify thymomas. The Masaoka system (Table 21-3) is the most frequently used classification system. It allows diagnosis and staging at the time of surgical intervention and appears to have the greatest correlation with mortality.

Thymectomy with resection of surrounding tissue is indicated for stage I thymomas. Postoperative adjunctive therapy is not necessary in the absence of capsular invasion and these patients have a 100% 5-year survival rate and a 0.9% risk of reoccurrence. Surgery is also indicated for stage II and III lesions. A preoperative course of chemotherapy may be

Table 21-3   Thymoma Staging System (Masaoka)
I. Macroscopically, completely encapsulated; microscopically, no capsular invasion
II. Macroscopic invasion into surrounding fatty tissue or mediastinal pleura; microscopic invasion into capsule
III. Macroscopic invasion into neighboring organs (pericardium, lung, and great vessels)
IVa. Pleural or pericardial dissemination
IVb. Lymphogenous or hematogenous metastases

indicated for patients with stage III lesions. Postoperative radiotherapy following complete resection reduces the reoccurrence rate from 28–36% to 0–5% for stage II and from 53% to 28% for stage III thymomas. Surgery for an invasive stage IVa thymoma involves resection of invaded local structures and may require major vascular resections, including removal and reconstruction of the superior vena cava, innominate vein, aortic arch, and pulmonary artery. Unilateral resection of the phrenic nerve, pericardial resection, and pleuropneumonectomy may also be indicated. Preoperative chemoradiation may be indicated to reduce tumor volume. Incomplete resection or debulking of a stage IVa thymoma combined with postoperative chemoradiation can improve survival rates in these patients. Treatment of stage IVb thymoma is limited to chemotherapy.

An anterior approach, utilizing a parasternal approach at the second or third intercostal space (ICS), is used for mediastinoscopic biopsies of the thymus. Surgical approach for a thymectomy is controversial and dependent on the degree of involvement of local tissues. For myasthenic patients, a video-assisted thoracoscopic surgery (VATS) or robotics-assisted thoracoscopic surgery (RATS) will allow a simple thymectomy. A complete resection of the thymus and surrounding tissues is necessary. An upper sternal split with division only of the manubrium or a transcervical approach similar to that used for a thyroidectomy will provide good surgical access for an early stage thymoma. With advanced stages of thymoma, a complete sternotomy is necessary for removal of all anterior mediastinal tissue that may have thymic metastasis.

Postsurgical complications associated with thymectomy includes:

- Unilateral phrenic nerve injury with short-term dyspnea upon exertion
- Pleural effusion
- Hemorrhage
- Respiratory insufficiency
- Postoperative thrombosis following dissection near the innominate vein
- Left recurrent nerve injury
- Vocal cord paralysis following dissection near the aortopulmonary window

Surgical mortality is < 2% and is frequently related to diseases such as MG and other autoimmune diseases. Thymectomy in adults does not have an effect on the immune system; in young children, it is associated with severe immunodeficiency and increased susceptibility to infection.

9. Analyze the major anesthetic considerations for an MG patient undergoing a thymectomy.

General endotracheal anesthesia (GETA) is required for a thymectomy. A double lumen tube and one-lung ventilation is required for a VATS or RATS technique. Patients with advanced stages of the disease or isolated bulbar involvement are at risk for aspiration and an awake fiberoptic intubation (FOI) is the safest technique for securing the airway.

With a 70% reduction in the number of nAChRs, myasthenic patients are generally resistant to the neuromuscular blocking effects associated with succinylcholine and higher doses are required for intubation. However, responses can be unpredictable and myasthenic patients are more likely to develop a phase II block, especially with repeat doses of succinylcholine. Preoperative anticholinesterase therapy or plasmapheresis may prolong the duration of succinylcholine. Myasthenic

patients are extremely sensitive to nondepolarizing neuromuscular blockers (NDMR) and it is best to avoid them. Even a small defasciculating dose prior to succinylcholine administration can result in respiratory distress and loss of airway protection. Sevoflurane or propofol and remifentanil can be used for induction and tracheal intubation. If muscle relaxants are required for intubation, succinylcholine is the best choice. Surgical muscle relaxation can be accomplished with a volatile anesthesia. Small doses of intermediate-acting relaxants (10–25% of the ED_{95}) such as cisatracurium have been used successfully in myasthenic patients but long-acting NDMR should be avoided. Due to the unique manner of degradation associated with cisatracurium, a combination of Hofman elimination, and ester hydrolysis, reversal may not be necessary. Use of a peripheral nerve stimulator (PNS) is mandatory; a control twitch should be assessed prior to the administration of an NDMR and a single twitch should be maintained during surgery. Use of an electromyelogram (EMG) or a mechanomyogram (MMG) is preferable for monitoring the neuromuscular function.

If an NDMR is used, the decision to reverse residual neuromuscular blockade at the end of surgery is controversial. Administration of an anticholinesterase and antimuscarinic will confound the differential diagnosis of a myasthenic crisis versus a cholinergic crisis. In addition, reversal of an NDMR block may be ineffective due to chronic pyridostigmine administration. Extubation following spontaneous recovery of neuromuscular function and consistent demonstration of acceptable respiratory parameters may be preferable to pharmacologic reversal of the neuromuscular blockade. A prolonged recovery from anesthesia should be anticipated if high concentrations of an inhalation agent were administered to provide muscle relaxation.

Other anesthetic concerns include the potential interactions between patient medications and anesthetic drugs. Anticholinesterases potentiate vagal responses and may require administration of atropine; they can also decrease the sensitivity to NDMR.

Inhibition of plasma cholinesterase activity can result in decreased metabolism of ester local anesthetics and succinylcholine. Azathioprine can inhibit phosphodiesterase and antagonize neuromuscular blockade, and cyclosporine is associated with prolonged neuromuscular blockade.

10. Identify the major side effect of radiation therapy.

Thymomas are highly radiosensitive and postoperative radiation therapy is frequently indicated following surgical resection of a large or invasive thymoma. Radiation is also synergistic with concurrent induction chemotherapy. Short-term side effects of radiotherapy include loss of hair and reddening, swelling, and blistering of the skin over the irradiated area. Effects on the skin resemble sunburn and the skin may become dry, flaky, or peel with resolution of the changes within a few weeks of finishing treatment. A dry cough and SOB, lasting for a few days or weeks, is not uncommon.

Long-term side effects of radiation therapy include radiation pneumonitis, an inflammatory response of the lungs that can occur 1–6 months following radiotherapy. It occurs in approximately 10% of chest-irradiated patients. Symptoms include a fever, cough, SOB, and CXR changes. It may be treated with a short course of steroids and usually resolves over time. Pulmonary fibrosis is also a risk of chest radiotherapy, with a reduction in the number and efficiency of functioning lung units within the irradiated region. CT scans of irradiated lungs reveal increased lung densities, decreased lung volume, pleural thickening, and severe vascular damage within the radiation beam boundaries. Bronchiolitis obliterans, pneumothorax, mesothelioma, and lung cancer may also occur with radiotherapy.

Irradiation of the mediastinum and left side of the chest can have serious side effects on the cardiovascular system including cardiomyopathy, premature coronary artery stenosis, ascending aortic calcification, pericardial disease, valvular injury, and conduction abnormalities. Radiation-induced heart disease is directly correlated with previous

chemotherapy and duration of radiation exposure. Formation of thymic cysts, calcified lymph nodes, esophageal damage, radiation-induced sarcomas, osteochondroma, and rib or clavicle fractures are also recognized risks of radiation therapy. A patient with a history of chest radiotherapy should be assessed for loss of skin integrity, pulmonary fibrosis, pericardial or pleural effusion, myocardial fibrosis, valvular disorders, and fistula formation.

11. Discuss the anesthetic concerns for patients who have had preoperative chemotherapy.

A preoperative course of chemotherapy may be indicated for patients with stage III and IVa thymomas. Commonly used agents include bleomycin (Blenoxane), cisplatin, (Platinol), cyclophosphamide (Cytoxan), doxorubicin (Adriamycin), lomustine (CeeNU), vincristine (Oncovin), and ifosfamide (Mitoxana). In varying degree of severity, all chemotherapeutic agents have a depressant effect on all rapid-turnover cells, resulting in hair loss; gastrointestinal distress including nausea, vomiting, anorexia, ulceration, and ileus; sensory loss and paresthesias; muscle waiting; neuritic pain; and myelosuppression, as evidenced by leucopenia, thrombocytopenia, and anemia. In general, these effects are dose dependent and reversible. Reactivation of hepatitis B (HBV) may also occur during systemic chemotherapy. Several antimetabolites have the potential to enhance radiation injury to tissues (radiation recall reactions), and recurrent injury to a previously radiated site can occur weeks to months following radiotherapy.

Several of the antimetabolites used in the treatment of thymic carcinoma present additional concerns for the anesthetist. Cisplatin is associated with renal toxicity, especially in the elderly population. Renal damage is greatest with high doses and repeated courses of the drug. Electrolyte abnormalities may be present, a function of the depressed renal function. Peripheral neuropathies are also reported with the use of cisplatin. A dose dependent cardiomyopathy is associated with doxorubicin and potentially fatal congestive heart failure (CHF) may occur months to years after treatment.

Approximately 10% of patients treated with bleomycin develop pneumonitis that can progress to pulmonary fibrosis. Symptoms include a dry, hacking cough, dyspnea, tachypnea, fever, and cyanosis; 20% of patients will have abnormal PFT results. Symptoms can appear in 1–3 months after treatment and death occurs in 1% of patients with bleomycin pneumonitis. Risk factors include: age > 70 years, preexisting pulmonary disease, coexisting renal failure, prior or concomitant thoracic radiation therapy, subsequent high-dose oxygen exposure, smoking, or previous exposure to bleomycin. Corticosteroids are used to treat bleomycin pneumonitis but are of questionable value once interstitial fibrosis has occurred.

Preoperative testing of patient with a history of chemotherapy should include a complete blood count (CBC), electrolytes, and renal and liver function tests. Patients with a history of doxorubicin treatment should also have an ECG and echocardiography (ECHO). A CXR and PFTs are indicated in patients who have received bleomycin. To decrease possible superoxide and free radical damage, the inspired oxygen concentration (FiO_2) should not exceed 28% during anesthesia. Blood and third space losses should be replaced with colloids to prevent the development of pulmonary interstitial edema. Due to the possibility of persistent immunosuppression in patients who have a recent history of chemotherapy, strict attention must be paid to infection control and the use of aseptic technique is mandatory during insertion of intravenous lines, arterial lines, airways, and nasogastric tubes during the perioperative period.

Postoperative Period

12. Discuss the implication of damage to the phrenic nerve during a thymectomy.
Injury to the phrenic nerve can occur during thymectomy, resulting in a temporary or permanent diaphragmatic paralysis. Phrenic nerve damage must be considered in any patient presenting with unexplained respiratory difficulty in the postoperative period. Symptoms of unilateral damage include dyspnea and atelectasis and a CXR will reveal elevation of the ipsilateral hemidiaphragm and pulmonary infiltrates on the affected side. Bilateral injury of the phrenic nerve causes paralysis of both hemidiaphragms resulting in a reduced vital capacity (VC), residual volume (RV), and total lung capacity (TLC). The resultant hypoxemia and hypercapnia mandates continuation of mechanical ventilation during the postoperative period. The transient neurapraxia that is seen with phrenic nerve injury usually resolves spontaneously within 7–10 days.

13. Review the postoperative management concerns for a patient with MG.
Patients who have MG have an increased risk of developing postoperative respiratory failure and approximately 50% will require prolonged postoperative ventilation following a transsternal thymectomy. Sustained respiratory muscle strength and resumption of spontaneous ventilation must be confirmed prior to extubation, especially in patients with bulbar and/or respiratory muscle weakness. Postoperative mechanical ventilation should be anticipated for patients presenting with:

- Long history (> 6 yrs) of MG
- Significant bulbar weakness
- History of other chronic respiratory disease
- Grades III and IV MG
- Preoperative vital capacity < 2.9 l
- Daily doses of pyridostigmine of ≥ 750 mg

Arterial blood gases (ABG) should be used to guide respiratory management; a CXR is indicated if aspiration is suspected.

Myasthenic patients should be closely monitored for muscular weakness in the postoperative period. Differential diagnosis of residual weakness includes myasthenic crisis, cholinergic crisis, and residual effects of anesthetics, or nonanesthetic drugs that interfere with neuro-muscular transmission, and a myasthenic or cholinergic crisis. Hypothermia and hypokale-mia may also increase muscle weakness in the postoperative period.

Postoperative pain management can be chal-lenging in the myasthenic patient as there is a sig-nificant risk of respiratory depression if potent opioids are administered. Postoperative pain can be successfully managed with a thoracic or lumbar epidural, especially for patients under-going a transsternal thymectomy. If inserted preoperatively, an epidural offers the additional advantage of intraoperative analgesia. Amide local anesthetics are preferable, as metabolism of ester local anesthetics may be prolonged by maintenance anticholinesterase therapy. The need for anticholinesterase medication is decreased in the postoperative period, approxi-mately 75% of the preoperative dose is required for the first few postoperative days. The benefits of thymectomy are usually delayed for months to years after surgery.

14. Discuss the long-term prognosis for patients with thymomas.

The majority of thymomas are associated with autoimmune disorders, and metastasis is usually limited to the pleura. Advanced stage thymomas are associated with pleura, kidney, bone, liver, and brain metastasis. Invasive thymomas are prone to recurrence and can reoccur 5–10 years after surgery; recurrence rates are significantly reduced with postoperative radiation therapy. Prognosis of this relatively indolent disease is good: the 10-year survival is 80–100% for stage I, 60–95% for stage II, 45–47% for stage III, and 30–47% for stage IV. Approximately 15% of patients with a thymoma will develop a second cancer. Patients with MG have a near-normal life expectancy.

REVIEW QUESTIONS

1. Thymic epithelial cells are associated with the development of:
   a. thymomas.
   b. non-Hodgkin lymphomas.
   c. Hodgkin disease.
   d. deficient humoral immunity.
2. Symptoms that are associated with myasthenic crisis are associated with:
   a. myosis.
   b. increased lacrimination.
   c. increased salivation.
   d. flaccid paralysis.
3. The most effective treatment for myasthenic crisis includes:
   a. prednisolone.
   b. plasmapheresis.
   c. atropine.
   d. thymectomy.
4. Thymomas are most often associated with which of the following conditions?
   a. Hyperthyroidism
   b. Anemia
   c. Small cell carcinoma
   d. Myasthenia gravis
5. In the pediatric patient, thymic dysfunction is associated with:
   a. DiGeorge syndrome.
   b. small cell carcinoma.
   c. myasthenia gravis.
   d. Cushing syndrome.

REVIEW ANSWERS

1. **Answer: a**
   Thymic lymphocytes give rise to called thymic lymphomas such as Hodgkin disease and non-Hodgkin lymphomas.
2. **Answer: d**
   Cholinergic crisis is associated with myosis and increased lacrimination and salivation.
3. **Answer: b**
   Neostigmine (Physostigmine) or pyridostigmine are also used for management of a myasthenic

crisis but steroids and surgery are indicated for chronic management of the myasthenic patient. Atropine is used in the treatment of a cholinergic crisis.

4. **Answer: d**

Thymomas are also associated with hypothyroidism and pernicious anemia. Lambert-Eaton myasthenic syndrome is associated with small cell carcinoma.

5. **Answer: a**

Partial DiGeorge syndrome is associated with an immune deficiency that improves over time. Complete DiGeorge syndrome is associated with athymia, severe immunodeficiency, and death before 2 years of age.

SUGGESTED READINGS

Augustin F, Schmid T, Sieb M, et al. Video-assisted thoracoscopic surgery versus robotic-assisted thoracoscopic surgery thymectomy. *Ann Thorac Surg* 2008; 85:768–771.

Bechard P, Letourneat L, Lacasse Y, et al. Perioperative cardiorespiratory complications in adult with mediastinal masses: Incidence and risk factors. *Anesthesiology* 2004;100:826–834.

Casey EM, Kiel PJ, Loehrer PJ. Clinical management of thymoma patients. *Hematol Oncol Clin North Am* 2008;22:457–473.

Girard N, Mornex F, Van Houtte P, et al. Thymoma: A focus on current therapeutic management. *J Thorac Oncol* 2009;4:119–126.

Gothard JWW. Anesthetic considerations for patients with anterior mediastinal masses. *Anesthesiol Clin* 2008;26:305–314.

Hilton-Jones D, Palace J. The management of myasthenia gravis. *Pract Neurol* 2005;5:18–27.

Kaiser LR. Surgical treatment of thymic epithelial neoplasms. *Hematol Oncol Clin North Am* 2008;22:475–488.

Markert ML, Alexieff MJ, Li J, et al. Postnatal thymus transplantation with immunosuppression as treatment for DiGeorge syndrome. *Blood* 2004;104:2574–2581.

Suster S, Moran CA. Thymoma classification: current status and future trends. *Am J Clin Pathol* 2006;125:542–554.

Tormoehlen LM, Pascuzzi RM. Thyoma, myasthenia gravis, and other paraneoplastic syndromes. *Hematol Oncol Clin North Am* 2008;22:509–526.

Organ
Procurement

VI

Multiorgan Procurement

22

Bernadette T. Higgins Roche

KEY POINTS

- An individual's signature on a driver's license or donor card attesting to their desire to be an organ/tissue donor is legally binding and does not require family permission.
- Absolute contraindications for organ donation include: age > 80 years, HIV infection, active metastatic cancer, prolonged hypotension or hypothermia, active infection, disseminated intravascular coagulation (DIC) sickle cell anemia, or other hemoglobinopathy.
- Aggressive donor management increases the number and quality of retrieved organs and improves both the number and outcome of subsequent transplantations.
- The most frequently transplanted organ is the kidney; the lung is the least transplanted organ.
- Anesthesia services are required for organ donation after brain death (DBD) but not for donation after cardiac death (DCD).

CASE SYNOPSIS

A 35-year-old man is admitted, unresponsive, to the emergency department following a gunshot injury to the head. Patient is intubated and mechanically ventilated. His Glasgow Coma Scale (GCS) score is 4 and a computed tomography (CT) scan reveals a large subdural hematoma and extensive cerebral edema with a midline shift.

PREOPERATIVE EVALUATION AND DEMOGRAPHIC DATA

Past Medical/Surgical History

- Healthy male
- Nonsmoker, no recreational drug use, no alcohol intake
- Appendectomy at age 22

List of Medications

- Ibuprofen

Diagnostic Data

- Hemoglobin, 11.4 mg/dl; hematocrit, 37%
- Glucose, 250 mg/dl
- Electrolytes: sodium, 158 mEq/L; potassium, 3.2 mEq/L; chloride, 106 mEq/L; carbon dioxide, 22 mEq/L
- Electrocardiogram (ECG): Sinus tachycardia, heart rate 154, with T inversion in multiple leads

Height/Weight/Vital Signs

- 180 cm, 86 kg
- Blood pressure, 100/60; heart rate, 154 beats per minute; room air oxygen saturation, 95%
- No spontaneous respirations; mechanical ventilation; tidal volume, 800; respiratory rate, 12 breaths per minute; inspired oxygen concentration, 40%

PATHOPHYSIOLOGY

The first solid organ transplant involved a kidney transplant between identical twins in 1954 followed by liver, lung, heart, and pancreas transplants in the 1960s. Cyclosporine, introduced in 1978, had a major impact on the growth and success of transplant surgery by decreasing the incidence of host rejection. Organs and tissues that can be transplanted include the heart, kidneys, lungs, pancreas, liver, intestines, corneas, skin, tendons, bone, and heart valves. Kidney and liver (whole organ or segmental) are the most frequently transplanted organs. Approximately 94,000 people are currently registered on national transplant lists; the largest number, 50,000, is waiting for kidneys. In contrast, there are only 29,000 solid organ transplants/year. The federally supported United Network for Organ Sharing (UNOS) links all organ procurement and transplant centers in the United States. When a donor is identified, individuals on waiting lists are matched and ranked via computer against the donor's characteristics. Ranking is based on blood type, tissue match, length of time on list, immune status, and geographical distance between donor and potential recipient. Other factors considered include: pediatric patients in specific age categories, reciprocal-sharing arrangements or payback agreements, dual-organ recipient, and acute failure of a recently transplanted organ. Medical urgency is considered for heart, liver, and intestinal transplantation.

Absolute contraindications to organ donation include age > 80 years, HIV infection, active metastatic cancer, prolonged hypotension or hypothermia, active infection, DIC, and hemoglobinopathy. Relative contraindications include malignancy other than in the central nervous system (CNS) or skin that is in remission, hypertension, diabetes mellitus, age > 70 years, hepatitis B or C, and a history of smoking.

The medical condition of the donor at the time of death determines the viability of retrieved organs. Following a cardiac arrest, the viability of the vital organs deteriorates quickly; whereas other tissues, such as bone, skin, heart valves, and corneas, can be donated within 24 hours after death. Minimizing the time interval (warm ischemic time) between cardiac death and perfusion of donor organs with cold preservation solutions increases the viability of the organs. The length of time is organ specific; the heart and liver must be retrieved within 30 minutes and kidneys and pancreas can be retrieved up to 60 minutes after cardiac death.

Classifications of Organ Donors

Living Organ Donors

A healthy individual who is between 18 and 60 years of age, and free from hypertension, diabetes, cancer, kidney disease, and heart disease can be considered for a living organ donation. Kidney donation is the most frequent type of living organ donation; individuals can also donate a lung or segments of the liver or pancreas. Some heart–lung recipients can donate their heart (domino transplant) if they have lung but not heart pathology. Living donors account for 44% of all donors and are frequently related to the recipients.

Deceased Organ Donors

The US Uniform Determination of Death Act (1980) defines death as the irreversible cessation of circulatory and respiratory functions, or of all functions of the entire brain, including the brain stem. Deceased organ donors include DBD and DCD. For DBD, causes of brain death include: severe head trauma, cerebral ischemia, infarction or hemorrhage, prolonged cardiopulmonary arrest, and intracranial tumors. Diagnosis of brain death is primarily based on clinical examination, but diagnostic tests are often used for confirmation. The patient is considered legally dead at the time that a physician determines that brain death has occurred.

In the event of cardiac death, also known as non-heart beating cadaver donation (NHBCD), the removal of transplantable organs occurs immediately after the patient has been declared dead using specific cardiac criteria. These patients are typically ventilator dependent, have a severe neurological injury following a cerebrovascular accident (CVA) or cerebral anoxia, a high spinal cord injury, or an end-stage neuromuscular disease. They do not meet brain death criteria but are not expected to recover, and the physician and family have decided to withdraw life support. The patient is considered legally dead at the time of asystole. In controlled DCD, organ procurement occurs immediately after withdrawal of life support and declaration of cardiac death, allowing retrieval of kidneys, liver, lungs, and pancreas. Hearts are rarely retrieved due to concerns about sustained ischemic injury following cardiac arrest. In uncontrolled DCD, the cardiac death is not anticipated and there may be a considerable time for warm ischemia to occur that limits retrieval to kidneys and nonvital tissues. DCD currently accounts for approximately 8% of all deceased donors and has significant potential for increasing the number of available organs.

SURGICAL PROCEDURE

State organ procurement organizations (OPOs) are to subject to regulations set forth by UNOS. Once a patient has been declared brain dead or a cardiac death is imminent, an OPO coordinator is sent to evaluate the patient and coordinate the organ procurement process. Surgical transplant teams are not involved until the donor is declared dead by the attending physician. Initially, the organs are allocated locally and then offered to other regional or state OPOs.

During organ procurement, surgical access is provided via a midline incision from the suprasternal notch to the pubis and a median sternotomy. The aortic arch, inferior vena cava (IVC), abdominal aorta, and portal vein or tributaries are cannulated for infusion of a cold preservative solution, and the heart, lung, liver, kidneys, and pancreas are dissected from supporting structures. Following administration of heparin 300 U/kg, the abdominal aorta is cross-clamped, a cold preservative solution is infused through the inferior aortic, portal, and cardiac cannulae, and the thoracic and abdominal cavities are packed with ice. The warm ischemic time must be minimized and organs are removed in order of susceptibility to warm ischemic damage; the heart is removed first, followed by the lungs, liver, pancreas, small intestines, and kidneys. An en bloc resection of organs may be utilized in which the organs are removed together and dissected in vitro either in the operating room or at the site of transplantation. Prior to transport, organs are flushed with a cold preservative solution, packed in wet ice, and stored at 4°C. Recipients are required to be at the transplant center within 4–6 hours of notification; for a heart or lung recipient, this time may be shortened.

ANESTHETIC MANAGEMENT AND CONSIDERATIONS

Preoperative Period

1. Identify the sources of consent for organ donation.

An individual's desire to be an organ donor can be documented on a driver's license, a donor card, a living will or durable power of attorney, or through verbal communication with family. Historically, family consent was required for organ donation, even in the presence of a signed driver's license or donor card. In states with first-person consent laws, an individual's signature is legally binding and does not require family permission. In the absence of a signed consent, the family, legal guardian, or medical coroner can agree to organ donation. Knowledge of the donor's wishes or families who had previous discussion regarding donation are more likely to agree to donate in the face of an unexpected terminal condition of a family member. To increase the number of donated organs, the Uniform Anatomical Gift Act (UAGA) was revised in 2007 granting new authority to OPOs over individuals with a signed driver's license or donor card. The OPO must be notified when a donor or potential donor is dead or near death; if necessary, the OPO will seek consent from family or authorized persons. The OPO can direct life-sustaining interventions before death to increase the viability of organs unless an advance directive specifically forbids them from doing so. The Act empowers a minor, eligible under other law to apply for a drive's license, to be a donor without family consent. The National Organ Transplant Act (1984) prohibits the sale of organs for transplantation.

2. Discuss the physiologic responses associated with brain death.

Brain death is a result of severe rostral–caudal ischemia. Intense sympathetic activity, an attempt to maintain cerebral perfusion pressure, is the initial response to cerebral ischemia and increased intracranial pressure (ICP). A mixed vagal and sympathetic response is seen with ischemia of the pons and Cushing response, hypertension, bradycardia, and altered respirations is present. Medullary ischemia causes an intense sympathetic response, loss of thermoregulatory control, and endocrinopathy due to hypothalamic and pituitary impairment. Catecholamine release causes a significant increase in systemic vascular resistance (SVR), increasing myocardial work and compromising cardiac function. Hypothermia can lead to myocardial depression, coagulopathy, and decreased oxygen (O_2) delivery to tissues. Disruption of the hypothalamic–pituitary axis results in adrenal insufficiency, loss of glycemic control, reduced antidiuretic hormone (ADH) secretion, and hypothyroidism. Brain stem herniation is associated with bradycardia, decreased SVR, low cardiac output (CO), pulmonary edema and dysfunction, and cardiopulmonary arrest. DIC may occur as the coagulation cascade is activated in response to the release of necrotic brain tissue. A systemic inflammatory response is associated with brain death; inflammatory mediators decrease SVR, increase lung injury, and may increase immune sensitivity following transplantation.

3. Discuss the preoperative management of an organ donor.

Hemodynamic instability can seriously compromise organ function; > 80% of organ donors require hemodynamic support and approximately 20% of potential donors are lost because of hemodynamic instability. Initial management includes aggressive fluid resuscitation with crystalloids and colloids; colloids are more effective than crystalloids in preventing pulmonary edema and congestion of other organs. Packed red blood cells (PRBCs) may be required to maintain a hemoglobin of > 10 mg/dl and fresh frozen plasma (FFP) is administered if the prothrombin time (PT) and partial thromboplastin time (PTT) are 1.5 times greater than control values.

Central venous pressure (CVP) or pulmonary capillary wedge pressure (PCWP) is used to guide fluid management. The infusion of inotropic medications is frequently indicated; dopamine 2–10 μg/kg/min is the initial drug of choice. Dobutamine 3–15 μg/kg/min, norepinephrine 0.5–5 μg/min, or epinephrine 0.1–1 μg/kg/min may also be required to maintain effective perfusion pressures. The goals of anesthetic management include: mean arterial pressure (MAP) > 60 mm Hg; CVP/PCWP < 12 mm Hg; SVR 800–1200 dyn·s/cm⁵; systolic blood pressure (SBP) > 100 mm Hg; and cardiac index (CI) > 2.5. Since the cardiac center is located within the medulla oblongata, when brain death occurs, functional myocardial denervation occurs and as a result atropine has a limited effect on increasing heart rate. Bradycardia is most effectively treated with isoproterenol, epinephrine, or cardiac pacing. Electrolytes are monitored frequently to maintain plasma sodium ≤ 150 mEq/dl and potassium ≥ 4.0 mEq/dl.

Brain death has a profound impact on lung function and lung recovery occurs in only 20% of actual donors. Neurogenic pulmonary edema occurs in response to the early elevation of SVR and left atrial and pulmonary capillary pressures. The inflammatory response and release of proteases, cytokines, and leukotrienes are associated with lung damage and decreased pulmonary function. The development of a coagulopathy may produce pulmonary microemboli. With brain stem death, the fall in SVR will increase ventilation/perfusion mismatch. In addition, aspiration, pulmonary contusion, excessive fluid resuscitation, atelectasis, and barotrauma negatively impact pulmonary function. Pulmonary management includes delivery of: large tidal volumes (12–15 mg/kg); low peak inspiratory pressure (PIP), ideally < 30 cm H_2O; positive-end expiratory pressure (PEEP) ≤ 7.5 cm H_2O; and an FiO_2 ≤ 40% in order to maintain arterial saturation (SaO_2) of ≥ 90%, arterial oxygen pressure (PaO_2) > 60 mm Hg, arterial carbon dioxide pressure ($PaCO_2$) 30–35 mm Hg, and arterial pH 7.35–7.45. Careful fluid management, chest physiotherapy,

frequent suctioning, and administration of antibiotics (cefazolin or equivalent) are also indicated to minimize lung trauma.

4. Discuss the common physiologic complications associated with brain death.

Donors are vulnerable to a variety of complications, especially endocrine dysfunction. Diabetes insipidus (DI) is caused by a lack of ADH production and/or release as a result of damage to the hypothalamus and/or pituitary gland. This syndrome is treated with vasopressin or desmopressin acetate (DDAVP [1-deamino-D-arginine vasopressin]) and the associated hypovolemia is corrected with hypotonic saline or dextrose and water, and electrolyte replacement as indicated. Thyroid dysfunction is characterized by low triiodothyronine (T_3), a result of decreased thyroid stimulating hormone (TSH) secretion and reduced conversion of thyroxine (T_4) to T_3. Anaerobic glycolysis and mitochondrial dysfunction are seen with T_3 deficiency, resulting in widespread acidosis. Sympathetically mediated hyperglycemia and depletion of insulin stores can contribute to hypovolemia (osmotic diuresis) and is best managed with an insulin infusion. A protocol for hormonal replacement for patients undergoing organ procurement is included in Table 22-1.

Table 22-1 Hormonal Replacement Protocol
Methylprednisolone: 15 mg/kg bolus every 24 hrs
Triiodothyronine (T_3): 4 mcg bolus followed by 3 mcg/hr infusion
Thyroxin (T_4): 20 mcg bolus, followed by 10 mcg/hr infusion
Arginine vasopressin: 1 unit bolus followed by 0.5–4 units/hr titrated to SVR of 800–1200 dyn·s/cm⁵ and urine output < 200 ml/hr or desmopressin 8 ng/kg, followed by 4 ng/kg/hr
Insulin infusion: 1 unit/hr titrated to maintain blood glucose 120–180 mg/dl

Table 22-2	Anesthetic Management for Organ Procurement: Rule of 100

Systolic blood pressure > 100 mm Hg

Heart rate < 100 beats per minute

Urine output >100 cc/hr

$PO_2 \geq 100$ mm Hg

The profound hypothermia that occurs with loss of thermoregulatory control is associated with cardiac depression, cold diuresis, coagulopathy, and reduced tissue oxygenation. Warming blankets, fluid warmers, and heated humidifiers are indicated to maintain core temperature greater than 34°C. Coagulation abnormalities are common due to release of thromboplastin, tissue plasminogen, and fibrinogen from necrotic brain tissue and reduced platelet aggregation secondary to hypothermia. A dilutional coagulopathy may occur if large amounts of crystalloids are used for resuscitation. Blood products, including FFP, platelets, and cryoprecipitate, are indicated to correct coagulation abnormalities. Immediate organ retrieval is indicated for severe fibrinolysis resistant to therapy.

Hypovolemia can result from fluid restriction for treatment of cerebral edema, DI, hemorrhage, hyperglycemic osmotic diuresis, cold diuresis, and decreased SVR. Crystalloids, colloids, and red blood cells are administered to maintain SBP > 100 mm Hg, urine output > 1 ml/kg/hr, hematocrit > 30%, and CVP < 12 cm H_2O. Cardiopulmonary management for organ procurement utilizing the rule of 100 is listed in Table 22-2.

5. List the criteria used to confirm brain death.
Diagnosis of brain death is primarily based on the absence of brain stem reflexes and respiratory effort. Optional confirmatory tests include an electroencephalogram (EEG), cerebral blood flow studies, and brain stem auditory evoked responses (BAER). Potentially reversible causes of coma (hypothermia, metabolic disturbances, mediations, hypoxia, or hypocarbia) must be corrected before brain death can be confirmed. The GCS provides an objective and reliable method of assessing the status of the CNS and the criteria is listed in Table 22-3. A fully awake patient will have a score of 15; a score ≤ 8 is indicative of a severe coma, 9–12 a moderate coma, and ≥ 13 a minor coma. The Pediatric GCS has a modified verbal response for assessment of young children.

- **Cerebral motor responses to pain**
  Cerebrally modulated motor responses of extremities to painful stimulation are abnormal with brain death. Eye opening, facial grimacing,

Table 22-3	Glasgow Coma Scale				
	SCORE 1	SCORE 3	SCORE 3	SCORE 4	SCORE 5	SCORE 6
Response of Eyes	Does not open eyes	Opens eyes in response to painful stimuli	Opens eyes in response to voice	Opens eyes spontaneously	N/A	N/A
Verbal Response	Makes no sounds	Incomprehensible sounds	Utters inappropriate words	Confused, disoriented	Oriented, converses normally	N/A
Motor Response	Makes no movements	Decerebrate posturing	Decorticate posturing	Flexion/ withdrawal to painful stimuli	Localizes painful stimuli	Obeys commands

and purposeful withdrawal of limbs from a noxious stimulus are an indication that consciousness is not greatly impaired. Asymmetric motor responses to pain or deep tendon reflexes may indicate a focal hemispheric lesion. Decorticate posturing is associated with damage to the cerebral hemispheres, internal capsule, and thalamus. A decerebrate response to pain indicates damage to the brain stem, midbrain, and cerebellum. Minor flexion of an extremity in response to painful stimulation of the same limb represents spinal cord reflexes and not cortical activity. Spinal automatism (Lazarus sign), limb flexion, gasping motions, and head turning also occur at the spinal cord level. It is more common in young adults and can occur spontaneously during apnea testing in the presence of hypoxia or hypotension or brisk neck flexion.

- **Brain stem reflexes**
  Pupillary response to light: Pupils may be round, oval, or irregularly shaped, and midsize (4–6 mm) but pupillary light reflex (constriction) is absent in brain death. Drugs such as atropine can influence pupillary size but not the response to light.

  Oculocephalic reflex (doll's eyes): When the head is rapidly turned from side to side, the eyes normally rotate to the opposite side. With brain stem death, there is no movement of the eyes and they remain fixed.

  Oculovestibular reflex (caloric reflex): Irrigation of both ear canals with iced saline or water will result in nystagmus and deviation of the eyes toward the side of irrigation. This reflex is absent in brain death. Several drugs can inhibit this reflex, including sedatives, tricyclic antidepressants, aminoglycosides, anticholinergics, and antiseizure agents.

  Corneal reflex (blink reflex): Normal closing of the eyelid in response to corneal stimulation is absent with brain stem death.

- **Apnea test**
  Following ventilation with 100% O_2 to normocapnia, the patent is disconnected from the ventilator but continues to receive O_2 by continuous positive airway pressure. The patient is observed for up to 10 minutes for signs of spontaneous breathing; arterial blood gases (ABGs) are drawn at the end of the observation period. A lack of spontaneous respirations and $PaCO_2 > 55–60$ mm Hg are indicative of brain death.

6. Discuss the laboratory evaluation for potential organ donors.
A variety of tests are required for the evaluation of potential DBD and DCD organ donors. These include a complete blood count (CBC); glucose; electrolytes; blood urea nitrogen (BUN); creatinine; ABG; ABO and human leukocyte antigens (HLA) typing; blood, sputum, and urine cultures; and venereal disease research laboratory (VDRL), human immunodeficiency virus (HIV), Epstein-Barr virus (EBV), cytomegalovirus (CMV), human T-cell leukemia virus type 1 (HTLV-1), and hepatitis B and C virus serologies. An ECG, chest x-ray (CXR), echocardiogram, creatine kinase (CK) and muscle and brain subunits (CK-MB), and troponin levels are required for heart donors; serial ABGs, CXR, and bronchoscopy for lung donors; serial blood glucoses and amylase and lipase levels for pancreas donors; and liver function tests (LFTs), PTT, and PT for liver donors.

7. Discuss the signs and management of diabetes insipidus (DI).
ADH (vasopressin) is produced by the hypothalamus and stored and released from the posterior pituitary gland. It increases water permeability in the renal collecting ducts and distal convoluted tubule where reabsorption of water maintains normovolemia. Central DI is caused by a deficiency of ADH secondary to autoimmune disease, malignancy, head trauma, intracranial tumor, infection, renal disease, and vascular disease. Signs of DI include: polyuria (urine output ≥ 25 ml/kg/hr) with a specific gravity of ≤ 1.005, lethargy, excessive thirst, hypernatremia, tachycardia, hypotension,

fatigue, vomiting, and seizures. DI that occurs from neurologic dysfunction is caused by damage of the hypothalamus and/or pituitary gland. In nephrogenic DI, the kidney fails to respond to ADH. Certain drugs such as lithium, amphotericin B, and demeclocycline and hypercalcemia can cause nephrogenic DI.

Diagnosis of DI is accomplished by restricting fluid and then monitoring the plasma and urine sodium and urine specific gravity. When ADH levels and kidney function are within normal limits, the urine output and plasma sodium levels will decrease, and urine specific gravity will increase. With DI, there is no change and the diagnosis of central DI is confirmed if the urine output decreases and specific gravity increases in response to ADH administration. Mild cases of central DI are treated with drugs that are used to stimulate ADH production such as chlorpropamide, carbamazepine, and clofibrate. Nephrogenic DI is treated with indomethacin, hydrochlorothiazide, or amiloride.

DI occurs in approximately 70–80% of DBD donors. If the donor is hemodynamically unstable, vasopressin is the preferred treatment; desmopressin can be used if the donor is hemodynamically stable. Electrolytes are monitored frequently and after correction of hypovolemia, the plasma sodium should return to normal without any additional intervention.

8. Discuss the role of steroids in the preoperative management of organ donors.

Steroids increase tissue oxygenation and attenuate the effects of proinflammatory cytokines that are released in response to brain death. They improve donor organ function, increase the number of organs transplanted from each donor, and improve graft survival, especially in heart and lung recipients. Methylprednisolone 15–30 mg/kg is administered every 24 hours. To protect the heart and lungs from ischemia, an additional 30 mg/kg may be administered 1–2 hours prior to actual organ procurement.

Intraoperative Period

9. Describe the requirements for declaring death in a DCD donor.

A variety of tools, such as the University of Wisconsin DCD Evaluation Tool, is used to predict DCD donors who will expire within 60 minutes following extubation. The DCD donor is transported to the operating room with O_2 and manual ventilation. Heparin is administered to prevent thrombi formation; vasodilators and antioxidants such as steroids, vitamin E, or N-acetylcysteine are also frequently administered. Large arteries and veins are cannulated to facilitate the rapid infusion of organ-preservation solutions and the donor is surgically prepped and draped. Analgesics and sedatives may be administered by the treating physician to prevent or relieve suffering during termination of life support but not with the intention of hastening death. The donor is extubated and all medications discontinued. The Institute of Medicine (IOM) recommends an observation period of 5 minutes to ensure lack of cardiac reanimation (flat ECG tracing, flat pressure arterial line tracing, absence of carotid pulse). The National Conference of Donation after Cardiac Death recommends > 2 minutes but < 5 minutes of observation. Once the patient is pronounced dead, a cold preservative solution is infused, and organ procurement is instituted immediately to limit the time of warm ischemia and increase organ viability. If death does not occur within 60 minutes after termination of life support, the procedure is cancelled and palliative care/life support is resumed for the patient; this occurs in approximately 20% of cases. Anesthesia services are not required for treatment of DCD donors.

10. Discuss the anesthetic requirements of a DBD donor during organ retrieval.

There is no perception of pain in the higher brain centers because of neuronal death and providing anesthesia with the intent of inhibition of cerebral function is not required for DBD donors. However, anesthesia services are required to manage the physiologic responses to surgical trauma, spinal cord reflexes, catecholamine release, and release of inflammatory mediators that can damage the vital organs before procurement. The American Society of Anesthesiologists Physical Status Category VI is used for DBD donors who require anesthesia care. In addition to standard monitors, an arterial line and CVP/PA catheter are used for pressure monitoring; warming blankets, fluid warmers, and heated humidifiers are necessary to prevent intraoperative hypothermia. The donor is mechanically ventilated with 100% O_2 unless lung retrieval is planned in which case a $FiO_2 \leq 0.4$ is indicated. Dopamine, norepinephrine, epinephrine, dobutamine, or vasopressin infusions are continued to support hemodynamics and organ perfusion during organ procurement. Hemodynamic responses to surgical stimulation occur at the spinal cord level and can be managed with alpha- and beta-blockers and/or volatile anesthetics. A long acting muscle relaxant is administered to provide maximal intrathoracic and intra-abdominal surgical exposure and to prevent donor movements that are also initiated by spinal reflexes. Heparin 20,000–30,000 IU is administered to prevent postmortem clotting. Other drugs that may be required include: mannitol, fluorsemide, allopurinol, methylprednisolone, and PGE_1. Following aortic cross-clamping, vasodilators, such as phentolamine, may be required to treat an increased SVR. Significant third space losses occur during multiple organ procurement and glucose-free crystalloids, colloids, and PRBCs are used to maintain normovolemia, SBP > 100 mm Hg and hematocrit > 30%. Colloids are preferable for lung and pancreas donors to increase viability of these organs. Serial evaluation of electrolytes, glucose, hemoglobin, hematocrit, and ABGs are monitored, especially for heart and lung donors. For liver and pancreas retrieval, a Betadine and amphotericin B solution is inserted via a nasogastric tube to decontaminate the intestinal tract (not gastrointestinal system).

Several surgical teams are involved in the organ procurement. Organs are removed in order of their susceptibility to ischemia, the heart first and the kidneys last. Anesthesia care is terminated when the aorta is cross-clamped and the heart removed (at that time mechanical ventilation and monitors are turned off and all medications discontinued). If lung retrieval is planned, mechanical ventilation is continued until the surgeon is ready to remove the lungs at which time the endotracheal tube is suctioned and removed. In the event of a premature cardiac arrest, cardiopulmonary resuscitation (CPR) is instituted to preserve viability of the organs; unsuccessful CPR will eliminate the heart and lungs for donation but rapid aortic cross-clamping and infusion of a cold preservative solution allow retrieval of liver, pancreas, and kidneys. The maximum time before organ transplantation must occur varies according to the different vital organs, ranging from 5 hours for the heart to 3 days for kidneys and this information is included in Table 22-4.

Table 22-4 Organ Preservation Times	
Heart	≤ 5 hours
Heart/lung	≤ 5 hours
Intestines	≤ 8 hours
Liver	≤ 18 hours
Pancreas	≤ 20 hours
Kidney	≤ 72 hours
Corneas	≤ 10 days
Skin	≥ 5 years
Bone	≥ 5 years
Heart valves	≥ 5 years

Postoperative Period

11. Discuss the long-term survival of transplant recipients.

In the US, there are over 163,000 individuals living with a functioning transplanted organ. One-year survival rates are highest for kidney and pancreas recipients (95–98%). One-year survival for liver, intestine, lung, and heart recipients is 81–91%. The lowest survival rate (75%) is seen with heart–lung recipients. Long-term graft survival of a DCD kidney is similar to a DBD kidney but the DCD liver graft survival is significantly less than a DBD liver.

12. Discuss the professional conflicts healthcare providers encounter with organ donation.

The majority of healthcare providers are supportive of organ donation, but some providers may feel conflicted when required to transfer the emphasis of care from the donor to the recipient. The family may question the ability of the providers to continue with quality end-of-life care for their family member. Physicians and nurses must continue to provide quality end-of-life care for the donor and should not be involved with the care of the recipient, or with the organ procurement or transplantation process. It is never appropriate for them to discuss organ donation or obtain a consent from the family. The OPO is responsible for evaluating the donor, verifying or obtaining consent, coordinating the procurement and transplantation procedures, and assisting the family with the bereavement process. The treating physician is responsible for declaring death using brain or cardiac criteria; the transplant team cannot participate in end-of-life care or the declaration of death. Anesthetists, who provide anesthesia care for organ procurement, are required to withdraw life support in the operating room, an action that may appear contrary to their professional standards of practice.

13. Compare a signed driver's license or organ donor card with a surgical consent.

An informed surgical consent advises the patient of what the procedure entails, the risks and benefits to be expected, and alternative options for care. A signed driver's license or donor card is a limited informed consent as the risks and benefits are not explained and the donor agrees to a procedure without knowing specific details. Most donors do not know that their end-of-life care may be significantly altered and that a third party, the OPO, and not their treating physician, may direct their care. Under the UAGA, the OPO can decide what premortem mediations and procedures (heparin, CVP and PA catheter, femoral cannulae) are implemented and when mechanical ventilation is discontinued. To restrict their end-of-life care solely to their personal physician, a voluntary donor must specify this directive in a living will.

REVIEW QUESTIONS

1. Which parameter is representative of the rule of 100 during organ procurement?
   a. Systolic blood pressure < 100 mm Hg
   b. Urine output < 100 ml/hr
   c. $PaO_2 \geq 100$ mm Hg
   d. Heart rate > 100 mm Hg
2. Which is true regarding diabetes insipidus?
   a. Rarely seen in donors who have sustained brain death
   b. Associated with hypovolemia, hypernatremia, and hypokalemia
   c. Causes hypertonic diuresis
   d. Best treated with intramuscular pitressin
3. Viability of harvested organs is primarily dependent on the:
   a. length of warm ischemic time.
   b. age of the patient.
   c. early administration of steroids.
   d. corrections of fluid deficits.

4. Anesthesia is required for DBD donors to prevent:
   a. recall.
   b. spinal reflexes.
   c. pain.
   d. parasympathetic activation.
5. An organ procurement organization can only direct end-of-life care and implement donor management protocols without family consent if the patient:
   a. has a signed driver's license or donor card.
   b. is $\geq$ 12 years old.
   c. has a living will that restricts end-of-life care to their treating physician.
   d. has signed a refusal that bars others from making a gift of their organs after death.

REVIEW ANSWERS

1. **Answer c**
   The rule of 100 includes a $PaO_2 \geq 100$ mm Hg. It also includes SBP > 100 mm Hg, urine output > 100 ml/hr, and a heart rate < 100 beats per minute.
2. **Answer b**
   Diabetes insipidus presents with hypovolemia, hypernatremia, and hypokalemia. It causes hypotonic urine formation, occurs frequently with brain death, and is treated with IV vasopressin or desmopressin.
3. **Answer a**
   Viability of harvested organs is primarily dependent on the length of warm ischemic time. Organs are removed in the order of susceptibility to warm ischemia.
4. **Answer b**
   Anesthesia is required for DBD donors to eliminate spinal reflexes, which are activated by surgical stimulation. There is no perception of pain or awareness with brain death.
5. **Answer a**
   The OPO can direct end-of-life care without family consent for an individual with a signed driver's license or donor card.

SUGGESTED READINGS

Abt PL, Fisher CA, Singhal AK. Donation after cardiac death in the US: History and use. *J Am Coll Surg* 2006; 203(2):208–225.

Baker J, Yost CS, Niemann CU. Organ transplantation. In Miller RD, ed. *Miller's Anesthesia.* 6th ed. Philadelphia: Elsevier, 2006:2231–2284.

Brockmann JG, Vaidya A, Reddy S, et al. Retrieval of abdominal organs for transplantation. *Br J Surg* 2006;93(2):133–146.

Mandell MS, Zamudio S, Seem D, et al. National evaluation of healthcare provider attitudes toward organ donation after cardiac death. *Crit Care Med* 2006; 34(12):2952–2958.

Mascia L, Bosma K, Pasero D, et al. Ventilatory and hemodynamic management of potential organ donors: An observational survey. *Crit Care Med* 2006;34(2): 321–327.

Petersen SR. Done vida-donate life: a surgeon's perspective of organ donation. *Am J Surg* 2007;194: 701–708.

Rosendale JD, Kauffman HM, McBride MA, et al. Aggressive pharmacological donor management results in more transplanted organs. *Transplantation* 2003;75: 482–487.

Steinbrook R. Donation after cardiac death. *N Engl J Med* 2007;357(3):209–213.

U.S. Organ Procurement and Transplantation Network and the Scientific Registry of Transplant Recipients. *2007 OPTN / SRTR Annual Report: Transplant Data 1997–2006.* Available online at http://www.optn .org/AR2007/default.htm. Accessed December 7, 2008.

Van Norman GA. A matter of life and death: What every anesthesiologist should know about the medical, legal, and ethical aspects of declaring brain death. *Anesthesiology* 1999;91:275–287.

Vascular Surgery

VII

Carotid Endarterectomy

23

Nancy A. Moriber

KEY POINTS

- Cerebrovascular accidents (CVA) are the third leading cause of death in the United States and costs the healthcare delivery system $14 billion a year.
- Patients presenting with a recent hemispheric transient ischemic attack (TIA) and high-grade stenosis (70–99%) have a 65% risk reduction for the development of an ipsilateral stroke within 2 years of carotid endarterectomy (CEA).
- Chronic essential hypertension is present in the majority of patients undergoing CEA and is associated with an increased incidence of postoperative stroke or death.
- Monitoring neurologic function under general anesthesia is necessary to detect for episodes of cerebral ischemia, hypoperfusion, and cerebral embolization.
- Regional anesthesia allows for the continuous monitoring of the patient's neurologic status but requires patient cooperation throughout the procedure.
- Hemodynamic instability occurs regardless of the anesthetic technique employed and requires prompt management to decrease the incidence of postoperative complications.
- Postoperative complications of CEA include hypertension, hypotension, myocardial ischemia/infarction, stroke, cerebral hyperperfusion syndrome, recurrent laryngeal nerve damage, hematoma, tension pneumothorax, and respiratory failure.

CASE SYNOPSIS

A 78-year-old woman presents with a recent history of a TIA with complete resolution of symptoms. Carotid angiography shows a 90% stenosis of the right carotid artery and 50% stenosis of the left carotid artery. She is scheduled for a right CEA.

PREOPERATIVE EVALUATION AND DEMOGRAPHIC DATA

Past Medical/Surgical History

- Hypertension
- Stable angina
- Percutaneous transluminal coronary angioplasty 1 year ago
- Smoker with 40 pack/year history
- History of TIA, no residual deficits

List of Medications

- Plavix
- Metoprolol
- Lisinopril

Diagnostic Data

- Hemoglobin, 12.1 g/dl; hematocrit, 36.2%
- International normalized ratio, 1.08
- Electrolytes: sodium, 140 mEq/l; sodium, 3.7; chloride, 104 mEq/l; carbon dioxide (CO_2), 23 mEq/l
- Glucose, 108 mg/dl

Height/Weight/Vital Signs

- 157 cm, 60 kg
- Blood pressure, 156/88; heart rate, 64 beats per minute; respiratory rate, 18 breaths per minute; room air oxygen saturation, 97%; temperature, 36.8°C
- Electrocardiogram (ECG): normal sinus rhythm, 1st degree AV block, nonspecific ST-T wave changes, evidence old inferior wall myocardial infarction
- Dobutamine stress test: normal left ventricular function, no evidence ischemia, normal study

PATHOPHYSIOLOGY

Each year in the United States over 700,000 individuals experience an adverse cerebrovascular event. Currently, 4.6 million stroke survivors are living in the United States with varying degrees of disability. Stroke is the third leading cause of death and the number one cause of major morbidity. Atherosclerotic disease accounts for approximately 30% of all of these strokes. It is estimated that 0.5% of individuals over the age of 60 and 10% of people over the age of 80 have carotid artery stenosis, accounting for the increased prevalence of stroke in the elderly population. CEA is, therefore, a prophylactic treatment, performed for individuals who are considered to be at increased risk of decreased cerebral perfusion.

Blood is supplied to the brain via the right and left internal carotid arteries and the vertebral arteries. The two internal carotid arteries are responsible for 80–90% of the blood supply and the remainder comes from the vertebrobasilar system. These vessels join to form the circle of Willis and the major intracranial vessels including the anterior cerebral arteries, the middle cerebral arteries, and the posterior cerebral arteries as is shown in Figure 23-1. Occlusion of a particular major cerebral vessel results in a predictable pattern of neurologic symptoms specific to the area of the brain supplied by the vessel.

Cerebral blood flow (CBF) is dependent on several factors, which are summarized in Table 23-1. CBF is normally autoregulated over a range of mean arterial pressures (MAP) from 50–150 mm Hg. Cerebral perfusion pressure (CPP) is calculated using Equation 23-1. The normal range for CPP is 80–100 mm Hg. In the absence of increased intracranial pressure (ICP) or an elevated central venous pressure, the major determinant of CPP is MAP.

In patients who have hypertension, the autoregulation curve is shifted to the right such that higher perfusion pressures are required to maintain consistent CBF. Normal cerebral metabolic requirements for oxygen ($CMRO_2$) range from 3.0–3.8 mL O_2/100 g brain tissue/minute. These requirements can be decreased by hypothermia, barbiturates, benzodiazepines, and volatile anesthetics. However, hyperthermia, seizure disorders, and ketamine all increase $CMRO_2$. Finally, CO_2 is a potent cerebral vasodilator such that CBF is increased 1 mL/100 g/minute for each 1 mm Hg increase in $PaCO_2$.

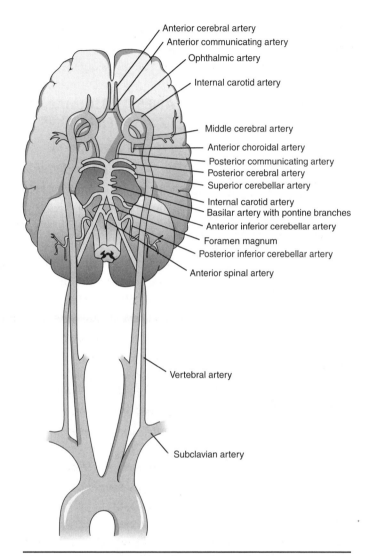

Figure 23-1 *The blood supply to the brain (circle of Willis).*

Table 23-1 Determinants of Cerebral Blood Flow
• Cerebral metabolic rate of oxygen and glucose consumption
• Cerebral perfusion pressure
• $PaCO_2$
• PaO_2
• Intracranial pathology
• Influence of concomitant drug therapy

Equation 23-1
CPP = MAP − ICP or CVP
Note: The value that is higher, ICP or CVP is used. CPP, cerebral perfusion pressure; CVP, central venous pressure; ICP, intracranial pressure; MAP, mean arterial pressure

Therefore, dramatic increases in CBF will occur in the presence of hypercarbia.

Carotid artery stenosis most frequently occurs where the common carotid artery bifurcates into the internal and external carotid arteries. This results in turbulent blood flow which leads to endothelial cell damage and plaque formation. Carotid plaques usually take one of two forms, homogeneous or heterogeneous. *Homogeneous plaques* are stable deposits of fatty streaks and fibrous tissues that rarely rupture and therefore patients may be asymptomatic. However, over time, the plaque becomes covered by a fibrous cap, which can rupture releasing the underlying debris into the cerebral circulation. Restabilization of the ruptured cap results in the development of *heterogeneous plaques* which are unstable and can rupture. Patients who are symptomatic are most likely to have heterogeneous plaques that are prone to acute disruption and spontaneous embolization which is the cause of the majority of strokes resulting from carotid artery stenosis. Carotid endarterectomy is recommended for symptomatic patients with greater than 70% carotid stenosis in the associated carotid artery.

SURGICAL PROCEDURE

CEA involves careful exposure of the common carotid artery including its bifurcation into the internal and external carotid arteries. Once exposure is complete the external, internal, and common carotid arteries are cross-clamped so that the carotid bifurcation can be isolated from the circulation. The artery is then opened through a longitudinal incision and the plaque is removed extending as far cephalad into the internal carotid as feasible. A synthetic patch graft is then utilized to close the vessel in order to increase the diameter of the artery and prevent restenosis. Several surgeons utilize an eversion CEA technique in which the carotid artery is completely transected and turned inside out in order to remove the plaque. A shunt may or may not be utilized. Regardless of the technique that is performed, it is essential that the surgeon remove all debris from the vessel intima in order to prevent embolization and postoperative neurologic sequelae.

ANESTHETIC MANAGEMENT AND CONSIDERATIONS

Preoperative Period

1. Discuss the indications for CEA including criteria for patient selection.

The American Academy of Neurology reviewed the indications for CEA and they have identified two groups of patients that are candidates for surgical treatment, symptomatic and asymptomatic patients. Symptomatic patients are considered when rupture of the plaque releases emboli into the cerebral circulation causing TIAs that produce reversible neurological effects. Asymptomatic patients have carotid artery stenosis but there is no history of a neurological event that is attributable to the carotid lesion.

Several large studies have compared patient outcomes after surgery and medical treatment. They found that for symptomatic patients with greater than 70%, stenosis there was an absolute risk reduction of 16% for perioperative death and subsequent stroke over the next 5 years. A reduction in the patients' risk was not observed in symptomatic patients with less than 70%, stenosis and no benefit was demonstrated in patients with 30–49% stenosis or total occlusion. CEA was shown to be harmful in patients who had less than 30% carotid artery stenosis. CEA is, therefore, recommended for symptomatic patients with greater than 70% carotid artery stenosis.

2. Discuss a minimally invasive surgical procedure used to treat carotid artery stenosis.

Carotid artery angioplasty and stent placement (CAS) is a nonsurgical alternative to CEA that has recently become available for the primary and secondary prevention of a CVA as a result of carotid artery stenosis shown in Figure 23-2. The results of outcome studies have been mixed but more recent studies have shown favorable results as technology

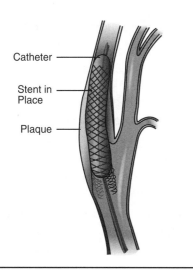

Figure 23-2   *Carotid artery stenting.*

has improved and distal embolic protection devices have been developed. The risk of adverse neurologic events appears to be higher with CAS particularly during catheterization and ballooning, but re-stenosis rates appear to be comparable to the traditional CEA technique.

Patient selection is based on a thorough evaluation of the vasculature to determine the feasibility of conducting the angiography and stenting procedures. All patients undergo an aortic arch, carotid, and cerebral angiogram or high resolution magnetic resonance imaging (MRI) in order

Table 23-2   Complications Associated with Carotid Artery Angioplasty and Stenting

- Stroke
- Myocardial infarction/ischemia
- Death
- Bradycardia and hypotension from stimulation baroreceptor reflex
- Stent thrombosis and embolization
- Carotid artery dissection from stent placement
- Cerebral hyperperfusion syndrome
- Horner syndrome
- Hemorrhage

to guide the choice of catheters, balloons, and stents to be employed. Hemodynamic changes are similar to those seen with CEA, including reperfusion hypotension due to baroreceptor dysfunction. Anesthesia services may be provided for sedation and hemodynamic monitoring. Complications associated with CAS are related to anticoagulation, balloon angioplasty, and the stent placement and are presented in Table 23-2.

3. Discuss the common coexisting disease states, preoperative medications, and factors that contribute to morbidity and mortality in patients undergoing CEA.

The majority of patients presenting for CEA suffer from significant atherosclerotic disease in both the coronary and peripheral vasculature and are at risk for developing myocardial ischemia and/or infarction. Most of these patients will be medically managed preoperatively utilizing a combination of beta-blockers, calcium channel blockers, antiarrhythmics, nitrates, diuretics, ACE inhibitors, and other antihypertensive drugs. In addition, some patients may be receiving antiplatelet therapy with aspirin (ASA) and/or clopidogrel (Plavix). Current recommendations are that all patients with carotid artery disease should be on low dose aspirin therapy on regular basis and it should be continued through the perioperative period. There is no evidence to support the continued use of other antiplatelet medications and these should be discontinued a week before surgery to ensure that platelet function has normalized.

The incidence of perioperative myocardial infarction has been reported to range from 0–4% and this complication is the leading cause of mortality following CEA. Patients presenting with both significant coronary artery disease and carotid artery disease requiring surgical intervention present a specific problem since it is unclear which surgical procedure to undertake first. Patients undergoing CEA before coronary revascularization are at significant risk for cardiac events. However, coronary revascularization prior to CEA may increase the incidence of post-operative CVA. Surgical management is, therefore, determined on an individual basis.

Chronic essential hypertension is highly associated with carotid artery stenosis and increases the morbidity and mortality for patients undergoing CEA.

- There is a significant association between post-operative stroke or death and a *preoperative* systolic blood pressure > 180 mm Hg.
- A *postoperative* systolic blood pressure > 220 mm Hg is associated with an increased risk of stroke or death following CEA.
- A preoperative systolic blood pressure of > 160 mm Hg is a risk factor for postoperative hypertension.
- It is recommended that blood pressure control be achieved preoperatively in patients with a systolic blood pressure > 180 mm Hg, who do not have severe bilateral carotid artery disease, and who are not having frequent adverse neurologic events.

The anesthetist must consider that cerebral autoregulation is shifted to the right requiring a higher mean arterial pressure in patients with hypertension and it is unknown how long it takes for the mechanism to reset. The concern is that patients with severe hypertension will be at increased risk for impaired cerebral perfusion during surgical correction. The preoperative risk factors associated with perioperative events during CEA are presented in Table 23-3.

Table 23-3	Preoperative Risk Factors Associated with Perioperative Events During CEA

- Chronic essential hypertension
- Coronary artery disease (CAD)
- Peripheral vascular disease
- Preexisting renal disease
- Symptomatic carotid artery stenosis in combination with severe CAD

4. Discuss the preoperative evaluation of the patient undergoing CEA including cardiac risk assessment.

Preoperative evaluation of the patient undergoing CEA should include the conduct of a comprehensive history and physical examination. All preexisting neurologic deficits should be documented in the patient's record. A careful cardiovascular assessment should be carried out since the possibility of cardiovascular disease is high. This should include a preoperative ECG, echocardiogram, or cardiac stress test as dictated by the patient's history and presentation. A careful assessment of preoperative blood pressure is also necessary since the risk of preoperative neurological events is high in the patient with hypertension. All patients undergoing CEA should be evaluated by a cardiologist prior to surgery.

In addition to the cardiac assessment, the patient's preoperative respiratory function should also be assessed to determine their pulmonary reserve. Information regarding the patient's smoking history is also essential as cigarette smoking is associated with a substantially significant increase in the risk of a stroke. Other preoperative factors associated with an increased risk of stroke include preexisting renal disease, diabetes mellitus, hyperlipidemia, and excessive alcohol consumption.

Intraoperative Period

5. Describe the various anesthetic techniques utilized for CEA.

Anesthesia for CEA can be provided utilizing both regional or general anesthesia. The choice of technique is dependent on the patient's, surgeon's, and anesthetist's preference, as well as familiarity with a particular technique and the patient's status. The advantages comparing regional and general anesthesia for CEA are listed in Table 23-4. Regardless of anesthetic technique, it is necessary to provide cerebral and cardiac protection, as well as control of blood pressure, heart rate, and the stress response to surgery. Standard monitoring includes an intra-arterial catheter for

Table 23-4 Advantages of Regional Versus General Anesthesia for CEA	
REGIONAL ANESTHESIA	**GENERAL ANESTHESIA**
• Superior perioperative neurologic assessment	• Does not require patient cooperation
• ↓ incidence mortality	• Anesthetic induced decreased in $CMRO_2$ may provide cerebral protection
• ↓ incidence perioperative stroke	
• ↓ intraoperative hemodynamic instability	
• Maintenance cerebral blood flow	
• ↓ rate of shunting	
• Decreased length of stay	

continuous beat-to-beat blood pressure monitoring, noninvasive blood pressure monitoring, ECG, pulse oximetry, and capnography. Patients with poor left ventricular function may benefit from a pulmonary artery catheter but the benefits must be weighed against the risks of accidental carotid puncture. When general anesthesia is employed, transesophageal echocardiography can be used.

General Anesthesia General anesthesia for CEA can be safely administered utilizing a variety of anesthetic agents. Comparisons of inhalation versus narcotic based techniques have shown no difference in outcome since both volatile anesthetics and narcotics decrease $CMRO_2$. If somatosensory evoked potentials (SSEPs) are to be monitored intraoperatively, inhalation anesthetics may have to be avoided because they have been shown to depress the amplitude and increase the latency of SSEP transmission. However, regardless of the anesthetic agents utilized, it is essential that hemodynamic stability be maintained and that emergence occurs promptly so that immediate assessment of postoperative neurologic functioning can occur in the operating room.

Regional Anesthesia Regional anesthesia for CEA can be accomplished using either local infiltration or superficial and/or deep cervical plexus block. The greatest advantage of this technique is the ability to assess the patient's neurologic functioning throughout the procedure. Signs of impaired neurologic function include:

• Dizziness
• Slurred speech weakness
• Dysphasia
• Altered level of consciousness

It has not been conclusively determined that regional anesthesia performed for CEA improves long-term outcomes. Since the patient is awake for the duration of the procedure, preoperative patient education is essential. Anxiety and fear can stimulate the stress response and create hemodynamic instability unrelated to the underlying surgical intervention. Mild sedation can be utilized but deep sedation can impair neurologic assessment and produce hypoventilation which increases CO_2. It is also difficult to convert to a general anesthetic because access to the patient's airway is limited. It is, therefore, essential to determine those candidates who are appropriate for regional anesthesia.

6. Discuss the rationale and methods for monitoring neurologic status during CEA.
Monitoring neurologic function under general anesthesia is necessary in order to detect episodes of cerebral ischemia, hypoperfusion, and cerebral embolization. These monitors are employed to identify patients who would benefit from the use of

Table 23-5 Methods of Monitoring for Cerebral Ischemia During CEA

- EEG: Monitors cortical events but does not disclose ischemia in deeper structures
- SSEP: Assessing the integrity of sensory pathways in both cortical and deep structures of the brain
- Near infrared spectroscopy (NIRS) or cerebral oximetry: Measures regional cerebral oxygenation
- Transcranial Doppler: Allows ultrasonic measurement of blood flow through the middle cerebral artery; can be used to monitor both cerebral hemodynamic and the occurrence of emboli.

a carotid artery shunt during carotid artery cross-clamping. A number of methods of monitoring are currently available and are outlined in Table 23-5:

- *Electroencephalogram* (EEG) can be used to monitor neurologic functioning under general anesthesia for CEA. While the technique is sensitive when detecting cerebral ischemia, the signal only reflects cortical events and does not detect ischemia in deeper structures of the brain. In addition, the raw EEG data is difficult to interpret.
- *Somatosensory evoked potentials* (SSEPs) have many advantages as compared to the EEG to detect cerebral ischemia. The information determined from SSEPs examines both cortical and deep brain structures because they assess transmission along the entire sensory nerve pathway. However, like the EEG, they are sensitive to the effect of global ischemia rather than regional ischemia. In addition, volatile anesthetics suppress the SSEP and if they are used, the agent concentration should be ≤ 0.5 minimum alveolar concentration (MAC).
- *Near infrared spectroscopy* (NIRS), also known as cerebral oximetry, provides information regarding regional cerebral oxygenation (rSO_2),

which is a composite measure of arterial, venous, and capillary oxygenation. The predominant influence on the value comes from the venous blood. Carotid cross-clamping is associated with decreases in rSO_2 but there are no well-defined parameters for the "normal" range of values. In addition, changes in rSO_2 can be related to changes in the regional distribution of blood flow as a result of anesthesia rather than a result of ischemia. This monitoring modality has been associated with a high false-positive rate.

- *Transcranial Doppler* measures velocity of flow through the middle cerebral artery by way of a probe placed on the thin petrous temporal bone. A marked reduction in velocity during carotid artery cross-clamping is an indication for the use of a carotid shunt. Studies assessing the efficacy of this technique are conflicting. Unlike other monitors utilized, the transcranial doppler is capable of detecting the presence of emboli. Since the majority of untoward neurologic events during CEA are embolic in nature, this technique provides advantages over those previously discussed.

7. Describe the methods available for providing cerebral protection and reducing the risk of neurologic injury during CEA.

Measuring Stump Pressures Before the introduction of more sophisticated forms of cerebral monitoring, stump pressures have been traditionally used to determine the need for shunt placement during carotid cross-clamping. Once the common carotid and external carotid arteries are clamped, the pressure measured within the internal carotid artery reflects the perfusion pressure within the circle of Willis, and thus the adequacy of collateral blood flow. A wide range of pressures (25–70 mm Hg) have been proposed as acceptable during carotid artery cross-clamping, and it has been determined that stump pressures tend to be specific (ability to detect true negatives) but not sensitive (ability to detect true positives) for the development of cerebral ischemia.

Carotid Shunting Frequently shunts are utilized during carotid cross-clamping to ensure the adequacy of CBF during CEA. A shunt is inserted in the proximal and distal aspects of the carotid artery. The surgeons dissect the plaque within the carotid artery as blood flows from the common carotid artery through the shunt, bypasses the surgical field, and enters the circle of Willis. While this technique would appear to be extremely useful to prevent postoperative neurologic sequelae, it is associated with risks. Complications of shunt insertion include air embolization, plaque embolization, tears of the vessel intima, and carotid dissection. In addition, there is an increased risk of local complications including the development of hematomas, infection, nerve injury, and carotid restenosis. Because up to 95% of postoperative neurologic deficits are the result of embolic events, many surgeons do not routinely shunt but place shunts selectively based on evidence of cerebral hypoperfusion in response to cross-clamping. Determining factors include measuring of stump pressures and assessing changes in neurologic monitoring parameters. Patients undergoing CEA with intraoperative EEG and SSEP monitoring who have selective shunting demonstrate a significantly reduced rate of developing a stroke. Patients who received selective shunting are thought to be more than seven times less likely to experience a perioperative stroke.

8. Discuss the rationale for anticoagulation during carotid cross-clamping.

Heparin is administered intraoperatively, prior to carotid artery cross-clamping, in order to reduce the risk of thromboembolic complications. Several different methods are employed by anesthetists to guide the dosing for heparin but 50–100 U/kg is commonly administered. A wide range of plasma concentrations with some patients being overdosed and others underdosed. This practice is also

associated with a trend toward a higher incidence of neurologic deficits in patients who have not been adequately anticoagulated as determined by the activated clotting time (ACT). Heparin administration on a Units/kg basis is associated with more consistent plasma levels and a lower risk for the development of postoperative hematoma. Redosing is determined based on the duration of anticoagulation needed and the amount of drug left in the body. The elimination half-time of heparin is 1.5 hours with a range of 1–2 hours. Despite the improved control achieved with weight-based dosing, no statistically significant advantage has been demonstrated in clinical studies to advocate for weight-based versus fixed dosing.

The decision to reverse the anticoagulation effects of heparin with protamine is made on an individual basis and depends on the presence of bleeding. There is an increased incidence of stroke associated with protamine administration but a decreased risk for postoperative hematoma requiring surgical decompression. The dose of protamine administered 1 mg/100 U of heparin assumed to be left in the blood at the time of reversal. Therefore, 25 mg of protamine should be sufficient to reverse the effects of a 5000 U-dose of heparin administered an hour prior to reversal.

9. Explain the importance of controlling the patient's blood pressure during CEA.

As previously stated, hypertension is present in the majority of patients presenting for CEA. In general, hypertensive patients suffer from profound blood pressure lability during the perioperative period, especially when general anesthesia is utilized. Cardiovascular instability is even more pronounced when these patients undergo CEA. Hypotension and/or hypertension can occur as a result of carotid sinus baroreceptor stimulation and manipulation. In addition, carotid artery cross-clamping is associated with marked increased in arterial pressure regardless of the anesthetic technique. The cardiovascular changes produced as a result of the combined effect of anesthesia and carotid sinus manipulation place the patients undergoing CEA at risk for negative perioperative cardiac and cerebrovascular events.

10. Describe the methods utilized for control of blood pressure during CEA.

Intraoperative blood pressure control begins during the preoperative period as outlined previously. The patient's cardiovascular and neurologic conditions should be optimized prior to surgical intervention. All antihypertensive medications should be continued throughout the perioperative period. Since there are multiple intraoperative events that can result in sympathetic stimulation including induction of anesthesia, incision, carotid cross-clamping, and emergence, short acting beta-adrenergic blocking agents should be readily available. Should hypertension be sustained, nitroglycerin and nitroprusside can be utilized for titratable control of blood pressure. Bradycardia associated with manipulation of the carotid sinus can be blocked with local infiltration of local anesthetic by the surgeon. The initial treatment for bradycardia that is caused by the baroreceptor reflex and results in severe hypotension is to notify the surgeon to release pressure on the carotid sinus. Sustained hypotension can be treated by administering intravenous fluids and vasopressors. Bradycardia that is unresponsive to local infiltration may require the administration of atropine sulfate.

Postoperative Period

11. Discuss the pathophysiology and treatment of commonly occurring postoperative complications that are associated with CEA.

The most frequently occurring postoperative complications associated with CEA are summarized in Table 23-6. Both hypertension and hypotension are common following CEA. It has been estimated that hypertension is seen in approximately 25% of patients and hypotension occurs in approximately 10% of patients, but

Table 23-6	Postoperative Complications Following CEA

- Hemodynamic instability (hypotension and hypertension)
- Myocardial ischemia/infarction
- Carotid sinus dysfunction
- Stroke
- Cerebral hyperperfusion syndrome
- Recurrent/superior laryngeal nerve damage
- Hematoma
- Tension pneumothorax
- Respiratory failure

the causes have not been completely explained. Unrecognized bleeding and/or inadequate intraoperative fluid replacement may cause postoperative hypotension. It has been hypothesized that postoperative hypertension results from a decreased baroreceptor reflex responsiveness as a result of mechanical injury during surgical manipulation. In addition, patients with bilateral carotid artery disease is been shown to exhibit more severe deterioration in baroreceptor function after surgery. Sustained systolic blood pressures > 180 mm Hg is associated with an increased risk of TIA, stroke, and myocardial infarction in the postoperative period. The intervention should be determined by the individual anesthetist but nitrates may be useful in this setting since they are more likely to maintain CBF.

Cerebral hyperperfusion syndrome occurs in 1–3% of patients undergoing CEA. These patients develop profound increases in CBF and often demonstrate an increased flow velocity in the middle cerebral artery estimated to be 100% greater than the values measured preoperatively. These patients develop an ipsilateral (operative side) headache, severe arterial hypertension, seizures, and, often, focal neurologic deficits. If left untreated, cerebral hyperperfusion syndrome can progress to cerebral edema, intracranial hemorrhage, and death. Preoperative risk factors for the development of cerebral hyperperfusion syndrome include decreased cerebrovascular reserve, preoperative hypertension, previous CVA, or surgery for > 90% carotid artery stenosis. Therefore, it is essential that blood pressure control be achieved before the day of surgery and throughout the perioperative period. Table 23-7 summarizes the risk factors associated with the development of cerebral hyperperfusion syndrome.

The development of a postoperative stroke is most commonly attributed to thrombus formation and embolization of plaque debris during the insertion of shunts and removal of the intimal plaque. Neurologic assessment is conducted within the operating room immediately after emergence in order to identify the presence of neurologic deficits.

Postoperative bleeding is infrequent but can occur after a CEA. When bleeding is significant, it can cause the development of an incisional hematoma that may be large enough to cause airway compromise. The initial intervention after a hematoma is discovered is to immediately notify the surgeon to evacuate the hematoma followed by airway management. This seems counterintuitive; however, the definitive treatment is to relieve the pressure on the structures of the neck. Normally viewed anatomic structures that are identifiable during direct laryngoscopy may not be visualized during subsequent

---

Table 23-7   Risk Factors for Developing of Cerebral Hyperperfusion Syndrome

- Diminished cerebrovascular reserve
- Preoperative uncontrolled hypertension
- Recent ipsilateral nonhemorrhagic stroke
- Previous ischemic cerebral infarction
- Surgery for > 90% ipsilateral carotid stenosis
- Intraoperative ischemia/embolization
- Postoperative hypertension
- Hyperperfusion lasting greater than several hours after CEA

---

attempts. It may also become difficult or impossible to ventilate the patient. Immediate reexploration of the surgical site is mandatory.

Tension pneumothorax can also occur in the postoperative period since the apices of the lungs extend above the clavicles and the pleural cavity may be inadvertently entered during surgical dissection of the neck. This will require immediate decompression.

12. Describe the neurologic cranial nerve assessment for a patient having a CEA.

During dissection and retraction of neck structures, it is possible for damage to occur to the underlying cranial nerves as they pass through the surrounding tissues. The postoperative evaluation of the patient's neurologic and cognitive function should include an assessment of the integrity of cranial nerves VII (facial), IX (glossopharyngeal), X (vagus), XI (spinal accessory), and XII (hypoglossal).

The facial nerve (VII) is a mixed sensory and motor nerve responsible for motor control to the muscles of the face and for the secretion of saliva. Damage to the facial nerve results in an asymmetric ipsilateral smile. Contralateral asymmetry may be indicative of a possible intraoperative CVA.

The glossopharyngeal nerve (IX) controls the pharyngeal muscles and the ability to swallow. Damage to this nerve will result in difficulty swallowing and ipsilateral Horner syndrome. Horner syndrome is associated with miosis, ptosis, and anhydrosis.

The vagus nerve (X) branches divides to form the superior and recurrent laryngeal nerves, which control the muscles of the larynx. Unilateral damage to the internal branch of the superior laryngeal nerve which innervates the cricothyroid muscle, will result in hoarseness. Unilateral damage to the recurrent laryngeal nerve which innervates the posterior and lateral cricoarytenoid muscles, can cause vocal cord paralysis on the operative side, hoarseness, impairment of the gag reflex, difficult vocalization, and respiratory difficulty especially in those patients with preoperative respiratory insufficiency.

Table 23-8 Assessment of Cranial Nerve Function Following CEA

CRANIAL NERVE	ABNORMAL ASSESSMENT
• Facial nerve	• Ipsilateral smile asymmetry
• Glossopharyngeal nerve	• Difficulty swallowing • Ipsilateral Horner syndrome
• Vagus nerve (recurrent and superior laryngeal nerves)	• Unilateral vocal cord paralysis • Hoarseness • Impairment of the gag reflex • Voice fatigue
• Spinal accessory nerve	• Ipsilateral weakness of the trapezius and sterno cleidomastoid muscles • Ipsilateral weakness of the neck and shoulder against resistance
• Hypoglossal nerve	• Ipsilateral tongue drift • Difficulty with speech • Difficulty with chewing

The spinal accessory nerve (XI) controls the sternocleidomastoid and the trapezius muscles. Damage to this nerve during CEA will result in ipsilateral weakness in the neck and shoulder. Patients will have difficulty turning their head or shrugging against resistance.

Finally, the hypoglossal nerve (XII) is responsible for control of the muscles of the tongue. Damage to this structure will result in ipsilateral drift of the tongue when patients are asked to stick out their tongue. In addition, patients may have difficulties with speech and chewing. A summary of the cranial nerves that should be assessed is included in Table 23-8.

REVIEW QUESTIONS

1. Which is a disadvantage of regional anesthesia administered for carotid endarterectomy?
   a. Results in an increased length of stay
   b. Associated with increased morbidity and mortality
   c. Requires patient cooperation
   d. Increases hemodynamic instability

2. Monitoring carotid artery stump pressures is:
   a. reflective of perfusion pressure in the internal carotid artery.
   b. highly sensitive for the development of cerebral ischemia.
   c. measured prior to the application of the carotid cross-clamp.
   d. sensitive indicator of cerebral hypoperfusion.

3. One hour after a dose of heparin, 7000 U have been administered. The appropriate initial dose of protamine for this patient who weighs 60 kg is:
   a. 70 mg.
   b. 50 mg.
   c. 35 mg.
   d. 15 mg.

4. Which is not caused by cranial nerve injury during carotid endarterectomy?
   a. Contralateral smile asymmetry
   b. Unilateral vocal cord paralysis
   c. Horner syndrome
   d. Ipsilateral tongue drift

5. The majority of postoperative neurologic deficits occur as a result of:
   a. perioperative hypertensive episodes.
   b. thromboembolic events.
   c. carotid dissection.
   d. cranial nerve injury.

REVIEW ANSWERS

1. **Answer c**
   Regional anesthesia requires that the patient be awake and able to cooperate for the duration of the surgical procedure. Careful patient selection and preoperative education is essential because heavy sedation increases the incidence of intraoperative complications.

2. **Answer d**
   Stump pressures show a high degree of specificity but not sensitivity for the detection of cerebral hypoperfusion and ischemia.

3. **Answer c**
   The elimination half-time of heparin is approximately 1 hour, so only 3500 U of heparin should be circulating in the body 1 hour after administration. Since the dose of protamine is 1 mg/100 U heparin left in the body, the initial dose of protamine that should be administered is 35 mg.

4. **Answer a**
   Ipsilateral smile asymmetry is the result of cranial nerve damage. Contralateral asymmetry is the result of an intraoperative cerebral vascular event.

5. **Answer b**
   Ninety-five percent of all postoperative neurologic deficits are the result of thromboembolic events during carotid endarterectomy.

SUGGESTED READINGS

American Heart Association. *Heart disease and stroke statistics: 2003 update.* Dallas, TX: American Heart Association, 2002.

Cao P, De Rango P, Verzini F, et al. Outcome of carotid stenting versus endarterectomy: a case-control study. *Stroke* 2006;37(5):1221–1226.

Chaturvedi S, Bruno A, Feasby T, et al. Carotid endarterectomy—an evidence-based review: report of the therapeutics and technology assessment subcommittee of the american academy of neurology. *Neurology* 2005;65(6):794–801.

Elisha S. Anesthesia for vascular surgery. In: Nagelhout JJ, Plaus KL, eds. *Nurse Anesthesia*, 4th ed. St. Louis, MO: Saunders Elsevier, 2010:528–559.

Ellis JE, Roizen MF, Mantha S, et al. Anesthesia for vascular surgery. In: Barash PG, Cullen BF, Stoelting RK, eds. *Clinical Anesthesia*, 5th ed. Philadelphia: Lippincott Wiliams & Wilkins, 2006:933–973.

Gonzalez M. Vascular disease. In: Hines RL, Marshall KE, eds. *Stoelting's Anesthesia and Coexisting Disease*, 5th ed. Philadelphia: Saunders Elsevier, 2008:135–160.

Howell SJ. Carotid endarterectomy. *Br J Anaesth* 2007;99(1):119–131.

Nouraei SA, Al-Rawi PG, Sigaudo-Roussel D, et al. Carotid endarterectomy impairs blood pressure homeostasis by reducing the physiologic baroreflex reserve. *J Vasc Surg* 2005;41(4):631–S637.

Wakhloo AK, Lieber BB, Seong J, et al. Hemodynamics of carotid artery atherosclerotic occlusive disease. *J Vasc Interv Radiol* 2004;15(1 Pt 2):S111–S121.

Woodworth GF, McGirt MJ, Than KD, et al. Selective versus routine intraoperative shunting during carotid endarterectomy: a multivariate outcome analysis. *Neurosurgery* 2007;61(6):1170–1176; discussion 1176–1177.

Acute Aortic Dissection and Repair

24

Marjorie A. Geisz-Everson

KEY POINTS

- The incidence of acute aortic dissection is rare and is estimated to be 5–30 cases per 1 million people per year in the United States.
- Aortic dissection is associated with a tear in the intimal layer of the aorta.
- An acute aortic dissection may involve the ascending and/or the descending aorta.
- The incidence of acute aortic dissection occurs more frequently in men than in women.
- The morbidity and mortality rate associated with acute aortic dissection even when treatment occurs is 90% within a 3-month period.

CASE SYNOPSIS

A 65-year-old man presents to the emergency room (ER) with severe sharp chest pain that radiates to his upper back. A transesophageal echocardiogram (TEE) reveals an acute ascending aortic dissection.

PREOPERATIVE EVALUATION AND DEMOGRAPHIC DATA

Past Medical/Surgical History

- Hypertension
- Coronary artery disease
- Coronary artery bypass grafting 1 year ago
- Right inguinal hernia repair 20 years ago

List of Medications

- Zestril (Lisinopril)
- Atorvastatin (Lipitor)
- Aspirin (80 mg)

Diagnostic Data

- Hemoglobin, 12.8 g/dl; hematocrit, 38.2%
- Electrolytes: sodium, 141 mEq/l; potassium, 3.7 mEq/l; chloride, 101 mEq/l; carbon dioxide, 19 mEq/l
- Electrocardiogram (ECG): normal sinus rhythm; heart rate, 95 beats per minute
- Chest x-ray: widening mediastinum, otherwise normal

Height/Weight/Vital Signs

- 183 cm, 85 kg
- Blood pressure, 165/100; heart rate, 95 beats per minute; respiratory rate, 18 breaths per minute; room air oxygen saturation, 96%; temperature, 98.5°F

PATHOPHYSIOLOGY

Acute aortic dissection is an uncommon yet life-threatening condition that involves a disruption of the intimal layer of the aorta. The aorta is exposed to constantly high pressure which creates shear stress on the intimal layer. The high degree of wall tension within the aorta can be described by law of Laplace. When patients have long-term untreated hypertension and plaque formation within the aorta, there is an increased incidence of dissection. Once the intimal layer is damaged, blood flows through the disruption between the intima and media creating a false lumen that separates the middle and outer layers of the aorta. The false lumen may eventually rupture.

There are numerous classification systems that exist to describe the location of the aortic dissection. The Stanford classification system is the most commonly used to differentiate between the regions of the aortic defect. This system divides aortic dissection into a Type A and a Type B as shown in Figure 24-1. The Type A dissection involves the ascending thoracic aorta with or without the involvement of the descending thoracic aorta. The Stanford Type B dissection involves the descending thoracic aorta. Aortic dissections can extend to the

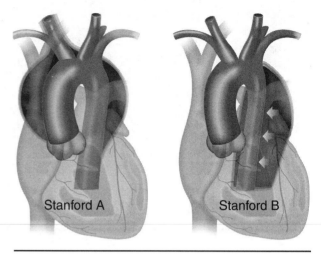

Figure 24-1 *Stanford Type A and Type B aortic dissections.*

aortic root and produce aortic valve insufficiency. Untreated aortic dissections have a 50% mortality rate in the first 48 hours and a 90% mortality rate within 3 months. The most common anatomic positions for an aortic dissection to occur include the aortic arch, distal to the left subclavian artery and immediately superior to the aortic root.

A Stanford Type A acute aortic dissection requires immediate medical treatment and surgical intervention. The Stanford Type B acute aortic dissection is most often treated with medical management unless the patient has uncontrolled hypertension, poor perfusion to the gastrointestinal tract or lower extremities, and rupture of the aorta. Surgical treatment is warranted in these cases.

Open surgical repair of the aorta is the usual procedure used to correct the Stanford Type B aortic dissection. Endovascular aortic repair (EVAR) is being explored as a treatment option for aortic aneurysms and recent evidence supports the effectiveness of this technique. It is estimated that 70% of patients who develop an aortic dissection have hypertension. Aneurysms of the aorta may or may not be present prior to aortic dissection. TEE is a first-line diagnostic tool used to identify the presence of an acute aortic dissection. The TEE can reveal the extent of the dissection into the aortic

Aortic Dissection and Surgical Repair

TYPE I DISSECTION EXTENDS,
CREATING A FALSE LUMEN

FALSE LUMEN OF DISSECTION CAN
DISRUPT FLOW TO GREAT VESSELS

DACRON AORTIC
GRAFT

Flap of vessel wall
narrows the
true lumen

False
lumen

Figure 24-2 *Repair of a dissection of the ascending aorta.*

root as well as the condition of the aortic valve. Computed tomography (CT) and magnetic resonance imaging (MRI) techniques provide definitive data as to the presence, location, and size of the aortic dissections. A repair of a dissection of the ascending aorta is illustrated in Figure 24-2.

MEDICAL MANAGEMENT

The Stanford Type B aortic dissection is routinely medically treated by administering beta-adrenergic blocking drugs. If the use of beta-adrenergic blocking drugs is contraindicated, then calcium channel blocking agents and sodium nitroprusside may be used. The goal of medical management is to avoid aortic rupture. Antihypertensive therapy is titrated to maintain the systolic blood pressure between 100 and 120 mm Hg which decreases the mechanical stress exerted on the aortic wall. Careful monitoring for aortic rupture is necessary. Obtaining data from serial TEE, CT scans, or MRI can be utilized to monitor for progressive increases or decreases in the size of the aortic dissection and aortic rupture.

SURGICAL MANAGEMENT

The Stanford Type A aortic dissection requires immediate surgery to resect the ascending aorta. It is necessary to use cardiopulmonary bypass, hypothermia, and circulatory arrest. If the dissection involves the aortic root and aortic valve,

Table 24-1 Stanford and DeBakey Classification Systems for Aortic Dissection

STANFORD CLASSIFICATION

- Type A dissection involves the ascending aorta.

- Type B dissection involves the descending aorta.

DEBAKEY CLASSIFICATION

- Type I dissection involves both the ascending and descending aorta.

- Type II dissection involves only the ascending aorta.

- Type III dissection involves only the descending aorta.

  - Type IIIA dissection involves the descending aorta between the left subclavian artery and the diaphragm.

  - Type IIIB dissection involves the descending aorta below the level of the diaphragm.

replacement with a prosthetic valve is usually performed due to the likelihood of developing aortic valvular pathology in the future. EVAR using endovascular stenting techniques are continuing to become more popular for elective and acute treatment of Stanford Type B aortic aneurysms. There is a decrease in the 30-day mortality rate associated with EVAR as compared to an open approach; however, the 1-year postoperatively mortality rates are similar for both surgical approaches. The anesthetic technique that is most often employed during EVAR is conscious sedation.

ANESTHETIC MANAGEMENT AND CONSIDERATION

Preoperative Period

1. Describe the most usual signs and symptoms associated with acute aortic dissection.
It is estimated that up to 50% of patients who develop an acute aortic dissection are initially misdiagnosed because the symptoms can be easily mistaken for other medical problems. The typical symptoms that occur include sharp, tearing, or ripping chest pain and hypertension or hypotension which is less common. The hypertension that ensues is thought to be caused by the release of catecholamines resulting from sympathetic nervous system predominance from decreased peripheral perfusion. Hypotension is suggestive of cardiac tamponade or hypovolemia resulting for partial or complete rupture of the aorta. Some patients have presented with epigastric pain or paraplegia. At times, only after an autopsy is the diagnosis of aortic dissection confirmed.

This patient has severe chest pain that radiates to his back which are symptoms of an acute aortic dissection. His chest x-ray revealed a widening of the mediastinum which may be indicative of an aortic dissection. A finding of a widening mediastinum should prompt further testing such as a CT scan, angiography, or TEE to confirm aortic dissection. A widening mediastinum can also be found with an aortic aneurysm, esophageal rupture, pericardial effusion, and other pathologies. A complete list of signs and symptoms associated with acute aortic dissection is listed in Table 24-2.

2. Examine the various coexisting disease processes that may be associated with patients presenting with an acute aortic dissection.
The most common comorbidities that are associated with aortic dissection in the order of frequency include hypertension, atherosclerosis, aortic aneurysm, and Marfan syndrome. Males are more likely to have acute aortic dissections. Chronic hypertension can cause thickening of arteries, atherosclerosis, and arterial aneurysms. Constant high blood pressure in thickened, atherosclerotic, or aneurismal arteries can predispose the patient to aortic dissection. Atherosclerosis causes decreased compliance of the arterial walls. This alteration will increase the patient's susceptibility to aortic dissection. Weakness in the aortic wall can lead to an aneurysm which is a "bulging" or "ballooning" of the vessel

Table 24-2	The Signs and Symptoms Associated with an Acute Dissecting Aneurysm

NEUROLOGIC

- Altered level of consciousness
- Syncope
- Cerebrovascular accident
- Paraplegia

CARDIOVASCULAR

- Hypertension and bounding peripheral pulses
- Hypotension and decreased peripheral pulses
- Congestive heart failure
- Acute aortic regurgitation
- Cardiac tamponade
- Sudden onset of severe chest pain (anterior and/or posterior)
- Jugular venous distention
- Widening pulse pressure
- Dysrhythmias
- Superior vena cava syndrome

RESPIRATORY

- Shortness of breath
- Bilateral rales
- Hemothorax
- Hoarseness caused by impingement on the left recurrent laryngeal nerve

Table 24-3	Coexisting Diseases That are Associated with Acute Aortic Dissection

- Pain
- Abdominal distention
- Bloating
- Constipation
- Nausea and vomiting
- Fever
- Leukocytosis
- Hemodynamic variability
- Intraluminal gas fluid within the lumen of segments proximal to the obstruction
- Free air present within the peritoneum (suggestive of bowel perforation)

wall, and with constant pressure the aneurysm may rupture. Inherited connective tissue disorders such as Marfan syndrome alter the normal physiology of arterial vessels and increase the probability of aortic dissection. A complete list of coexisting disease factors that are related to acute aortic dissection are listed in Table 24-3.

3. Discuss the preoperative preparation and monitoring considerations for this patient.

- If patient is hemodynamically unstable, then the time available for a thorough preoperative history and physical may be limited.

- Control hemodynamic variability with vasopressors and vasodilators.
  - Treatment for hypertension: beta-adrenergic antagonists, nitroprusside, nitroglycerin
  - Treatment for hypotension: phenylephrine, dopamine, dobutamine, epinephrine
- Large-bore IV lines
- Right side radial arterial line. The left subclavian artery provides perfusion to the left radial artery. During aortic cross-clamp application, impingement of the left subclavian artery will decrease the effectiveness of arterial monitoring if the left radial artery is cannulated. Insertion of femoral arterial lines may be used but the femoral arteries should be spared for the arterial cannulation associated with cardiopulmonary bypass.
- Central venous catheter to infuse fluid/blood and monitor central venous pressure
- Pulmonary artery catheter to assess the cardiac output
- Cell saver and rapid transfusion devices
- TEE
- Packed red blood cells, fresh frozen plasma, and platelets

Intraoperative Period

4. Describe common surgical corrections of acute aortic dissection.

The most common procedure used to correct acute aortic dissection is the Stanford Type A and this is accomplished by performing a sternotomy utilizing cardiopulmonary bypass, deep hypothermia, and circulatory arrest. If aortic cannulation for cardiopulmonary bypass is unable to be achieved due to the dissection, the right axillary artery and the right femoral artery can be used. Intraoperative electroencephalography (EEG) and TEE are commonly used to evaluate neurologic function and cardiac function, respectively. Preservation of neurologic function is accomplished by administering barbiturates, utilizing cerebral perfusion via the cardiopulmonary bypass machine, and instituting deep hypothermic circulatory arrest (DHCA). These measures decrease the cerebral metabolic rate of oxygen consumption and protect the brain during periods of decreased perfusion. Repair of the acute aortic dissection may include replacement of the aortic root (with reimplantation of coronary arteries), replacement of aortic root and aortic valve (with reimplantation of coronary arteries), replacement of the aortic root keeping the native valve, ascending aortic graft, and ascending aortic graft with aortic valve replacement.

5. Identify the key components of anesthetic management for the patient with an acute aortic dissection.

- The induction of anesthesia should provide cardiovascular stability while ensuring loss of consciousness.
- It is vital that all attempts should be made to keep the patient hemodynamically stable.
- The systolic blood pressure should remain between 100 and 120 mm Hg.
- Maintenance of anesthesia can be accomplished by administering narcotics, inhaled anesthetic agents, and neuromuscular blocking agents.

- The information gained from the TEE will guide vasodilator and vasopressor therapy.
- Ideally a baseline EEG tracing will be established prior to the induction of anesthesia. The EEG will be continuously monitored throughout case. Burst suppression should be achieved during DHCA.
- Initiation of cardiopulmonary bypass and cooling to between 18° and 25°C.
- Barbiturate administration can occur prior to DHCA; however, there is a lack of definitive clinical evidence that this intervention offers additional cerebral protection.
- Steroid administration is warranted prior to DHCA for brain and multiorgan protection.
- Mannitol may be given to preserve renal function and to decrease cerebral edema. DHCA is initiated when surgeon is ready to repair the aorta.
- Selective cerebral perfusion may be used during aortic dissection repair to protect the brain and to prolong circulatory arrest time to 45 minutes while decreasing the potential for neurologic damage. Infusion of cold, oxygenated blood can be achieved by antegrade and/or retrograde cannulation. Antegrade cannulation is commonly accomplished via the innominate and left carotid arteries. Retrograde cannulation usually occurs in the superior vena cava.

6. Discuss the deep hypothermic circulatory arrest.

DHCA has been utilized since the 1970s to protect the brain during surgery when cerebral perfusion is compromised. Cardiopulmonary bypass is initiated and the patient is cooled. Once hypothermia is achieved and the surgeon is ready to repair the aorta, circulatory arrest is initiated. The method by which circulatory arrest occurs is by turning the cardiopulmonary bypass machine off and thereby stopping perfusion to the entire body. Circulatory arrest should only be employed for 30 minutes or less because increased time can result in organ ischemia. Retrograde and/or antegrade perfusion is continued during circulatory arrest to provide additional cerebral protection. The head may be packed in ice to provide additional cooling. Care must be taken to protect exposed skin surfaces to the ice and to avoid the development of frostbite. Once the aorta has been repaired or replaced, cardiopulmonary bypass is reinitiated and incremental warning begins. The glucose level should be monitored to avoid global cerebral ischemia. Allowing the blood pH to be more alkaline as hypothermia is accomplished helps to preserve cerebral autoregulation. The rewarming process should be slow because cerebral hyperthermia results in increased metabolic demands and may result in cerebral injury.

7. List the physiologic alterations associated with deep hypothermia.
- Decreased cerebral metabolic rate of oxygen consumption
- Decreased organ metabolic rate of oxygen consumption
- Increased blood viscosity
- Coagulopathy
- Hemorrhage
- Thrombocytopenia
- Peripheral vasoconstriction
- Impaired renal and liver function

Postoperative Period

8. Identify the postoperative anesthetic concerns after acute aortic dissection repair.
Following the surgical procedure, patients remain intubated and are transferred to the intensive care unit. Careful monitoring of the blood pressure, urine output, and bleeding are required. The patient should also be assessed for other potential complications related to the surgery such as stroke, ventricular dysrhythmias, myocardial infarction, and

renal failure. If the patient remains hemodynamically stable, they should be extubated as soon as possible in order to assess for adequate neurologic integrity. Decreasing the amount of vasoactive medication should be accomplished as expeditiously if possible.

REVIEW QUESTIONS

1. Which intervention is used to prolong the amount of time that deep hypothermic circulatory arrest can be used?
   a. Administration of sodium pentothal
   b. Administration of steroids
   c. Retrograde cerebral perfusion
   d. Selective antegrade perfusion
2. A TEE reveals that a patient has an aortic dissection that extends to the aortic root and the aortic arch. Which Stanford classification type is consistent with these findings?
   a. Type A
   b. Type B
   c. Type C
   d. Type D
3. Retrograde cerebral perfusion is accomplished by cannulating the:
   a. right axillary artery.
   b. right carotid artery.
   c. internal jugular vein.
   d. left subclavian vein.
4. The most common comorbid factor that is associated with an acute aortic dissection is:
   a. an aortic aneurysm.
   b. hypertension.
   c. atherosclerosis.
   d. deep vein thrombosis.
5. Which complication is associated with deep hypothermia circulatory arrest?
   a. Hyperoxia
   b. Thrombocytopenia
   c. Deep vein thrombosis
   d. Atherosclerosis

REVIEW ANSWERS

1. **Answer: d**
   Selective antegrade perfusion is utilized to prolong the amount of time that deep hypothermic circulatory arrest can be used.

2. **Answer: a**
   Stanford Type A aortic dissections include the aortic root, ascending aorta, and aortic arch.

3. **Answer: c**
   The internal jugular vein is usually cannulated for retrograde cerebral perfusion.

4. **Answer: b**
   Hypertension is the most common comorbidity present in the patient with acute aortic dissection.

5. **Answer: b**
   Thrombocytopenia is a complication associated with deep hypothermic circulatory arrest.

SUGGESTED READINGS

Banoub M. Anesthesia for thoracic aortic surgery. In: Estafanous FG, Barash PG, Reeves JG, eds. *Cardiac Anesthesia Principles and Clinical Practice*, 2nd ed. Philadelphia: Lippincott Williams & Wilkins, 2001: 767–856.

Elisha S. Vascular surgery. In: Nagelhout JJ, Zaglaniczy KL, eds. *Nurse Anesthesia*, 3rd ed. St Louis, MO: Elsevier Saunders, 2005: 485–501.

Golledge J, Eagle KA. Acute aortic dissection. *Lancet* 2008;372:55–64.

Henly WS. Acute aortic dissection and visceral ischemia. *JMDHVC* 2008;4:12–13.

Kocher AA, Bonaros N, Nagiller J, et al. Acute aortic dissection mimicking cholecystitis. *Eur Surg* 2007;39:203–205.

Pantin EJ, Cheung AT. Thoracic aorta. In: Kaplan JA, Reich DL, Lake CL, Konstadt SN, eds. *Kaplan's Cardiac Anesthesia*, 5th ed. Philadelphia: Saunders Elsevier, 2006:723–764.

Patel PD, Arora RR. Pathophysiology, diagnosis, and management of aortic dissection. *Ther Adv Cardiovasc Dis* 2008;2:439–468.

Raghupathy A, Nienaber CA, Harris KM, et al. Geographic differences in clinical presentation, treatment, and outcomes in Type A acute aortic dissection (from the international registry of acute aortic dissection). *Am J of Cardiol* 2008;102:1562–1566.

Skubas N, Lichtman AD, Sharma A, et al. Anesthesia for cardiac surgery. In: Barash PG, Cullen BF, Stoelting RK, eds. *Clinical Anesthesia*, 5th ed. Philadelphia: Lippincott Williams & Wilkins, 2006:886–932.

Tsai T, Evangelista A, Nienaber CA, et al. Long-term survival in patients presenting with type A acute aortic dissection: Insights from the International Registry of Acute Aortic Dissection (IRAD). *Circulation* 2006;114(1):350–356.

Thoracic Aneurysm Repair

25

Cliff Roberson

KEY POINTS

- Significant comorbidities are prevalent in patients with atherosclerotic lesions of the thoracic aorta. These include hypertension, coronary artery disease, chronic obstructive pulmonary disease (COPD), renal insufficiency, and cerebrovascular disease.
- Mortality rates for open repairs of thoracic aortic aneurysms (TAA) are approximately 8% in centers with concentrated experience and may approach 20% for all cases in the United States.
- One-lung anesthesia is typically required to facilitate surgical access to the descending thoracic aorta.
- Monitoring and regulation of proximal and distal perfusion during aortic cross-clamping of the thoracic aorta are central to the anesthetic management of patients undergoing aneurysm repair.
- Aortic reconstruction that is performed superior to the level of the renal arteries poses an increased risk of temporary or permanent spinal cord injury. The incidence of paraplegia associated with thoracic aortic surgery range from 2 to 16%.
- Aneurysmal leakage, rupture, and aortic dissection increase the risk for intraoperative hemorrhage and massive transfusion.

CASE SYNOPSIS

A 67-year-old man has been diagnosed with a descending TAA that was discovered on a recent history and physical examination for a chronic cough and mild interscapular back pain. He is scheduled for an open repair of the aneurysm under general anesthesia.

PREOPERATIVE EVALUATION AND DEMOGRAPHIC DATA

Past Medical/Surgical History

- Hypertension, COPD, cigarette smoking
- Inguinal hernia repair under local/monitored anesthesia care

List of Medications

- Atenolol, lisinopril, atorvastatin (Lipitor), budesonide and formoterol (Symbicort), albuterol

Diagnostic Data

- Complete blood count: white blood cells, 4.31 K/mcl; red blood cells, 5.28 K/mcl; hemoglobin, 14.1 g/dl; hematocrit, 42.3%; platelets, 285 K/mcl
- Coagulation: prothrombin time, 11.2 s; international normalized ratio, 1.1; partial thromboplastin time, 29.2 s
- Electrolytes: sodium, 139 mmol/l; potassium, 4.1 mmol/l; chloride, 105 mmol/l; carbon dioxide, 38 mmol/l
- Glucose, 98 mg/dl
- Blood urea nitrogen, 28 mg/dl; creatinine, 1.4 mg/dL
- Electrocardiogram: sinus rhythm, nonspecific ST abnormalities
- Chest x-ray: widened mediastinum consistent with a TAA; no infiltrates
- Pulmonary function testing: moderate COPD; $FEV_1/FVC = 68\%$ predicted
- Echocardiogram: no wall motion abnormalities; ejection fraction, 61%
- Computed tomography (CT) scan: 5.2 cm TAA just distal to the left subclavian artery

Height/Weight/Vital Signs

- 185 cm, 87 kg
- Blood pressure, 147/82; heart rate, 76 beats per minute; respiratory rate, 18 breaths per minute; room air oxygen saturation, 94%

PATHOPHYSIOLOGY

A TAA is defined as a permanent dilation in any area of the aorta above the diaphragm that measures at least 1.5 times the expected normal diameter as shown in Figure 25-1. The majority of TAAs are caused by atherosclerotic degenerative disease,

Figure 25-1   *Thoracic aortic aneurysm.*

but the aneurysm may also develop from chronic aortic dissection, connective tissue disease, infection, trauma, or following surgical procedures that require aortic cannulation or cross-clamping. Aortic aneurysms are also seen in congenital disorders of metabolism, such as Marfan syndrome and Ehlers-Danlos syndrome. Regardless of etiology, a TAA arises from a weakening of the aortic wall which results in a progressive dilation of all three structural layers of the vessel (*intima*, *media*, and *adventitia*). The increased diameter of the aortic lumen compromises aortic blood flow, compresses surrounding structures, and increases arterial wall tension, placing the patient at risk for aortic rupture, exsanguination, and death.

TAA constitute 30–40% of all aortic aneurysms and may develop in one or more anatomic segments along the course of the aorta within the thorax. The thoracic aorta originates from the aortic root and encompasses the ascending aorta, the aortic arch, and the descending thoracic aorta. The descending aorta originates distal to the left subclavian artery and terminates at the diaphragm as shown in Figure 25-2. Thoracic lesions can also extend below the level of the diaphragm into the abdominal aorta in the form of thoracoabdominal aneurysm as is illustrated in Figure 25-3. The majority of all TAAs involve the aortic root and/or the ascending aorta. Approximately 40% of all TAAs

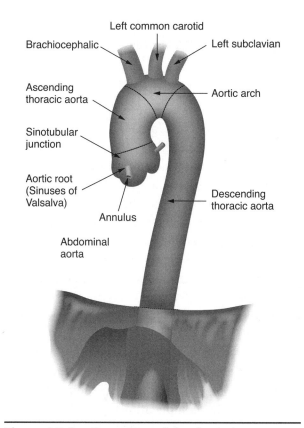

Figure 25-2 *Segments of the thoracic aorta.*

involve areas of the descending aorta. Dissections of the thoracic aorta are also classified with reference to their anatomic location. Dissections occur when a tear in the intima allows blood to enter the medial layer, creating an extraluminal channel (false lumen) that can course along the length of the aorta.

The clinical presentation varies with the location of the TAA and the mechanism of vessel dilation. Many patients are asymptomatic; however, the aneurysm may be discovered as an incidental finding while investigating an unrelated problem. Degenerative lesions are less likely to cause symptoms than those caused by dissection, from which up to 85% of patients may be symptomatic. A common symptom is back pain, often interscapular. Pain may also be felt in the neck and jaw, the precordium, or the left thoracic region. The aneurysm can often be localized by symptoms that result from its expansion at the expense of surrounding structures. Compression of the left mainstem bronchus can cause dyspnea, coughing, wheezing, and stridor, as well as tracheal deviation. Aneurysm expansion near the esophagus produces dysphagia and even weight loss. The left recurrent laryngeal nerve is situated around the aortic arch and impingement from the aneurysm manifests hoarseness and unilateral left sided vocal cord paralysis. Horner syndrome can be precipitated by encroachment in the area of the stellate ganglia. Compression of the vena cava can produce facial edema and may occasion dyspnea and other symptoms consistent with a superior vena cava syndrome. Aortic root and ascending thoracic aneurysms may give rise to symptoms of congestive heart failure produced by aortic valve dilation and regurgitation. A local mass effect in the aortic root may provoke myocardial ischemia due to compression or dissection of the coronary arteries. Finally, patients with a ruptured TAA may present with profound hypovolemia and hemorrhagic shock, as well as the signs and symptoms of hemothorax or hemopericardium.

SURGICAL PROCEDURE

Repair of the descending thoracic aorta is usually performed with the patient positioned in right lateral decubitus. Rotation of the hips up to 45 degrees

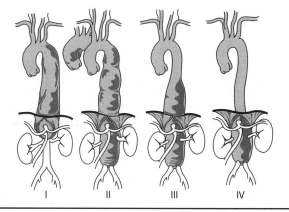

Figure 25-3 *Types of thoracoabdominal aneurysms.*

Figure 25-4 *Aortic cross-clamp placement and tube graft repair.*

is necessary to facilitate access to the descending aorta and the femoral vessels. Once the lesion is isolated, the repair is often accomplished with a tube graft. The aneurysm may be either excised or oversewn around the completed aortic graft. The repair requires clamping of the thoracic aorta normally above and below the area of the lesion. The proximal clamp is most commonly placed just distal to the left subclavian artery as is shown in Figure 25-4. The distal clamp may be placed sequentially along the aorta with the goal of minimizing visceral ischemia.

In addition to the aortic cross-clamp, procedures that are performed on the descending thoracic aorta may require the placement of shunts or extracorporeal support with partial cardiopulmonary bypass (CPB) in order to maintain lower body perfusion and to provide adequate spinal cord and visceral blood supply distal to the clamp. Complete CPB is indicated for ascending and aneurysms that involve the aortic arch. For descending aorta aneurysms, aortic clamping techniques with or without shunts or partial distal bypass are most commonly employed. The intercostal or segmental spinal arteries may be incorporated into the graft or reimplanted into the descending aorta to prevent ischemic spinal cord injury after excision of the aneurysm. Visceral branches (celiac, mesentery, renal arteries) must be preserved and these arteries are incorporated into the aortic graft.

ANESTHETIC MANAGEMENT AND CONSIDERATIONS

Preoperative Period

1. Describe the comorbidities associated with atherosclerotic lesions of the thoracic aorta and the measures to evaluate the extent of coexisting disease in the preoperative period.

Most patients with atherosclerotic lesions of the thoracic aorta are of advanced age and have significant comorbidities. The scope of the preoperative evaluation will depend on the urgency of the surgical procedure. TAAs that are leaking, or dissecting or have ruptured should be repaired immediately, and the limited preoperative time allows for a rapid assessment of the patient's condition. For elective surgery, a complete health history and thorough assessment of all systems is warranted in order to reveal the extent of coexisting disease, to optimize the patient's preoperative condition, and to help reduce the risk of perioperative complications.

Atherosclerosis is a systemic disease that can cause degenerative changes in the entire arterial system which may cause coronary artery disease, cerebrovascular disease, and renal dysfunction. Chronic hypertension is another key risk factor for aneurysm formation and is usually evident preoperatively. Patients often have a long history of cigarette habituation; significant COPD is a very common finding. Preoperative renal dysfunction may be present in up to 30% of patients, particularly with descending aortic aneurysms when the lesion extends to the renal arteries.

Cardiac status is evaluated by electrocardiography (ECG) to detect myocardial ischemia and/or infarction, conduction abnormalities, and ventricular hypertrophy; by echocardiography to evaluate the size and location of the TAA, ventricular function, and valvular competence. Angiography is performed to assess the dimensions and location of the TAA, the coronary vascular anatomy, and cardiac function. Pulmonary status may be assessed with arterial blood gas analysis, chest radiography, and pulmonary function testing. Airway obstruction caused by the aneurysm can be detected by pulmonary function testing. A thorough neurologic history may be supplemented in some patients by carotid artery angiography or carotid duplex studies, as well as a neuropsychoiogical consultation to establish a baseline for postoperative assessment. Routine preoperative measurement of blood urea nitrogen (BUN) and creatinine will help identify the presence of renal dysfunction.

2. Discuss the natural history and strategies used to treat thoracic aortic aneurysms.

Atherosclerotic TAAs generally develop over time and the destruction of the supporting matrix of the aorta causing vessel dilation at a rate of 0.5 cm or less per year. Patients who are asymptomatic and have TAAs whose anteroposterior diameter is less than 5 to 6 cm may be managed medically. As the risk of rupture increases with elevations in diastolic blood pressure and obstructive lung disease, medical management focuses on risk factor modification, including the strict control of blood pressure, low sodium diet, and cessation of smoking. A TAA that is ≥ 6 cm in diameter increases the potential for rupture by fivefold. The natural course of luminal expansion results in aortic rupture or dissection and death. Surgical intervention is warranted in large aneurysms, as well as in acutely symptomatic patients, in rapidly expanding lesions and in Type B dissections. The risk of death for descending TAA surgery is about 8% in centers with concentrated experience and may reach 20% nationally.

3. Explain the mechanism for airway compromise for patients who have a thoracic aneurysm.

Expansion of a TAA may distort the airway due to the proximity of anatomic structures along the course of the thoracic aorta. Ascending TAAs may compress the right mainstem bronchus, whereas descending TAAs may cause tracheal deviation and compression of the left mainstem bronchus.

Airway compression may cause dyspnea or stridor. Larger ascending thoracic aneurysms can create a mediastinal mass effect and complicate induction and intubation. These patients may not be able to breathe if they are placed supine. Prolonged compression of airway structures can lead to tracheomalacia. Aneurysms may also leak into the airways precipitating hemoptysis.

4. Discuss spinal cord vascular anatomy and perfusion in the context of thoracic aneurysm surgery.

The spinal cord receives its blood supply from three principal sources: the anterior spinal artery (75%) and two posterior spinal arteries (25%). The anterior spinal cord receives supplementation of blood flow by way of the spinal branches of the intercostal arteries in the thorax and the lumbar arteries in the abdomen. These collateral vessels originate in the posterior aorta, the most important of which is the artery of Adamkiewicz (greater radicular artery). This artery's origin is positioned on the left in 80% of the population and joins the anterior spinal artery in 60% of patients at the T9-T12 vertebral segments, at the T5-T8 vertebral segments in 15%, and at L1-L2 vertebral segments in 25% of the population. As the anterior spinal artery tapers in the thorax, the artery of Adamkiewicz provides the majority of blood supply to the anterior, lower two-thirds of the spinal cord. Thus, spinal cord ischemia can occur to anterior portion of the spinal cord which is involved in motor function from hypotension, aortic cross-clamping, and interruption of segmental arteries. The incidence of paraplegia has been estimated to be approximately 20% after elective surgery and as high as 40% during aortic reconstruction for dissecting or ruptured TAAs.

5. Describe the potential for blood loss and list techniques for venous access in patients undergoing repair of the descending thoracic aorta.

The risk of major hemorrhage is substantial during repair of a TAA. The estimated blood loss ranges from 5000–8000 ml. This is particularly true if only proximal clamping of the aorta is used, which causes retrograde blood flow and bleeding from visceral vessels. Sudden and catastrophic blood loss from aortic rupture is also possible throughout the surgical procedure. Insertion of one or two large-bore (14–16 gauge) peripheral intravenous catheters is routine along with the placement of central introducer cannulae (7–9 French) in the internal jugular, subclavian, or femoral veins.

6. Describe the requirements for fluid, blood, and blood product requirements necessary for thoracic aortic surgery.

The incision for thoracic aorta surgery is extensive and exposes both the thoracic and abdominal cavities to the extracorporeal environment. As a result, insensible fluid losses from evaporation are large. Due to the potential for major hemorrhage, the availability of sufficient blood products and systems for their infusion is imperative. Eight to 15 units of packed red blood cells (PRBCs) should be readily accessible in the operative suite. The administration of fresh frozen plasma (FFP) and platelets should also be anticipated as massive fluid resuscitation and the development of an intraoperative coagulopathy is common. A rapid infusion or cell salvage system and fluid warming capabilities should be primed and in place prior to the beginning of surgery. Intraoperative assessment of hematological and coagulation lab values is imperative.

Intraoperative Period

7. Describe the cardiovascular and hemodynamic monitoring modalities for thoracic aorta surgery.

The dynamic nature of patient responses during TAA and the risk of complications due to existing comorbidities and intraoperative events make hemodynamic monitoring a complex and critical process. Standard ECG with ST segment analysis in leads II and V5 is indicated for the detection of

myocardial ischemia, injury, and dysrhythmias. The risk of a myocardial infarction is considerable and it is the major cause of perioperative mortality.

Dramatic and precipitous changes in hemodynamics during thoracic aorta repairs are very common due to aortic cross-clamping/unclamping and ongoing major blood loss. These changes necessitate placement of an arterial catheter for beat-to-beat monitoring of blood pressure. Serial sampling of blood for laboratory analysis is likewise facilitated. The *right radial artery* is the preferred site for blood pressure assessment during a descending aorta repair. This is due to the fact that aortic cross-clamping is occasionally required proximal to the left subclavian artery, making the left upper extremity unsuitable for arterial pressure monitoring. A right brachial arterial line is considered a safe alternative. Pulse oximetry and plethography should be avoided in the left upper extremity for the same reason. Femoral artery blood pressures may be monitored in order to determine the adequacy of distal perfusion during the aortic cross-clamping. The assessment of femoral arterial pressures allows timely interventions to be made for low distal perfusion, which may reduce overall spinal and renal ischemia.

In contrast to the descending aorta, repairs of the ascending aorta require monitoring of arterial blood pressure in the *left upper extremity*, as the innominate (brachiocephalic) artery may be clamped. Noninvasive blood pressure cuffs can also be placed on both arms to document differences in upper extremity perfusion. Pulmonary artery (PA) catheter placement has been frequently advocated for use in thoracic aorta surgery to assess cardiac function, volume status, and mixed venous oxygen saturation. The insertion of PA catheters is associated with complications such as pneumothorax, intrathoracic bleeding, inadvertent carotid artery puncture, dysrhythmias, pulmonary artery ischemia, and infection. Pulmonary artery occlusion pressures (PAOP) may substantially overestimate the left ventricular end-diastolic pressures (LVEDP) during one-lung anesthesia. Moreover, the usefulness of mixed venous oxygen saturation as an indicator of cardiac output during cross-clamping of the aorta has been questioned.

Transesophageal echocardiography (TEE) has become a routine modality for intraoperative monitoring during thoracic aorta surgery. It is a minimally invasive technique used to assess biventricular function, volume status, and the development of myocardial ischemia. The information obtained from the TEE assessment has been found to be more accurate in estimating preload than PA catheters and more effective in detecting early myocardial ischemia than ECG monitoring. The TEE is an important tool in the diagnosis of acute aortic dissection and can confirm proper placement of central access devices. Passage of the TEE probe may cause injury to the oropharynx and esophagus, precipitate rupture of the aneurysm, and compression can make placement difficult.

8. Explain induction techniques for thoracic aorta surgery that serve to minimize the hypertensive response and the risk of aneurysm rupture.

The goals for the induction of anesthesia in thoracic aorta surgery focus primarily on myocardial preservation and the prevention of hemodynamic stress on the aortic lesion. Tachycardia and hypertension are the principal concerns, especially during laryngoscopy and endotracheal intubation. Tight control of heart rate and blood pressure during induction helps decrease the potential for myocardial ischemia or infarction. Tachycardia and hypertension may also trigger the rupture of an aneurysm or may extend an aortic dissection by increasing the shearing forces present within the aorta. Adequate anesthesia depth is essential.

The hemodynamic stability that is associated with etomidate is desirable for induction agent prior to TAA repair. High-dose narcotic techniques have been advocated, but must be used with caution prior to the establishment of mask ventilation due to the risk of chest wall rigidity and consequent sympathetic stimulation. Careful titration of narcotics, such as fentanyl or sufentanil, is preferred and is considered a safe and effective method to blunt the hemodynamic effects of airway manipulation. Beta-adrenergic antagonists, particularly short-acting agents such as esmolol, are useful adjuncts in treating tachycardia and hypertension during induction. Treatment of hypertension may require the administration of vasoactive agents; nitroglycerine or sodium nitroprusside may be helpful in reducing blood pressure in the context of a normal heart rate.

9. Discuss the potential problems during management of one-lung anesthesia for repair of descending thoracic aneurysms.

The use of a double-lumen endotracheal tube (DLT) is a standard practice for surgeries of the descending thoracic aorta that are performed through a left thoracotomy incision. Lung separation and the subsequent collapse of the left lung facilitate exposure of the thoracic aorta and reduce iatrogenic trauma to the left lung from surgical retraction. One-lung anesthesia (OLA) for thoracotomy typically makes use of a left-sided DLT, although airway distortion of the left bronchus from a large descending lesion may make placement difficult. Fiberoptic examination of the left bronchus may facilitate proper left endobronchial intubation; findings of pulsatile compression or frank erosion within the left bronchus warrant the use of a right-sided DLT in order to avoid complications. Proper positioning of the right-sided DLT should be confirmed fiberoptically to ensure adequate right upper lobe ventilation with OLA. Following surgery, DLTs are generally changed to single-lumen devices for postoperative ventilatory support. An alternative to using a DLT for OLA is a single-lumen tube with a retractable bronchial blocking device. If the patient requires postoperative ventilation, then the DLT should be replaced by a standard endotracheal tube.

Patients undergoing OLA during thoracic aorta surgery are at substantial risk for developing hypoxemia. Collapse of the nondependent lung creates a significant right-to-left shunt, which may be further exacerbated in those with preexisting lung disease. Maintenance of 100% oxygen may lower the incidence of hypoxemia with OLA, as hypoxic pulmonary vasoconstriction (HPV), which shunts blood from the nonventilated left lung to the ventilated right lung is inhibited. The effectiveness of HPV may be diminished by the administration of potent vasodilators, such as inhalation of anesthetic agents, nitroglycerin, and sodium nitroprusside. Effective measures in addressing hypoxemia during OLA include use of 100% oxygen, application of 5 to 10 cm H_2O continuous positive airway pressure (CPAP) to the collapsed left lung, positive end-expiratory pressure (PEEP) to the ventilated right lung, intermittent reinflation and ventilation of both lungs, and ligation of the pulmonary artery to the collapsed lung. High peak airway pressures (greater than 30 cm H_2O) may also counteract the beneficial effects of HPV and can be managed with slight reductions in tidal volume (6 to 8 ml/kg) and increases in respiratory rate in order to maintain minute ventilation at a lower pressure.

10. Describe the physiologic and hemodynamic impact of aortic clamping/unclamping during repair of a TAA.

Application of a cross clamp to the descending aorta causes significant hemodynamic alteration. Acute occlusion of the aorta increases afterload, resulting in a reduction of ventricular ejection and a rise in LVEDP. Preload is augmented by a redistribution of blood from vessels below the clamp. Ventricular contractility may be enhanced by increased filling and by catecholamine release in response to clamping. These changes may precipitate acute left ventricular failure or myocardial ischemia, especially in patients with preexisting cardiac disease. Proximal to the clamp, arterial blood pressure dramatically increases and often requires active intervention when bypass techniques are not utilized. Vasodilators, such as sodium nitroprusside and nitroglycerin, may be used. Higher concentrations of inhalation anesthetics may be helpful in lowering proximal blood pressure in patients with normal ventricular function. Esmolol may be administered to control proximal hypertension without compromising spinal cord perfusion. Peripheral perfusion is significantly decreased distal to the aortic clamp, causing severe reductions in end-organ blood flow and autoregulation, notably to the kidneys, the abdominal viscera, and the distal spinal cord. Impaired perfusion to organs and tissues results in anaerobic metabolism with lactic acid production and metabolic acidosis. Reduced hepatic blood flow impairs lactate clearance and exacerbates acidosis.

Unclamping of the aorta causes profound hemodynamic instability. Systemic vascular resistance and blood pressure may be reduced by 50%, creating a "declamping shock" state. Arterial hypotension is most likely caused by massive peripheral vasodilation, made worse by the redistribution of blood from the upper to lower body. Myocardial depression, central hypovolemia, and the systemic effects of ischemic metabolites exacerbate the reduction in blood pressure. Reperfusion of ischemic tissues causes inflammatory mediators and oxygen free radicals which cause cellular damage are produced and released. In anticipation of this profound hypotension, aggressive volume loading may be instituted, along with decreasing the anesthetic depth and stopping the infusion of vasodilators. A staged or slow removal of the aortic clamp by the surgeon may reduce the intensity of the response, but hypotension is usually unavoidable. The minute ventilation may be increased and sodium bicarbonate administered to counter the acidosis. Once the clamp is removed, the administration of vasopressors, such as phenylephrine, may be necessary to stabilize the blood pressure, as well as calcium chloride to correct hypocalcemia if present. Hypertension should be avoided as it may place stress on the suture lines of the graft and cause bleeding.

11. List techniques for lower body perfusion during repair of the descending thoracic aorta.

Distal perfusion techniques are generally indicated for complex repairs of the descending aorta that may require prolonged aortic cross-clamping. They are designed to maintain lower body perfusion, to reduce ischemic injury, and to decrease the incidence of paraplegia and renal failure. Distal perfusion techniques can also attenuate the proximal hypertension associated with the placement of the clamp, the development of metabolic acidosis during clamping, and the profound hypotension that occurs with unclamping.

The least complex technique for lower body perfusion utilizes a conduit that diverts blood flow from the proximal descending aorta or the left ventricle to the distal aorta. Blood flows through the shunt passively using the pressure in the proximal source as its driving force. The Gott shunt is heparin coated, which eliminates the need for systemic heparinization. The most common technique for distal aortic perfusion is partial bypass or left-heart bypass, which uses a centrifugal pump to direct blood from the left atrium to the left femoral artery. Other proximal sites with partial bypass include the aortic arch, the proximal descending aorta, or the pulmonary vein. The bypass circuits are also coated with heparin, so a reduced dose of systemic heparin may be given (100 U/kg). The pump allows for adjustments in blood flow to be made during aortic cross-clamping to correct alterations in preload or afterload and to control proximal hypertension. Both radial and femoral blood pressure monitoring are indicated with partial bypass techniques in order to assess pressures above and below the aortic cross-clamp. Finally, extracorporeal support for lower body perfusion can also be achieved with a femoral vein–femoral artery bypass, which provides retrograde perfusion below the clamp. This approach requires an oxygenator, a roller clamp, and systemic heparinization.

Distal perfusion techniques reduce visceral and renal ischemia and may decrease the risk of paraplegia during descending aortic surgery. The provision of perfusion to the lower body prevents metabolic acidosis and the accumulation of hypoxia-induced metabolites. Bypass techniques provide an effective means for controlling proximal hypertension during aortic cross-clamping and for preventing post-clamp hypotension. Their large cannulae supply access for rapid volume infusion; their flexible configuration allows for extracorporal oxygenation and temperature manipulation. The disadvantages of distal perfusion techniques include bleeding, dislodgement, increased operative time, and injury to anatomic structures. As with all extracorporeal support, there is an increased risk of air emboli and embolic stroke. The anticoagulation required for many techniques increases the risk of hemorrhage and adverse medication reactions from heparin and protamine.

12. Compare and contrast modalities used to monitor the integrity of the spinal cord during thoracic aortic surgery.

The integrity of the spinal cord may be assessed by neurophysiologic monitoring using evoked potentials. Evoked potentials refer to the electrical activity of the nervous system that is elicited in response to a stimulus. With this form of monitoring, a stimulus is generated and the evoked waveform is measured in terms of amplitude (strength) and latency (delay). The pathways between the brain and the peripheral nervous system or vice versa, including the spinal cord, may be continually evaluated in this manner. Decreases in amplitude and increases in latency may indicate an alteration in neuronal function, which is most likely caused by hypotension, hypothermia, or spinal cord ischemia. Somatosensory evoked potential (SSEP) monitoring involves the initiation of a signal in the periphery, usually at the posterior tibial or peroneal nerves, and the measurement of the cortical response in the brain by means of scalp electrodes. SSEP monitoring reflects the integrity of ascending sensory pathways in the lateral and posterior tracts of the spinal cord. Motor evoked potential (MEP) monitoring is achieved by stimulation of the motor cortex of the brain and measurement of the motor neuron response in the periphery or at the level of the spinal cord itself. MEP reflects the integrity of the descending motor pathways in the anterior tracts of the spinal cord.

Both SSEPs and MEPs have been used to monitor spinal cord integrity during thoracic aortic surgery. SSEPs reliably deteriorate from impaired perfusion to the cord during aortic cross-clamping or hypotension, but this deterioration may not predict permanent spinal cord injury with any degree of certainty. There does appear to be a strong correlation between the aortic cross-clamp time and the loss of SSEPs. While the preservation of evoked potentials during surgery presumes adequate spinal cord perfusion, postoperative paraplegia has been observed despite normal intraoperative SSEPs. This suggests that monitoring of the posterior sensory tracts may be of less clinical significance than that of the anterior motor tracts, given the nature of thoracic spinal perfusion and the vulnerability of the distal anterior cord during thoracic aortic surgery. MEPs may be better suited to detect clinically relevant spinal cord ischemia with greater sensitivity and specificity. Aortic cross-clamp placement and spinal cord protective measures can be directed, in part, by neurophysiologic monitoring. Identification of collateral vessels that may be critical to the perfusion of a specific segment of the spinal cord can also be facilitated by evoked potential data, allowing the surgeon to revascularize the area by reimplantation of segmental arteries or by endarterectomy.

Evoked potential monitoring may be impacted by a number of factors. The type and depth of anesthesia can alter both SSEP and MEP monitoring. All volatile anesthetic agents interfere with evoked potential monitoring causing dose-related reductions in amplitude and increases in latency. Avoidance of these agents or reduction of delivered concentrations is necessary; the use of isoflurane at 0.5 MAC with 60% nitrous oxide, for example, is felt to be compatible with effective SSEP monitoring. Intravenous anesthetic agents depress the SSEP waveform, although ketamine and etomidate may actually increase the amplitudes of both SSEP and MEP by reducing inhibitory mechanisms. Opioids have a minimal effect on both SSEP and MEP. Muscle relaxants profoundly inhibit MEPs; complete blockade renders the modality useless as a monitor of ventral tract integrity. It is recommended that muscle twitches in response to neuromuscular blockade monitor be maintained at a minimum of 30% of baseline to avoid interference with MEP. Patient parameters, such as temperature, hematocrit, and oxygen saturation, can also adversely affect evoked potential monitoring.

13. Outline intraoperative methods that may be used to protect the spinal cord from ischemic injury during the repair of the descending thoracic aorta.

Aortic cross-clamping of the descending thoracic aorta poses a risk for spinal cord ischemia and injury due to the resultant hypoperfusion. Paraparesis and paraplegia are the most devastating consequences of this iatrogenic impairment of spinal perfusion. The reported incidences of postoperative neurologic deficits in thoracic aortic surgery vary widely; rates for paraplegia average 2 to 16%. Risk factors for spinal cord injury include advanced patient age, the urgency of the procedure, the presence of rupture or dissection, as well as the level and the duration of aortic cross-clamping. A history of preoperative renal dysfunction is also an important risk factor for the development of spinal cord ischemia during thoracic aortic surgery. Spinal cord integrity may also be impaired by perioperative hypotension and hypoxemia, elevations in cerebrospinal fluid (CSF) pressure, and surgical transection of spinal arteries.

The management of perfusion distal to the aortic clamp is a key element in spinal cord protection. Foremost, the limitation of clamp time may help reduce the overall risk of spinal deficits by reducing the total ischemic time, although cases of paraplegia have been reported when the aortic clamp time is less than 20 minutes. The provision of distal perfusion during aortic cross-clamping by means of shunts or bypass techniques attempts to prevent end-organ ischemia, including the spinal cord. No one surgical intervention, however, has proven to be totally protective. The modulation of acute changes in CSF pressure after cross-clamping has been advocated, as spinal cord perfusion pressure (SCPP) is a function of the difference between mean arterial pressure (MAP) and CSF shown in Equation 25-1. Attenuation of CSF pressure increases may be achieved with the placement of a lumbar catheter and the drainage of CSF fluid, which serves to increase SCPP by lowering CSF pressure. Risks of lumbar drainage include cerebral herniation, spinal headache, meningitis, and epidural hematoma.

Hypothermia provides a reliable method of neuronal protection and prolongs cross-clamp time even with the use of mild hypothermia (34°C). It can be achieved systemically prior to clamping with passive cooling or partial bypass, or regionally by means of local spinal cord cooling through epidural or spinal catheters. A number of pharmacologic interventions have been studied, including systemic administration of corticosteroids, mannitol, thiopental, magnesium, and naloxone, with varying degrees of spinal cord protection. Intrathecal papaverine has been used to improve the perfusion through spinal arteries by vasodilation.

Equation 25-1

$$SCPP = MAP - CSF$$

CSF, cerebrospinal fluid; MAP, mean arterial pressure; SCPP, spinal cord perfusion pressure.

14. Discuss strategies to monitor and maintain renal perfusion during repair of thoracic aneurysm surgery.

Urinary output is measured with a Foley catheter, which provides an indirect, albeit inconsistent means of assessing volume status and renal perfusion. Renal dysfunction following repairs of the descending thoracic aorta can be as high as 14% and is associated with a substantially increased mortality rate. Advanced age, preoperative renal dysfunction, operative complexity, and prolonged aortic cross-clamp times predispose patients to perioperative renal failure. The mechanism of renal injury is most commonly ischemia caused by reduced renal perfusion due to aortic cross-clamping or hemodynamic instability. Oxygen free radicals and other inflammatory compounds impact the renal vasculature and may play an important role as well.

Renal protective strategies begin with the minimization of aortic cross-clamp time. Adequate renal perfusion should likewise be assured through the maintenance of intravascular volume and the avoidance of arterial hypotension during the perioperative period. Distal hypoperfusion during cross-clamping should be avoided and may be obviated by the use of shunts or bypass. Hypothermia, either systemic or regional, reduces renal oxygen requirements and metabolism and can protect the kidneys during ischemia. Pharmacologic interventions are varied and a matter of considerable debate. Mannitol may improve renal blood flow and glomerular filtration during ischemia and diminish the impact of reperfusion injuries through its capacity for oxygen free radical scavenging. Low-dose dopamine (3 mcg/kg/min) acts as a vasodilator on the renal vasculature to improve blood flow and exerts a natriuretic effect by inhibiting sodium transport. There is no evidence that dopamine decreases renal failure during ischemia. Other drugs that increase renal blood flow and natriuresis include furosemide, prostaglandin E1, and fenoldopam, a dopamine-1 selective agonist.

15. Describe sources of altered coagulation function in descending thoracic aortic surgery and outline methods of treatment.

The development of coagulopathies is common during thoracic aortic surgery, especially when extreme intraoperative blood loss and massive fluid resuscitation occurs. Patients may require replacement of several blood volumes during repair of descending thoracic aneurysms. Alterations in normal coagulation function can occur from hypothermia, heparinization, acidemia, as well as dilutional thrombocytopenia. Profound hypoperfusion may cause disseminated intravascular coagulation (DIC). Visceral ischemia may initiate fibrinolysis; liver ischemia may result in reduced production of coagulation factors. In addition to monitoring of the patient's hematocrit and hemoglobin, frequent assessment of the prothrombin time (PT), partial thromboplastin time (PTT), fibrinogen, and platelets is warranted during massive transfusions. Early administration of FFP and platelets may be effective in preventing severe derangements in coagulation. Cryoprecipitate may be necessary to correct coagulopathies that occur in the context of volume overload from massive fluid resuscitation. The use of antifibrinolytics, such as tranexamic acid, are associated with decreased perioperative bleeding during thoracic aortic surgery. Aprotinin, another fibrinolytic, is no longer used because of adverse renal, cardiac, and neurologic outcomes.

Postoperative Period

16. List the potential complications following thoracic aortic surgery.

Myocardial infarction
Respiratory failure
Renal failure
Bleeding
Paraplegia
Cerebrovascular accident

Spinal cord injury in the immediate postoperative period presents with paraparesis or flaccid paralysis. An anterior spinal artery syndrome may be present with a loss of motor function and pin-prick sensation but sparing of vibratory sensation and proprioception. The delayed onset of neurologic deficits is most likely caused by postoperative hypotension in patients with severe atherosclerotic disease.

17. Explain strategies for postoperative pain management in patients undergoing TAA.

The large incision required for descending thoracic aortic surgery creates significant postoperative pain. Both the thoracic and abdominal components of the incision require transection of major muscle groups. The posterolateral thoracotomy may entail removal of one or more ribs. Pleural chest tube sites are another source of patient pain and discomfort. The use of thoracic epidural analgesia following descending TAA repair is common but a matter of some controversy.

The potential benefits of pain relief and the reduction of pulmonary and cardiac morbidity must be weighed against the risks of hypotension and epidural hematoma formation after anticoagulation. Early recognition of an anterior spinal artery syndrome may be delayed by the use of neuraxial local anesthetics. Parenteral narcotics administered by intermittent bolus, continuous infusion, or patient-controlled analgesia may also be used for pain management, but must be titrated carefully to prevent excessive respiratory depression. Coughing and deep breathing are essential to avoid developing postoperative pneumonia which requires adequate analgesia.

18. Discuss emerging evidence for the advantages and disadvantages of endovascular techniques for repair of thoracic aneurysms.

EVAR has become an alternative to open techniques for the repair of aneurysms of the thoracic aorta. Endovascular stenting avoids the extensive surgical exposure required for an open repair and the protracted cross-clamping of the thoracic aorta. Preliminary data suggest that endovascular repairs have a lower incidence of neurologic complications in patients with descending TAAs and a significantly reduced perioperative mortality rate. A reduction in hospital and critical care stay may be an additional benefit of endovascular techniques. Endovascular stenting may be unsuitable for anatomically complex lesions and endograft longevity has not been fully established.

REVIEW QUESTIONS

1. The inability of a patient to tolerate the supine position during a preoperative evaluation before thoracic aortic surgery is suggestive of aneurysmal compression of the:
    a. stellate ganglia.
    b. superior vena cava.
    c. left mainstem bronchus.
    d. esophagus.
2. The anterior spinal artery is most commonly supplemented in thoracic region by which blood vessel?
    a. Vertebral artery
    b. Artery of Adamkiewicz
    c. Basilar artery
    d. Celiac artery
3. The preferred site for placement of an arterial cannula to monitor blood pressure in surgery on the descending thoracic aorta is the:
    a. right radial artery.
    b. left radial artery.
    c. left femoral artery.
    d. right femoral artery.
4. Evoked potential monitoring during surgery on the descending thoracic aorta would be least affected by:
    a. isoflurane.
    b. hypothermia.
    c. hypotension.
    d. fentanyl.
5. Spinal cord perfusion pressure (SCPP) is defined as the difference between the mean arterial blood pressure and which of the following measures?
    a. Central venous pressure
    b. Diastolic blood pressure
    c. Cerebrospinal fluid pressure
    d. Thoracic pleural pressure

REVIEW ANSWERS

1. **Answer: c**
    Compression of the conducting airways by a thoracic aneurysm may create a mediastinal mass effect and intolerance of the supine position. Such symptoms may have life-threatening consequences during induction of anesthesia. Careful evaluation and planning prior to surgery is imperative.
2. **Answer: b**
    The anterior spinal artery is most commonly supplemented in the thoracic region by the artery of Adamkiewicz, a greater radicular artery which supplies the majority of blood flow to the lower two-thirds of the anterior spinal cord.
3. **Answer: a**
    The right radial artery is the preferred because aortic cross-clamping is sometimes required proximal to the left subclavian artery during descending aortic repairs, making it impossible to use the left upper extremity for blood pressure monitoring.
4. **Answer: d**
    Hypotension, hypothermia, and volatile anesthetics all produce decreases in amplitude and increases in latency with evoked potential monitoring, potentially mimicking spinal ischemia. Narcotics, including fentanyl, have a minimal inhibitory effect on evoked potential monitoring.
5. **Answer: c**
    SCPP is defined as the difference between mean arterial pressure (MAP) and cerebrospinal fluid (CSF) pressure.

SUGGESTED READINGS

Gonzales M. Vascular disease. In: Hines RL, Marschall KE, eds. *Stoelting's Anesthesia and Coexisting disease*, 5th ed. Philadelphia: Churchill Livingstone, 2008: 135–160.

Kahn RA, Stone ME, Moskowitz DM. Anesthetic considerations for descending thoracic aortic aneurysm repair. *Semin Cardiovasc Vasc Anesth* 2007;11:205–223.

Makkad B, Pilling S. Management of thoracic aneurysm. *Semin Cardiovasc Vasc Anesth* 2005;9:227–240.

Moskowitz DM, Kahn RA, Reich DL. Anesthesia for the surgical treatment of thoracic aortic disease. In: Thys DM, Hillel Z, Schwartz AJ, eds. *Textbook of Cardiothoracic Anesthesiology*. New York: McGraw-Hill, 2001:680–710.

Norris EJ. Anesthesia for vascular surgery. In: Miller RD, ed. *Miller's Anesthesia*. Vol. 2. Philadelphia: Churchill Livingston, 2005:2051–2125.

O'Connor CJ, Rothenberg DM. Anesthetic considerations for descending thoracic aortic surgery: part I. *J Cardiothorac Vasc Anesth* 1995;9:581–588.

O'Connor CJ, Rothenberg DM. Anesthetic considerations for descending thoracic aortic surgery: part II. *J Cardiothorac Vasc Anesth* 1995;9:734–747.

Oliver WC, Nuttall G, Murray MJ. Thoracic aortic disease. In: Kaplan JA, ed. *Cardiac Anesthesia*, 4th ed. Philadelphia: WB Saunders, 1999:821–860.

Silvay G, Stone ME. Repair of thoracic aneurysms, with special emphasis on the preoperative work-up. *Semin Cardiovasc Vasc Anesth* 2006;10:11–15.

Walsh SR, Tang TY, Sadat U, et al. Endovascular stenting versus open surgery for thoracic aortic disease: systematic review and meta-analysis of perioperative results. *J Vasc Surg* 2008;47:1094–1098.e3.

Abdominal Aortic Aneurysm Repair

26

Rachel Polazzi

KEY POINTS

- Risk factors for developing an abdominal aortic aneurysm (AAA) include: male gender, increasing age, smoking, elevated plasma cholesterol levels, hypertension, and a family history of AAAs.
- A thorough preoperative evaluation is essential in this patient population due to the presence of multiple underlying comorbidities.
- Coronary artery disease is the single most significant risk factor that influences long-term outcomes and a definitive cardiac evaluation is vital prior to an elective repair.
- Surgical repair utilizing an open or endovascular technique remains the only definitive treatment.
- Hemodynamic changes from the application and removal of the abdominal aortic cross-clamp are one of the most challenging aspects of patient management for the anesthetist.
- Myocardial dysfunction is the single most likely cause of morbidity following vascular surgery.

CASE SYNOPSIS

A 65-year-old man presents for surgical repair of a 6-cm AAA. He is scheduled for an open abdominal repair procedure.

PREOPERATIVE EVALUATION AND DEMOGRAPHIC DATA

Past Medical/Surgical History

- 42 pack/year smoking history
- Hypertension
- Hypercholesteremia

List of Medications

- Lovastatin
- Atenolol
- Hydrochlorothiazide

Diagnostic Data

- Hemoglobin, 14 g/dl; hematocrit, 42%
- Glucose, 107 mg/dl
- Blood urea nitrogen, 10 mg/dl; creatinine, 0.8 mg/dl
- Electrolytes: sodium, 142 mEq/l; potassium, 3.6 mEq/l; chloride, 104 mEq/l; carbon dioxide, 26 mEq/l
- Coagulation studies: prothrombin time, 12 s; international normalized ratio, 1.0; partial thromboplastin time, 28 s

Height/Weight/Vital Signs

- 183 cm, 80 kg
- Blood pressure,142/84; heart rate, 61 beats per minute; respiratory rate, 18 breaths per minute; room air oxygen saturation, 98%; temperature, 36.8°C
- Electrocardiogram (ECG): normal sinus rhythm; heart rate, 61
- Cardiac Doppler ultrasound: mild left ventricular hypertrophy, estimated ejection fraction, 50%
- Chest x-ray: within normal limits

PATHOPHYSIOLOGY

The proposed pathophysiology associated with the development of an AAA is complex and multifaceted. AAA is defined as a weakening of the aortic wall which results in progressive dilatation that can eventually rupture. The most common site of an AAA is infrarenal (> 90%) as shown in Figure 26-1; however, the aneurysm may occur in a juxtarenal or suprarenal position. AAAs affect approximately 5% of elderly men and are estimated to account for about 2% of all deaths within the United States. However, it is believed that the incidence is an underestimation due to sudden death that is caused by cardiac disease as compared to an undiagnosed AAA. Even though the reason has not been elucidated, the incidence of AAA is increasing. Potential causes may include increased incidence of obesity and atherosclerosis or improved detection and diagnostic screening modalities. The pathophysiologic process associated with AAA remains unclear but it is believed that they develop from the combination of lipid deposition within that aortic adventitia. Cytokines and proteolytic enzymes degrade the elastin and collagen causing inflammation and atherosclerosis. This pathophysiologic process involved with the development and progression of AAA is present in Figure 26-2.

SURGICAL PROCEDURE

Surgical repair of a AAA is recommended once the aneurysm expands to > 5 cm in cross-section dimension, if the AAA is between 4.0 and 5.0 cm with expansion of > 0.5 cm within 6 months, if the patient

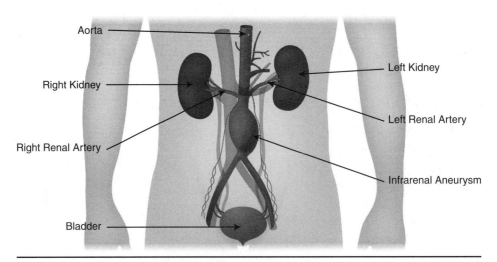

Figure 26-1 *Anatomic representation of infrarenal aneurysm.*

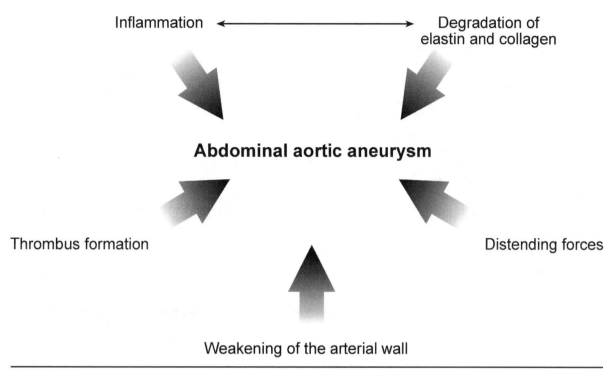

Figure 26-2 *Pathophysiologic process for development and progression of AAA.*

is exhibiting signs and symptoms associated with AAA, or if the aneurysm is dissecting or has ruptured. Traditionally, the procedure is done via open abdominal incision and the patient is placed in the supine position. The operation may also be performed via a retroperitoneal approach. Once the aorta is exposed, the aortic cross-clamp is applied above the aneurysm and the aneurysm is dissected and removed. A Dacron graft replaces the diseased portion of the aorta. It is sewn into the normal proximal and distal aorta.

Recent advances in endovascular procedures have now made AAA repair less invasive. An endograft is placed inside the lumen of the aorta at the level of the aneurysm. The deployment device is advanced via the femoral arteries. The position of the endograft is assessed under fluoroscopy prior to final placement. Since the surgeon does not have to cross-clamp the aorta, the dramatic cardiac and metabolic manifestations associated with this process does not occur. Endovascular aortic repair (EVAR) is associated with a decreased incidence of cardiovascular, pulmonary, and renal complications as compared to a traditional

open approach. However, there is no significant difference in the long term survivability when comparing these two surgical techniques to AAA repair. A complication that is specific to EVAR is known as endoleak. Blood from the proximal aorta leaks around the graft into the aneurysm sac and can cause aortic aneurysm rupture. There are several interventions that can be performed if this circumstance occurs such as placement of a graft extension, use of a coil or fibrin glue to seal the entrance to the aneurysm sac, or removal of the graft and direct aortic repair via an open approach. A comparison of these surgical techniques is represented in Figure 26-3.

ANESTHETIC MANAGEMENT AND CONSIDERATIONS

Preoperative Period

1. Discuss the risk factors associated with the development of an AAA.

The occurrence of AAAs is greater in men than women at an incidence of approximately 9:1. AAAs

Figure 26-3 *Comparison of an open versus EVAR technique for AAA repair.*

are more frequently diagnosed in men over the age of 55, and women at age 65. Ethnicity may play a role in the development of an AAA and this disease has been reported to be more common in whites than blacks. In patients that develop an AAA, 90% have a history of current or previous smoking. Smoking is the strongest independent risk factor for development of an AAA. Hypertension is present in 60% of patients with AAA and other risk factors are listed in Table 26-1.

2. Describe the components of a comprehensive preoperative evaluation for a patient with an AAA.

Three-fourths of patients are asymptomatic when they are diagnosed with an AAA. Typically, the diagnosis is made either on a radiologic exam or physical exam which reveals a pulsatile epigastric mass. Patients that do experience symptoms usually complain of vague abdominal pain, back pain, or rarely gastrointestinal or ureteral obstruction. Symptoms associated with a ruptured AAA include persistent, severe pain that radiates to the back and groin. Coronary artery disease (CAD) is present in 30–40% of patients who have AAA. Aortoiliac or peripheral arterial occlusive disease manifests as tissue ischemia such as claudication of the lower extremities.

For elective repair of an AAA, the most common imaging studies performed, ultrasound and computerized tomography (CT), reveal the location and size of the aneurysm. The size of the aortic aneurysm is the most important determining factor for rupture. Further imaging studies completed prior to elective repair includes chest radiograph and ECG. If a patient is identified as having symptomatic CAD, further cardiac evaluation is recommended. The most dependable diagnostic tool in determining the extent of CAD is coronary angiography. A thorough preoperative evaluation

Table 26-1	Pathophysiologic Conditions Associated with AAA

- Family history
- Coronary artery diseases
- History of myocardial infarction
- Hypertension
- Hyperlipidemia
- Peripheral vascular disease
- Obesity
- Smoking
- Chronic obstructive pulmonary disease
- History of stroke
- Renal insufficiency
- Gender (male > female)
- Elevated C-reactive protein

and an appreciation of the anticipated postoperative outcomes are essential when providing anesthetic care for patients with an AAA.

3. Differentiate between a suprarenal, juxtarenal, and infrarenal AAA and the associated anesthetic management concerns.

Approximately 90% of AAAs are infrarenal. Juxtarenal aneurysms are found at the level of the renal arteries, but do not extend into the orifice of the renal arteries. Suprarenal aneurysms are located above the renal arteries and may involve some of the visceral vessels. Thus, renal failure, though possible with aortic cross-clamping at any level, occurs more frequently with suprarenal aortic occlusion due to decreased renal perfusion. Anesthetic management aimed to counter this effect would include maintaining adequate intravascular volume, administration of osmotic diuretics prior to clamp application (mannitol), and a loop diuretic (Lasix). A low-dose dopamine infusion (2–5 mcg/kg/min) may also help to preserve renal perfusion. The most significant predictor of postoperative renal failure following AAA repair is determined by the presence or absence of preoperative renal impairment. Ultimately, the effects of aortic cross-clamping are similar for all types of abdominal aneurysms, but the cardiovascular and hemodynamic alterations are more dramatic as the clamp is placed more proximally.

4. Contrast the advantages and disadvantages of open AAA repair versus EVAR.

The first successful elective open repair of an AAA occurred in 1952. Since then, great advances have been made in improving outcomes and decreasing morbidity and mortality. However, the elective open repair is a highly invasive procedure that is costly to not only the patient's physical well-being, but also to the healthcare system. The average intensive care stay for a patient undergoing an open repair is 2.58 days and an overall hospital stay of 19 days. The physiologic stress that the patient must endure is immense. On average, a patient will lose 2000–5000 ml of blood. The list of potential adverse complications associated with the traditional AAA repair is present in Table 26-2. However, the durability of AAA repair is superior as compared to EVAR. In addition, patients must meet specific anatomic requirements such as the

Table 26-2	Potential Complications Associated with an Open AAA Repair

- Hemorrhage
- Myocardial ischemia/infarction
- Cerebral ischemia/infarction
- Thrombolization/embolization
- Mesenteric traction syndrome
- Organ ischemia
- Wound infection
- Renal failure
- Graft failure/thrombosis/infection
- Respiratory insufficiency
- Lower extremity ischemia

size and distance from the aneurysm to the renal arteries in order to be an acceptable candidate for the EVAR procedure.

In 1991, the introduction of EVAR for AAA repair has drastically changed the manner in which this disease can be surgically managed. It has been demonstrated that EVAR reduces the time spent in the intensive care unit to 0.33 days, hospital stays to 6 days, and blood loss to 200–500 ml. However, EVAR is also associated with unique complications such as endoleak, stent graft migration and collapse, and endograft limb occlusions. As a result, contrast-enhanced CT scans must be performed frequently in order to monitor the stent graft. Therefore, decreased renal function from graft migration and renal artery occlusion is a risk associated with EVAR.

5. Distinguish between the transperitoneal versus retroperitoneal approach for surgical repair of the AAA.

Most commonly, open repair of AAAs are carried out via the transperitoneal approach. This technique involves a large midabdominal incision with the patient in the supine position. The retroperitoneal approach involves the patient being in the right lateral decubitus position. The skin is then incised from the lateral edge of the left rectus muscle to the bottom of the 12th rib. The benefits of the retroperitoneal position include decreased postoperative ileus, reduced pulmonary complications, and minimized postoperative incision pain.

6. Identify the contraindications to elective repair of AAA.

For patients in which the aneurysm diameter measures less than 5 cm are medically managed as the benefit of repair is outweighed by the risks of the procedure.

Contradictions to elective repair of AAAs include recent myocardial infarction, pulmonary insufficiency/disorders, unstable angina pectoris, and chronic renal insufficiency.

7. Describe the nonsurgical management of AAA.

In patients in which repair of the AAA is contradicted or deferred, the nonsurgical management is similar to that of a patient with CAD. These interventions help to reduce the rate of aneurysm expansion. Modifiable lifestyle changes are among the most important treatment modalities. Smoking cessation is crucial as nicotine abuse is not only a factor in developing an AAA, but it also increases the expansion, risk for rupture, and worsens the prognosis of an AAA. Medically, research demonstrates that the control of hypercholesteremia with statin drugs, combined with angiotensin II inhibitors, macrolides, and anti-inflammatory agents reduce the production of proteolytic enzymes and cytokines. Treatment of hypertension and sodium restriction is also vital.

Intraoperative Period

8. Identify appropriate intraoperative anesthetic monitoring techniques for open repair of an AAA.

Appropriate intraoperative monitoring for patients undergoing AAA repair is crucial in order to detect changes in hemodynamic status. Cardiac morbidity is of the utmost concern during this procedure. ECG monitoring of leads II and V5 will detect approximately 80% of ischemic events. Arterial monitoring is essential for continuous assessment of the blood pressure, fluctuations in hemodynamics due to aortic cross-clamping, and access for blood sampling. Central line placement and central venous pressure assessment can help guide fluid resuscitation. Due to the wide fluctuations in systemic vascular resistance that result from the aortic cross-clamp, pulmonary artery catheters may also utilized to monitor left-heart filling pressures. Transesophageal echocardiography (TEE) can also be used to monitor cardiac function.

9. List other pharmacologic agents that are utilized during anesthetic management of AAA.

Heparin 100 U/kg is administered approximately 5 min before the application of the cross-clamp in order to inhibit thrombus formation. If the clamp time is prolonged, additional doses may be needed. After the clamp is removed, protamine can be given to inhibit the anticoagulant effects of heparin. Protamine should not be administered faster than 50 mg/min in order to avoid hypotension.

10. Discuss acceptable anesthetic techniques for induction and maintenance for this patient.

It is most important when formulating an anesthetic plan to tailor the plan individually to each patient. However, most patients presenting for abdominal aortic reconstruction are elderly with coexisting morbidities. Titration is essential because not every patient will require the same amount of medications. Premedication is used if the patient is hemodynamically stable. An epidural catheter placed before induction can provide adequate analgesia during the intra- and postoperative periods. It also allows for a combined epidural and general technique which lowers the level of volatile agents consumed, decreases spinal cord sensitization, and causes vasodilation which decreases the blood pressure during aortic cross-clamping. The disadvantage of infusing local anesthesia into the epidural catheter during the intraoperative period is that if severe hypotension occurs from hemorrhage or myocardial dysfunction, then treating the hypotension may be more difficult. Also, concerns regarding the development of an epidural hematoma are warranted due to systemic anticoagulation.

Induction should be carried out in a manner in which the patient's hemodynamics remain as close to baseline as possible. Hypertension and tachycardia should be avoided. For maintenance of general anesthesia, patients who have a poor myocardial performance may develop hypotension when exposed to moderate or severe myocardial depression caused effects by inhalation agents. In this instance, it may be prudent to administer lower concentrations of inhalation agents ($\leq$ 1 MAC) and greater amounts of narcotics. Overall, constant vigilance combined with accurate interpretations and interventions are the keys to a successful anesthetic regardless of the anesthetic technique that is employed.

11. Describe the hemodynamic changes that occur with the application and removal of the aortic cross-clamp.

The initial response to aortic cross-clamp application is arterial hypertension that results from an increased systemic vascular resistance and increased impedance to aortic flow. In the majority of patients who undergo aortic reconstruction, the cross-clamp is placed below the level of the renal arteries due to the high prevalence of infrarenal aneurysms. The organs above the clamp experience a redistribution of blood volume, and blood flow to the pelvis and lower extremities will cease. With infrarenal cross-clamping, the arterial blood pressure can increase 7–10% above the clamp. In general, patients with normal cardiac reserve can tolerate this increase. However, in patients with significant cardiac dysfunction, even the slightest change in pressure will precipitate heart failure and ischemia. Table 26-3 outlines the hemodynamic changes that occur in response to aortic cross-clamp application.

Table 26-3   Hemodynamic Changes That Occur in Response to Aortic Cross-clamping

CARDIOVASCULAR VARIABLE	RESPONSE TO AORTIC CROSS-CLAMP
Mean arterial pressure	Increases
Systemic vascular resistance	Increases
Cardiac output	No change or decreases
Pulmonary artery occlusion pressure	Increases

The removal of the aortic cross-clamp is not a benign process and constant communication between the surgeon and anesthetist is vitally important. The clamp should be removed incrementally in order to avoid drastic reductions in blood pressure due to the abrupt decrease in systemic vascular resistance combined with the release of metabolites such as lactate which is created due to reperfusion of the ischemic lower extremities. Adequate fluid administration combined with vasoconstrictors generally offsets this response.

These metabolites cause vasodilation and myocardial depression. Hypotension can be treated with by infusing a fluid bolus, decreasing the depth of anesthesia, and administering medications that cause vasoconstriction such as phenylephrine or norepinephrine. The surgeon should also reclamp the aorta as needed in case of severe and persistent hypotension. Interestingly, patients who have occlusive disease develop collateral circulation which can continue to perfuse the patient's lower extremities during cross-clamping. Thus, these patients may experience less dramatic hemodynamic changes during the procedure.

12. Discuss appropriate pharmacologic responses to the changes in hemodynamic parameters that occur during AAA repair.

The appropriate pharmacologic therapies utilized in the management of the patient undergoing aortic aneurysm reconstruction require a comprehensive understanding by the anesthetist. In anticipation of the application of the aortic cross-clamp, the anesthetist should have the patient at a deep level of anesthesia. Once the clamp is applied, the main goal is to decrease afterload with arterial dilators (nitroprusside) and to maintain preload with venodilators (nitroglycerin). There is increased incidence of acute renal dysfunction when the mean arterial pressure is < 60 mm Hg for longer than 15 minutes.

Postoperative Period

The total resection time for this surgery was 270 minutes. In the postanesthesia care unit, the patient exhibits the following acute symptoms: restlessness, pain, shivering, blood pressure of 178/86, respiratory rate 28, sinus tachycardia rate 102, oxygen saturation 98%, temperature 35.4°C, lungs clear to auscultation, and decreased urine output.

13. Examine the patient's vital signs; what would be an appropriate treatment?

Administration of a fluid bolus would be appropriate at this time. Aggressive volume administration to allow for third-space loss in the first 12 hours postoperatively is recommended. However, in the patient with limited cardiac reserve, careful fluid resuscitation is warranted in order to prevent heart failure. Shivering dramatically increases myocardial oxygen consumption and meperidine (Demerol) can be administered to decrease this response. If the patient has an epidural catheter in place, a test dose may be given to assess proper placement, then local anesthesia can be administered in order to provide pain relief. Blood should be drawn to assess the hemoglobin value, electrolyte and coagulation status, and an arterial blood gas to determine the adequacy of ventilation

14. Identify the potential postoperative complications following AAA repair.

The mortality rate for an elective repair of an AAA is approximately 2–5%, for emergent repair this rate dramatically increases to 50%. There are multiple complications that can occur postoperatively. These complication rates are increased parallel to the number of comorbidities that may already exist in each patient. The most common postoperative morbidity is myocardial infarction with a reported rate of 10–15%. Continuous cardiac monitoring is recommended for at least 48 hours after surgery to monitor for ischemic events. Respiratory and renal complications may also occur postoperatively.

Adequate pain relief should be ensured, but not at the expense of adequate ventilation. Postoperative atelectasis commonly leads to pneumonia in this patient population. Urine output should be maintained at 1 ml/kg/hr. The administration of fluid and diuretics may be necessary. Other less common complications include bleeding, leg ischemia, and stroke.

15. Discuss the development and treatment associated with acute renal insufficiency.

Reports of acute renal injury in patients undergoing abdominal aneurysm repair vary with estimates between 2–22%. Most patients that experience acute renal dysfunction have preoperative elevated plasma creatinine levels. Intrarenal aortic cross-clamp placement can decrease renal blood flow by as much as 40%. Also, in response to the cross-clamp, it is believed that the kidneys respond by activating the renin–angiotensin system. These combined factors can exacerbate renal insufficiency postoperatively. Fortunately, the reported incidence of renal failure requiring dialysis postoperatively is 0.6%. Mannitol is frequently given 20 to 30 minutes prior to the application of the cross-clamp in order to preserve renal function. However, adequate fluid replacement is the best prophylaxis for avoiding acute renal failure.

Furosemide (Lasix), a loop diuretic, may be given postoperatively, but an adequate fluid and electrolyte status must be maintained. Low-dose dopamine (1–3 mcg/kg/min) may be instituted in order to increase renal blood flow and glomerular filtration rate. However, research has provided limited concrete evidence that these interventions prevent acute renal failure.

16. Discuss the anesthetic management of a ruptured AAA.

Ruptured abdominal aneurysms are associated with a mortality rate as high as 94% and is the 10th leading cause of mortality in White men over the age of 65. Patients typically present with abdominal discomfort, pulsatile abdominal mass, decreased distal pulses, back pain, and hypotension.

A patient who has a ruptured AAA is taken to the operating room for immediate surgical exploration. A brief preoperative exam is conducted and venous access as well as arterial line and central line placement are rapidly accomplished. Etomidate is the drug of choice for induction for these patients. Fluid resuscitation should be carried out with crystalloid and colloid solutions until blood and blood products are available. The patient's hemodynamic response to the application and removal of the aortic cross-clamp is frequently more extreme. Postoperative mechanical ventilation postoperatively due to the large volumes of fluid and blood replacement required throughout the procedure.

Endovascular grafting techniques have been used to treat dissecting and ruptured AAAs. The use of EVAR to treat ruptured aortic aneurysms is being studied and is still under investigation; however, the initial results appear to be promising.

REVIEW QUESTIONS

1. Which independent risk factor is most highly correlated with the development of an AAA?
   a. Hypertension
   b. Smoking
   c. Coronary artery disease
   d. Diabetes

2. Which is the initial hemodynamic consequence that occurs in response to application of the aortic cross-clamp?
   a. Hypotension
   b. Hypertension
   c. Increased cardiac output
   d. Decreased pulmonary artery occlusion pressure

3. Which statement best describes reactive hyperemia?
   a. Elevation in body temperature
   b. Chemical reaction involving the kidneys
   c. Transient vasodilation secondary to the restoration of blood flow to ischemic tissue
   d. Muscle spasms that occur in response to application of aortic cross-clamp

4. Which postoperative complication is associated with the highest morbidity rate after AAA repair?
   a. Renal failure
   b. Graft rupture
   c. Myocardial infarction
   d. Deep vein thrombosis
5. Which is an advantage to the EVAR as compared to the open approach for AAA repair?
   a. Absence of aortic cross clamping
   b. Increased postoperative pain
   c. Potential for endoleak
   d. Higher incidence of renal insufficiency

REVIEW ANSWERS

1. **Answer: b**
   Smoking is the single most independent risk factor for the development of AAA. It has been reported that 90% of all AAA patients have a history of nicotine abuse.
2. **Answer: b**
   The initial response to aortic cross-clamping is arterial hypertension. Sodium nitroprusside, an arterial vasodilator, is the pharmacologic agent of choice. The anesthetist may also deepen the anesthetic agents to aid in decreasing the blood pressure.
3. **Answer: c**
   Reactive hyperemia causes a transient decrease in blood pressure that results from the restoration of blood flow to ischemic tissues.
4. **Answer: c**
   Myocardial infarction accounts for the highest postoperative morbidity in patients undergoing abdominal aortic aneurysm repair.

5. **Answer: a**
   One major advantage associated with EVAR as compared to an open approach to AAA repair is that it is unnecessary to apply an aortic cross clamp.

SUGGESTED READINGS

Elisha S. Vascular surgery. In: Nagelhout JJ, Plaus KL, eds. *Nurse Anesthesia*, 4th ed. St. Louis, MO: Elsevier Saunders, 2009:528–546.

Golledge J, Muller J, Daugherty A, et al. Abdominal aortic aneurysm: pathogenesis and implications for management. *Arterioscler Thromb Vasc Biol* 2006;26:2605–2613.

Guessous I, Periard D, Lorenzetti, D, et al. The efficacy of pharmacotherapy for decreasing the expansion rate of abdominal aortic aneurysms: a systematic review and meta-analysis. *Plos ONE* 2008;3(3):1–10.

Lederle FA. Screening for AAA in the USA. *Scand J Surg* 2008;97:139–141.

Lovegrove RE, Javid M, Magee TR, et al. A meta-analysis of 21178 patients undergoing open or endovascular repair of abdominal aortic aneurysm. *Brit J Surg* 2008;95:677–684.

Powell JT. Non-operative or medical management of abdominal aortic aneurysm. *Scand J Surg* 2008;97:121–124.

Sadat U, Boyle JR, Walsh SR, et al. Endovascular vs open repair of acute abdominal aortic aneurysms—A systematic review and meta-analysis. *J Vasc Surg* 2008;48:227–236.

Tallgren M, Niemi T, Poyhia R, et al. Acute renal injury and dysfunction following elective abdominal aortic surgery. *Eur J Vasc Endovasc Surg* 2007;33:550–555.

Wozniak MF, LaMuraglia GM, Musch G. Anesthesia for open abdominal aortic surgery. *Int Anesthesiol Clin* 2005;43:61–78.

Zankl AR, Schumacher H, Krumsdorf U, et al. Pathology, natural history and treatment of abdominal aortic aneurysms. *Clin Res Cardiol* 2007;96:140–151.

Cardiac Surgery

VIII

Minimally Invasive Coronary Artery Bypass Graft

27

Gayne Brenneman

KEY POINTS

- Extracardiac procedures, such as coronary artery bypass grafting (CABG), are often performed while the heart is beating.
- Intracardiac CABG is accomplished while using cardiopulmonary bypass.
- The surgery is performed via a minithoracotomy or a ministernotomy.
- Thoracoscopic video-assisted surgery, often with robotic assistance, necessitates prolonged one-lung ventilation to optimize exposure.
- Adequate flow during cardiopulmonary bypass may increase the risk of air emboli.
- Limited exposure of the heart during surgery poses surgical and anesthetic challenges which include arrhythmias, hemostasis, myocardial protection, and de-airing at the end of surgery.
- Patient selection is important to avoid intraoperative and postoperative complications. Prolonged one-lung ventilation, incomplete revascularization in hybrid procedures, and limited access for rapid intervention pose challenges with patient management.
- Conversion to sternotomy that may be required and extension of the laparoscopic portals extended over several dermatome segments mandate the need for postoperative analgesia.

CASE SYNOPSIS

A 53-year-old man with diabetes with new onset chest pain underwent cardiac catheterization, following a positive cardiac stress test study. He is scheduled for a minimally invasive direct CABG (MIDCABG).

Past Medical/Surgical History

- Hypertension
- Obesity
- Diabetes
- Hyperlipidemia

- Peripheral neuropathy
- Anterior cruciate ligament reconstruction on right knee; no anesthetic complications

List of medications

- Atenolol
- Simvastatin
- Insulin regular
- Aspirin
- Lisinopril

Laboratory and Diagnostic Data

- Chest x-ray: cardiomegaly is stable; prominent pulmonary vasculature centrally without interstitial edema
- Electrocardiogram (ECG): normal sinus rhythm with first degree AV block; heart rate, 74 beats per minute; possible left arterial enlargement (LAE)
- Cardiac catheterization: proximal left anterior descending artery occlusion; mild proximal occlusion of the circumflex artery; proximal right coronary artery occlusion; ejection fraction 65%; biatrial enlargement is present; right ventricle, left ventricle, and aortic root are of normal size; the tricuspid and mitral are of normal appearance; right ventricular systolic function is normal
- Adenosine myocardial perfusion study: overall, moderately abnormal myocardial perfusion study; consistent with prior infarct involving the inferior wall with moderate peri-infarct ischemia; consistent with mild stress induced myocardial ischemia involving the mid-to-distal anterior/anterolateral wall.
- Hemoglobin, 14.7 g/dl; hematocrit, 41.5%; white blood cells, 5.8 mm³; platelets, 176/mm³; hemoglobin A1C, 6.0%
- Cholesterol, 141 mg/dl; high-density lipoproteins, 34 mg/dl; triglycerides, 143 mg/dl; ALT 30 U/ml.
- Blood urea nitrogen (BUN), 14 mg/dl; creatinine, 0.9 mg/dl

- Electrolytes: sodium, 139 mEq/l; potassium, 3.8 mEq/l; serum bicarbonate, 24 mEq/l; chloride, 103 mEq/l; international normalized ratio, 1.1
- Glucose, 121 mg/dl; fasting glucose, 105 mg/dl

Height/Weight/Vital Signs

- 183 cm, 152.862 kg
- Blood pressure, 176/68; heart rate, 68 beats per minute; respiratory rate, 18 breaths per minute; room air oxygen saturation, 99%; temperature, 97.9°F
- Tobacco use, never; alcohol use, never

PATHOPHYSIOLOGY

Coronary artery disease (CAD) is the narrowing of the coronary arteries (the blood vessels that supply oxygen and nutrients to the heart muscle), caused by accumulation of fatty material within the walls of the arteries. This buildup causes the inside of the arteries to become rough and narrowed, limiting the supply of oxygen-rich blood to the heart muscle as is shown in Figure 27-1.

One method used to treat the blocked or narrowed coronary arteries is to bypass the blocked portion of the coronary artery with another piece of blood vessel. Blood vessels, or grafts, used for

Figure 27-1   *Endovascular pathologic changes associated with atherosclerosis.*

the bypass procedure may be pieces of a vein taken from the legs or an artery in the chest. One end of the graft is attached above the blockage and the other end is attached below the blockage. Thus, the blood is rerouted around, or bypasses, the blockage through the new graft to reach the heart muscle. This bypass of the blocked coronary artery can be done by performing CABG surgery.

Traditionally, in order to bypass the blocked coronary artery in this manner, the chest is opened in the operating room and the heart is stopped so that the surgeon can perform the bypass. In order to open the chest, the breastbone (sternum) is cut in half and spread apart. Once the heart is exposed, tubes are inserted into the heart so that the blood can be pumped through the body during the surgery by a cardiopulmonary bypass machine (heart–lung machine). The bypass machine is necessary to pump blood while the heart is stopped and kept still in order for the surgeon to perform the bypass operation.

While the traditional "open heart" procedure is still performed and often preferred in many situations, newer, less invasive techniques have been developed to bypass blocked coronary arteries. "Off-pump" procedures, in which the heart does not have to be stopped, were developed in the 1990s. Other minimally invasive procedures, such as keyhole surgery (performed through very small incisions) and robotic procedures (performed with the aid of a moving mechanical device), are also in development.

SURGICAL PROCEDURE

Minimally invasive direct coronary artery bypass graft (MIDCABG) surgery is an option for patients who require a left internal mammary artery bypass graft to the left anterior descending artery. A small, 2- to 3-in incision is made in the chest wall between the ribs, whereas the incision made during traditional CABG surgery is about 6 to 8 in long and is made down the center of the sternum (breastbone). Keyhole approaches

or port-access techniques are also available for some types of surgery.

The patient is intubated with a double-lumen endotracheal tube and transesophageal echo-cardiography is used to position coronary sinus cardioplegia and pulmonary artery vent catheters. This procedure can be performed either without cardiopulmonary bypass while the heart remains beating or with cardiopulmonary bypass. After the patient has been positioned in the supine position with the right side of the chest elevated, the femoral vessels are exposed. The right lung is then deflated and the endoscope of the da Vinci Robotic Surgical System is inserted through a 12-mm port placed in the fourth or fifth intercostal space at or just medial to the right anterior axillary line. The 30 degrees up endoscope with the "wide angle" da Vinci camera is moved manually to confirm access to the mediastinum. The handle of the atrial septal retractor is then inserted through a 16 French (F) introducer set in the same intercostal space as the endoscope just lateral to the right internal thoracic artery. The endoscope is removed and a 37-mm service port incision is made in the same intercostal space 20 to 30 mm lateral to the endoscope port. With the surgeon's finger in this service port to protect intrathoracic structures, trocars for the robotic instrument arms, 14-gauge angiocatheters for traction sutures and infusion of carbon dioxide, and a 20 F DLP cardiac sump for left atrial suction are inserted as shown in Figure 27-2. Heparin is administered and the femoral vessels are cannulated for port access. A 20-mm flexible port is temporarily placed in the service port incision.

Cardiopulmonary bypass is initiated, endoaortic balloon occlusion is achieved, and cardioplegic solution is administered. All knot tying is performed extracorporeally by the assistant using a shafted knot pusher. Approaching the mediastinum from the more lateral chest allows more working space for peri-cardiotomy and placement of traction sutures

Figure 27-2   *Position of instruments used for MIDCABG.*

before initiating cardiopulmonary bypass. Since the surgical approach is endoscopic, the surgical field can be enhanced by pressurizing the right pleural space by insufflation of carbon dioxide. This technique also has the advantage of creating high carbon dioxide levels in the left cardiac chambers, potentially reducing the risk of air embolism. Cutting and suturing can be performed by the console surgeon, who has three-dimensional vision and intracorporeal robotic wrists, while suctioning of blood, retraction, and suture retrieval can be simultaneously performed by the patient-side assistant. This technique uses retrograde femoral artery perfusion and is contraindicated for *patients with advanced atherosclerosis or marked tortuosity of the aorta.*

In order to avoid a median sternotomy scar, an arterial inflow cannula is placed in a femoral artery and the venous outflow cannula is placed through a femoral vein. A catheter with a balloon is advanced up the aorta and the balloon is inflated in the ascending aortic arch. Cardioplegia is then delivered antegrade to the coronary arteries which have been separated from the systemic circulation by the ascending aortic arch balloon.

A catheter is advanced from the internal jugular vein into the pulmonary artery for venting the left ventricle. The patient is placed on fem-fem bypass and cardioplegia established. A single vessel CABG is then performed either through a minithoracotomy or thoracoscopically. One of the major morbidities associated with traditional CABG surgery is postoperative neuropsychiatric disorders and strokes caused by extracorporeal circulation.

A minithoracotomy without using bypass can be accomplished by stabilizing the heart by placing latex sutures under the left anterior descending (LAD) artery proximal and distal to the site of the anastomosis. Blood flow is stopped in the target vessel by the stabilizing sutures. The technique requires improved technical skill on the part of the surgeon in that the heart is moving (contraction as well as movement of the chest wall during ventilation). It also requires increased technical skill on the part of the anesthetist because an area of the myocardium is ischemic, nonfunctional, and prone to reperfusion arrhythmias. The advantage of the operation includes reduced cost (no extracorporeal circulation, reduced hospitalization time) and reduced risk of stroke (no extracorporeal circulation).

ANESTHESTIC MANAGEMENT AND CONSIDERATIONS

Preoperative Period

1. Identify the major obstacles that are experienced during anesthetic management for minimally invasive CABG.

- Preservation of ventricular function and systemic perfusion
- Detection and treatment of myocardial ischemia
- Prevention of hypothermia in coronary artery bypass grafting on the beating heart
- Intermittent selective ventilation of the collapsed lung using continuous positive airway pressure (CPAP) in case of limited thoracotomy (to prevent hypoxemia)

Table 27-1 Type and Frequency of Comorbidities Associated with CAD	
• Hypertension	75.1%
• ≥ 65 years of age	57.1%
• Obesity	66.2%
• Smoker	25.1%
• Diabetes mellitus	24.7%
• Coronary artery disease	28.8%
• Chronic kidney disease	25.3%
• Congestive heart failure	16.5%
• Peripheral arterial disease	10.9%

2. Discuss the type and frequency of comorbidities associated with coronary artery disease.
See Table 27-1.

3. Identify the cardiovascular risk associated with diabetes.
Cardiovascular disease is the primary cause of morbidity and mortality among patients with diabetes. Although microvascular pathologies, including retinopathy and nephropathy, have been shown to be strongly associated with glycemic control, macrovascular complications, including heart disease and cerebrovascular disease, appear to be less responsive to glycemic control. Strategies to reduce the risks associated with diabetes are focused on controlling other risk factors such as hypertension, hyperlipidemia, smoking, and obesity.

It is estimated that over three quarters of diabetic patients are diagnosed with hypertension. Patients with type 2 diabetes develop subclinical left ventricular dysfunction characterized by reduced myocardial functional reserve. This influence becomes quantitatively more pronounced in the presence of coexistent CAD and hypertension. The coexistence of type 2 diabetes and hypertension appears to have additive negative effects on both systolic and diastolic left ventricular function, even in the absence of CAD.

Table 27-2 Comorbidities Associated with Obesity

- Cancer (kidney, colorectal, prostate, ovarian, uterine/endometrial, esophageal, pancreatic, and breast)
- Type 2 diabetes
- Cardiovascular disease (hypertension, coronary artery disease, congestive heart failure, pulmonary embolism, stroke, dyslipidemia)
- Gallbladder disease
- Chronic back pain
- Osteoarthritis
- Asthma
- Obstructive sleep apnea

4. Identify the comorbidities that are associated with obesity.

There are numerous comorbidities associated with obesity that present specific anesthetic challenges and these factors are listed in Table 27-2.

5. Discuss how gender, race, and age affect cardiovascular health.

Increasing age is positively associated with all cardiovascular comorbidities. Male sex is associated with a higher incidence and prevalence of all comorbidities except hypertension. Disparities associated with race/ethnicity vary categorically. Non-Hispanic whites have lower rates of hypertension than African Americans but higher rates of heart disease, especially myocardial infarctions. Asians and Hispanics had more favorable outcomes on several measures.

6. Discuss the link between hypertension and concentric left ventricular hypertrophy in this patient.

Compared with normotensive participants, prehypertensive and hypertensive participants have hypertrophic interventricular septal and left ventricular (LV) wall thickness. The LV internal dimension and relative wall thickness are increased and

as a result, LV mass was greater in patients with prehypertension and hypertension. The prevalence of LV hypertrophy was twofold higher in the prehypertensive group and threefold higher in the hypertensive group compared with the normotensive group. Concentric LV hypertrophy, which was rare in this age population, showed a slightly higher prevalence in the prehypertensive and hypertensive groups, but the prevalence of eccentric LV hypertrophy was two- and threefold higher in the prehypertensive and hypertensive groups, respectively.

7. Explain the mechanism of action and the side effects associated with this patient's medication regimen.

Atenolol (Tenormin) can be used to treat cardiovascular diseases and conditions such as *hypertension, CAD, arrhythmias, angina*, and reduces the risk of heart complications following myocardial infarction. Beta-blocking medications have cardioprotective properties because they increase myocardial oxygen supply by decreasing heart rate which increases diastolic filling time and decreases demand by inhibiting heart rate, contractility, and cardiac conduction. Atenolol is a β_1-selective (cardioselective) drug that exerts greater inhibitory effect on myocardial β_1-adrenergic-receptors as compared to β_2-adrenergic receptors which among other places in the body are located in the lungs. The β_2-adrenergic receptor inhibition can result in bronchospasm and for this reason caution should be exerted if atenolol is administered to patients with asthma. Unlike most other β-blockers, atenolol is excreted almost exclusively by the kidneys.

Simvastatin decreases lipid concentrations and this medication can decrease low density lipoprotein (LDL) levels by up to 50%. It has become apparent that simvastatin and other statin medications inhibit the progression of atherosclerosis beyond their effects on LDL. Many explanations have been proposed such as an inhibitory effect on macrophages that are present within the athero-sclerotic plaque lesions. All statins act by inhibiting 3-hydroxy-3-methylglutaryl coenzyme A (HMG-CoA) reductase, the rate-limiting enzyme of the HMG-CoA reductase pathway. This metabolic pathway is responsible for the endogenous production of cho-lesterol. However, statins reduce cardiovascular dis-ease events and total mortality irrespective of the initial cholesterol concentration. A rare but serious side effect associated with simvastatin is rhabdomy-olysis and this complication is enhanced if amioda-rone is concomitantly administered. Common side effects ($>1\%$ incidence) may include abdominal pain, diarrhea, indigestion, and a general feeling of weakness. Rare side effects include joint pain, memory loss, and muscle cramps.

Insulin is a hormone that has extensive effects on metabolism and other body functions, such as vascular compliance. Insulin causes cells in the liver, muscle, and fat tissue to absorb glucose from the blood and storing it as glycogen in the liver and muscle. When insulin is absent (or low), glucose is not transported into body cells, and the body begins to use fat as an energy source, for example, by transfer of lipids from adipose tissue to the liver for mobilization as an energy source. Patients with type 1 diabetes mellitus depend on external insulin (most commonly injected sub-cutaneously) to survive because the hormone is no longer produced by the islets of Langerhans within the pancreas. Patients with type 2 diabetes mellitus are insulin resistant, and because of such resistance, may suffer from a *relative* insulin defi-ciency. Some patients with type 2 diabetes may eventually require insulin when other medications fail to control blood glucose levels adequately.

Aspirin (acetylsalicylic acid) is a salicylate drug, often used as an analgesic to relieve minor aches and pains, as an antipyretic to reduce fever, and as an anti-inflammatory medication. Additionally, aspirin causes anticoagulation due to the drug's antiplatelet effects by inhibiting thromboxane and decreasing prostaglandin synthesis. As a result, aspirin is admin-istered for long periods, in low dosages to prevent heart attacks, strokes, and thromboembolism. Low-dose aspirin may be given immediately after myo-cardial infarction to reduce the risk of another heart attack or of the death of cardiac tissue. The main side effects associated with aspirin are gastrointesti-nal ulcers, stomach bleeding, and tinnitus, which is more likely to occur is high dosages are given.

Lisinopril is an angiotensin converting enzyme (ACE) inhibitor that is primarily used in treatment of hypertension, congestive heart failure, heart attacks, and also in preventing renal and retinal complications associated with diabetes. This drug has a long half-life that allows for once a day dosing which aids patient compliance. Lisinopril causes the kidneys to reabsorb potassium, which may lead to hyperkalemia. A severe and rare allergic reaction can occur that rarely can affect the inter-nal lumen of the bowel causing abdominal pain.

8. Explain the presence of cardiomegaly on this patient's chest x-ray and the association with obesity.

The cardiomyopathy associated with morbid obe-sity is characterized by:

- cardiomegaly
- LV dilatation
- myocyte hypertrophy without interstitial fibrosis

Cardiomyopathy is the most common cause of sudden cardiac death in these patients. Dilated car-diomyopathy is the most frequent cause of sudden cardiac death, followed by severe coronary athero-sclerosis, concentric LV hypertrophy without LV dilatation, pulmonary embolism, and hypoplastic coronary arteries.

9. Explain why an adenosine perfusion study was chosen instead of a stress treadmill in order to assess his cardiac function.

The dobutamine stress echocardiography has been the gold standard for myocardial stress procedures. Now with the use of tissue velocity echocardiography

(TVE), is associated with superior quantification of the longitudinal LV wall motion with improved sensitivity and specificity to diagnose CAD is possible. There has been continued interest in this technique for assessing subclinical myocardial systolic and diastolic function for patients who have diabetes, hypertension, and chronic kidney disease.

Intraoperative Period

10. Why was a MIDCABG procedure chosen in this particular case?
A MIDCABG approach is easier on the patient and is probably less expensive as compared to the traditional CABG. Exposure to the heart is limited and completion of the coronary artery anastomosis is more difficult. Significant myocardial ischemia leading to hemodynamic compromise may occur.

11. Discuss the concerns regarding gastroesophageal reflux disease and transesophageal echocardiography.
Gastroesophageal reflux disease (GERD), which is defined as acid regurgitation that occurs more often than twice per week, can cause inflammation of the esophagus. This condition can also exacerbate asthma, chronic cough, insomnia, and pulmonary fibrosis. If left untreated, GERD is considered a relative contraindication to the use of transesophageal echocardiography, since the probe is inserted into the esophagus. There is a risk of esophageal perforation, which can lead to leakage of acids from the esophagus into the chest, sepsis, and death.

12. Is the need for a three-vessel bypass a contraindication to performing MIDCABG?
A three-vessel bypass can be performed using a MIDCABG technique. However, aortic atherosclerotic disease is a definite contraindication for this operation. An arterial inflow cannula is placed in a femoral artery and the venous outflow is placed through a femoral vein. A catheter with a balloon is advanced up the aorta and the balloon inflated in the ascending aortic arch. Therefore, *aortic*

Table 27-3　Advantages of a Thoracic Epidural for MIDCABG

- Inhibition of sympathetic nervous system hyperactivity
- Cardiac sympathectomy
- Inhibition of inflammatory mediator release
- Postoperative analgesia without causing respiratory or gastrointestinal depression
- Improved respiratory function

atherosclerotic disease is an absolute contraindication for this operation.

13. Discuss the anesthetic intervention for cardiac fibrillation.
External defibrillation pads should be placed and sterile paddles should be available in the operating room. Prophylactic medications for arrhythmias include: magnesium 1 g mixed with lidocaine 100 mg. The medication should be infused at 2 mg/min. Amiodarone can also be used to treat cardiac fibrillation.

14. Describe the advantages for placing a thoracic epidural as an adjunct to general anesthesia.
See Table 27-3.

15. Explain the major advantages associated with avoiding cardiopulmonary bypass.
Patients who undergo MIDCABG have a significant reduction in the systemic inflammatory response, postoperative morbidity, and hospital stay compared with patients who undergo conventional CABG with cardiopulmonary bypass.

16. Explain the major advantages and disadvantages associated with MIDCABG.
The advantages associated with minimally invasive cardiac surgery include:
- Reduced surgical trauma
- Decreased morbidity
- Lower procedural costs

- Increased patient satisfaction
- Decreased infusion of blood and blood products
- If cardiopulmonary bypass is not used, the absence of complications associated with extracorporeal circulation
- Shortened hospitalization ad return to activities of daily living

The disadvantages associated with minimally invasive cardiac surgery include:

- Technically challenging
- Increased risk of graft occlusion
- Limited to vessels on the anterior aspect of the heart
- Inability for vessel bypass on the posterior aspect of the heart
- Learning curve prior to proficiency

Postoperative Period

17. List the most significant postoperative complications for a patient with diabetes and obesity following median sternotomy.

- Wound infection
- Pain control
- Prolonged intubation
- Prolonged hospitalization period

18. List emerging innovative surgical methods for performing CABG.

The technological advancements improve the equipment and the operating conditions that are used for MIDCABG. However, the physical limitations by which access to the heart is minimized remains problematic. One of the first problems to address is to formulate an intervention if and when ventricular fibrillation occurs. If the surgical plan consists of a small thoracotomy, what will occur when ischemia caused by the stabilizing sutures or reperfusion arrhythmias caused by releasing the sutures progresses to ventricular fibrillation?

If the surgical and anesthesia teams can continue to develop strategies to overcome the technical challenges (motion, bleeding, arrhythmias, hemodynamic variability, decreased cardiac exposure),

this technique could continue to emerge as a viable option for patients who need coronary artery revascularization.

REVIEW QUESTIONS

1. Which is an advantage of minimally invasive cardiac surgery for CABG?
   a. Larger surgical incision
   b. Increased postoperative pain
   c. Improved wound healing
   d. Higher incidence of cerebrovascular accident
2. Which factor increases the risk of cardiovascular disease?
   a. Diabetes
   b. Osteoarthritis
   c. Gastroesophageal reflux disease
   d. Asthma
3. Which condition is an absolute contraindication for having a MIDCABG?
   a. Ejection fraction of 42%
   b. Triple vessel disease
   c. Aortic atherosclerotic disease
   d. History of myocardial infarction
4. Which condition disqualifies the use of transesophageal echocardiography?
   a. Carotid artery stenosis
   b. Esophageal varices
   c. Chronic renal insufficiency
   d. Obstructive sleep apnea
5. Which is true regarding the physiologic effects associated with atenolol (Tenormin)?
   a. Decreases myocardial oxygen supply
   b. Causes bronchodilation
   c. Enhances the effects of angiotensin converting enzyme
   d. Inhibits myocardial contractility

REVIEW ANSWERS

1. **Answer: c**
   Improved wound healing occurs due to the minimally invasive nature of the surgery and relatively small incisions as compared to a traditional sternotomy.

2. **Answer: a**

   The microvascular and macrovascular changes that are associated with diabetes predispose the patient for developing cardiovascular disease.

3. **Answer: c**

   From these choices, aortic atherosclerotic disease is the only absolute contraindication to MIDCABG.

4. **Answer: b**

   Employing transesophageal echocardiography for a patient with esophageal varices can result in severe esophageal hemorrhage and/or esophageal perforation.

5. **Answer: d**

   Atenolol (Tenormin) is a beta-adrenergic receptor blocking drug which causes increased myocardial oxygen supply, decreased myocardial oxygen demand, decreased myocardial contractility, and potentially bronchoconstriction from inhibition of B_2-adrenergic receptors in the lungs.

SUGGESTED READINGS

Caffarelli AD, Robbins, RC. Will minimally invasive valve replacement ever really be important? *Curr Opin Cardiol* 2004;19:123–127.

Casselman FP, Slycke SV, Helge D, et al. Endoscopic mitral valve repair: feasible, reproducible, and durable. *J Thorac Cardiovasc Surg* 2003;125:273–282.

Douglas AM, Miller JS, Langford DA, et al. Endoscopic robotic mitral valve surgery: surgery for Acquired Cardiovascular Disease. *J Thorac Cardiovasc Surg* 2002;132(4):781–790.

Felger JE, Chitwood WR, Nifong LW, et al. Evolution of mitral valve surgery toward a totally endoscopic approach. *Ann Thorac Surg* 2001;72:1203–1209.

Grossi EA, Galloway AC, LaPietra A, et al. Minimally invasive mitral valve surgery: a 6-year experience with 714 patients. *Ann Thorac Surg* 2002;74:660–664.

Martens S, Dietrich M, Doss M, et al. Optimal carbon dioxide application for organ protection in cardiac surgery. *J Thorac Cardiovasc Surg* 2002;124:387–391.

Nifong LW, Chu VF, Bailey M, et al. Robotic mitral valve repair: Experience with the da Vinci System. *Ann Thorac Surg* 2003;75:438–443.

Savage EB, Ferguson TB, DiSesa VJ. Use of mitral valve repair: analysis of contemporary United States experience reported to the Society of Thoracic Surgeons National Cardiac Database. *Ann Thorac Surg* 2003;75:820–825.

Scarabelli CC. Beating-heart coronary artery bypass graft surgery: indications, advantages, and limitations. *Crit Care Nurse* 2002;22:44–58.

Wallace A. Anesthesia for minimally invasive cardiac surgery: MID-CABG. *Ann Thorac Surg* 1998;65:420–424.

Neurosurgery

IX

Intracranial Tumor Debulking

28

Mark D. Welliver

KEY POINTS

- The composition of the cranial vault is comprised three components: brain tissue (80%), blood (12%), and cerebrospinal fluid (CSF) (8%) which together determines intracranial pressure (ICP).
    - Brain: 1300 grams (3 lbs or 2% of total body wt)
    - Blood: 15–20% of cardiac output, 750 ml/min
    - CSF: 150 ml total in cranium and spinal cord, 75 ml in cranium at any given time
- Normal ICP is ≤ 10 mm Hg.
- CSF production by choroid plexuses in lateral ventricles makes approximately 400 ml/day.
- The circle of Willis allows bilateral communication of internal carotid and vertebral artery blood flow.
- Tumor locations are generally described as supratentorial or infratentorial.

CASE SYNOPSIS

A 50-year-old woman with a 1-year history of fatigue, depression, memory loss, and headaches presented with an acute onset severe headache, syncope, nausea and vomiting, followed by a seizure. Computerized axial tomography (CT scan) revealed hydrocephalus with displacement of the lateral and third ventricles by a large intracranial mass. Stereotactic biopsy confirmed a diagnosis of glioblastoma. A ventriculostomy drain is placed and it drains clear CSF.

PREOPERATIVE EVALUATION AND DEMOGRAPHIC DATA

Social History

- Smoker 1 pack/day for 25 years
- Drinks alcohol socially (< 2 glasses wine/week)
- Denies illicit drug use

Past Medical/Surgical History

- Controlled hypertension
- Migraine headaches
- Severe gastroesophageal reflux disease (GERD)
- Appendectomy at age 19, splenectomy at age 40, no anesthetic complications

List of Medications

- Phenytoin (Dilantin)
- Propanolol (Inderal)
- Esomeprazole magnesium (Nexium)
- Oxycodone (Percocet)
- Zolpidem tartrate (Ambien)

Diagnostic Data

- Hemoglobin, 13.5 g/dl; hematocrit, 40.1%
- Glucose, 110 mg/dl; blood urea nitrogen, 11 mg/dl; creatinine, 0.9 mg/dl
- Electrolytes: sodium, 142 mEq/l; potassium, 4.0 mEq/l; chloride, 100 mEq/l; carbon dioxide, 26 mEq/l
- Chest x-ray: normal chest x-ray, normal heart size, no evidence of infiltrates or consolidations
- CT scan: Hydrocephalus with displacement of the lateral and third ventricles by an intracranial mass measuring 5 × 4 cm. Diffuse edematous tissues surrounding mass with suspected patchy necrotic infiltrates.

Height/Weight/Vital Signs

- 165 cm, 67 kg
- Blood pressure, 133/78; heart rate, 62 beats per minute; respiratory rate, 18 breaths per minute; room air oxygen saturation, 97%; temperature, 36.6°C
- Electrocardiogram (ECG): sinus bradycardia; heart rate, 58 beats per minute

Cerebral Physiology

CSF Flow Through the Brain

CSF, produced by the choroid plexus located in the two lateral ventricles, flows through the interventricular foramen of Monro and into third ventricle. The CSF flow then proceeds from the third ventricle through the aqueduct of Sylvius and then into fourth ventricle. From the fourth ventricle, CSF moves through foramen of Magendie and two foramina of Luschka into the cerebellomedullary cistern (cistern magna) and then into the subarachnoid space and spinal column. The CSF is absorbed in the subarachnoid space by arachnoid villi of venous system. Figure 28-1 illustrates the structures and flow of CSF through the brain.

Cerebral Blood Flow (CBF)

- Average: 50 ml/100 Gm/min (Total 750 ml/min) (Range: 10–300 ml/100 Gm/min)
- Gray matter (neuronal bodies): 80 ml/100 Gm/min
- White matter (axons): 20 ml/100 Gm/min

Alterations in CBF may be detrimental by decreasing blood flow to ischemic areas or beneficial by providing more blood, and hence oxygen, to ischemic areas. Table 28-1 lists factors that can affect CBF. CBF occurs through the circle of Willis which is included in Figure 28-2.

Determinants of CBF

- **$PaCO_2$**: Linear relationship, 1 mm Hg↑ $PaCO_2$ = ↑1–2 ml/100 g/min CBF
- **PaO_2**: Profound increase in CBF only at PaO_2 < 50 mm Hg
- **Cerebral perfusion pressure** (CPP) = mean arterial pressure (MAP) − ICP (or central venous pressure [CVP])
  - Normal CPP 100 mm Hg
  - CPP < 50 mm Hg = electroencephalogram (EEG) slowing
  - CPP = 25–40 mm Hg = EEG flat
  - CPP < 25 mm Hg = permanent brain damage
- **Autoregulation**: Cebrovascular autoregulation occurs by vasoconstriction or vasodilation that occurs between MAP 60 and 160 mm Hg as shown in Figure 28-3. If the MAP is less than 60 mm Hg or exceeds 160 mm Hg, additional vasoconstriction or vasodilation in order to maintain constant CBF will not occur. Blood flow

Figure 28-1 *Cerebrospinal fluid flow.*

Table 28-1 Alterations in Cerebral Blood Flow

1. Luxury perfusion: Perfusion in excess of metabolic needs. Luxury perfusion may be beneficial in healthy brains but may cause a "steal phenomenon" in brains which have ischemic areas. Examples include:

   a. Tumor metabolites that cause vasodilatation in surrounding tissues.

   b. Inhalation anesthetic agents decrease $CMRO_2$ and increase CBF.

2. Steal phenomenon: Detrimental. Increased PCO_2 or VAA globally "steal" blood flow from ischemic areas of the brain by causing vasodilatation in healthy areas of the brain. Ischemic brain tissue, which already has maximally dilated vessels due to released vasodilator substances, loses luxury perfusion benefit due to global shunting of blood flow.

3. Inverse steal or Robin Hood phenomenon: Decreased PCO_2 constricts normal vessels but not necessarily in ischemic areas due to vasomotor paralysis. This is one rationale for hyperventilating patients with intracranial tumors associated with increased ICP especially when administering VAAs which cause vasodilatation.

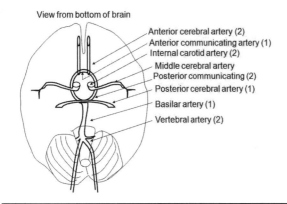

Figure 28-2   *Circle of Willis.*

becomes solely dependent on pressure as the vasculature cannot further constrict or dilate to maintain CBF. The autoregulation curve is sifted to the right for patients with chronic hypertension. Therefore, these patients require a higher MAP to maintain CBF.

- **Volatile anesthetic agents** (VAAs): All of the VAAs increase CBF in a dose-dependent manner.

Cerebral Metabolic Rate of Oxygen Consumption (CMRO$_2$)

- Cerebral metabolic rate is expressed as ml of oxygen consumed per 100 g of brain tissue per minute.

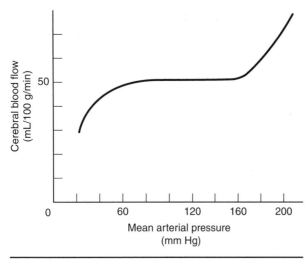

Figure 28-3   *The influence of autoregulation on cerebral blood flow.*

- CMRO$_2$ = 3–3.8 ml O$_2$/100 g/min
- Coupling is the direct linear relationship of CMRO$_2$ to CPP. As CMRO$_2$ increases (or decreases), CPP will correspondingly increase (or decrease).
- The direct linear relationship between CMRO$_2$ and CBF can be modified and altered by anesthetics and anesthetic management.
- All VAAs, barbiturates, and benzodiazepines decrease CMRO$_2$.
- VAAs decrease CMRO$_2$ while increasing CPP disrupting the relationship of CMRO$_2$ to CPP.
- Glucose is the main energy substrate used by the brain. Glucose consumption averages 5 mg/100 g/min.

Determinants of CMRO$_2$

- Coupling: As metabolic demands increase, so does CBF and vice versa.
- Temperature: For each 1°C decrease in temperature, there is a corresponding 7–8% decrease in CMRO$_2$. At 20°C body temperature, an EEG is flat showing no brain activity.
- Seizures increase CMRO$_2$.

Intracranial Pressure (ICP)

- Normal ICP is ≤ 10 mm Hg. Temporary elevated ICP occurs during coughing, Valsalva maneuver, and hypertensive episodes.
- Sustained elevated ICP > 15 mm Hg decreases CPP and increases the risk of cerebral ischemia. Severely increased ICP may lead to brainstem herniation through the foramen magnum.
- Intracranial tumors are space occupying lesions and, depending on their size and location, may increase ICP.
- Preventing increases in ICP is a primary anesthetic concern.
- Hyperventilation decreases CBF by causing cerebral vascular vasoconstriction which decreases CBF.
- Decreasing cerebral blood volume (CBV) decreases ICP.

- Diuretics decrease brain tissue water content thereby decreasing ICP.
- Ventriculostomy and intrathecal catheters allow CSF to drain which decrease ICP.

PATHOPHYSIOLOGY

Glioblastomas are tumors that rapidly expand and arise from white or gray matter usually in the frontal or temporal regions of the brain. Often these tumors are surrounded by inflammatory and necrotic tissue. Glioblastomas can become large rapidly prior to the patient developing significant symptoms. Tumors which infiltrate or displace the ventricles may cause obstructive hydrocephalus. Treatment includes tumor debulking, CSF diversion, chemotherapy, and radiation to the affected site. Despite these treatments, survival remains low.

Intracranial tumors may not cause serious symptoms initially because of compensatory physiologic mechanisms that help maintain normal ICP. Glioblastomas often develop rapidly and cause increases in ICP. When CPP requirements exceed the arterial pressure, hypothalamic sympathetic reflex increases blood pressure to restore CBF. The increased blood pressure stimulates carotid bodies which lowers the heart rate by initiating Cushing reflex. Cushing reflex is one of the bodies most potent physiologic responses that, when stimulated, dramatically increases sympathetic nervous system predominance. The cardiovascular response includes *hypertension* and *bradycardia*. Bradycardia is the result of baroreceptor stimulation in response to increased systemic vascular resistance. If ICP continues to increase, for which the Cushing reflex cannot adequately compensate, pressure on the brain stem causes irregular respiration. Cushing triad, which includes *hypertension*, *bradycardia*, and *irregular respirations*, reflect severe increases in ICP and severe cerebral ischemia and impending herniation of the brain stem down through the foramen magnum can occur. It is estimated that up to 33% of patients with elevated ICP display all three components of Cushing triad.

SURGICAL PROCEDURE

The planned surgical procedure is an open craniotomy for tumor debulking utilizing a parietal approach with the patient in the lateral position. An intraoperative biopsy for tumor confirmation and identification will be performed. Prior to surgical closure, tumor boundaries (margins) will be biopsied to assess the absence of tumor tissues. Complete removal of the tumor is desired as tumor remnants may regrow.

Differences between supratentorial as compared to infratentorial tumors

- Supratentorial tumors occupy the area of the midbrain and cerebral cortex.
- Infratentorial tumors occupy the area of the vital centers of the cerebellum and brain stem.

The location of the tentorium is illustrated in Figure 28-4.

- The location of an intracranial tumor necessitates specific positioning for surgical access. Unique surgical positioning requirements are sometimes associated with increased risks. It is important to note that complications such as venous air emboli (VAE), nerve injuries, and

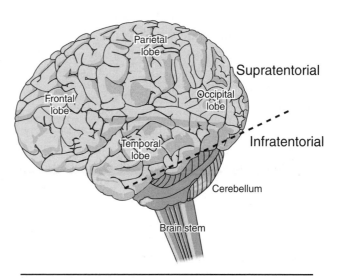

Figure 28-4   *Location of tentorium.*

postoperative vision loss (POVL) can occur when the patient is placed in any position.

- Sitting position: Increased VAE risk.
- Lateral oblique position: Brachial plexus injury.
- Prone position: POVL risk associated with lengthy prone position cases and intraoperative hypotension, especially in diabetic patients.
- Supine position: May have head and neck rotation or extension; may have cranial pinning/fixation in head tongs.

ANESTHETIC MANAGEMENT AND CONSIDERATIONS

Preoperative Period

1. Discuss the goals associated with anesthetic management that is associated with intracranial tumor debulking.

The preoperative goals include maintaining, or achieving, normal ICP and maintaining CPP (minimum 70 mm Hg) to optimize cerebral circulation and oxygenation. Maintenance of adequate CPP limits ischemia around the tumor and during intraoperative brain retraction. If there are no changes in mental status, midazolam 0.025–0.05 mg/kg IV may be given to attenuate increases in blood pressure and ICP related to anxiety. Other preoperative interventions include:

- Place at least one large bore IV access preoperatively and another after induction.
- Avoid narcotics preoperatively as these agents depress respiratory function and raise PCO_2 causing cerebral vessel dilation and corresponding increases in ICP.
- Administer antibiotics and corticosteroids (dexamethasone 4–10 mg IV) per surgeon preference prior to induction. Dexamethasone given prior to induction has an antiemetic effect in addition to attenuating inflammatory responses intraoperatively and postoperatively.

2. List the signs and symptoms of elevated ICP.

The signs and symptoms that are associated with elevated ICP progress on a continuum from mild to severe. Symptoms may include headache, diffi-culty concentrating, memory disturbances, vision disturbances, vertigo, syncope, nausea, vomiting, severe headache, Cushing reflex, and triad, seizures, or coma.

3. Do all intracranial tumors cause increases in ICP?

No. Small tumors and larger slow growing tumors associated with cerebral physiologic compensation may present with delayed increases in ICP. The compensation that occurs includes the nonlinear compliance of cerebral tissues with CSF and CBV displacement out of the cranial vault. Once ICP is increased due to a tumor, small increases in MAP can result in profound elevations of ICP. Intracranial tumors are often identified after compensatory mechanism can no longer maintain normal ICP. Additionally, any tumor that obstructs the flow of CSF from the cranial vault to spinal canal (obstructive hydrocephalus) will raise ICP. Pituitary tumors are usually small and rarely associated with increased ICP.

4. Discuss the most prevalent location of intracranial tumors, infratentorial or supratentorial.

The location of most neurosurgical procedures for tumor resection is supratentorial and involves the cerebral hemispheres. The cerebral hemispheres are divided by the medial longitudinal fissure. The right and left hemispheres are connected by a bundle of nerve fibers called the corpus callosum. The cerebral cortex is composed of the frontal, parietal, temporal, and occipital lobes. Infratentorial refers to the location of the brain stem consisting of the midbrain, medulla, cerebellum, and pons; it contains major motor and sensory pathways and the cranial nerve nuclei.

5. Explain how the location of an intracranial tumor influences patient positioning.

Infratentorial tumors usually require a prone or lateral position for surgical access. Supratentorial tumors are often resected while the patient is positioned supine or lateral. Lateral or semilateral positions may use foam supports or a bean bag vacuum mattresses to support the patient. The sitting position is associated with the increased risk of VAE and excessive neck flexion. Venous drainage from the head is impeded by neck flexion. Mild head elevation (reverse Trendelenburg) may be done with any surgical position. The patient's head may be held by a horseshoe-shaped support, a foam support, or pinned in tongs which fixes the skull to a support frame. Discussion of the patient and operating room table position should be discussed preoperatively in order to plan for intraoperative airway and invasive line access.

Intraoperative Period

6. Discuss the anesthetic concerns during induction for a patient with elevated ICP.

Hypoxia, hypercarbia, hypertension, and hypotension are the primary concerns during induction. A smooth induction is appropriate with hyperventilation by proper mask ventilation; however, since this patient has severe GERD, a rapid sequence induction is indicated. Continuous blood pressure monitoring is important, and placement of an arterial line at this time may be beneficial in order to assess an accurate MAP. Arterial blood pressure monitoring before induction should be considered.

Induction agents may depress cardiac function and cause hypotension and, conversely, laryngoscopy may cause sympathetic stimulation and hypertension. Hypotension decreases CBF and risks further ischemic injury to brain tissue. Hypertension can increase ICP and impede adequate cerebral circulation. Inducing an adequate depth of anesthesia before direct laryngoscopy should be assured to prevent sympathetic stimulation and the associated increases in blood pressure.

7. What are the primary intraoperative goals of anesthesia care for the patient with elevated ICP?

- Decreasing intracranial volume to prevent further increases in ICP
- Maintaining adequate CPP by manipulating the blood pressure
- Decreasing $CMRO_2$

8. Describe various methods that can be used to decrease $CMRO_2$.

Intravenous agents: The intravenous agents sodium thiopental, etomidate, and propofol all lower $CMRO_2$ and CBF. The modulation of GABA receptors by these agents lowers neuronal activity which corresponds with lower cerebral oxygen consumption. Barbiturate coma is sometimes induced to maximally suppress $CMRO_2$ and is reflected by an isoelectric EEG.

Volatile anesthetics agents (VAAs): VAAs decrease $CMRO_2$ and increase CBF. VAAs decrease neuronal activity which lowers oxygen and glucose consumption by brain tissue. The vasodilatory effects of VAAs may provide additional oxygen to brain tissue.

Temperature: Some anesthetists allow a mild decrease in body temperature to help lower $CMRO_2$. Each 1°C decrease in body temperature corresponds to a 7–8% decrease in $CMRO_2$. The rationale for hypothermia is to lower $CMRO_2$ and metabolite formation in order to protect brain tissue, but this practice remains controversial. Presently, there is no conclusive objective data that supports the use of hypothermia as an independent variable that decreases morbidity and mortality for patients with space occupying lesions. Although hypothermia may or may not provide benefit, hyperthermia should be avoided as it has been found to be detrimental.

9. Explain the term "coupling" in relationship of $CMRO_2$ to CBF.

Coupling is the direct relationship of $CMRO_2$ and CBF. An increase in one corresponds to an increase in the other. During normal functioning, increases in cerebral metabolic activity will correlate with an increase in CBF. Decreases in cerebral metabolic activity require less oxygen and glucose and CBF decreases accordingly. Benzodiazepines, barbiturates, and propofol all decrease $CMRO_2$ and allow normal regulatory decreases in CBF (coupling). VAAs disrupt or "uncouple" this relationship by decreasing $CMRO_2$ while increasing CBF. The term "uncoupling" is controversial in its definition. VAAs change the direct relationship of $CMRO_2$ and CBF to an inverse relationship. Some refer to this as uncoupling. Others assume a more stringent definition of uncoupling that requires a proportionally inverse relationship. All VAAs to varying degrees, and in a dose-dependent manner, decrease $CMRO_2$ while increasing CBF due to their vasodilating effects.

A decrease in $CMRO_2$ is beneficial to ischemic brain tissue, but increases in CBF may cause detrimental increases in ICP and possibly divert blood flow away from ischemic areas to nonischemic areas. This is known as "steal phenomenon" and this physiologic effect is listed in Table 28-1.

10. Describe the methods used to lower ICP.
Methods used to lower ICP address the need to decrease one or more of the three components of the cranial vault producing ICP: brain, blood, and CSF. Decreasing the volume of these components reduces ICP. Specific interventions used to decrease ICP are reviewed in Table 28-2.

11. Describe the rationale for each method that decreases intracranial volume.
1. ***Brain***: Diuretics are administered to decrease blood and brain volume. These agents shrink the brain size and therefore lower ICP.
   - Furosemide is a loop diuretic and lowers blood volume.

- Mannitol is specifically used for its osmotic diuretic effect which extracts fluid from brain tissues thereby decreasing its volume. Unfortunately, mannitol also increases renal excretion of water causing hypovolemia which contributes to hypotension.
- Hypertonic saline administration may be a better option to osmotically decrease brain water content without causing hypovolemia. Hypertonic saline causes water to be held intravascularly with minimal renal effects compared to mannitol. This improves maintenance of MAP intraoperatively. Hypertonic saline administration is guided by serum sodium (target 155–157 mEq/l) and serum osmolality (target 310–315 mOsm/l).
- Corticosteroids block inflammatory responses and may prevent further brain edema. The effectiveness of high-dose steroids has come under question; no definitive studies have shown improved outcomes with their use.

2. ***Blood***: An effective method used to decrease intracranial blood volume is hyperventilation; decreases PCO_2 causing cerebral vasoconstriction.
   - Hyperventilation ($PCO_2 < 30$ mm Hg) causes cerebral vasoconstriction thereby lowering

Table 28-2 Methods to Lower Intracranial Volume and ICP	
COMPONENT	**INTERVENTION TO INTRACRANIAL VOLUME AND ICP**
Brain	Diuretics: loop (furosemide 10–100 mg) and osmotic (mannitol 12.5–50 g)
	Hypertonic saline (3%) at 20 ml/hr or 20-ml bolus (23.2%)
	Corticosteroids (dexamethasone 10–20 mg; methylprednisone [solumedrol] 1+ g)
Blood	Hyperventilation (PCO_2 25–30 mm Hg)
	Limit intravenous fluids (< 1 l)
	Elevate head of bed (30 degrees)
CSF	Ventriculostomy
	Subdural drain
	Lumbar drain (rarely)

the amount of blood (CBV) within the cranial vault at any given moment. Lowering the PCO_2 to 25–30 mm Hg is effective for lowering the ICP, but this action occurs for approximately 24 hours. Prolonged hypocarbia is associated with increased mortality in patients with increased ICP due to vasoconstriction mediated hypoperfusion.

- Limiting intravenous fluid prevents increases in intravascular volume and increases in hydrostatic pressure. Intraoperative fluid administration is often limited to 1–1.5 l or less until the intracranial tumor is removed. This may make it difficult to maintain adequate blood pressure. Hypotension caused by hypovolemia can be attenuated by the administration of hypertonic saline which increases intravascular volume by establishing an osmotic gradient. Elevating the head of the bed and maintaining a neutral head position facilitates venous drainage.

3. **CSF**: CSF drainage removes volume from the cranial vault and aids in lowering ICP. A ventriculostomy or lumbar drain may be placed preoperatively or intraoperatively to drain CSF. The level of the CSF drain and amount of CSF drained should be discussed with the surgeon and closely monitored throughout the perioperative period.

12. Describe how hyperventilation is beneficial for patients with increased ICP.
Hyperventilation is a universal treatment for acute increases in ICP because hypocarbia causes cerebral vessel constriction which decreases the amount of blood within the cranial vault. Vasoconstriction is thought to occur in areas of the brain that are not ischemic. Injured areas of brain tissue contain ischemic mediated vasodilator substances and are not likely to respond to hyperventilation with vasoconstriction. Theoretically, this mechanism inhibits the benefits of the inverse steal or Robin Hood phenomenon in which CBF is diverted toward ischemic areas of brain and away from adequately oxygenated

areas. A growing body of evidence suggests that hyperventilation may indeed worsen existing ischemia in acutely injured brain tissues. With this in mind, the use of hyperventilation should be thoroughly assessed and discussed with the surgeon. No conclusive evidence exists regarding the benefit or detriment of hyperventilation and ischemic tissue perfusion. Hyperventilation decreases CBF with resultant decrease in overall intracranial volume. This effect lowers ICP, improving global CBF, and improves surgical exposure and visualization. An ICP of greater than 20 mm Hg impedes CBF to such a great extent that the potential risks of hyperventilation are outweighed by the benefits. Hyperventilation starts to lose its effectiveness to cause cerebral vasoconstriction after 6–8 hours.

13. Analyze the need for neuromuscular blockade (NMB) during tumor debulking procedures.
Adequate NMB is important for immobility. Neurologic patients are often taking medications such as phenytoin which induces the hepatic enzymes causing increased metabolism of certain drugs such as aminosteroidal and neuromuscular blocking agents. Increased doses of NMBs may be required for motor function suppression. Neuromuscular monitoring by peripheral twitch monitor or accelerometry is prudent. Patient movement during intracranial procedures may have devastating consequences. Coughing or "bucking" against positive pressure ventilation also risks cervical injury when the head is fixed in tongs. NMB also prevents shivering which may occur. Shivering increases metabolic requirements of oxygen and interferes with surgical visualization, especially during cases using visual magnification. Maintaining 1 out of 4 twitches on train of four (TOF) monitoring often provides adequate NMB with the ability to reverse the paralysis with a cholinesterase inhibitor.

14. Discuss intraoperative monitoring for a patient undergoing intracranial tumor debulking.
Standard AANA monitoring should be used as with all general anesthetic procedures. An arterial line, for

continual blood pressure monitoring and serial arterial blood gasses, should be placed before or immediately after induction. Note the correlation of arterial carbon dioxide ($PaCO_2$) to end-tidal carbon dioxide ($ETCO_2$) ($PaCO_2$ 5–10 mm Hg higher than $ETCO_2$).

EEG, evoked potentials (EP), brain tissue oxygen ($PtiO_2$), and transcranial perfusion monitoring may also be used. These neurologic monitoring modalities, though used more often before and after surgery, may be used intraoperatively. An EEG reflects an increase or decrease in brain activity, whereas EP monitoring provides more specific data regarding sensory and motor functions. Stimulation of a peripheral nerve and measuring the time (latency) and degree (amplitude) of brain response is the basis of EP monitoring. In general, increases in latency and decreases in amplitude reflect impaired neurologic function. VAAs increase latency and decrease amplitude in a dose-dependent manner. A minimum alveolar concentration (MAC) of 0.5% is often acceptable; above this concentration significant suppression may occur. Monitoring brain tissue oxygenation is specific to the area of the brain that surrounds a sensor probe. The probe uses a polarographic sensor that measures the diffused oxygen from local brain tissues. Ongoing studies are exploring the specific interpretations that may be made regarding the correlation of $PtiO_2$ to CBF and $CMRO_2$. It appears that $PtiO_2$ increases with regional increases of CBF although $PtiO_2$ will also increase with increased inspired oxygen (FiO_2).

15. Analyze the intravenous fluids that are acceptable for use in patients with elevated ICP.
Normal saline and lactated Ringers solution are superior to other fluids that contain higher percentages of free water. Infusion of free water must be avoided as it lowers the osmotic pressure and promotes increased extravascular volume resulting in swelling. Dextrose containing solutions are also avoided because metabolism of the glucose will lower the osmotic pressure of the fluid. Dextrose containing solutions also oppose the goal of decreasing cerebral metabolism. Glucose is the main energy substrate used by the brain and increases cerebral metabolism which risks further ischemic insult.

16. Cite the specific concerns associated with positioning for intracranial tumor resection.
Head fixation: Movement or coughing while in tongs risks catastrophic injury. Assure adequate anesthetic depth and neuromuscular blockade unless surgeon requires intact motor function for neurophysiologic monitoring. The risks associated with placement of the patient's head in tongs include excessive neck flexion, airway swelling, cervical cord compression, and decreased venous outflow. The cranial nerves IX, X, XI, and XII, which control airway patency, respiration, and hemodynamics, are at particular risk with excessive neck flexion and during posterior fossa surgery. A list of these cranial nerves and their function is included in Table 28-3. The potential of injury to these cranial

Table 28-3	**Cranial Nerve Functions**
CRANIAL NERVE	**INNERVATION/FUNCTION**
IX: Glossopharyngeal nerve	Tongue, larynx; swallowing, larynx elevation
X: Vagus nerve	Most larynx and pharyngeal muscles, thoracic and abdominal organs; airway patency, parasympathetic effects, hemodynamics
XI: Accessory nerve	Neck and upper shoulders; some respiratory accessory muscle function, swallowing
XII: Hypoglossal	Tongue/airway patency, swallowing

nerves and swelling of the brain stem requires thorough discussion and assessment with the surgeon prior to the decision to extubate the patient.

Venous air embolism: VAE can occur due to the entrainment of air into the open venous system which is above the level of heart in sitting position. As the air enters the venous system, it travels to the right atria and ventricle entering the pulmonary arterioles. A right ventricular airlock is created and can cause hypoxemia, CO_2 retention, decreased $ETCO_2$, and heart failure. Additionally, reflex pulmonary and bronchial constriction due to the release of endothelial mediators causes pulmonary hypertension and increased peak inspiratory pressures. Venous bleeding decreases the risk for VAE as the venous pressure likely exceeds atmospheric pressure, air will not be entrained into the venous system.

17. Evaluate the methods used to detect VAE.
The most sensitive to least sensitive monitoring modalities that are used to determine if a VAE has occurred include: transesophageal echocardiography, precordial Doppler, $ETCO_2$, pulmonary artery catheter, cardiac output, central venous pressure, ECG changes, blood pressure changes, and a precordial stethoscope. When air is present in the right atrium, the sound is described as a "millwheel" murmur and it is distinctly different from baseline heart sounds.

18. Construct a systematic treatment for VAE.
Upon detection of VAE, notify surgeon to flood surgical area with saline, saline soaked sponges, or gel foam to prevent further venous entrainment of air. If possible, lower the patient's head to increase venous pressure and slow air entrainment. Immediately aspirate blood and air with a 60-ml syringe from the central line that has been placed preoperatively. The distal end of the central line catheter is optimally positioned at the entrance to the right atria. It is prudent to discontinue the use of nitrous oxide as it will diffuse into the venous air bubble, increase the size, and worsen the condition.

19. Describe the main goals associated with the anesthetic management of patients for tumor debulking.
The main anesthetic goals for tumor debulking patients are cerebral protection and facilitation of surgical exposure. The reduction of ICP and $CMRO_2$ to reestablish adequate cerebral oxygenation are the main goals. Elevation of ICP above 20 mm Hg is associated with increased morbidity and mortality. Anesthetic management of increased ICP focuses on decreasing the amount of the three main constituents of the cranial vault: blood, brain, and CSF.

20. List the three main components of the cranial vault and differentiate how interventions focused on each of the three components of the cranial vault may affect ICP.
Blood component: Hyperventilate in order to lower $PaCO_2$ which decreases CBV. Attempt to minimize stimuli to avoid elevations in blood pressure by administering narcotics and beta blockers.

Brain component: Decrease brain fluid content by administering mannitol and/or furosemide. Limit IV fluids to prevent increases in brain fluid and, therefore, brain volume. Administer barbiturates to decrease $CMRO_2$ by suppressing neuronal activity. Corticosteroids may also be given preoperatively for extended anti-inflammatory effects and reduction of brain tissue water content (vasogenic edema).

CSF component: A ventriculostomy for supratentorial, or a lumbar CSF drain for infratentorial skull base lesions may be placed to drain CSF. At any given time, 75 ml of CSF is located in the cranial vault, and drainage aids in lower ICP. Elevating the head facilitates venous outflow and helps reduce ICP.

21. Explain appropriate methods for treating intraoperative hypertension.
Medications that have a rapid onset of action and a short duration are often best for treating intraoperative episodes of hypertension. Hypertension increases blood volume in the cranial vault which

elevates ICP and can increase bleeding. Hypertension may also make surgical exposure and visualization more difficult. Intravenous beta blockers, such as esmolol and labetalol, are beneficial. Direct-acting vasodilators will increase CBF, whereas enalapril, an angiotensin-converting enzyme inhibitor, has been found to have little effect on CBF. The short-acting calcium channel blocker nicardipine is useful for treating hypertensive periods. Calcium channel blockers have been shown to effectively lower hypertension, to decrease the potential for cerebrovascular spasm, and to be neuroprotective. Intermittent boluses of propofol or narcotic may aid in attenuating increases in blood pressure related to noxious stimuli. Acute perioperative hypertension is associated with specific periods of noxious stimuli including intubation, skin incision, outer periosteal scraping of the skull bone, skin closure, and emergence. Increasing the anesthetic depth prior to surgical stimulation attenuates sympathetic discharge. Hypotension should also be avoided as a decrease in CBF dilates cerebral vessels which increase CBV. Maintenance of an appropriate MAP is important to preserve an adequate CPP. Often recommended is a CPP of at least 60 mm Hg (preferably 70 mm Hg).

22. Differentiate Cushing response and Cushing triad.

Cushing response is the periodic increase in blood pressure and reflex bradycardia that occurs when the ICP exceeds 30 mm Hg. The associated decrease in CBF causes cerebral ischemia leading to further edema and elevating the ICP. This is a vicious cycle than leads to Cushing triad. Cushing triad is hypertension, bradycardia, and respiratory variability that occur with sustained elevations in ICP. Cushing triad is a hallmark feature of severe elevated ICP which can lead to herniation through the foramen magna.

23. Discuss the different intravenous anesthetic agent choices for use in tumor debulking procedures in reference to CBF and $CMRO_2$.

Barbiturates, propofol, and etomidate all lower CBF and $CMRO_2$ in a dose-dependent fashion. Cerebral autoregulation as well as CO_2 responsiveness are maintained with these agents at anesthetic doses. Barbiturates also maintain autoregulation and CO_2 responsiveness at doses that induce coma. Total intravenous anesthesia (TIVA) using propofol has been used for intracranial procedures. The advantages of TIVA include:

- Decreases CBF and $CMRO_2$
- Lowers CBV
- Lowers ICP
- Possible neuroprotection from antioxidant activity, activation of GABA type A receptors, and alterations in glutamate uptake and release
- Easily titratable
- Attenuates evoked potential monitoring waveforms less than VAAs
- Metabolizes rapidly allowing for quick emergence and assessment

Propofol lowers MAP and therefore will lower CPP. Care must be taken to maintain adequate CPP. Benzodiazepines decrease CBF and $CMRO_2$ and also possess anticonvulsant properties. Dexmedetomidine is used during intracranial tumor debulking procedures because of its sedative effects and its ability to cause cerebral vasoconstriction and decreases CBF. The growing body of literature suggests that dexmedetomidine decreases CBF but not $CMRO_2$.

Ketamine increases CBF and $CMRO_2$. Increases in ICP associated with ketamine can be attenuated with hyperventilation. Cerebral autoregulation as well as CO_2 responsiveness are maintained. Ketamine, like etomidate, does not cause seizure activity but may promote seizures in epileptic patients. The use of ketamine is not advised for intracranial procedures.

Narcotics have little to no direct effect on ICP, CBF, and $CMRO_2$ but will attenuate sympathetic response to noxious stimuli. Narcotics are a useful adjunct to volatile and intravenous anesthetic agents. Shorter acting narcotics, such as remifentanil and alfentanil, facilitate quick emergence.

24. Evaluate the effect of emergence on ICP.

Emergence from anesthesia is associated with increases in heart rate and blood pressure. Increased cardiac output increases CBF, which in turn increases ICP. Increased cerebral activity also increases $CMRO_2$ which further increases CBF. Bucking or coughing causes increased intrathoracic pressures which impedes cerebral venous drainage and causes spikes in ICP. Smooth emergence with normal blood pressure and heart rate is desirable. Elevated ICP is usually no longer a significant concern after tumor debulking, but hemorrhage remains a potential risk. Extubation of the patient "deep" while still anesthetized but with adequate respiratory function, is beneficial unless other contraindications exist.

25. Formulate a plan to accomplish a smooth emergence in patients after a craniotomy for tumor debulking.

VAAs that have low blood–gas solubility are beneficial for quick emergence after general anesthesia. Titration of narcotics and intravenous lidocaine has been helpful at attenuating the stimulatory effects of an endotracheal tube but may slow awakening and delay the time before the patient is fully alert. Laryngeal tracheal anesthesia (LTA) provided by administering lidocaine spray is helpful at the time of intubation but its duration of effect is approximately 90 minutes. The lidocaine can be instilled into the endotracheal cuff at the time of intubation to help anesthetize the trachea and improve tolerance of the endotracheal tube during periods of light anesthesia such as emergence. This technique's duration of effect is quite long, as lidocaine has been shown to diffuse through the polyvinylchloride membrane over time. Switching from one agent, such as a VAA, to a propofol drip, or vice versa, has not been proven to speed emergence.

Postoperative Period

26. Discuss goals associated with the recovery phase of anesthesia.

Pain control and maintenance of adequate blood pressure is important postoperatively. If the patient is extubated, the anesthetist should observe for changes in mental status or any signs and symptoms which may suggest an intracranial event such as increased ICP, vasospasm, or hemorrhage. Central nervous system depressants such as propofol, benzodiazepines, and barbiturates are usually avoided postoperatively because they promote hypoventilation and decrease the patient's level of consciousness. If the patient is to remain intubated, sedation using central nervous system depressant medications is imperative.

REVIEW QUESTIONS

1. Which is not considered a component of the cranial vault?
   a. Blood
   b. Brain
   c. Bone
   d. CSF
2. Which factor can decrease ICP?
   a. Hypoxia
   b. Hyperventilation
   c. Delivery of VAAs
   d. Hypercarbia
3. Which is not a potential consequence of elevated ICP?
   a. Confusion or lethargy
   b. Cushing response
   c. Cushing syndrome
   d. Cushing triad
4. Which is the mechanism of action by which mannitol protects brain tissue?
   a. Venous engorgement and increased permeability
   b. Osmotic diuresis and free radical scavenging
   c. Hypotension and decreased tissue perfusion
   d. Osmotic diuresis and decreased $CMRO_2$
5. Which events cause physiologic stimulation during a tumor debulking procedure?
   a. Induction, intubation, skin incision, bone sawing, brain tissue resection
   b. Intubation, skin incision, skull periosteal scraping, brain tissue resection

c. Intubation, skin incision, skull periosteal scraping, emergence

d. All events during tumor debulking are equally stimulating

REVIEW ANSWERS

1. **Answer: c**
The cranial vault consists of bone and establishes a fixed space in which blood, brain, and CSF occupy. Increases in blood, brain, or CSF volume will increase ICP. Decreasing the volume of any or all of these components will lower ICP.

2. **Answer: b**
Hyperventilation causes cerebral vasoconstriction which lowers the total amount of blood in the cranial vault. The lower cranial vault blood volume lowers ICP. Hypoxia, hypercarbia, and VAAs cause cerebral vasodilatation, increasing the cranial vault volume which increases ICP.

3. **Answer: c**
Cushing syndrome (hypercortisolism) is a hormonal disease marked by excessive cortisol. Cushing reflex is a physiologic response (increased blood pressure and reflexive decreased heart rate) to elevated ICP in reestablish adequate CPP. Cushing triad is marked by the addition of irregular respirations to the Cushing reflex of hypertension and bradycardia. Confusion and lethargy are associated with elevated ICP.

4. **Answer: b**
Mannitol is an osmotic diuretic which pulls water out of intracellular and interstitial tissues into the vascular space for excretion. This lowers the amount of brain water (edema) and shrinks the volume of brain tissue lowering ICP. Mannitol is also a free radical scavenger. Mannitol has a greater affinity for free radicals and readily binds to them, thereby protecting tissues from the damaging effects.

5. **Answer: c**
The events associated with the greatest noxious stimulation are: intubation, skin incision, glial resection and scraping, and emergence. The glial lining is the mesh of nerves and connective tissue that covers the skull under the scalp flap. Resection and scraping of this tissue is stimulating and may be associated with increased heart rate and blood pressure as seen with other noxious events. Brain tissue is devoid of sensory nerve fibers and is not a stimulating procedure by itself. Skin closure is another noxious event and may unmask light anesthesia if anesthetics are weaned early, otherwise emergence is the last event associated with noxious stimulation.

SUGGESTED READINGS

Adembri C, Venturi L, Tani A, et al. Neuroprotective effects of propofol in models of cerebral ischemia. *Anesthesiology* 2006;104:80–90.

DeAngelis LM. Brain tumors. *N Engl J Med* 2001;344:114–123.

Hans P, Bonhomme V. Why we still use intravenous drugs as the basic regimen for neurosurgical anaesthesia. *Curr Opin Anaesth* 2006;19:498–503.

Hoffman W, Charbel F, Edelman G, et al. Thiopental and desflurane treatment for brain protection. *Neurosurgery* 1998;43:1050–1053.

Menon D, Wheeler D. Neuronal injury and neuroprotection. *Anaesth Int Care Med* 2005;6:184–188.

Mishra LD. Cerebral blood flow and anaesthesia: a review. *Indian J Anaesth* 2002;46:87–95.

Rozet I, Vavilala MS. Risks and benefits of patient positioning during neurosurgical care. *Anesthesiol Clin* 2007;25:631–653.

Smith M. Perioperative uses of transcranial perfusion monitoring. *Anesthesiol Clin* 2007;25:557–577.

Stocchetti N, Maas AIR, Chieregato A, et al. Hyperventilation in head injury: a review. *Chest* 2005;127:1812–1827.

Summors AC, Gupta AK, Matta BF. Dynamic cerebral autoregulation during sevoflurane anesthesia: a comparison with isoflurane. *Anesth Analg* 1999;88:341–345.

Transsphenoidal Hypophysectomy

29

John Cavitt

KEY POINTS

- A thorough preoperative evaluation is necessary to identify abnormalities resulting from abnormal pituitary hormone secretion or mass effect of the pituitary tumor.
- Vigilant postoperative observation is needed to identify life-threatening complications.
- Perioperative complications of a transsphenoidal hypophysectomy include hemorrhage, increased intracranial pressure (ICP), cranial nerve palsy, diabetes insipidus (DI), and syndrome of inappropriate antidiuretic hormone secretion (SIADH).
- Intubation by direct laryngoscopy will be difficult in 12–30% of acromegalic patients as a result of physiologic changes that occur to the airway.

CASE SYNOPSIS

A 36-year-old man, who recently moved to the United States, has been diagnosed with acromegaly. Presently, he has received no treatment. He is scheduled for transsphenoidal hypophysectomy.

PREOPERATIVE EVALUATION AND DEMOGRAPHIC DATA

Past Medical/Surgical History

- Acromegaly diagnosed outside the United States several years prior

List of Medications

- None

Diagnostic Data

- Imaging studies
    - Pituitary mass identified on magnetic resonance imaging (MRI)

- Physical assessment
  - Hypertrophy of facial and cranial bones
  - Macroglossia, prognathism, and enlarged hands and feet
  - Deep voice without hoarseness
  - Mallampati Class 2, thyromental distance > 6 cm, and no limitations in range of motion of neck and temporomandibular joint
- Laboratory testing
  - Plasma growth hormone (GH), 12.1 ng/ml (normal 0.7–6.0 ng/ml; level may be within normal limits as secretion is pulsatile)
  - Insulin-like growth factor 1 (IGF-1), 1282 ng/ml (normal 100–402 ng/ml)
  - Hemoglobin, 15.9 g/dl; hematocrit, 48.4%
  - Platelet count, 299,000/mm^3
  - Electrolytes: sodium, 139 mEq/l; potassium, 4.2 mEq/l; chloride, 101 mEq/l; serum bicarbonate, 22 mEq/l

Height/Weight/Vital Signs

- 185 cm, 128 kg, body mass index (BMI) 37 kg/m^2
- Blood pressure, 147/87; heart rate, 72 beats per minute; respiratory rate, 18 breaths per minute; temperature, 36.3°C; room air oxygen saturation, 99%
- Electrocardiogram (ECG): Normal sinus rhythm

PATHOPHYSIOLOGY

The pituitary gland, consisting of a large anterior lobe, the adenohypophysis, and a smaller posterior lobe, the neurohypophysis, is located at the base of the brain and is confined to a bony depression in the base of the skull called the sella turcica. The floor of the sella turcica and anterior wall adjoin the sphenoid air sinus. Its lateral walls are adjacent to the cavernous sinuses, which house the internal carotid arteries and cranial nerves III, IV, V, and VI as seen in Figure 29-1.

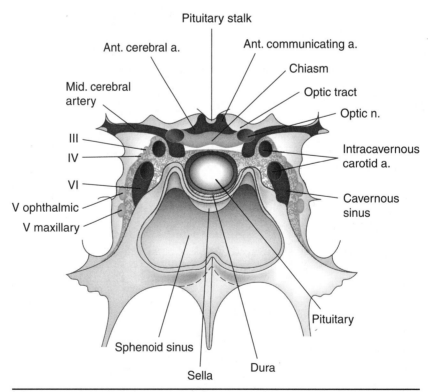

Figure 29-1 *Pituitary gland, sella turcica, and surrounding anatomic structures.*

The anterior portion of the pituitary gland secretes six hormones, each by a specific cell type: prolactin, secreted by lactotrophs; adrenocorticotropin, secreted by corticotrophs; growth hormone, secreted by somatotrophs; follicle-stimulating hormone and luteinizing hormone, both secreted by gonadotrophs; and thyroid stimulating hormone, secreted by thyrotrophs. The secretion of these hormones is regulated by the hypothalamus. The posterior portion of the pituitary gland which is also regulated by the hypothalamus, secretes vasopressin and oxytocin. The hormones of the pituitary influence target organs, which are therefore affected by pathology of the pituitary.

Almost all pituitary tumors originate in the anterior lobe and most are benign adenomas. Seventy-five percent of these adenomas cause an inappropriate amount of hormone secretion. Pituitary adenomas are most commonly found in adults in their fourth to sixth decade of life, and they are classified as to their size and functionality. Functioning tumors usually consist of a single cell type and therefore secrete a single hormone, defining the disease process, such as acromegaly and Cushing disease. Nonfunctioning tumors do not secrete excess hormones and are therefore usually not discovered until they are larger. When these tumors reach a critical mass, they impinge on adjacent structures which leads to specific symptomatology directly related to the structures affected. Pressure on the optic chiasm can lead to vision changes. Numerous other effects can occur as a result of pituitary tumor including headache, increased ICP due to obstruction of the third ventricle, cranial nerve palsy, and neurologic changes due to vascular occlusion. Tumors may also impinge on the normal pituitary tissue and cause a decrease in hormone secretion.

Acromegaly and Cushing disease are conditions that have many significant implications for the management of anesthesia. Acromegaly results from an excess production of growth hormone when the individual develops the condition in adulthood, and gigantism if the condition develops before epiphyseal closure. The most common cause of acromegaly is a pituitary somatotroph adenoma that releases growth hormone. An excessive amount of growth hormone stimulates the production of IGF-1 by the liver. Supraphysiologic concentrations of these two hormones contributes to the signs and symptoms of the disorder, characterized by increased growth, and increased carbohydrate, fat, and protein metabolism. The onset of the defining characteristics can evolve over 10 years before fully developing. As a result, the signs and symptoms of acromegaly may be very subtle which makes this endocrine disorder difficult to correctly diagnose.

Excessive amounts of growth hormone cause an overgrowth of the bony and soft tissues, which can be seen in the mouth, tongue, and laryngeal cartilages. The resulting prognathism, macroglossia, and enlargement of the uvula can hinder ventilation and intubation. Other anatomic changes associated with acromegaly include thickening of the vocal cords, reduced size of the laryngeal aperture, and hypertrophy of the periepiglottic folds. Obstructive sleep apnea (OSA) is seen in 60–75% of individuals who have acromegaly. Recurrent laryngeal nerve palsy has been observed and attributed to tissue overgrowth and the subsequent tension exerted on the nerve. Compression of the trachea as a result of an enlarged thyroid has also been described. Hypertension is seen in 30% of acromegalic patients and is commonly associated with myocardial hypertrophy. Diabetes mellitus is observed in 25% of these patients and can drastically impact perioperative care.

The pituitary gland secretes adrenocorticotrophic hormone (ACTH or corticotropin), which causes cortisol secretion by the adrenal gland. Cushing syndrome results from excessive secretion of cortisol. The etiology of Cushing syndrome includes medications that stimulate the production of glucocorticoids, adrenal tumors, ectopic ACTH production, and Cushing disease, resulting from ACTH-secreting pituitary tumors. Hypersecretion of cortisol has dramatic and systemic effects on the body which include truncal obesity, redistribution of fat ("moon face"), proximal myopathy, osteoporosis, hypertension, left ventricular hypertrophy, hypernatremia, hypervolemia, hypokalemia, sleep apnea, gastrointestinal reflux, glucose intolerance, insomnia, and depression.

The diagnosis of Cushing syndrome is based on assessing free cortisol levels which is measured in urine (> 250 mcg/24 hours). Other assays that are used to measure plasma corticotropin are utilized to differentiate between corticotropin-dependent and corticotropin-independent hypercortisolism. Nearly 70% of the cases of corticotropin-dependent hypercortisolism are the result of Cushing disease. The diagnosis of an ectopic cortisol source can be excluded by using a high-dose dexamethasone suppression test.

SURGICAL PROCEDURE

The treatment of choice for a well-circumscribed pituitary tumor is a transsphenoidal hypophysectomy, which accounts for approximately 20% of the intracranial surgeries done in academic institutions. This procedure debulks the pituitary mass and, as a result, endocrine function improves. Access to the pituitary gland is best achieved via the transsphenoidal approach, although this technique may not be possible if very large tumors exist. This technique is achieved either from a sublabial or endonasal approach. It minimizes surgical trauma to the brain and has the least incidence of complications. Once the sphenoid sinus is traversed, access to the sella turcica is achieved by removing the inferior portion. The surgeon is able to remove the tumor using a microscope. The imaging techniques that are employed include fluoroscopy, ultrasound, frameless stereotaxy, three-dimensional computer-assisted neuronavigation, or MRI. The free space created by excision of the tumor can be packed with synthetic reabsorbing material, fat, fascia, or muscle that is harvested from the abdomen or thigh. This graft also seals the dura. The bone fragment from the floor of the sella turcica and the sphenoid sinus is packed.

ANESTHETIC MANAGEMENT AND CONSIDERATIONS

Preoperative Period

1. Discuss the preoperative evaluation of a patient with a pituitary tumor.
Evaluation of the prolactin concentration, thyroid function test, and an MRI should be performed preoperatively. Although thyroid gland dysfunction is rarely caused by a pituitary adenoma, it is important to determine if the patient is euthyroid. An MRI yields superior results as compared to a computed tomography (CT) scan because of its capability for differentiating soft tissues. This difference allows the surgeon to identify the presence of microadenomas. Depending on the disease process, a more in-depth evaluation should be performed based on the target organs affected, such as the musculoskeletal, cardiovascular, and respiratory systems.

2. Discuss the neurologic abnormalities possible in a patient with a pituitary tumor.
Functional tumors rarely extend beyond the sella turcica and, therefore, they seldom produce symptoms by mass effect. Nonfunctional tumors are usually not diagnosed until the tumor is outside the sella, causing impingement on adjacent structures. A pituitary tumor is the most common cause of bitemporal hemianopsia due to its close proximity to the optic chiasm. The cavernous sinuses exist lateral to the sella and contain cranial nerves III, IV, V, and VI as shown in Figure 29-1. Cranial nerve palsy can result from compression of these nerves. Increased ICP due to the tumors mass may cause symptoms such as headache, papilledema, and altered level of consciousness.

3. Discuss the anatomic airway abnormalities and associated anesthetic implications that are observed in a patient with acromegaly.

Distinct abnormalities in the airway anatomy of patients with acromegaly was first described in 1896, when a dying patient was described to have respiratory failure. The autopsy of this patient described a narrow glottic opening, thickened laryngeal cartilages, and soft tissue hypertrophy. Further investigation shows the presence of laryngeal stenosis, subglottic narrowing, and vocal cord paralysis, resulting from recurrent laryngeal nerve stretching. These changes, in conjunction with prognathism, macroglossia, and hypertrophy of the lips and epiglottis, can make airway management challenging. It has been estimated that 12–30% of acromegalic patients will be difficult to intubate by direct laryngoscopy. It has been suggested that glottic or subglottic involvement can be suspected if hoarseness, stridor, or OSA is observed. These findings strongly suggest the need for alternative airway management strategies such as an awake intubation. The use of a smaller endotracheal tube than what would be expected is prudent to avoid soft tissue trauma, bleeding, and subsequent edema.

Intraoperative Period

4. Describe the positioning considerations for transsphenoidal hypophysectomy.

Since the approach of a transsphenoidal hypophysectomy involves either a sublabial or endonasal approach, the surgeon must have access to the upper lip and nose. The operating table and patient are rotated 180 degrees. The patient's head is slightly elevated and secured in a headrest. This head position increased the potential for a venous air embolus to occur. The surgeon typically stands to the left of the patient and the patient's head is therefore turned to the left. The endotracheal tube should be secured to the left side of the mouth and taped to the patient's cheek or lower lip.

5. Discuss the potential cardiovascular abnormalities for a patient with acromegaly and Cushing disease.

Half of all untreated acromegalic patients die before the age of 50 and the increased mortality is attributed to cardiac disease. Approximately half of normotensive patients with acromegaly have left ventricular hypertrophy. Increases in cardiac output and stroke volume may also be observed in conjunction with the increased ventricular mass. Diastolic dysfunction, evidenced by decreased left ventricular compliance and resulting in increased left ventricular filling pressure is characteristic of acromegalic cardiomyopathy. Large proximal coronary arteries are rarely affected in acromegalic patients, but distal branches may become stenotic. An increased incidence of supraventricular and ventricular ectopy with exertion has been described in this patient population. ECG abnormalities associated with acromegaly include bundle branch block, ST segment depression, and T-wave abnormalities.

It is estimated that nearly 80% of all patients with Cushing disease have hypertension, and 50% of those untreated have a diastolic blood pressure greater than 100 mm Hg. In light of these findings, ECG abnormalities are common, such as high voltage quick release system (QRS) complexes, inverted T waves, and left ventricular hypertrophy as evidenced by strain patterns. Diastolic dysfunction is prevalent in over 40% of patients with Cushing disease.

6. Discuss the intraoperative anesthetic considerations when caring for the patient with Cushing disease.

OSA is present in over one half of all patients with Cushing disease. Hyperglycemia frequently occurs and intraoperative blood glucose assessment is imperative. One third of patients with Cushing disease exhibits exophthalmos, which predisposes these patients to develop corneal abrasions. Thinning skin, resulting from hypercortisolism, leads to the presence of superficial veins which can make vascular cannulation difficult. Pathologic fractures occur in approximately 20% of these patients due to the development of osteoporosis. Therefore, careful positioning and padding all pressure points is vital. Due to protein catabolism, muscle hypermetabolism resulting in weakness occurs. The dose of muscle relaxant medication should be decreased and subsequently dosed based on the response to peripheral nerve stimulation. The presence of hypokalemia should be corrected preoperatively to avoid the untoward cardiac effects and inhibit further skeletal muscle weakness.

7. Describe the anesthetic complications that can be encountered during a transsphenoidal hypophysectomy.

Since vital neurologic structures exist within close proximity of the pituitary gland, adequate muscle relaxation should be maintained throughout surgery to avoid inadvertent patient movement and subsequent trauma. Such trauma may produce cranial nerve damage, injury to the optic chiasm, or vascular injury. The internal carotid arteries exist lateral to the pituitary gland and massive hemorrhage can occur as a result of accidental dissection. In the event of internal carotid hemorrhage, deliberate hypotension may be necessary during surgical repair. The expected blood loss is usually minimal, but may be significant if the tumor is large or involves the suprasellar region. The surgeon may request a Valsalva maneuver to assess for a cerebrospinal fluid (CSF) leak. If a CSF leak is discovered, the sella turcica is often packed with autologous fat.

Postoperative Period

8. Explain the anesthetic considerations related to emergence and extubation for a patient undergoing transsphenoidal hypophysectomy.

A significant amount of blood can passively enter into the patient's stomach during surgery. Since blood has known emetogenic effects, it should be removed at the conclusion of the case by orogastric suctioning. An oral airway should be placed before emergence to encourage the patient to breath through his or her mouth since the nasal cavity is packed. Although deep extubation can be performed in neurosurgical patients, awake extubation is most often appropriate, especially if ventilation and intubation were difficult. If airway management was difficult, extubation can occur using an endotracheal tube changer. Pharyngeal suctioning should occur prior to emergence to avoid excessive stimulation and coughing. During emergence, intravenous lidocaine can be administered to blunt hyperreactive airway reflexes.

A postoperative assessment of the patient's neurologic status needs is performed expeditiously. This can be facilitated by administering drugs that produce short clinical effects, such as propofol and remifentanil, and inhalation agents with low blood solubility, such as sevoflurane.

9. Explain the importance of a comprehensive neurologic examination postoperatively.

An in-depth neurologic assessment needs to be done postoperatively to evaluate the involvement of structures in close proximity to the surgical site such as the internal carotid arteries; cranial nerves III, IV, V, and IV; and the optic chiasm. Complications involving these structures include carotid artery spasm and hemorrhage, cranial nerve damage, and visual changes, respectively. Postoperative bleeding may impinge on the brain stem causing visual changes and altered level of consciousness. If deficits or abnormalities are discovered, an immediate direct assessment utilizing CT, MRI, or reexploration, are indicated.

10. Discuss the postoperative complications that may have a delayed onset after transsphenoidal hypophysectomy.

Complications involving neuroendocrine abnormalities may not be detectable in the immediate postoperative period. Disruption of the posterior pituitary can lead to DI or SIADH. These conditions usually become evident in the first 24–48 hours after surgery and are rarely seen in the immediate postoperative period. DI occurs in approximately 25% of these patients; however, DI is usually transient. A Foley catheter may be placed intraoperatively and maintained postoperatively for assessment of urinary output. Treatment of DI includes fluid and electrolyte replacement and administration of vasopressin.

Assessing the patient for the presence of fluid draining into their throat, frequent swallowing, or continuous drainage can be indicative of a CSF leak. Nausea and vomiting occurs in nearly 40% of neurosurgical patients and can have detrimental consequences on increased ICP. The use of prophylactic antiemetic medication should be incorporated into the plan of care. Hypopituitarism can also occur in the postoperative period. Plasma cortisol levels may decrease significantly after microadenomectomy, and this situation will require corticosteroid administration in order to avoid the development of acute adrenal crises.

REVIEW QUESTIONS

1. Which statement regarding an acromegaly is false?
   a. The etiology is excess secretion of growth hormone.
   b. The signs and symptom develop rapidly.
   c. A narrow glottic opening and subglottic stenosis should be anticipated.
   d. A gradual change in voice occurs.
2. Which comorbid factor is uncommon in a patient with acromegaly?
   a. Biventricular hypertrophy
   b. Obesity
   c. Insulin resistance
   d. Sleep apnea
3. Which complication is least frequently observed in immediate postoperative period following transsphenoidal hypophysectomy?
   a. Diabetes insipidus
   b. Altered level of consciousness
   c. Cranial nerve palsy
   d. Visual changes

4. Which anesthetic intervention is warranted for a patient having transsphenoidal hypophysectomy?
   a. Muscle relaxation should be used to avoid patient movement
   b. Placement of a laryngeal mask airway is suggested to avoid coughing on emergence
   c. Long acting analgesics are beneficial to ensure a smooth emergence and analgesia in the postoperative period
   d. Either an oral or nasal endotracheal tube is acceptable
5. Which cardiovascular abnormality is least likely associated with Cushing disease?
   a. Aortic stenosis
   b. Diastolic dysfunction
   c. Inverted T waves
   d. Hypertension

REVIEW ANSWERS

1. **Answer: b**
   Acromegaly typically develops over a period of years and its onset of symptoms is gradual and subtle, making the initial diagnosis difficult.
2. **Answer: b**
   Biventricular hypertrophy, insulin resistance, and sleep apnea are commonly occurs in patients with acromegaly. Excess grown hormone does not lead to fat deposition and obesity.
3. **Answer: a**
   DI and SIADH may occur within the first 24–48 hours after surgery. Cranial nerve palsy, visual changes, and an altered level of consciousness can occur in the immediate postoperative period. These signs and symptoms are indications for the need for reexploration, CT scanning, or MRI.
4. **Answer: a**
   Muscle relaxation should be used to ensure immobility and, for this reason, the use of a laryngeal mask airway is precluded. In the case of an acromegalic patient, laryngeal mask airway

placement may be difficult because of anatomic changes. Short-acting medications should be used to expedite emergence so that an assessment can be performed immediately after extubation. Due to the prevalence of obstructive sleep apnea in this patient population, narcotics and benzodiazepines should be administered with caution. Transsphenoidal hypophysectomy involves a sublabial or endonasal approach, and access to the upper lip and nose is necessary. This is best achieved by placement of an oral endotracheal tube.

5. **Answer: a**

Nearly 80% of patients with Cushing disease have hypertension, and 50% have a diastolic blood pressure greater than 100 mm Hg. In light of these findings, ECG abnormalities are common and include high-voltage QRS complexes and inverted T waves, possibly due to left ventricular strain and hypertrophy. Diastolic dysfunction is seen in over 40% of patients. The development of aortic stenosis is not specifically related to Cushing disease.

SUGGESTED READINGS

Holdaway IM, Rajasoorya CR, Gamble GD. Factors influencing mortality in acromegaly. *J Clin Endocrinol Metab* 2004;89:667–674.

Keegan MT, Atkinson JL, Kasperbauer JL, et al. Exaggerated hemodynamic responses to nasal injection and awakening from anesthesia in a cushingoid patient having transsphenoidal hypophysectomy. *J Neurosurg Anesthesiol* 2000;12(3): 225–229.

Nemergut EC, Dumont AS, Barry UT, et al. Perioperative management of patients undergoing transphenoidal pituitary surgery. *Anesth Analg* 2005;101: 1170–1181.

Nieman LK, Ilias I. Evaluation and treatment of Cushing's syndrome. *Am J Med* 2005;118(12):1340–1346.

Russell TW. Endocrine disease. In: Hines RL, Marschall KE, eds. *Stoelting's Anesthesia and Co-Existing Disease*, 5th ed. Philadelphia: Churchill Livingstone, 2008: 394–395, 402–404.

Saussez S, Mahillon V, Chantrain G, et al. Acromegaly presented as a cause of laryngeal dyspnea. *Auris Nasus Larynx* 2007;34(4):541–543.

Schmitt HS, Buchfelder M, Radespiel-Troger M, et al. Difficult intubation in acromegalic patients. *Anesthesiology* 2000;93:110–114.

Schubert A, Deogaonkar A, Lotto M, et al. Anesthesia for minimally invasive cranial and spinal surgery. *J Neurosurg Anesthesiol* 2006;18(1):47–56.

Seidman PA, Kofke WA, Policare R, et al. Anaesthetic complications of acromegaly. *Br J Anaesth* 2000;84: 179–182.

Smith M, Hirsch NP. Pituitary disease and anaesthesia. *Br J Anaesth* 2000;85(1):3–14.

Spiekermann BF, Stone DJ, Bogdonoff D, et al. Airway management in neuroanaesthesia. *Can J Anaesth* 1996;43:820–834.

Asleep-Awake Craniotomy

30

C. Wayne Hamm

KEY POINTS

- Asleep-awake craniotomies are necessary in only a small percentage of patients, those in whom seizure focus may be suppressed during general anesthesia or may be adjacent to "eloquent" cortex.
- The eloquent cortex is defined as areas of cortex that—if removed—will result in loss of sensory processing or linguistic ability, minor paralysis, or paralysis.
- The most common areas of eloquent cortex are in the left temporal and frontal lobes for speech and language, bilateral occipital lobes for vision, bilateral parietal lobes for sensation, and bilateral motor cortex for movement.
- When these conditions exist, an awake craniotomy may be the best/only option to identify the seizure focus and minimize brain injury.
- One of the most important elements for a successful asleep-awake craniotomy is a highly motivated and well-informed patient.
- Factors that mitigate the successful conduct of an asleep-awake craniotomy include intraoperative confusion, nausea, and seizures.

CASE SYNOPSIS

A 59-year-old White woman presents with a left frontal oligodendroglioma tumor that has reoccurred in various areas of the eloquent cortex. She has also experienced several recent seizures. Due to the recurrence in eloquent cortex and seizure history, the neurosurgeon elects to proceed with an asleep-awake craniotomy with intraoperative mapping of eloquent cortex and electrocorticographic identification of seizure nidus.

PREOPERATIVE EVALUATION AND DEMOGRAPHIC DATA

Past Medical/Surgical History

- Hypertension
- Seizures
- Smoking history of 25 years

- Left frontal craniotomy with partial tumor resection in 1986 under general anesthesia; no anesthetic complications
- Gamma knife treatment of tumor recurrence in 2000

List of Medications

- Phenytoin
- Depakote
- Metoprolol
- Dexamethasone
- Famotidine

Diagnostic Data

- Hemoglobin, 12.8 g/dl; hematocrit, 38%
- Glucose, 176 mg/dl (week before surgery)
- Electrolytes: sodium, 132 mEq/l; potassium, 3.6 mEq/l (week before surgery)
- Phenytoin level, 12 mcg/dl; Depakote level, 86 mcg/ml (week before surgery)

Height/Weight/Vital Signs

- 160 cm, 81 kg
- Blood pressure, 164/88; heart rate, 58 beats per minute; respiratory rate, 21 breaths per minute; room air oxygen saturation, 96%; temperature, 37.1°C

PATHOPHYSIOLOGY

In 2005, the United States Central Brain Tumor Registry reported an annual incidence of oligodendroglial tumors of 0.35 cases per 100,000 individuals. Representing 9.4% of all primary brain and central nervous system tumors, oligodendroglioma is a well-differentiated, diffusely infiltrating tumor that occurs in adults and is typically located in the cerebral hemispheres. These tumors are predominantly composed of cells that morphologically resemble oligodendroglia. In 50–80% of the cases, patients with oligodendrogliomas present with seizures reflective of increased intracranial pressure. Because of the typically slow growth of oligodendrogliomas, the elapsed time between the initial symptoms and clinical diagnosis may vary from 1 week to 12 years. Oligodendrogliomas, like all other infiltrating gliomas, have a very high rate of recurrence. Historically, surgery has been the mainstay of treatment for oligodendrogliomas. The extent of resection depends in large part on the location of the tumor and its proximity to eloquent cortex. If possible, the goal is total resection of the tumor. In patients who undergo total gross resection, no further treatment may be necessary, but the patient must be followed up for clinical or radiologic recurrence. Figure 30-1 depicts a magnetic

Figure 30-1 *Functional MRI scan of recurrent left frontal oligodendroglioma. (See Color Plate.)*

Figure 30-2 *Ojemann cortical stimulator. (See Color Plate.)*

resonance imaging (MRI) scan of a patient with a recurrent left frontal oligodendroglioma.

SURGICAL PROCEDURE

The removal of an oligodendroglioma recurrence is accomplished by a left frontotemporal craniotomy. After adequate exposure of the cortical surface is achieved, mapping of areas which, when stimulated via Ojemann stimulator, produce aphasia is accomplished. Ojemann stimulation results in an inability to speak and this apparatus which is shown in Figure 30-2, is marked with numbered plastic indicators and recorded (areas of aphasia). Following the mapping of the areas of aphasia, Ojemann stimulation is

Figure 30-3 *Anatomic areas are mapped that represent aphasia and anomia. (See Color Plate.)*

Figure 30-4 *Use of Ojemann cortical stimulator in concert with electrocorticography for identification of spike wave and seizure activity. (See Color Plate.)*

used to identify areas where stimulation results in an inability to name the playing card shown to the patient while stimulation is occurring (areas of aphasia and anomia) as depicted in Figure 30-3. Placement of cortical electrodes are used to electrocortigraphically identify areas of seizure activity as is shown in Figure 30-4. Surgical removal of tumor is guided by the boundaries identified by cortical mapping and includes areas identified by electrocorticography.

ANESTHETIC MANAGEMENT AND CONSIDERATIONS

Preoperative Period

1. Discuss the role, contents, and timing of preoperative education surrounding asleep-awake craniotomy.

It is essential that preoperative education for a patient undergoing an asleep-awake craniotomy be thorough, frank, and conducted in such a manner that both the patient and the anesthetist believe that the anticipated procedure should and can be accomplished in an awake state. The anesthetist who is directly responsible for the conduct of the asleep-awake craniotomy and will be present throughout the procedure should meet with the patient at a date prior to the surgery.

The preoperative education should allow first for the anesthetist to assess the suitability of the patient for an asleep-awake craniotomy. Only those patients with the ability to clearly understand risks and benefits and who, in the opinion of the neurosurgeon and the anesthetist, will cooperate during surgery should be considered as candidates for an asleep-awake craniotomy. The preoperative education of the patient should focus on what the patient is to expect from a sensory standpoint. Visually, they are to be instructed in what to expect in the operating room, what they will be seeing when they emerge under the drapes, who they will see, and how they will be dressed. The odors can be especially offensive to some patients and should be explained, especially regarding use of the electrocautery. Tastes regarding use of airway devices and medications should also be explained. The sensation of feeling and touch should focus on how the patient will be positioned and the use of the Mayfield/pinion head holder, the awkward body positioning with the need for minimal movement and the potential for significant discomfort. Special emphasis should be placed on the sounds that may be heard. Usually patients are emerging from anesthesia during removal of the bone flap. The drilling sound is conducted directly to the ear and can be quite loud and disturbing to the patient. The preoperative education should focus next on the required activities of the patient during the surgery.

The mapping of aphasia and anomia should be clearly explained to the patient with attention for the potential of Ojemann stimulation to result in temporary aphasia and anomia. The preoperative education should next focus on how intraoperative issues will be addressed. The patient's seizure history should be thoroughly addressed to assess presence of "aura," time of day when most seizures occur, and medications. The anesthetist must have a clear understanding of the type of seizure the patient has historically and its presentation.

The patient should be fully informed of all plans for dealing with seizures encountered during the procedure. The potential for emergent intubation and general anesthesia should the patient become uncooperative have persistent seizure activity, airway compromise, or hemodynamic instability occur should also be discussed. All additional questions should be addressed and a written outline of all of these details should be provided to the patient for further review. Arguably, the single most important element in the successful awake craniotomy is the well-motivated, well-informed patient.

Intraoperative Period

2. Describe the induction of and maintenance of the "asleep" portion of the awake craniotomy

The purpose of the "asleep" portion of the awake craniotomy is to minimize patient discomfort and facilitate placement of invasive monitoring, patient positioning, local anesthetic injection, and removal of the cranium. This patient is given appropriate prophylactic antibiotics prior to arrival in the operating room. Ondansetron is administered prior to the induction of anesthesia to decrease the potential for nausea and vomiting.

After monitors are placed, induction is accomplished using propofol followed by a remifentanil and propofol infusion. A laryngeal mask airway (LMA) is placed and secured. The patient is manually ventilated to achieve a rate and tidal volume that is sufficient to produce an end-tidal carbon dioxide ($ETCO_2$) representative of low normocarbia ($ETCO_2$ 28-32 mm/Hg). Increases in CO_2 levels above normal concentrations regardless of whether the patient is awake or asleep, will cause and increase in cerebral blood flow that will increase intracranial pressure (ICP). Anesthesia is maintained with the propofol and remifentanil infusion while all invasive monitoring is accomplished.

The patient is placed in a Mayfield headrest after local infiltration, secured to the operating table with straps across the chest, hips, and legs. The surgical field is infiltrated with local anesthesia, surgical prepping and draping are accomplished, and surgery is initiated. Careful attention is placed to the head positioning to assure:

- Access to the airway is maintained at all times
- The LMA is secured and positioned such that it can be rapidly reinserted should the need arise
- The patient can see the anesthetist and is able to see the pictures/playing cards necessary for anomia mapping
- Patient comfort is maximized
- Careful attention to assure that the patient's joints are flexed and the body is secured to avoid movement when turning the table from side to side

A light is placed under the drapes and positioned in such a manner as to provide light to the patient at all times. At this time an arterial blood gas, electrolyte levels, and antiseizure medication levels are collected and treated as indicated.

3. Cite various methods that can be used to reduce intracranial pressure during an awake craniotomy.

Controlling ICP is vitally important during an awake craniotomy. The primary method that is used to reduce ICP in awake craniotomies is accomplished by using osmotic diuretics and hypertonic saline. Immediately after the central line is secured and the urinary catheter has been placed, 1–1.25 gm/kg of mannitol is administered. Additionally, 150 ml of 7.5% saline are also administered over a 2-hour period. Both of these medications facilitate the movement of fluid from the extravascular space into the intravascular space which decreased the total brain fluid volume and ICP.

These patients often develop cerebral edema associated with the lesion and dexamethasone 10 mg every 4–6 hours is also administered at induction. It is prudent to avoid medications/techniques which increase ICP, and these are listed in Table 30-1.

Table 30-1	Factors That May Increase Intracranial Pressure
• Hypercarbia
• Hypoxia
• Coughing/straining
• Venous outlet obstruction from improper positioning
• Trendelenburg position
• Hypertension
• Fluid overload

4. Describe the interventions that can be used to treat intraoperative nausea, confusion, and seizures during an awake craniotomy.

Any anesthetic plan for an asleep-awake craniotomy must account for management of nausea, confusion, and seizures.

- **Nausea:** Treatment of intraoperative nausea focuses on avoiding factors that contribute to nausea such as hypotension, pain, and medications that are especially emetogenic. Rapid movement of the patient subsequent to the administration of anesthetic agents can result in nausea. Moving the patient during the course of the procedure should be done slowly after requesting that the patient close their eyes prior to movement. Additional prophylaxis for nausea includes the administration of ondansetron prior to induction, the use of propofol for anesthesia induction and maintenance, and administration of dexamethasone and the use of ephedrine to treat nausea related to hypotension. Acute episodes of nausea that are unrelated to hypotension may be treated with additional doses of ondansetron. If hypotension occurs, additional doses of ephedrine or vasopressor agents can be administered.
- **Anesthetic management:** Local anesthesia is the primary anesthetic during the awake phases of the operation. The local anesthesia

that is injected subcutaneously contains epinephrine which causes vasoconstriction of local vessels and, after absorption, the systemic effects include tachycardia and increased blood pressure can occur. The maintenance of anesthesia during the period when the skull cap is removed is accomplished by using short-acting anesthetic agents so that hemodynamic instability can be rapidly treated and emergence can occur quickly. Pain can be alleviated by administering short-acting narcotics and augmentation of the field block by the surgeon.

- **Level of consciousness:** Treatment of confusion focuses on avoiding anesthetic agents that contribute to amnesia and can often cause confusion. Medications such as benzodiazepines (midazolam), hypnotics such as diphenhydramine, haloperidols such as droperidol or Haldol, and phenothiazines such as Phenergan or Thorazine should be avoided if possible. Appropriate preoperative preparation is crucial for preventing confusion. Since most patients having an awake craniotomy are emerging from general anesthesia during the bone removal of bone flap, explaining to the patient that there will be noise from surgical interventions such as drilling is imperative. Additionally, it is well recognized that any preoperative focal neurologic deficits will be enhanced immediately upon emerging from general anesthesia.

  This patient exhibited difficulty with verbal expression soon after emergence; however, she was prepared that expressive aphasia, receptive aphasia, or both might occur. Immediately upon emergence, she was unable to speak although she would hold up fingers appropriately. This possibility had been discussed with the patient preoperatively and resulted in minimal discomfort.

- **Seizures:** The treatment of all intraoperative seizures is predicated on the assumption that the potential for seizures have been adequately treated preoperatively as evidenced by therapeutic blood concentra-

tions of antiseizure medications. Blood should be drawn immediately after the induction of anesthesia to determine the phenytoin and Depakote concentrations. Also, cold irrigating fluid placed on the brain by the surgeon has been used to inhibit seizure activity.

This patient's phenytoin level is low, 5 mcg/dl (normal range 10–20 mcg/dl) and after induction he was treated with phenytoin 500 mg prior to emergence. The diagnosis and treatment for intraoperative active seizures must address the following:

- Is the activity being exhibited a seizure?
- Is it a focal seizure or consistent with the seizures reported in the preoperative visit?
- Is the seizure progressing to a grand mal seizure?

During the course of Ojemann stimulation, it may be difficult to determine the onset of aphasia as compared to "absence" seizure activity. The treatment for seizures is to stop the stimulation and frequently no further treatment is routinely necessary. A thorough preoperative seizure history will also determine the presence of any "aura" which the patient is instructed to report to the anesthetist if they occur. The treatment of the aura is the same as for a seizure, stopping brain stimulation. Should the twitching continue, 10–20 mg of propofol may be given. If the seizure activity is inconsistent with that reported preoperatively and/or appears to be progressing to uncontrollable movements of the head and neck after withdrawal of stimulation, application of cold saline to the cortical surface by the neurosurgeon is indicated. If seizure activity continues, administration of propofol 100–200 mg and reinsertion of the LMA is indicated.

The major concerns if a grand mal seizure occurs and is sustained during awake craniotomy is that the violent movement may result in cervical trauma or the head springing free from the Mayfield apparatus and lacerating the scalp on the sharp pins. Also, the increased cerebral neuronal activity will increase the cerebral metabolic rate of oxygen consumption and can also result in swelling of the brain and increase ICP.

5. Describe one technique for awakening the patient while their head is in a Mayfield headrest.

When the patient emerges from general anesthesia, they are in a confined, draped, and dark environment. Their movements are restrained by multiple straps and their head is fixed in the three pins of the Mayfield headrest. Because it takes longer to emerge from propofol than remifentanil, after completing the skin flap, during the creation of burr holes, the propofol infusion is discontinued and the remifentanil drip is decreased and then stopped. The patient emerges from general anesthesia and the LMA is removed just prior to the bone flap removal. Continuation of the propofol and remifentanil infusions until the bone flap is removed can result in hypoventilation causing hypercarbia, and the brain can become swollen at the dural incision.

6. Discuss appropriate sedation techniques after the awake-data has been gathered.

When the neurosurgeon determines that patient participation is no longer essential, sedation may be established. The use of medications and dosages that can contribute to confusion and dysphoria should be avoided. If sedation is to be established prior to dural closure, respiratory depression will result in cerebral edema and closure of the dural will be difficult. Nausea can be triggered by use of narcotics such as morphine and are avoided. Tailoring the depth of sedation should be determined by the individual's current level of anxiety and discomfort. Administering dexmedetomidine may be useful to produce sedation without causing significant respiratory depression.

7. Develop an anesthetic plan for airway management during an asleep-awake craniotomy.

Any plan for managing the airway during an asleep-awake craniotomy must take into account the three distinct times of the surgery: *the asleep phase, the awake phase, and the sedation phase.*

The asleep phase of the surgery must account for the physiologic stimulation that occurs during fixation of the head in the Mayfield headrest. Coughing and bucking during extubation while the patient's head is fixed to this apparatus is prohibitive. Since the LMA is situated above the vocal cords, subglottic nociceptive reflexes are minimally stimulated and bucking may be minimized as compared to an endotracheal tube.

The awake and sedation phases of the procedure do not frequently require airway manipulation. The placement of a nasal cannula with $ETCO_2$ monitoring is sufficient during these phases. Airway obstruction is usually associated with a medication overdose and this situation is easily relieved by pulling the chin forward. Talking to the patient and simply requesting that they take a breath may be sufficient. If the patient will require sustained hyperventilation and muscle relaxation, usually an unforeseen surgical event has occurred. In this instance, additional anesthesia personnel will be needed. Reinsertion of the LMA should be accomplished as soon as possible. When the surgical events permit, an endotracheal tube should be placed using a fiberoptic approach, or if removal of the head from the Mayfield headrest is permitted, under direct vision. If the LMA is not able to be reinserted, the patient must be removed from the Mayfield headrest immediately and bag-mask ventilation established. An induction agent and muscle relaxant is indicated during intubation in order to rapidly facilitate airway management and avoid increases in ICP.

Postoperative Period

8. Discuss the potential causes of nausea, confusion, and seizures during the immediate postoperative period.

Upon the completion of surgery, the patient's head is removed from the Mayfield headrest and the drapes are removed. The patient should be cautioned against exaggerated head movement. Due to the removal of the tumor and associated tissue, intracranial volume is decreased. Shearing of cerebral venous complexes can lead to the development of a subdural hematoma. Nausea, confusion, and lethargy can be a symptom associated with a subdural hematoma. The presence of iatrogenic intracranial pathology should be excluded during the evaluation.

Presentation of seizures immediately postoperatively should be evaluated and managed as in the intraoperative portion of the procedure. Auras and small focal seizures consistent with preoperative history and intraoperative experience should be observed, noted, and reported to the surgeon. The decision to administer supplemental antiseizure medication during the postoperative period is at the discretion of the surgeon. If focal seizures occur and progress to grand mal seizures, administration of an induction dose of propofol should be administered and airway management initiated. Valsalva maneuvers and jerking movements can lead to intracerebral bleeding and cerebral edema which both increase ICP.

REVIEW QUESTIONS

1. The single most important factor in a successful awake craniotomy is:
   a. a low-grade tumor in Broca's area.
   b. maintaining normocarbia.
   c. decreasing ICP.
   d. a highly motivated, well-informed patient.
2. All of the information should be discussed during preoperative education except:
   a. the patient's seizure history.
   b. the limitations regarding the head being placed in a fixed position.
   c. the options communicated by the surgeon should the asleep-awake option fail.
   d. the activities that the patient will be required to perform while they are awake.
3. A patient undergoing an awake craniotomy experiences a focal seizure which is resistant to 2 small doses of propofol which then progresses

to generalized tonic/clonic seizures. The most appropriate initial intervention includes:
   a. instilling cold irrigation solution to the brain.
   b. increasing the dose of ketamine.
   c. administering diazepam.
   d. administering succinylcholine.
4. The patient emerging from the "asleep" part of the "asleep-awake" craniotomy, if properly prepared, will encounter all of the following except:
   a. their head fixed to a rigid frame.
   b. a loud drilling noise.
   c. a dark and confined space.
   d. a sharp pain on left side of the chest.
5. The indications for awake craniotomy include:
   a. patients with receptive aphasia.
   b. patients with tumors in areas of eloquent cortex.
   c. patients without an opinion as to whether they have general or local anesthesia.
   d. patients who have very high pain tolerance.

REVIEW ANSWERS

1. **Answer: d**
   Arguably, the single most important element in the successful asleep-awake craniotomy is a highly motivated, well-informed patient.
2. **Answer: c**
   The anesthetist should determine the patient's wishes with regard to abandoning the asleep-awake technique for a general anesthetic.
3. **Answer: a**
   Cold irrigating solution applied to the cortex has been shown to stop seizure activity.
4. **Answer: c**
   A light is placed under the drapes at the beginning of surgery to avoid the patient awakening in a dark and confined space.
5. **Answer: b**
   Asleep-awake craniotomies are necessary in only a small percentage of patients, those in whom seizure focus may be suppressed during general anesthesia or may be adjacent to an "eloquent" cortical function.

SUGGESTED READINGS

Boulton M, Bernstein M. Outpatient brain tumor surgery: innovation in surgical neurooncology. *J Neurosurg* 2008;108(4):649–564.

Dinsmore J. Anesthesia for elective neurosurgery. *Br J Anaesth* 2007;99(1):68–74.

Erickson KM, Cole DJ. Anesthetic considerations for awake craniotomy for epilepsy. *Anesthesiol Clin* 2007;25(3):535–555.

Frost EA, Booij LH. Anesthesia in the patient for awake craniotomy. *Curr Opin Anaesthesiol* 2007;20(4):331–335.

Manninem PH, Mrinalini B, Lukitto K, et al. Patient satisfaction with awake craniotomy for tumor surgery: a comparison of remifentanil and fentanyl in conjunction with propofol. *Anesth Analg* 2006;102(1):237–242.

Olsen KS. The asleep-awake technique using propofol-remifentanil anaesthesia for awake craniotomy for cerebral tumours. *Eur J Anaesthesiol* 2008;25(8):662–669.

Palese A, Skrap M, Fachin M, et al. The experience of patients undergoing awake craniotomy: in the patients' own words. A qualitative study. *Cancer Nurs* 2008;31(2):166–172.

Petrovich Brennan NM, Whalen S, deMorales Branco D, et al. Object naming is a more sensitive measure of speech localization than number counting: converging evidence from direct cortical stimulation and fMRI. *Neuroimage* 2007;37 Suppl 1:S100–S108.

Piccioni F, Fanzio M. Management of anesthesia in awake craniotomy. *Minerva Anestesiol* 2008;74(7–8):393–408.

Sarang A, Dinsmore J. Anaesthesia for awake craniotomy—evolution of a technique that facilitates awake neurological testing. *Br J Anaesth* 2003;90(2):161–165.

Ophthalmic Surgery

X

Retinal Surgery

31

Sarah E. Giron

KEY POINTS

- Retinal detachments (RDs) are the result of three main causes which include, but are not limited to:

  1. A hole, break, rip, or tear in the neuronal layer.
  2. Exudation of fluid into the subretinal space from retinal vessels.
  3. Traction of adhesions between the vitreous gel and the retina.

- Patients presenting for RD surgeries frequently have a constellation of coexisting diseases.
- Many factors influence the type of anesthesia given to the RD patient and a team approach between the patient, surgeon, and anesthetist is imperative for a successful intraoperative course.
- Nitrous oxide (N_2O) use during general anesthesia will increase the size and pressure of intravitreal tamponading agents.

CASE SYNOPSIS

A 73-year-old woman experienced a spontaneous loss of vision in her right eye is scheduled for a vitrectomy.

PREOPERATIVE EVALUATION AND DEMOGRAPHIC DATA

Past Medical/Surgical History

- Obesity, body mass index (BMI) of 38 kg/m^2
- Tobacco use history of 70+ pack/year
- Poor exercise tolerance
- Hypertension
- Noninsulin-dependent diabetes
- Gastroesophageal reflux disease (GERD)
- Previous surgeries: bilateral cataracts
- She had no anesthetic problems, blood transfusions, and has no familial anesthetic problems.

List of Medications

- Amlodipine (Norvasc)
- Metformin (Glucophage)
- Pantoprazole (Protonix)

Diagnostic Data

- Hematocrit, 39.1%; platelets 240,000/μl; prothrombin time, 11.1 seconds; partial thromboplastin time, 28 seconds; international normalized ratio, 1.0
- Electrolytes: sodium, 135 mEq/l; potassium, 4.2 mEq/l; chloride, 108 mEq/l; bicarbonate, 31 mEq/l; blood urea nitrogen, 20 mg/dl; creatinine, 1.3 mg/dl; glucose, 190 mg/dl
- Finger stick blood glucose was 187 mg/dl on the morning of surgery
- Electrocardiogram (ECG): normal sinus rhythm with nonspecific T-wave abnormalities
- Stress echocardiogram left ventricular ejection fraction of 50% with no wall motion abnormalities
- Chest x-ray: small right pleural effusion

Height/Weight/Vital Signs

- 165 cm, 104 kg
- Blood pressure, 149/87; heart rate, 89 beats per minute; respiratory rate, 18; temperature, 36°C; room air oxygen saturation, 97%

PATHOPHYSIOLOGY

Approximately 1 in 10,000 patients will develop an RD in any given year, with odds of 1 in 300 over a lifetime, and a broad spectrum of symptoms can occur. Most patients will report sensations of flashing lights (related to retinal traction), vision loss, shadows, clouds, or a curtainlike blackness that comes into the field of vision. It can occur spontaneously, when the patient reportedly was straining (working out, running, etc.) or as a result of a trauma such as a motor vehicle accident. Figure 31-1 represents the anatomic structures that comprise the retina. Approximately 40–50% of patients presenting with RDs are myopic, 30–40% have had cataract extractions, and 10–20% have incurred a direct ocular trauma.

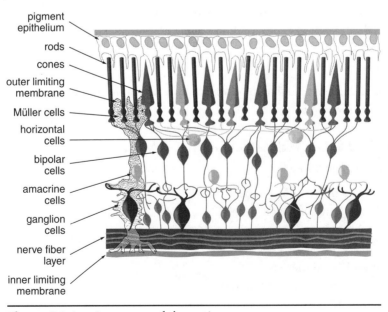

pigment epithelium
rods
cones
outer limiting membrane
Müller cells
horizontal cells
bipolar cells
amacrine cells
ganglion cells
nerve fiber layer
inner limiting membrane

Figure 31-1 *Anatomy of the retina.*

Predisposing factors for the development of an RD include:

- Advanced age (66% of people over 70 years of age will develop an RD)
- Prior eye surgery (especially cataract extraction with or without lens implantation)
- Vitreal diseases such as glaucoma
- RD in the opposite eye
- Metabolic disorders such as diabetic retinopathy
- Vascular disorders such as sickle cell disease
- Tumors
- Myopia

There are three different types of RDs that are based on the etiology of retinal damage: *rhegmatogenous, exudative,* or *tractional.* Rhegmatogenous RDs are the most common form of RD in which a hole, break, rip, or tear in the neuronal layer allows fluid that is present in the vitreous cavity to separate the sensory and retinal pigment epithelium (RPE) layers. Exudative (serous) detachments occur when subretinal fluid accumulates and causes a detachment without a break or tear in the retina. Tractional RDs occur as a result of adhesions between the vitreous gel and the retina and mechanical forces that cause the separation of the retina from the RPE without a retinal break. If a greater concentration of adhesions exist, then there is a higher incidence that a tear or break may occur in the retina. Figure 31-2 represents the cross-sectional anatomy of eye with an associated enlarged retina.

SURGICAL PROCEDURE

The primary surgical goal of an RD is to restore and/or preserve vision in the affected eye. Two types of surgical procedures, a vitrectomy or scleral buckle, are used to repair RDs and can be utilized separately or in combination, depending on the type and severity of detachment, etiology, or disease process.

A vitrectomy is an intraocular procedure in which three 19–25 gauge openings are made into the vitreous cavity. The opening in the inferotemporal quadrant is used to infuse a balanced salt solution throughout the case, while the openings at 10 and 2 o'clock are used to insert a fiberoptic

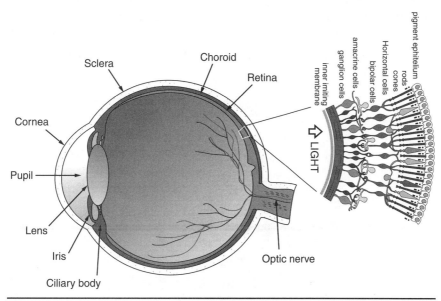

Figure 31-2 *Cross-sectional anatomic representation of eye with enlargement of retina.*

light source and other instruments such as scissors, picks, forceps, and suction. This operation is performed using a microscope with a lens that is either sutured into or held in place over the eye. Once the retina is repaired, a tamponade is needed to rehabilitate sight by securing the retina in proper orientation. An internal tamponading gas bubble is introduced during a vitrectomy to seal a retinal detachment when a scleral buckle alone is not adequate for the repair. These patients must sometimes remain in the prone position postoperatively for several days to facilitate improved retinal reattachment. Silicone oil is utilized as a long-term tamponading agent and it is injected only in those patients that are at increased risk of developing another retinal detachment. The oil will be removed several months later during a second operation. Silicone oil does not usually necessitate a prone position to elicit its tamponading effect and, therefore, is particularly useful in patients who cannot cooperate with a prone postoperative position (i.e., children). Surgical instrumentation used for a vitrectomy is shown in Figure 31-3.

A scleral buckle involves localizing and repairing retinal breaks with a cryoprobe or laser and supporting the damaged retina with an extraocular scleral buckle that consists of a solid or sponge silicone piece. For surgical optimization, a rectus muscle is severed to gain access to the sclera. The retinal tear is then repaired, the silicone buckle is sewn onto the sclera to create an indentation or buckle effect inside the eye, and the muscle is then repaired over the buckle. The buckle is positioned so that it pushes in on the diseased retina (an external tamponading effect), causing the tear to close. Once the break is closed, the subretinal fluid will usually spontaneously resolve over a few days. Sometimes the surgeon elects to drain the subretinal fluid at the time of surgery. Figure 31-4 illustrates a scleral buckle procedure.

ANESTHETIC MANAGEMENT AND CONSIDERATIONS

Preoperative Period

1. Define the types of retinal detachments, the coexisting diseases, and anesthetic concerns associated with retinal surgery.

Rhegmatogenous, exudative, and tractional are the three different types of RDs commonly seen in patients that require treatment. *Rhegmatogenous* RDs can occur from stressful activities, straining, or advanced age. *Exudative* RDs occur as a result of inflammatory processes or tumors. *Tractional* RDs are usually associated with diabetic retinopathy and sickle cell disease. All patients presenting

Figure 31-3 *Surgical instrumentation orientation for a vitrectomy.*

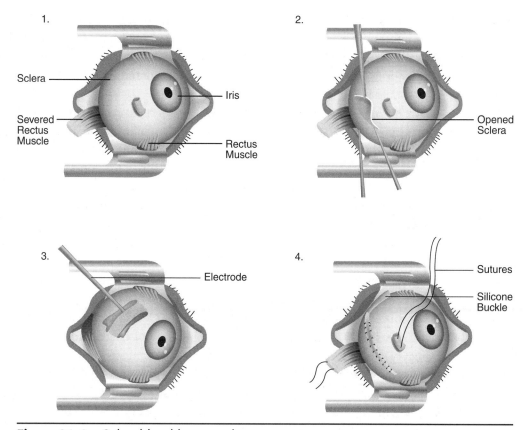

1.

Sclera

Iris

Severed
Rectus
Muscle

Rectus
Muscle

2.

Opened
Sclera

3.

Electrode

4.

Sutures

Silicone
Buckle

Figure 31-4 *Scleral buckle procedure.*

for repair of RDs, emergently or not, should have a thorough preoperative exam.

It is important to evaluate the patient's cardiovascular status due to the physiologic stress associated with general endotracheal anesthesia (GETA), medications utilized during ophthalmic surgery, and the side effects that can occur with regional blocks. An in-depth preoperative evaluation may be indicated, if time permits, to establish a thorough understanding of any cardiac disease state or altered functional capacity. Many patients with tractional RDs present with diabetes; blood glucose levels should be considered when monitoring throughout the perioperative period. Depending on the patient's normal glucose levels, preoperative optimization in glucose readings may be indicated. Since no absolute consensus has been determined as an ideal glucose value, a range of 90–180 mg/dl is an appropriate goal. The risks and benefits associated with the administration of high dose steroids for preventing postoperative nausea and vomiting (PONV) or edema should also be considered when dealing with diabetic patients as these medications can dramatically increase blood glucose levels. The anesthetist should also keep in mind that diabetic patients are at increased risk for silent myocardial ischemia (MI). A continuous ECG should be monitored for ischemic changes throughout the perioperative period. Measures such as preoperative aspiration prophylaxis and rapid sequence induction (RSI) should be considered to prevent aspiration caused by diabetic gastroparesis.

Renal and hepatic function must be considered when dealing with patients who have RD. An electrolyte panel is prudent for any patient, especially those that may have renal disease. Several of the medications used in ophthalmic procedures can drastically alter electrolytes and lead to cardiac dysrhythmias including severe sinus bradycardia, atrial flutter and fibrillation, supraventricular tachycardia, junctional rhythms, and sinus arrest. Altered metabolism and potentially prolonged effects of anesthetics and analgesics should be considered in patients with increased cytochrome P450 enzyme induction or decreased liver function.

Hematological factors should be considered when coagulopathies are present or specifically with patients who have sickle cell disease. Coagulopathies, either pharmacologically induced or because of a disease state, need to be discussed with the surgical team to determine if a regional technique would be contraindicated due to the risk of hematoma with needle placement.

The patient's level of anxiety needs to be assessed, considered, and treated appropriately. When faced with the possibility of vision loss, many patients develop high levels of anxiety and apprehension. Additionally, they are anxious about the possibility of being conscious or aware during a procedure, can become claustrophobic under the operating room (OR) drapes, or are afraid of the pain they might feel during the operation. It is estimated that up to 90% of patients having a vitrectomy experience visual sensations without pain during their procedure that they found frightening if they were not properly informed that these experiences could occur. Appropriate education and preparation, with proper reassurance from both the anesthesia and surgical teams is indicated before any regional technique.

2. Identify drugs commonly used during retinal detachment surgery that may affect coexisting diseases in this patient population.

The effects of several drugs that are important for the ophthalmologist must be used with caution for patients who present for retinal surgery. Topical phenylephrine, when used in the concentrated 10% solution, may cause severe hypertension and should be used with caution or avoided in patients with severe coronary artery disease, history of myocardial infarction, dysrhythmias, or those

with cerebral aneurysms. Patients with borderline renal and cardiovascular function should be evaluated before an infusion of mannitol, an osmotic diuretic, is administered. Large doses of mannitol can be used to decrease intraocular pressure (IOP), but this intervention can also result in serious side effects such as renal failure, congestive heart failure, pulmonary congestion, electrolyte imbalances, extremes in blood pressures, MI, and allergic reactions. Acetazolamide (Diamox) is a carbonic anhydrase inhibitor used to decrease aqueous humor production and lower IOP. Its use is relatively contraindicated in patients with renal and hepatic dysfunction due to its propensity to cause electrolyte imbalances and metabolic acidosis. These patients may develop cardiac dysrhythmias from electrolyte abnormalities. Patients with chronic lung diseases and CO_2 retention may develop severe acidosis from administration of Diamox. The pharmacologic agents commonly used in retinal surgery and their physiologic effects and anesthetic concerns are listed in Table 31-1.

Intraoperative Period

3. Discuss the differences between anesthetic techniques for retinal detachments and the challenges each pose for the anesthetist.

Regional techniques are increasingly popular because they offer increased safety for high-risk patients. They decrease operating room time, provide patients with prolonged analgesia, and are associated with rapid recovery time. Regional techniques, such as retrobulbar, peribulbar, and sub-Tenon's nerve blocks, are reserved for vitrectomies lasting less than 2 hours. The use of regional anesthesia varies according to the patient's willingness to participate, communicate, and cooperate; the patient's coagulation status; and the surgeon's preference. Squinting of the eyes can raise IOP over 25 mm Hg. A facial nerve block can be placed in addition to the regional technique to block these effects by anesthetizing the orbicularis oculi muscle. Topical anesthetic drops, used as the only

Table 31-1	Pharmacologic Agents Commonly Used During Retinal Surgery			
NAME AND ROUTE	**CLASS OF DRUG**	**MECHANISM OF ACTION**	**SIDE EFFECTS**	**INTENDED USE**
Diamox (IV)	Carbonic anhydrase inhibitor	Acts on sodium pump that is part of the mechanism of aqueous humor secretion	Potassium depletion, transient choroidal congestion, diuresis	Decreases IOP
Mannitol (IV)	Osmotic diuretic	Increases plasma oncotic pressure relative to aqueous humor	Transient choroidal congestion, renal failure, congestive heart failure, pulmonary congestion	Decreases IOP
Atropine (Topical)	Anticholinergic	Blocks acetylcholine at ciliary and circular muscles of the iris	Tachycardia, agitation, flushing	Causes mydriasis and cycloplegia
Phenylepherine (Topical)	α-Adrenergic agonist	Capillary decongestion	Tachycardia, palpitations, hypertension	Causes mydriasis
Epinephrine (Topical)	Sympathetic agonist	Decreases aqueous secretion, improves aqueous humor outflow	Tachycardia, hypertension, palpitations	Decreases IOP
Cyclogel (Topical)	Anticholinergic	Blocks acetylcholine at ciliary and circular muscles of the iris	Central nervous system toxicity, incoherence, slurred speech, hallucinations, convulsions in children	Short acting mydriatic and cycloplegia

anesthetic in other anterior segment ophthalmic procedures, unfortunately does not provide the akinesis necessary for a vitrectomy and is frequently used as an additional adjunct for perioperative pain control. Once a retrobulbar block is in place, control of anxiolysis and any necessary supplementation of analgesia should be continued with caution. Because the patient's airway is not readily accessible to the anesthetist, caution should be used to avoid oversedation and airway obstruction. Conversely, a semi-awake, disoriented who is moving, poses a risk of serious damage to the surgical site and can make it impossible to utilize a microscope to repair the detached retina. Intraoperative expectations of the surgical and

anesthesia teams, as well as the patient, need to be discussed preoperatively in order to devise a safe and smooth plan of intraoperative care.

General endotracheal anesthesia is usually reserved for vitrectomies requiring muscle paralysis (as is the case with some scleral buckles) and when the length of the surgery will exceed the estimated duration of local anesthetic action. Other indications for general anesthesia include the inability of patients to remain motionless, patients who refuse a regional technique, and the surgeon's preference. The overall goal of the anesthetist during GETA for repair of an RD should be to minimize hemodynamic variability, maintain normocarbia, and avoid abrupt increases in IOP by providing a smooth anesthetic induction, maintenance, and emergence. The anesthetist should administer medications that inhibit PONV and minimize the use of emetogenic agents, if possible, because vomiting dramatically raises IOP. Patients should be adequately premedicated with an anxiolytic and should take chronically prescribed calcium channel blocker or β-blocker medications to control heart rate and blood pressure. If gastroparesis is a possibility, administering metoclopramide and an H_2-antagonist during the preoperative period is prudent.

The "time-out" procedure should be followed prior to induction to identify and mark the correct surgical eye. Caution should be used when applying the mask for preoxygenation and during ventilation via the mask so as not to apply pressure on the affected globe. A smooth anesthetic induction with an appropriate intravenous (IV) agent, administration of a nondepolarizer muscle relaxant for paralysis, and the use of 4% lidocaine administered using a laryngeal tracheal anesthesia (LTA) kit prior to placement of a preformed right-angle oral Ring-Adair-Elwyn (RAE) endotracheal tube (ETT) is recommended. If N_2O is administered during the case, its use should be discontinued a minimum of 15 minutes before a tamponading gas agent is injected, since continued N_2O use may increase the size of the gas bubble and result in an increase in IOP. Intraoperative antiemetics such as dexamethasone, droperidol, and ondansetron are medications that can help in the prevention of postoperative retching and vomiting that can raise IOP to greater than 40 mm Hg. Intraoperative insertion of a nasogastric tube to empty the stomach may possibly reduce the incidence of PONV. The use of IV lidocaine upon emergence should also be considered to decrease the incidence of coughing during the return of airway reflexes, providing a smooth emergence and thus avoid a subsequent rise in IOP. Table 31-2 lists specific challenges associated with anesthesia management for retinal surgery.

Table 31-2	Challenges Associated with Anesthesia Management for Retinal Surgery
•	Patient safety and preference
•	Akinesia of the eye
•	Appropriate levels of analgesia, amnesia, and anxiolysis
•	Minimal bleeding
•	Maintenance of normal IOP and hemodynamics
•	Smooth induction and emergence
•	Postoperative course void of PONV
•	No access to the patient's airway intraoperatively

4. Discuss whether retinal detachment surgery should be considered an emergency.

While there are time-sensitive surgical concerns associated with this surgery, it is of paramount importance that a cautious approach is undertaken when dealing with these ophthalmologic emergencies. The patient's safety is the primary goal, and life-threatening risks associated with common comorbidities must be minimized prior to proceeding with anesthesia to preserve eyesight. The urgency of the surgery and the risk to vision should be discussed with the surgical team to devise a plan for safe anesthesia within a timeframe that is conducive to preserving the patient's sight.

If it is not possible to perform a regional technique for a patient with a full stomach, then a modified RSI for control and protection of the airway during GETA is indicated. It is not recommended to insert a nasogastric tube in patients with RD who are awake because of the distress and increase in IOP that may occur. Preoperative blood glucose should be corrected if necessary in patients with diabetes mellitus and β-blockers titrated as indicated in patients with cardiovascular disease. Once all standard monitors are applied, preoxygenation should be implemented without the mask compressing the affected globe. Cricoid pressure should be applied during induction using a rapid acting IV hypnotic and muscle relaxant of choice tailored to the individual patient. Muscle relaxation monitoring is useful to ensure that full paralysis is present before direct laryngoscopy (DL) to prevent coughing which can dramatically increase IOP. The use of succinylcholine for RSI in urgent cases is still controversial because of the transient rise in IOP caused by fasciculations. In the closed eye RD patient, succinylcholine has been shown to increase IOP 6 to 8 mm Hg for 1–4 minutes after administration. IOP returns to baseline in 5 to 7 minutes. Although the rise in IOP may be mild and abrupt, the use of succinylcholine should only be used after collaboration with the surgeon to avoid patient injury.

5. What monitors are imperative to patient safety during retinal detachment repairs and why?
Regardless of whether a regional or GETA technique is utilized to correct an RD, all standard monitors should be implemented.

- An ECG is imperative to monitor for ischemic changes, the oculocardiac reflex (OCR), as well as any changes indicative of electrolyte imbalances caused by coexisting illnesses or medications commonly used for ophthalmic purposes.
- Blood pressure measured frequently via an automated cuff must be continually monitored to assess for adequate perfusion and effects on IOP. Studies have shown ocular ischemia and retinal artery occlusion can occur if low systolic blood pressures are allowed to persist throughout the case. Heart rate and blood pressure deviations from baseline can be used to monitor for increasing anxiety or lightening levels of anesthesia.
- Pulse oximetry is essential to assure adequate oxygenation considering the distance and inaccessibility of the patient's airway.

- Continual end-tidal carbon dioxide ($ETCO_2$) monitoring will help avoid hyper- or hypoventilation, important because of the effect hypercarbia has on IOP as well as serving as a safety monitor for airway/circuit disconnects.
- Neuromuscular blockade monitoring should be utilized to assure adequate muscle relaxation and to prevent acute IOP increases from "bucking" or coughing in GETA cases.
- Bispectral index (BIS) monitoring provides information to help the anesthetist assess the patient's depth of anesthesia by evaluating the electromyelogram to determine central nervous system activity.

6. Discuss the effect of ocular physiology on IOP.
The normal range for IOP varies between 10 and 22 mm Hg and increases by several mm Hg in the supine position, varies 1–2 mm Hg with each cardiac contraction and changes 2–5 mm Hg during sleep and upon awakening. IOP contributes to the shape and optic properties of the eye and is determined by many anatomic and physiologic factors including a balance between production and drainage of aqueous humor and by changes in intraocular blood volume.

Aqueous humor is similar to blood plasma and occupies the anterior chamber, or front third of the eye. In addition to helping shape the eye, it also serves to nourish structures such as the cornea and lens, but also carries away waste materials with drainage through the trabecular network, Schlemm's canal, the episcleral venous system, and a system of venous pathways that lead to the superior vena cava. Aqueous humor is formed at a rate of 2 μl/min and drains at a similar rate through the venous system. When venous congestion increases, such as during a Valsalva maneuver or upon coughing, the outflow of aqueous humor is impeded and IOP rises significantly. Changes in venous pressure have been shown physiologically to have the most profound effect on IOP.

Intraocular blood volume is controlled by vessel dilation and contraction of the choroid layer that lies between the retina and the sclera. As choroidal arterioles dilate in response to hypercapnia and constrict in response to hypocapnia, intraocular pressure and volume fluctuate.

Minimal changes in IOP occur when normocarbia is maintained. Hypoxemia may minimally increase IOP through choroidal dilation. Changes in arterial blood pressure also have minimal effects on IOP, although abrupt hypertension and/or profound induced hypotension can affect IOP. It is an elevation in venous pressure that most profoundly increases IOP through an increase in intraocular blood volume and distention of the orbital vessels. Physiologic factors that effect IOP are listed in Table 31-3. Vigilance in maintaining hemodynamic stability with a venous pressure consistent with baseline values is crucial for successful retinal surgery.

7. Describe the effect of anesthetic agents on IOP.

Most general anesthetic agents cause a decrease in IOP. Potential explanations for the decrease in IOP include:

- Reduced choroidal blood volume from a decreased blood pressure.
- Decreased extraocular muscle tension from muscle relaxation resulting in a lower ocular wall tension.
- An increase in papillary muscle constriction that increases aqueous outflow.

Succinylcholine raises IOP up to 8 mm Hg for a total of 7 minutes after administration secondary to prolonged extraocular muscle contraction and its use is controversial during RSI for RD surgery. A summary of the effects of anesthetic medications on IOP is listed in Table 31-4.

Table 31-3 Physiologic Influences on Intraocular Pressure

PHYSIOLOGIC VARIABLE	EFFECT ON INTRAOCULAR PRESSURE
Central Venous Pressure	
Increase	Marked increase
Decrease	Marked decrease
Arterial Blood Pressure	
Increase	Mild increase
Decrease	Mild decrease
PaCO$_2$	
Increased through hypoventilation	Moderate increase
Decreased through hyperventilation	Moderate decrease
PaO$_2$	
Increase	No effect
Decrease	Mild increase
Coughing/Bucking	Marked increase
Vomiting	Marked increase
Deep Inspiration	Mild decrease

Table 31-4	Anesthetic Medications and Their Effects on Intraocular Pressure
DRUG	**EFFECT ON INTRAOCULAR PRESSURE**
Inhaled Anesthetics	
Volatile	Moderate decrease
N_2O	Mild decrease
Intravenous Agents	
Barbiturates	Moderate decrease
Benzodiazepines	Moderate decrease
Ketamine	Controversial
Narcotics	Mild decrease
Propofol	Decrease
Etomidate	Controversial because of myoclonus
Muscle Relaxants	
Depolarizers	Moderate increase
Nondepolarizers	0-Mild decrease

8. Discuss the oculocardiac reflex(OCR), possible causes, and treatment.

The OCR is a response caused by traction on ocular muscles or by pressure exerted on the globe. The afferent pathway is initiated through the trigeminal nerve (CN V) from the ciliary ganglion to the ophthalmic division of the trigeminal nerve through the gasserian ganglion. The main sensory nucleus is located in the fourth ventricle of the brain. Activation of the efferent pathway via the vagus nerve (CN X) can cause cardiac dysrhythmias that can include sinus arrest, heart block, bradycardia, and asystole. This reflex can be stimulated by any number of surgical maneuvers, most commonly during the administration of a retrobulbar block or during muscle manipulation during a vitrectomy.

Attempts to block the OCR with anticholinergics prior to retrobulbar blockade is controversial. Pretreatment has not been shown to consistently be effective, safe, or reliable for blocking the OCR. However, it should be noted that the OCR will usually stop after repeated traction on the rectus muscles due to reflex fatigue. Treatment for the oculocardiac reflex is presented in Table 31-5.

9. List the anesthetic implications for gases that are utilized for retinal tamponading.

Several agents are used as tamponading agents and are included in Table 31-6. When using N_2O during general anesthesia, it is imperative that N_2O be discontinued at least 15 minutes before the gas tamponading agent is injected. If N_2O is not discontinued prior to the gas injection, the gas bubble

Table 31-5	Treatment for Initiation of the Oculocardiac Reflex

- Immediately notify the surgeon to temporarily stop the surgical stimulus until heart rate increases.
- Confirm adequate ventilation and oxygenation of patient.
- Treat with anticholinergic if conduction disturbances continue.
- Ask for surgical application of local anesthetics to rectus muscles for persistent episodes.

	Table 31-6 Retinal Tamponading Agents		
AGENT	**BLOOD:GAS PARTITION COEFFICIENT**	**AVOID N$_2$O**	
Air	Nitrogen in air 0.015	5 days	
Sulfurhexafluoride (SF$_6$)	0.004	10 days	
Perfluoropropane	0.00125	30 days	

will increase in size. This occurs because the N$_2$O is significantly more soluble than nitrogen or other molecules in the tamponading agent, the N$_2$O molecules diffuse into the gas bubble and increase its size. If the bubble continues to increase in size after the eye is surgically closed, IOP increases and may decrease the effectiveness of the retinal repair by jeopardizing ocular perfusion. Additionally, once N$_2$O molecules diffuse from the tamponading bubble postoperatively, the enlarged gas tamponade bubble will shrink, which increases the potential for RD due to the variability of intraocular pressure gradient.

Postoperative Period

The surgery was performed utilizing a retrobulbar block with monitored anesthesia care (MAC), with minimal hemodynamic changes throughout 42 minutes of surgery. Six hours following surgery, the patient was still in the recovery room and was complaining of severe pain. Her vital signs include blood pressure, 168/90; heart rate, 101; and respiratory rate, 28.

10. Discuss possible explanations for the patient's current status.

Pain is the most likely cause of the patient's change in hemodynamic status. The most probable causes of pain after RD surgery include:

- Pain from a distended bladder and inability to urinate.

- Pain in the lower extremities from a deep vein thrombosis.
- Chest pain from MI, angina, shortness of breath from a pulmonary embolism, or other thromboembolic event.

Unlikely causes of the pain because of the delay in symptoms are:

- Pain in the eye from the injected antibiotics and steroids placed at the end of the case.
- Pain in the orbit from a retrobulbar hemorrhage.

It is most important to determine the specific cause of the patient's pain and then to provide interventions that treat the distinct problem.

REVIEW QUESTIONS

1. Which is the initial intervention if the oculocardiac reflex is suspected?
   a. Administer an anticholinesterase drug
   b. Wait for the reflex to fade and a normal rhythm to resume
   c. Immediately intubate the patient
   d. Notify the surgical team and request that they stop surgery
2. During general anesthesia for a retinal detachment repair using sevoflurane, 50% air and 50% oxygen, and vecuronium, one could expect:
   a. increased venous pressure.
   b. increased incidence of the oculocardiac reflex.
   c. increased IOP in healthy individuals.
   d. ocular akinesia.
3. A patient emergently comes to the OR for an appendectomy after undergoing a vitrectomy with a tamponading agent 1 week ago. Which is the best choice of inhalational maintenance during the case to maintain a safe anesthetic?
   a. 50% air, 50% O$_2$ with 1 MAC of sevoflurane
   b. 70% air, 30% O$_2$ with 0.3 MAC of desflurane
   c. 50% N$_2$O, 50% O$_2$ with 0.7 MAC isoflurane
   d. 70% N$_2$O, 30% O$_2$ with 0.5 MAC sevoflurane

4. Which is true regarding tamponading agent reabsorption?
   a. Air is reabsorbed in 5 days.
   b. Sulfurhexafluoride (SF_6) is reabsorbed in 30 days.
   c. Silicone oil is reabsorbed in 10 days.
   d. Perfluoropropane is absorbed in 10 days.
5. Which factor increases IOP to the greatest degree?
   a. Lying in the supine position
   b. Decrease in central venous pressure
   c. Use of succinylcholine
   d. Deep inspiration

REVIEW ANSWERS

1. **Answer: d**
   The initial intervention for treating OCR is to notify the surgical team immediately and have the surgeon release traction or pressure, which frequently extinguishes the response.

2. **Answer: d**
   During general anesthesia there will be a decrease in IOP and venous pressure and the eye will be relaxed. There is no drug that can reliably inhibit the OCR nor can the incidence of OCR be predicted.

3. **Answer: a**
   Regardless the volatile anesthetic used, 1 MAC if the hemodynamic status permits is preferable for maintenance to prevent intraoperative patient awareness. If a patient has had RD repair with an unknown tamponading agent, it is prudent to avoid N_2O in order to prevent another RD or an increase in IOP.

4. **Answer: a**
   Air is reabsorbed in 5 days, SF_6 in 10 days, and perfluoropropane is absorbed in 30 days. Silicone oil is never reabsorbed and usually requires a second procedure to be removed.

5. **Answer: c**
   Lying in the supine position and the administration of succinylcholine are the only options that increase IOP. Administration of succinylcholine raises IOP by 6 to 8 mm Hg, whereas lying in the supine position only increases IOP by 2 to 4 mm Hg. Both decreases in central venous pressure and deep inspiration decrease IOP.

SUGGESTED READINGS

Ahmad S. Sedation techniques in ophthalmic anesthesia. *Ophthalmol Clin North Am* 2006;19:193–202.

Charles S, Fanning GL. Anesthesia considerations for vitreoretinal surgery. *Ophthalmol Clin North Am* 2006; 19:239–243.

Dayani PN, Grand MG. Maintenance of warfarin anticoagulation for patients undergoing vitreoretinal surgery. *Arch Ophthal* 2006;124:1558–1565.

Fang ZT, Keyes MA. A novel mixture of propofol, alfentanil, and lidocaine for regional block monitored anesthesia care in ophthalmic surgery. *J Clin Anesth* 2006;18:114–117.

Kudlak TT, Donlon JV. Jr. Open-eye injury. In: Yao FF, ed. *Yao and Artusio's Anesthesiology*, 5th ed. Philadelphia: Lippincott Williams and Wilkins, 2003:917–933.

McCannel CA, Nordlund JR, Bacon D, et al. Perioperative morbidity and mortality associated with vitreoretinal and ocular oncologic surgery performed under general anesthesia. *Trans Am Ophthalmol Soc* 2003;101: 209–213.

McGoldrick KE. Anesthesia and the eye. In: Barash PG, Cullen BF, Stoelting RK, eds. *Clinical Anesthesia*, 4th ed. Philadelphia: Lippincott Williams and Wilkins, 2001:969–988.

Subramanian ML, Topping TM. Controversies in the management of primary retinal detachments. *Int Ophthalmol Clin* 2004;44:103–114.

Sugisaka E, Shinoda K, Ishida S, et al. Patients' descriptions of visual sensations during pars plana vitrectomy under retrobulbar anesthesia. *Am J Ophthalmol* 2007;104:245–251.

Vann MA, Ogunnaike BO, Joshi GP. Sedation and anesthesia care for ophthalmologic surgery during local/regional anesthesia. *Anesthesiology* 2007;107:502–508.

Ruptured Globe

32

Charles Griffis and Erica J. McCall

KEY POINTS

- There is an increased incidence of ruptured globe injuries in young athletic patients and elderly patients with multiple comorbidities.
- A traumatic accident that results in a ruptured globe may be associated with an acute head injury, cervical spine instability, and thoracoabdominal disruption requiring immediate resuscitation and stabilization.
- Increased intraocular pressure (IOP) can occur during the perioperative period as a result of coughing, straining, and pressure. There is an increased risk of leakage of vitreous humor and intraocular contents during the induction of anesthesia and intraoperative repair of the ruptured globe.

CASE SYNOPSIS

An 88-year-old woman has fallen at home resulting in the following injuries: ruptured left globe, fractured left hip, and fractured right mandible. The patient is admitted to the emergency department. She is evaluated by ophthalmology, orthopedics, oral maxillofacial, and medicine services. The patient specifically denied loss of consciousness before or after the injury, and described the cause of the fall as tripping over a rug. The first surgical procedure that the patient will undergo is repair of left ruptured globe.

PREOPERATIVE EVALUATION AND DEMOGRAPHIC DATA

Past Medical/Surgical History

- Essential hypertension
- Hypothyroidism
- History of breast cancer with resulting left breast mastectomy
- Bilateral total hip replacements

Medications

- Aspirin
- Vicodin
- Synthroid
- Fexofenadine (Allegra)
- Escitalopram (Lexapro)

Laboratory Values and Diagnostic Data

- Hemoglobin, 11.2 g/dl; hematocrit, 34.4%; glucose, 100 mg/dl; blood urea nitrogen, 24 mg/dl; creatinine, 0.9 mg/dl
- Electrolytes: sodium, 140 mEq/l; potassium, 4.5 mEq/l; chloride, 108 mEq/l; carbon dioxide, 23 mEq/l
- Electrocardiogram (ECG): normal sinus rhythm without abnormality
- Chest x-ray (CXR): no acute disease
- Left hip x-ray: fractured femoral head
- Interpretation of the computed axial tomography of head:
  1. Acute fracture at junction of right mandibular head and neck with displacement from the mandibular fossa.
  2. Biconvex well-circumscribed area of hyperdensity in the left lateral globe suggests subretinal hemorrhage; area of irregular density in the left globe likely vitreous hemorrhage; intact intraocular muscles and optic nerve. There is no evidence of cerebral hematoma or other abnormalities.

PATHOPHYSIOLOGY

It is estimated that more than 2 million people per year within the Unites States sustain ocular injuries involving the globe, which results in visual impairment or complete loss of vision in approximately 2% of this patient population. Approximately 33% of childhood blindness occurs as a result of trauma to structures of the eye. There is an increased incidence of ocular injuries associated with young male patients who engage in sports and strenuous physical activities.

A ruptured globe can be defined as loss of the integrity of the outer membranes of the eye. Globe rupture commonly occurs as a result of traumatic injury to a normal eye. Impact from blunt objects can cause anterior-posterior compression of the globe which raises IOP (normally 10–20 mm Hg) high enough to cause rupture of the ocular tissues. The rupture typically occurs in regions where the scleral covering is most thin, including the insertion points of the extraocular muscles, limbus, and around the optic nerve. An anatomic diagram of globe and the associated structures is included in Figure 32-1. Perforation of the globe can occur as a result of impalement by sharp objects and the severity of the injury is proportional to the velocity of the penetrating object. Foreign bodies may remain within the globe. The anterior or posterior segment of the globe may lose surface integrity following eye surgery if external pressure is exerted on the eye.

Since trauma to the globe is often caused by a forceful blow to the head, there is the potential for concurrent injuries such as acute head injuries that may be associated with neurologic damage. Contusions and fractures of orbital and facial bones can occur. Dental fractures can cause bleeding in oral structures and can become dislodged, complicating airway management. Patients who sustain head trauma should have a comprehensive evaluation to determine if cervical spine disruption has occurred prior to nonemergency airway manipulation. If the eye injury is associated with falling down, the patient's body should be surveyed for the presence of injuries to the thorax, abdomen and bony skeleton.

SURGICAL PROCEDURE

Ruptured globe injuries require surgical repair. Basic first aid measures include gentle cleansing of the periorbital area with an antiseptic, irrigation of the globe with sterile saline, followed

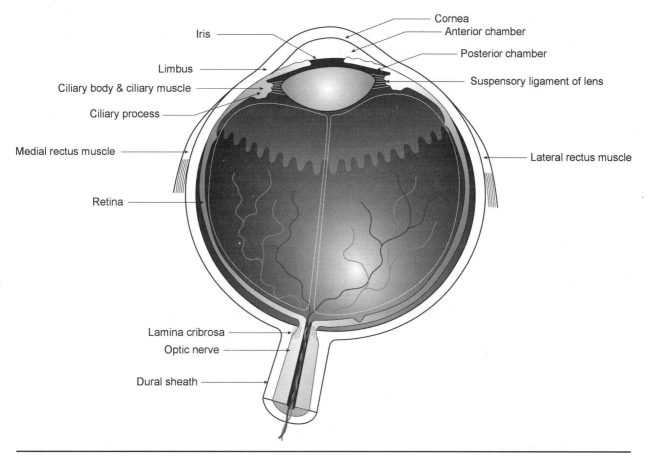

Figure 32-1 *Anatomic representation of the structures that comprise the globe.*

by application of a dressing and shield to prevent external ocular pressure. Patients are counseled to avoid coughing, sneezing, or initiating the Valsalva maneuver to limit the potential for increased IOP.

During surgery, the globe will be gently fixated with the lids elevated. Every effort will be made to avoid exerting pressure on the globe to prevent extrusion of intraocular contents. The eye will be thoroughly examined for the location and extent of injuries. Meticulous assessment and methodical repair of the structures of the globe will occur. These structures include the following: conjunctiva, cornea, sclera, anterior and posterior chambers, iris, lens, and retinal structures (see Fig. 32-1).

ANESTHETIC MANAGEMENT AND CONSIDERATIONS

Preoperative Period

1. Discuss the type and frequency of various coexisting diseases that are associated with patients presenting for repair of ruptured globe.

The presence of coexisting diseases is dependent on the circumstances of injury and the patient population that is affected. In young, athletic patients injured during sports or high-risk physical activities, medical health is likely, but coexisting neurologic, orthopedic, and organ damage is possible, depending on the nature and extent of the traumatic injury. The comorbidities and injuries associated with a ruptured globe are listed

Table 32-1   Comorbidities and Injuries Associated with Ruptured Globe

- Orbital bone fractures
- Head injuries: intracerebral hemorrhage, neurologic trauma
- Neck and cervical spine injuries
- Skeletal fractures
- Cardiac arrhythmias
- Recent eye surgery

in Table 32-1. In elderly patients with a ruptured globe following intraocular eye surgery or a fall, a more extensive list of coexisting medical disease processes associated with the ocular disorders are common.

2. Examine the basic anatomy of the intact eye (anterior and posterior segments); the physiology of aqueous fluid generation, pressure, and flow; and the motor, sensory, and autonomic innervation of the eyeball and its associated muscles.

Understanding the underlying ophthalmologic motor, sensory, and autonomic structure and function will assist the anesthetist to understand the anesthetic implications of the planned surgical repair. The eye is a globular structure, consisting of fluids, intricate internal membranes, and a proteinaceous crystalline lens, surrounded by a tough outer fibrous coat of tissue and muscle, nestled within the protective cavity of the bony orbit (Figs. 32-1 and 32-2).

There are multiple extraocular structures that surround the globe. The eyelids protect and

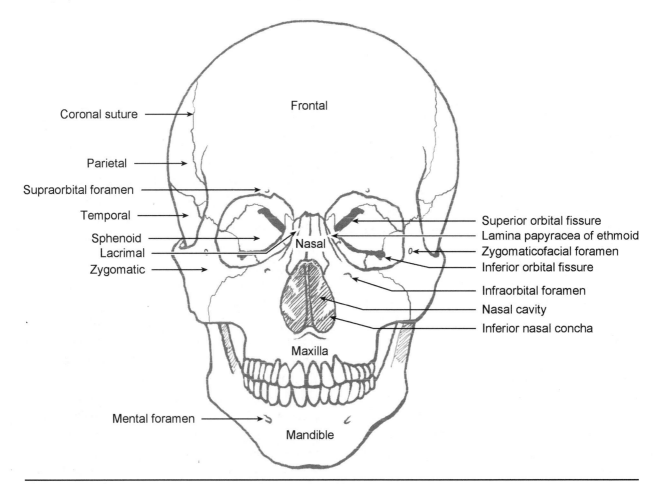

Figure 32-2   *The cranium with emphasis on the bony orbital structures.*

lubricate the eye and consist of thin skin supported by a fibrous layer called the tarsal plate which helps maintain the lids' shape and strength. Various muscles contribute to eyelid movement, including the orbicularis oculi and levator palpebrae. The outermost covering of the eye is a mucous membrane called the conjunctiva that extends from the edge of the cornea to the posterior aspect of the eye, looping back to form the inside of the eyelids. Accessory glands in the eyelids produce most of the liquid tears, which keep the eye moist and drain through the puncta into the nose.

The globe itself is divided into two segments. The anterior segment includes structures that lie anterior to the vitreous humor, a sphere of clear, gel-like material in the posterior globe. Comprising approximately 33% of the eye, the anterior segment includes the cornea (clear front surface of the eye), iris (the colored part of the eye that controls the pupil opening size), ciliary body (membranes derived from the pupil that control lens shape by tension on the lens zonules and secrete nutrient-containing aqueous humor bathing anterior segment structures), and lens. There are two fluid-filled spaces: the anterior chamber lying between the cornea and iris and the posterior chamber between iris and vitreous, containing the lens. The lens is a protenacious structure that consists of three layers: a tough outer capsule, a middle cortex, and a hard nucleus, all of which are suspended by zonule ligaments.

The posterior segment of the globe, which comprises 66% of the eye, consists of the anterior hyaloid membrane, the gel-like vitreous body, retina, choroid layers, and the optic nerve. The vitreous body is surrounded by a clear hyaloid membrane. Vitreous is actually a microfibrillar net-like structure; the gel consistency derives from mucopolysaccharides and hyaluronate acid components. This consistency serves to keep the retina firmly engaged against the lower layers of the eye and maintains the shape of the globe. The retina, the innermost surface, is an extension of the optic nerve, which corresponds to the pia mater meningeal membrane. This region converts light into electrical impulses that are relayed to the brain for interpretation. The choroid layer, immediately inferior to the retina, corresponds to the arachnoid mater meningeal membrane and supplies the retina with oxygen and nutrients. The outermost covering of the eye, called the sclera, corresponds to the dura mater in other areas of the central nervous system (CNS). Thus, the optic nerve sheathe is an extension of the CNS bathed in cerebrospinal fluid. Medications that are injected into this sheathe are rapidly transported to the brain.

Aqueous humor is the major determinant of the IOP which normally ranges from 10 to 20 mm Hg. This fluid is formed by the ciliary body in the posterior chamber by passive filtration from blood vessels and by an active process requiring the enzyme carbonic anhydrase. The fluid moves through the pupil into the anterior chamber and there it is drained via numerous interconnected venous channels associated with the canal of Schlemm. Thus, any factor that obstructs this drainage—elevated venous pressure from coughing or straining, or the mechanical obstruction associated with glaucoma—will cause acute elevations in the IOP. If increases in IOP are extreme, then nutrient supply to the avascular structures of the globe such as the lens and retina can become compromised.

The innervation to the eye is comprised of motor, sensory, and autonomic functions. There are six extraocular muscles controlling movement of the eyeball: the superior, medial, and inferior rectus muscles are all controlled by the oculomotor nerve (cranial nerve [CN] III); the lateral rectus, controlled by the abducens nerve (CN VI); the superior oblique nerve, controlled by the trochlear nerve (CN IV); and the inferior oblique innervated by oculomotor nerve (CN III). Eyelid motor function is controlled by branches of the facial nerve (CN VII). Sensory innervation to the periorbital area and eye structures is derived from the ophthalmic division of the trigeminal nerve

(CN V). The oculomotor nerve sends parasympathetic fibers to the ciliary ganglion that constricts the pupil (miosis), and sympathetic fibers arising from the superior cervical sympathetic ganglion and carotid plexus cause pupillary dilation (mydriasis). The "light reflex" refers to pupillary constriction in response to increased light exposure via oculomotor nerve activation of the preganglionic parasympathetic fibers which originate in the Edinger-Westphal nucleus of the rostral midbrain.

3. Discuss the preoperative evaluation of the patient with a ruptured globe.

The patient should undergo an in-depth interview in which the significant past medical history is elicited and special attention should be directed toward the CNS, cardiovascular (CV), and respiratory systems. The existing disease processes and their severity and treatment should be investigated, along with any previous difficulties with anesthesia and surgery. The cause of the ruptured globe should be thoroughly investigated. Patient falls that are accompanied by loss of consciousness may be associated with CNS or CV abnormalities that can affect the anesthetic management. A patient should be subjected to a thorough physical examination. An airway assessment should be accompanied by a search for occult neck or head injury. A general survey of the body should be undertaken to rule out previously unsuspected injuries, especially when the ruptured globe was caused by trauma. Information gathered from the medical history and physical assessment, appropriate laboratory tests, electrocardiogram, chest x-ray, and other diagnostic tests that should be obtained and interpreted prior to the induction of anesthesia in order to ensure a safe and individualized plan of care.

Intraoperative Period

4. Describe the controversial issues associated with anesthetic management for patients with ruptured globe.

Patients who have sustained a ruptured globe as a consequence of a traumatic accident are not good candidates to receive retrobulbar or peribulbar nerve blocks. Regional anesthesia is relatively contraindicated for several reasons. Insertion of the needle into the infraorbital foramen may cause further damage to traumatized tissue and increase the size and density of a hematoma. This event could result in increased IOP and extrusion of the intraocular contents. Additionally, a regional block may provide inadequate anesthesia as periorbital blood ameliorates the effectiveness of the local anesthetic by preventing the diffusion of sufficient anesthetic molecules to cause blockade of sensory nerves. These patients may sustain associated injuries including orbital fractures, soft tissue contusions or lacerations, and periorbital hematomas. Therefore, this patient will receive general anesthesia.

Patients with open globe injury requiring general anesthesia have two primary airway considerations: potential for pulmonary aspiration

Table 32-2 Effects of Anesthetic Agents on Intraocular Pressure	
DRUG	**EFFECT ON INTRAOCULAR PRESSURE**
Induction agents, benzodiazepines, opioids	Decreases IOP
Ketamine	No effect on IOP with lower doses (3 mg/kg); increases IOP in high doses (6 mg/kg)
Succinylcholine	Increases IOP (5–8 mm Hg) due to prolonged contraction of extraocular muscles
Inhaled anesthetics	Decreases IOP
Nondepolarizing muscle relaxants	Decreases IOP

Table 32-3 Effects of Various Anesthetic Interventions on Intraocular Pressure

INTERVENTION/PHYSIOLOGIC ALTERATION	EFFECT ON INTRAOCULAR PRESSURE
Airway instrumentation	Increases IOP with light levels of anesthesia
Hypoventilation, hypoxemia	Increases IOP
Coughing, vomiting, Valsalva maneuver	Increases IOP
Deep plane of anesthesia	Decreases IOP
Decreased sympathetic nervous system activation	Decreases IOP

with lack of fasting, and potential for increased IOP during laryngoscopy. In considering appropriate measures to secure the airway in nonfasted patients for emergent repair, prevention of aspiration is a priority; if airway examination reveals significant abnormality with potential inability to intubate or ventilate following induction, then awake fiberoptic intubation can be considered with excellent topicalization and appropriate sedation to reduce coughing and increased IOP.

If asleep orotracheal intubation is deemed appropriate in the nonfasted patient, there is some controversy surrounding the use of succinylcholine as a component of a rapid sequence induction. This depolarizing muscle relaxant is associated with an elevation in IOP of approximately 8 mm Hg lasting 5–7 minutes. Several mechanisms are hypothesized to explain this effect: specific tonic response of unique morphologic structures in the extraocular muscles; drug effects on cerebral blood flow; and alterations in the formation of aqueous humor. Regardless, there are no case reports of eye damage attributable to succinylcholine use. Nondepolarizing muscle relaxants lower IOP, thus are the paralytic drugs of choice for these cases, if deemed safe to use for intubation. A summary of the effects of anesthethic agents on IOP is included in Table 32-2.

5. Describe factors that influence intraocular pressure during anesthetic management.
Various anesthetic interventions and the alterations in physiology associated with general anesthesia can have pronounced effects on IOP as listed in

Table 32-3. The most profound effect is a rise that can be associated with direct laryngoscopy and intubation due to sympathetic nervous system stimulation. In general, patients should receive adequate anesthesia prior to airway instrumentation. It is imperative that intraoperative ventilation is adequate in order to avoid hypercarbia and hypoxemia because both of these factors will increase IOP.

6. Discuss the rationale for using intraoperative neuromuscular blockade.
Patients with "open-eye" conditions—a physical opening between the atmosphere and inner eye—are at risk for loss of intraocular contents with coughing, straining, or Valsalva when IOP increases due to increased sympathetic tone and increased venous pressure in periorbital veins. Thus during general anesthesia, such patients should receive nondepolarizing neuromuscular blockade to prevent sudden increases in IOP.

7. Develop an anesthetic care plan to include management of fluid therapy, changes in vital signs, oculocardiac reflex, and appropriate monitoring.
Fluid therapy for patients with ruptured globe should meet patient needs identified on preoperative assessment; the ophthalmologic injury and surgery for repair are not associated with fluid shifts or blood loss. Patients may be hypo- or hypervolemic due to coexisting injury or medical comorbidities, and crystalloid or colloid administration should be titrated to euvolemia.

Basic intraoperative monitors as recommended by the American Association of Nurse Anesthetists (AANA) (ECG, blood pressure, pulse oximetry, end-tidal CO_2) are usually sufficient. Regional anesthesia via retro- or peribulbar block may be associated with unintended intravascular or subarachnoid administration of local anesthetic drug, requiring resuscitation from unconsciousness, seizure, or hypotension. Intraoperative administration of local anesthetic block to patients receiving general anesthesia may be associated with hypotension due to decreased surgical stimulus. Vasodilation associated with potent inhaled anesthetics may produce hypotension requiring vasopressor treatment. Nitrous oxide (N_2O) should be avoided if the surgeon plans intravitreal gas injection; N_2O molecules will diffuse into the bubble, producing increased IOP.

Tension on the extraocular muscles during injury repair may serve as an afferent stimulus arc, via the ciliary ganglion to the ophthalmic branch of the trigeminal nerve, for the oculocardiac reflex. Efferent vagal discharge produces bradycardia, which can be profound. Treatment consists of stopping the stimulus, administration of anticholinergic drugs, and infiltration of periorbital local anesthetics if appropriate.

8. Examine the indications for antiemetic therapy in the patient with a ruptured globe.

The Society for Ambulatory Surgery has issued consensus guidelines on the prevention and management of postoperative nausea and vomiting (PONV), and several risk factors were identified that potentially apply to this specific patient population. Increased risk of PONV is associated with the use of volatile anesthetics, strabismus (extraocular muscle) repair, maxillofacial surgery, and the use of intra- and postoperative opioids. Furthermore, the guidelines state that preventative measures were appropriate in patient populations in which PONV might pose a risk to surgical outcome, and increases in IOP associated with retching and vomiting may well pose a risk to the surgical repair of intraocular structures. Thus, prophylactic treatment for the prevention of PONV should be considered in all patients with ruptured globe. Though numerous medications are available, a combination of dexamethesaone at outset of anesthesia combined with a 5-hydroxytryptamine (5-HT) receptor-blocking medication at conclusion of surgery would appear to be reasonable choices with minimal side effects.

9. Discuss issues related to extubation of the patient with a ruptured globe with or without a full stomach.

Extubation is ideally accomplished without straining or coughing to avoid increases in IOP. In fasting patients, "deep" extubation prior to reflex return is ideal in the absence of airway abnormality or aspiration risk. At the conclusion of surgery, inhaled anesthetics are maintained at surgical levels while administering 100% oxygen, muscle relaxants are reversed, and following return of spontaneous respiration IV lidocaine is administered to inhibit the cough reflex. Following oropharyngeal suctioning, the endotracheal tube cuff is slowly emptied, and the endotracheal tube is removed gently. The patient may be transferred to the postanesthesia recovery area with insufflated oxygen, positioned on his side to allow for secretion drainage.

In a nonfasting patient, a variation of this technique may avoid excessive coughing and straining, yet assure adequate reflex return prior to extubation. All steps outlined in the previous paragraph are followed. At the conclusion of oropharyngeal suctioning, a soft catheter is left in the oropharynx. The patient's head is elevated to 45 degrees, the inhalation agent is discontinued, and the patient is not disturbed again until he is responsive, at which time the pharynx is suctioned and the tube is removed.

10. Case management: induction, maintenance of anesthesia, emergence, and extubation.

The patient was induced with etomidate using a modified rapid sequence induction sequence with cricoid pressure. She was paralyzed with vecuronium and intubated atraumatically using the Glidescope Video Laryngoscope (Verathon; Bothell, Washington). Anesthesia was maintained with N_2O and sevoflurane, a brief period of hypotension was treated with ephedrine and a fluid bolus, and vecuronium was titrated to a single twitch on nerve stimulator. Fentanyl was administered incrementally for analgesia. Ondansetron was administered for emetic prophylaxis. Following surgery completion, residual relaxation was reversed with neostigmine and glycopyrrolate, spontaneous respiration resumed, lidocaine was administered with 100% oxygen, and the oropharynx was suctioned. When the patient opened her eyes to command, the endotracheal tube was removed without coughing and she was transported to the postanesthesia recovery area.

Postoperative Period

11. List the potential complications following repair of ruptured globe.

Acute increases in IOP can occur due to edema, intraocular, or periorbital hemorrhage, which may manifest as pain and nausea or sudden decrease in vision in the affected eye. Periorbital hemorrhage may occur from unsuspected orbital trauma or fracture, resulting in exophthalmos, swelling, and epistaxis. Emesis associated with pain and PONV may result in damage to the surgical repair through acute increases in IOP associated with retching.

12. Discuss the management of postoperative pain in this patient population.

Postoperative pain may be effectively prevented and treated by perioperative peri- or retrobulbar block. When local anesthetic block is contraindicated, pain may be persistent, severe, and associated with PONV. Patients should receive opioid analgesic drugs intraoperatively, and in the postoperative anesthesia care unit to decrease postoperative pain. Antiemetic prophylactic therapy should be administered intraoperatively to help prevent PONV. The head of bed should remain elevated to facilitate venous drainage and prevent excessive swelling, and an ice pack may be applied to operative eye. Severe and persistent postoperative pain that is resistant to high-dose opioid therapy is indicative of increased IOP or periorbital hemorrhage. These findings warrant immediate surgical evaluation, and possible reexploration of the globe to prevent damage to the eye.

13. Explain the pathophysiology related to increased intraocular pressure that occurs in the postoperative period after ruptured globe repair.

One of the most serious postoperative complications associated with repair of a ruptured globe is increased IOP. Increased pressure in the globe can rapidly compress vessels supplying oxygen and nutrients to intraocular structures. The pain is likely caused by a release of acidic metabolites and other mediator molecules. Neurons in trigeminal ganglia project onto emetogenic nuclei in the vagal nucleus tractus solitarius in the brain stem. Facial and eye pain can cause nausea and vomiting via this pathway.

REVIEW QUESTIONS

1. Why is the use of succinylcholine controversial in the anesthetic management of the patient with ruptured globe injury?
   a. The possibility of abnormal pseudocholinesterase may lead to prolonged neuromuscular blockade.
   b. Global rupture may lead to hyperkalemia in susceptible patients.
   c. Prolonged contraction of extraocular muscles may cause elevated IOP.
   d. Fasciculations may lead to decreases in IOP.

2. Which is a contraindication to the use of regional anesthesia for repair of a global rupture?
   a. Periorbital hemorrhage
   b. Decreased IOP
   c. Fractured mandible
   d. Decreased vision in affected eye

3. Neuromuscular blockade during anesthetic management of patients with ruptured globe injury ensures:
   a. adequate retinal perfusion.
   b. successful surgical repair.
   c. control of retinal hypoperfusion due to hemorrhage.
   d. prevention of IOP increases due to Valsalva.

4. Which of the intervention may interrupt the oculocardiac reflex?
   a. Relaxing tension on the extraocular muscles
   b. Pressure on the globe
   c. Tetracaine topical anesthesia on the globe
   d. Irrigation of the periorbital space

5. Deep extubation is often not possible because after repair of a ruptured globe because:
   a. regional anesthesia is usually employed.
   b. hypotension may ensue.
   c. of the risk of aspiration.
   d. IOP may increase.

REVIEW ANSWERS

1. **Answer: c**
   Succinylcholine is associated with a transient rise in IOP, which may theoretically cause loss of intraocular contents.

2. **Answer: a**
   The presence of blood in the periorbital space may ameliorate the effect of local anesthetic by interfering with diffusion of molecules to the sensory nerves, and the volume of local anesthetic may elevate IOP.

3. **Answer: d**
   Coughing or straining, which can be prevented by neuromuscular blockade, is associated with acute increases in IOP.

4. **Answer: a**
   By relaxing the traction on extraocular muscles, the afferent limb (via the ophthalmic branch of CN V) is interrupted, decreasing vagal efferent impulses to the heart.

5. **Answer: c**
   Many patients with open globe injury present for emergent surgical repair of the eye, and may not have been fasting prior to induction of anesthesia. These patients are at risk for aspiration of stomach contents if they are extubated prior to return of protective reflexes.

SUGGESTED READINGS

Barash, PG, Cullen, BF, Stoelting, RK. *Handbook of Clinical Anesthesia*, 5th ed. Philadelphia: Lippincott Williams & Wilkins, 2001.

Bell D. Anesthesia for ophthalmic procedures. In: Nagelhout JJ, Zaglaniczy KL, eds. *Nurse Anesthesia*, 3rd ed. St. Louis, MO: Elsevier Saunders, 2005:881–907.

Drummond PD, Granston A. Painful stimulation of the temple induces nausea, headache and extracranial vasodilation in migraine sufferers. *Cephalalgia* 2005;25:16–22.

Gan, TJ, Meyer, TA, Apfel, CC, et al. Society for Ambulatory Anesthesia Guidelines for the Management of Postoperative Nausea and Vomiting. *Anes Analg* 2007; 105:1615–1628.

Nissman SA, Pasternak JF. Delayed-onset expulsive choroidal hemorrhage attributed to an acute elevation in systemic blood pressure following traumatic globe rupture. *Opthalmic Surg Lasers Imaging* 2005;36(4):340–342.

Rahman, I, Maino A, Devadason D, et al. Open globe injuries: factors predictive of poor outcome. *Eye* 2006; 20(12):1336–1341.

Rozentsveig V, Yagev R, Wecksler N, et al. Respiratory arrest and convulsions after peribulbar anesthesia. *J Cataract Refract Surg* 2001;27(6):960–962.

Scott IU, Mccabe CM, Flynn HW, et al. Local anesthesia with intravenous sedation for surgical repair of selected open globe injuries. *Am J Ophthalmol* 2002; 134(5):707–711.

Vachon CA, Warner DO, Bacon DR. Succinylcholine and the open globe. *Anesthesiology* 2003;99:220–223.

Vinik HR. Intraocular pressure changes during rapid sequence induction and intubation: a comparison of rocuronium, atracurium, and succinylcholine. *J Clin Anes* 1999;11(2):95–100.

Gynecologic Surgery

XI

Open and Laparoscopic Approaches for Hysterectomy

33

Loretta Kitabjian

KEY POINTS

- For many patients, gynecologic procedures may bring about feelings such as fear, shame, anxiety, guilt, and embarrassment regarding the surgical procedure.
- Patients undergoing hysterectomy are at high risk for postoperative nausea and vomiting (PONV).
- Nerve injuries associated with positioning can occur during open and laparoscopic hysterectomy.
- Creation of a pneumoperitoneum using carbon dioxide (CO_2) may cause pronounced physiologic changes such as decreased respiratory compliance, increased airway pressure, and impaired cardiac function.
- Complications such as venous gas embolism (VGE), endobronchial intubation, extraperitoneal insufflation, and pneumothorax may occur during a laparoscopic hysterectomy.

CASE SYNOPSIS

A 49-year-old African American woman has developed painful uterine fibroid tumors. She has been scheduled by her gynecologist for a laparoscopic vaginal hysterectomy.

PREOPERATIVE EVALUATION AND DEMOGRAPHIC DATA

Past Medical/Surgical History

- Past medical history unremarkable; no previous surgical history

Medication List

- No routine medications
- No history of smoking, denies alcohol and recreational drug use

Diagnostic Data

- Human chorionic gonadotropin (hCG) urine pregnancy test, negative
- Hemoglobin, 13 g/dl; hematocrit, 39%; platelets, 240,000/mm^3

- Electrolytes: sodium, 139 mEq/l; potassium, 4.1 mEq/l; chloride, 104 mEq/l; CO_2, 23 mEq/l
- Type and screened for 2 units blood of packed red blood cells

Height/Weight/Vital Signs

- 163 cm, 102 kg
- Blood pressure, 128/64; heart rate, 72 beats per minute; respiratory rate, 20 breaths per minute; room air oxygen saturation, 99%; temperature, 36.8°C
- Electrocardiogram (ECG): normal sinus rate, no abnormalities

PATHOPHYSIOLOGY

Uterine leiomyomas (fibroids) are the most common benign tumor that occur in women; indications for a hysterectomy are listed in Table 33-1. These tumors may grow rapidly, particularly in the perimenopausal age woman. Fibroids may cause excessive uterine size, ureteral obstruction, and occasionally, first-trimester miscarriage. The most common symptoms associated with fibroids are menorrhagia, pelvic pain, or abdominal pressure. Fibroids may develop in any one of three uterine locations: (1) submucosal (within the innermost layer of the uterus); (2) intramural (within the myometrial layer); (3) subserosal (within the outermost uterine layer).

Table 33-1	Common Indications and Prevalence for a Hysterectomy

- Leiomyoma 38%
- Malignancy 15%
- Ovarian tumors 10%
- Abnormal bleeding 13%
- Adenomyosis 9%
- Pelvic pain or adhesions 5%
- Endometriosis 3%
- Uterine prolapsed 1%

Although the exact cause is unknown, genetic alterations and hormones such as estrogen and progesterone may be factors in the growth of fibroids. For patients older than 45 years of age, bilateral salpingo-oophorectomy (BSO) is often performed simultaneously during a hysterectomy to decrease the potential for ovarian cancer. Figure 33-1 provides an illustration of fibroids within the uterus.

SURGICAL PROCEDURE

There are two surgical approaches that are possible when performing a hysterectomy: vaginal and abdominal. The specific technique may be further divided into variations according to the specific disease process, the patient's individual anatomic characteristics, and the surgeon's preference. The vaginal approach is performed with the patient in a dorsal lithotomy position with steep head-down tilt (Trendelenburg). This procedure is advantageous due to surgical visibility, and it is associated with decreased morbidity and mortality. Recovery time is more rapid, is associated with less pain, and is a lower rate of complications involving the surgical site as compared to the abdominal approach. Its use is limited by anatomic and pathophysiologic factors such as uterine size, pelvic adhesions, or the presence of gynecologic cancer all of which may require an abdominal approach. A laparoscopic assisted vaginal hysterectomy (LAVH) is a variation in which the hysterectomy is initially accomplished via a laparoscopic technique, but the remainder of the surgery performed vaginally. Figure 33-2 illustrates the anatomic structures and removal of the uterus during vaginal hysterectomy.

The abdominal approach is performed with the patient in the supine position. Factors such as uterine size and possible need for lymph node dissection will determine if a Pfannenstiel or low midline is used. The abdominal hysterectomy approach may be further delineated into (1) subtotal or supracervical, (2) total, or (3) radical. A subtotal

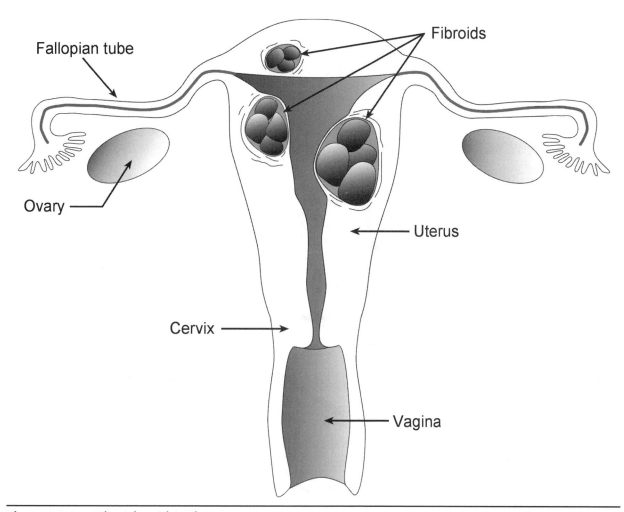

Figure 33-1 *Fibroids within the uterus.*

hysterectomy is the removal of part or all of the uterine fundus with the preservation of the lower uterine segment or uterine cervix. A total hysterectomy includes removal of the uterus and the uterine cervix but not the removal of fallopian tubes or ovaries. A total hysterectomy as compared to a subtotal hysterectomy is performed whenever possible because it decreases the possibility of cervical cancer that may occur in the future. A radical hysterectomy is accomplished if cancer is present and it involves the removal of the uterus, upper vagina, and all the parametrial tissues to the pelvic side wall. Figure 33-3 provides an illustration of the functional anatomy and surgical intervention during an abdominal hysterectomy.

ANESTHETIC MANAGEMENT AND CONSIDERATIONS

Preoperative Period

1. Discuss the potential psychological components for patients having a hysterectomy.

Fear, anxiety, embarrassment, shame, and guilt may be associated with gynecologic surgery. Patients who have chronic pain may have concerns regarding postoperative pain management. Women who have urinary incontinence may be embarrassed about their condition and those who have a pelvic mass may have anxiety or fear of disfigurement and concern over loss of sexual function and desirability. In addition, religion, ethnicity, family

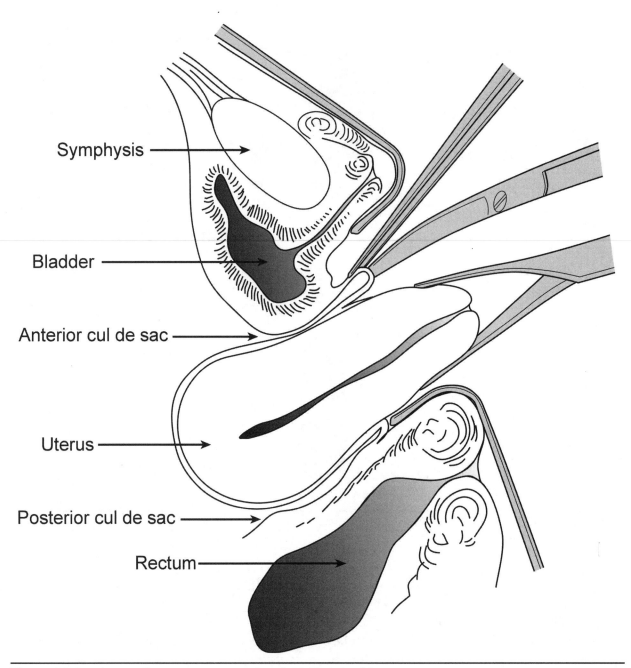

Figure 33-2   *Anatomic structures associated with vaginal hysterectomy.*

dynamics, educational level, gender identity, and the value placed on a woman's reproductive ability all may have an effect on the patient's thought process. The potential psychological ramifications of the surgery should be acknowledged, respected, and managed with sensitivity.

2. Identify the available anesthetic techniques for abdominal or vaginal hysterectomy.

General anesthesia is the most commonly used technique for patients having a hysterectomy. Regional anesthesia offers advantages such as rapid recovery, a decreased incidence of PONV, postoperative

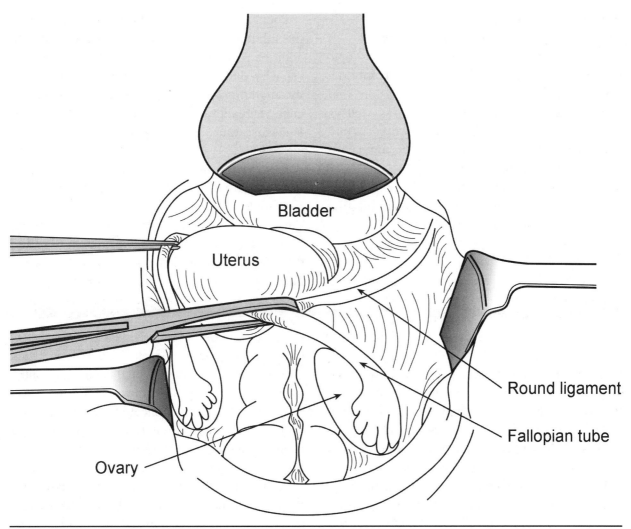

Figure 33-3 *Functional anatomy and surgical intervention during an abdominal hysterectomy.*

pain management, shorter postoperative stay, cost effectiveness, and decreased hemodynamic variability. However, the use of regional technique may be limited by factors such as surgical requirements and surgeon and/or patient preference. Spinal, epidural, or combined spinal-epidural (CSE) anesthesia is appropriate for patients undergoing simple hysterectomy through a Pfannenstiel's incision or vaginal hysterectomy. Spinal anesthesia may be less desirable in the younger population due to the increased propensity for postdural puncture headache (PDPH). If spinal anesthesia is used, a pencil-point needle should be used to decrease the incidence of PDPH.

A blockade of the T4-T6 sensory level is sufficient to provide anesthesia for uterine procedures.

3. Determine the anesthetic technique most commonly used for a laparoscopic hysterectomy.

General anesthesia with neuromuscular blockade is most commonly utilized. The airway is maintained and protected by an endotracheal tube. Neuromuscular blockade allows for maximal insufflation of the abdomen during pneumoperitoneum and results in lower intraabdominal pressures (IAPs) and improved surgical visualization and access.

4. Summarize the disadvantages of nitrous oxide during a laparoscopic hysterectomy.

The use of nitrous oxide (N_2O) during laparoscopic surgery is controversial. Since N_2O is highly diffusible, concerns about bowel distension that will limit surgical vision and access as well as potentially increasing the incidence of PONV are limitations. There is limited scientific data that definitively helps link the use of N_2O to these disadvantages. The decision to include or omit N_2O from a general anesthetic is best determined by the individual anesthesia provider.

Intraoperative Period

5. Describe the pertinent physiological changes that are associated with the lithotomy position.

The lithotomy position is often associated with Trendelenburg (head of the surgical table tilted downward) during a hysterectomy to increase visualization of the perineum and to improve the surgical access. Elevation of the legs above the thorax acutely increases venous return. Mean arterial blood pressure (MAP) and cardiac filling pressures such as central venous pressure (CVP) and pulmonary artery pressure (PAP) increase.

In patients with normal cardiovascular functioning, vascular physiologic reflexes compensate for these transient increases in filling pressures. However, those patients who have cardiovascular disease states may not tolerate the lithotomy or Trendelenburg positions. Patients who have peripheral vascular insufficiency can develop venous stasis and peripheral ischemia. Those patients with a hiatal hernia, gastroesophageal reflux disease, or who are obese, may have decreased lower esophageal sphincter tone and gastric barrier pressure, increasing the risk for regurgitation and aspiration of gastric contents. Acute and significant hypovolemia may not be observed during lithotomy position due to increased venous return. Lowering of the legs into the supine position is accompanied by a redistribution of blood volume which can result in severe hypotension.

Pulmonary side effects that are associated with the lithotomy position are minimal but with the addition of Trendelenburg, functional residual capacity (FRC) is decreased. Obese patients and those who are having general anesthesia experience ventilation-perfusion (VQ) mismatching and atelectasis thus decreasing lung aeration.

6. Discuss risk factors associated with positioning and nerve injury during laparoscopic hysterectomy.

The most common reason of nerve injuries during laparoscopy are caused by pressure that is applied directly on peripheral nerves. Risk factors which may lead to injury from pressure or stretching of the nerves include the length of surgery, the type of leg support used to place patients in the lithotomy position, and preexisting systemic diseases that decrease peripheral blood flow such as diabetes. The "candy cane" stirrup offers minimal control over the positioning of the hips and the lower legs. This device has been implicated with an increased incidence of lower extremity nerve injuries, especially common peroneal nerve. The use of leg supports ("boot-type" stirrups) that hold the entire posterior aspect of the leg are currently used more frequently. Slender patients or those with body mass index (BMI) of less than 20 kg/m^2 are thought to be at increased risk due to lack of subcutaneous tissue padding from external pressure.

7. Assess the various types of nerve injuries that are associated with laparoscopic and open abdominal hysterectomy.

- *Brachial plexus injuries* are the most commonly reported peripheral nerve injury related to positioning. During laparoscopy, the risk of brachial plexus injury is increased for patients with outstretched arms or when they are placed in steep Trendelenburg position. These injuries result in sensory deficits extending to the medial aspect of the hand, forearm, and arm.

- *Femoral nerve injury* is the most commonly reported nerve injury after gynecologic surgery. The damage is presumed to be caused by pressure related surgical instrument retraction on the femoral nerve during an open hysterectomy. However, during laparoscopy the femoral nerve can be injured as a result of protracted nerve stretching during the lithotomy position as a result of prolonged hip flexion, abduction, and external rotation. This injury may be decreased by positioning the patient in low lithotomy and using "boot-type" stirrups. Since the femoral nerve contains both sensory and motor components, nerve injury often results in a loss of sensation over the anterior thigh and medial aspect of lower leg and motor weakness of the quadriceps muscle and decreased patellar reflexes.

- *Lateral femoral cutaneous nerve injury* is similar to femoral nerve injury because of its near-identical anatomic path. In contrast to the femoral nerve which has mixed sensory and motor function, it is solely a sensory nerve. Injury to this nerve causes numbness or pain on the proximal-lateral aspect of the thigh.

- *Obturator nerve injury* results from prolonged hip flexion in the lithotomy position. This nerve has both sensory and motor function. Damage may lead to loss of sensation in the medial aspect of the thigh. Obturator nerve injury that causes weakness of the adductor muscle group and results in an impaired ability to walk is a rare event.

- *Sciatic nerve injury* may result from excessive abduction and external rotation of the hip in combination with flexion of the knee. The sciatic nerve supplies both the motor innervation to the hamstring muscle as well as providing motor and sensory transmission to the lower leg through the common peroneal nerve. Sciatic nerve injury may manifest as a loss of sensation over the calf and on the sole, dorsum, and lateral side of the foot. Foot drop is

also possible due to anterior and lateral compartment muscle weakness.

- *Common peroneal nerve injury* may result from direct pressure such as from the use of candy cane stirrups and excessive stretch due to prolonged flexion of the knee. Excessive external rotation of the hip may also increase risk of injury. The common peroneal nerve contains both sensory and motor functions. Injury may be manifested as loss of cutaneous sensation in the lateral and anterior aspect of the lower leg. More serious injuries may result in foot drop.

8. Describe the pertinent cardiovascular effects associated with a pneumoperitoneum.

Abdominal insufflation alters MAP and heart rate (HR). The extent of these and other cardiovascular changes are multifactorial and are dependent on the IAP that is achieved, the volume of CO_2 that is absorbed systemically, the intravascular volume, and mode and pressure during artificial ventilation. However, one of the most important determinants of cardiovascular function during laparoscopy is IAP. At an IAP below 15 mm Hg, cardiac output is increased due to increased venous return and increased cardiac filling pressures. At IAP values greater than 15 mm Hg, venous return decreases leading to a decrease in cardiac output which may result in hypotension. An increase in systemic vascular resistance (SVR), MAP, CVP, and mean PAP are associated with a pneumoperitoneum for laparoscopic hysterectomy.

Bradyarrhythmias such as bradycardia, atrioventricular dissociation, and asystole can occur during the creation of a pneumoperitoneum and traction on the abdominal viscera or intraperitoneal structures during an open hysterectomy. These phenomena have been attributed to vagal stimulation which initiates the celiac reflex caused by insertion of the Veress needle or trochar, pneumoperitoneum-induced peritoneal stretch, or CO_2

embolization. Conversely, tachyarrhythmias may occur due to increased concentrations of CO_2 and catecholamines.

9. Describe the pertinent respiratory effects of pneumoperitoneum.

Changes in respiratory function during laparoscopic surgery include a reduction in lung volume, increased peak airway pressures and decreased pulmonary compliance due to increased IAP and patient positioning. Elevated IAP reduces diaphragmatic excursion and shifts the diaphragm cephalad, leading to early closure of smaller airways (increased closing capacity) causing atelectasis and decreased FRC. This upward shift of the diaphragm may lead to preferential ventilation of the nondependent portions of the lung which results in V/Q mismatch and increased of intrapulmonary shunting.

10. Relate the use of CO_2 for creation of pneumoperitoneum.

Carbon dioxide gas is most commonly used during laparoscopic surgery because it is nonflammable, rapidly absorbed from the vascular space and easily excreted from the respiratory system. CO_2 is readily available and inexpensive. The disadvantages that are associated with the use of CO_2 gas for the pneumoperitoneum include increased risk of hypercarbia resulting respiratory acidosis. It is theorized that that CO_2 causes peritoneal and diaphragmatic irritation, which has been linked to postoperative shoulder pain. Air and oxygen both support combustion when bipolar diathermy or lasers are used. Nitrogen, argon, and helium have been studied but are considered more hazardous due their low blood gas solubility and potential to create a VGE.

11. List four respiratory complications associated with a pneumoperitoneum.

- **Endobronchial intubation** may occur due to cephalad displacement of the diaphragm and the carina during pneumoperitoneum and migration in the ETT during Trendelenburg positioning. The result may include decreased oxygen saturation, increased peak airway pressure, and the potential for bronchospasm from stimulation of the carina from the distal end of the ETT. The treatment for this situation involves manual ventilation with 100% oxygen; assessing the adequacy of bilateral, equal, and clear breath sounds; and finally, manipulating the ETT into the proper position.

- **Extraperitoneal insufflation** may be diagnosed by identifying a dramatic increase in end-tidal CO_2 ($ETCO_2$) and the presence of subcutaneous emphysema. Treatment includes immediately notifying the surgeon and exsufflation until the CO_2 is eliminated. This complication frequently resolves rapidly after surgery. The anesthetist should be cautious and determine if subcutaneous emphysema is present in the neck region. If so, ventilation and reintubation may be difficult or impossible to accomplish.

- **Venous gas embolism (VAE)** is a rare complication, but it can result in death. Carbon dioxide gas enters the venous system by placement of a trochar into a vein or an abdominal organ. An "air lock" is created at the junction between the inferior vena cava and the right atrium which disrupts blood flow into the heart. It may manifest as a sudden loss of $ETCO_2$, tachycardia, arrhythmias, hypotension, hypoxia, increased CVP, altered heart tones (mill-wheel murmur), and cardiovascular collapse. The treatment for VAE includes exsufflation, ventilation with 100% oxygen, aspiration from a CVP line, placing the patient in a head-down left lateral position to increase blood flow into the heart, and administration of fluids and vasopressors to augment the patient's blood pressure.

- A **pneumothorax** may occur due to diaphragmatic or pleural trauma, or though a defect in the aortic or esophageal hiatus. Increased airway pressures, absence of breath sounds over the affected lung, precipitous oxygen desaturation, hypoxemia, hypercarbia, and hemodynamic instability may be seen. The definitive treatment used for a pneumothorax that causes physiologic compromise is immediate thoracentesis.

Postoperative Period

12. Compare various pharmacologic and nonpharmacologic methods used to attenuate PONV.

Various nonpharmacologic methods are used to minimize the potential for developing PONV and these strategies are listed in Table 33-2.

Traditional antiemetic drugs used for the prevention of PONV include anticholinergics (atropine, scopolamine), antihistamines (cyclyzine, diphenhydramine), and phenothiazines (promethazine, prochlorperazine). Other commonly used antiemetics include:

- Benzamide (metoclopramide) which blocks dopamine receptors centrally within the vomiting center and chemoreceptor trigger zone (CTZ) as well as peripherally in the gastrointestinal tract. The drug also increases gastric emptying, increases lower esophageal sphincter tone, and lowers gastric fluid volume. Rapid IV administration may cause abdominal cramping, dystonia, and extrapyramidal reactions. Metoclopramide is contraindicated in patients with intestinal obstruction and should be avoided in patients with Parkinson disease.
- Butyrophenones (droperidol and haloperidol) act as a dopamine receptor antagonist within the CTZ. Droperidol has an onset of action from 30 to 60 minutes after administration and also an extended duration of action from 4 to 24 hours. However, the use of droperidol has been limited due to the US Food and Drug Administration (FDA) black box warning because of reports of QTc prolongation and torsades des pointes. This warning contained administration guidelines which include:
- Droperidol should not be given to those patients with known or suspected QTc prolongation.
- It is also held in those patients at risk for QTc prolongation such as congestive heart failure, bradycardia, cardiac hypertrophy, hypokalemia, hypomagnesemia, or those taking medications which may increase QTc.
- If droperidol is to be given, a 12-lead ECG is to be done prior to treatment to determine QTc interval.

Table 33-2   Methods Used to Decrease the Potential for PONV

- Use of regional anesthesia technique if possible
- Administration of medications used for PONV prophylaxis
- Gastric decompression with oral or nasogastric tube
- Adequate perioperative IV hydration
- Avoid/minimize use of N_2O
- Minimize use of neostigmine if muscle relaxation is necessary
- Pain control using nonsteroidal anti-inflammatory drugs, local anesthesia infiltration

- Post-droperidol administration, continuous ECG monitoring for 2–3 hours is necessary to observe for arrhythmias.
- The lowest dose of droperidol is to be given, with small increases to effect.
- Haloperidol has an onset of 30 minutes after administration with duration of about 4 hours. Adverse effects to butyrophenones include extrapyramidal side effects, orthostatic hypotension, neuroleptic malignant syndrome, and serious ECG changes.
- Dexamethasone is a synthetic steroid that is frequently used as a prophylactic measure against PONV. The exact mechanism by which dexamethasone exerts an antiemetic effect has not been determined; however, it may have an inhibitory effect on prostaglandin synthesis or antagonize neurokinin type 1 receptors present in the CTZ. It is most efficacious when given concomitantly with other antiemetic medications. Due to its slow onset of action (2 hours) and long half life (46–72 hours), dexamethasone is most efficacious if it is administered early in the perioperative phase and the antiemetic effects prolonged.
- Hydroxytryptamine type 3 receptor antagonists ($5HT_3$) such as ondansetron, dolasetron, and granisetron are medications that are commonly used for PONV prophylaxis. Ondansetron has a half-life of 3–4 hours and is thus best given toward the completion of surgery for PONV coverage. The time of administration of dolasetron has not been shown to decrease PONV. All $5HT_3$ antagonists have similar efficacy at equipotent doses and the side effects include headache, abdominal pain, increased liver enzymes, and possible QT prolongation.

13. Discuss the mechanism of shoulder pain commonly seen after laparoscopic surgery.
Shoulder pain is a common type of discomfort that is experienced on the first postoperative day following laparoscopic surgery. The visceral-like pain that is reported by patients is thought to be caused by the pneumoperitoneum rather than use of trochars in the peritoneal space. The pneumoperitoneum is thought to induce pain by distension of the peritoneum and abdominal wall leading to traction of the nerves and injury to blood vessels. Carbon dioxide contributes to pain by decreasing the intraperitoneal pH leading to acidosis. The resulting inflammation is believed to irritate the phrenic nerve which is perceived as shoulder pain. Ketorolac (Toradol) is an effective treatment for shoulder pain after laparoscopic surgery.

REVIEW QUESTIONS

1. Which nerve injury results in a loss of sensation over the anterior thigh and medial aspect of lower leg and motor weakness of the quadriceps muscle?
   a. Common peroneal
   b. Lateral femoral cutaneous
   c. Obturator
   d. Femoral

2. Sensory blockade at the ____ dermatome should be achieved if a spinal or epidural anesthetic technique is administered for hysterectomy?
   a. T4-T6
   b. T6-T8
   c. T1-T2
   d. T8-T10

3. Which hemodynamic parameter is decreased with creation of a pneumoperitoneum?
   a. Mean arterial pressure
   b. Stroke volume
   c. Systemic vascular resistance
   d. Pulmonary artery pressure

4. Which of the following respiratory parameters is increased with pneumoperitoneum?
   a. Peak inspiratory pressure
   b. Functional reserve capacity
   c. Vital capacity
   d. Pulmonary compliance

5. Which best describes the mechanism of action associated with metoclopramide?
   a. Enhances release of acetylcholine
   b. Inhibits prostaglandin synthesis
   c. Antagonizes hydroxytryptamine type 3 receptors
   d. Blocks dopaminergic receptors in the vomiting center, CTZ, and gastrointestinal tract

REVIEW ANSWERS

1. **Answer: d**
   Femoral nerve injury results in a loss of sensation over the anterior thigh and medial aspect of lower leg and motor weakness of the quadriceps muscle.

2. **Answer: a**
   Blockade of the sensory dermatome at T4-T6 provides adequate anesthesia for an open hysterectomy.

3. **Answer: b**
   Stroke volume is the only parameter of those listed that is decreased after creation of a pneumoperitoneum.

4. **Answer: a**
   Peak inspiratory pressure is the only parameter of those listed that is increased after creation of a pneumoperitoneum.

5. **Answer: d**
   Metoclopramide acts by blocking dopaminergic receptors located in the vomiting center, CTZ, and gastrointestinal tract.

SUGGESTED READINGS

Barnett JC, Hurd WW, Rogers RM Jr, et al. Laparoscopic positioning and nerve injuries. *J Minum Invasive Gynecol* 2007;14:664–672.

Gerges FJ, Kanazi GE, Jabbour-khoury SI. Anesthesia for laparoscopy: a review. *J Clin Anesth* 2006;18:67–78.

Giarrusso KA. Gynecology/infertility surgery. In: Jaffe RA, Samuels SI, eds. *Anesthesiologist's Manual of Surgical Procedures*, 3rd ed. Philadelphia: Lippincott Williams & Wilkins, 2004:647–651, 690–693.

Ho KY, Gan TJ. Postoperative nausea and vomiting. In: Lobato EB, Gravenstein N, Kirby RR, eds. *Complications in Anesthesiology*. Philadelphia: Lippincott Williams & Wilkins, 2008:571–580.

Lawler KM. Laparoscopic surgery. In: Karlet M, ed. *Nurse Anesthesia Secrets*. St. Louis, MO: Elsevier Mosby, 2005:347–353.

Monti-Siebert EJ, Dorman L, Hill D. Positioning for anesthesia and surgery. In: Nagelhout JJ, Zaglaniczny KL, eds. *Nurse Anesthesia*, 3rd ed. St. Louis, MO: Elsevier Saunders, 2005:398–399.

Nguyen, NT, Wolfe BM. The physiologic effects of pneumoperitoneum in the morbidly obese. *Ann Surg* 2005; 241(2):219–226.

Smith JC, Wright EL. Haloperidol: an alternative butyrophenone for nausea and vomiting prophylaxis in anesthesia. *AANA J* 2005;73:273–275.

Tsen LC. Anesthesia for obstetric care and gynecology surgery. In: Longnecker DE, Brown DL, Newman MF, et al., eds. *Anesthesiology*. New York: McGraw Hill Medical, 2008:1489–1497.

U.S. Food and Drug Administration. FDA Talk Paper *Dear Healthcare Professional*. Available online at http://www.fda.gov/medwatch/SAFETY/2001/inapsine.htm. Accessed April 24, 2009.

Waters E. Anesthesia for laparoscopic surgery. In: Nagelhout JJ, Zaglaniczny KL, eds. *Nurse Anesthesia*, 3rd ed. St. Louis, MO: Elsevier Saunders, 2005:705–713.

Dilation and Curettage

Donna Jasinski

34

KEY POINTS

- Dilation of the cervix and the curettage of the uterine lining is a common gynecologic procedure performed for diagnostic or therapeutic indications.
- Most patients who have a dilation and curettage (D&C) are discharged on the same day as the procedure.
- Risks associated with a D&C include a perforated uterus.

CASE SYNOPSIS

A 43-year-old woman with infertility and intervention with in vitro fertilization (IVF) 7 weeks ago has been experiencing vaginal bleeding for the past 2 weeks. She is scheduled by her gynecologist to have a D&C procedure.

PREOPERATIVE EVALUATION AND DEMOGRAPHIC DATA

Past Medical/Surgical History

- No significant past medical history
- D&C for spontaneous abortion 2 years ago

List of Medications

- Prometrium (fertility drug)
- Serophene (fertility drug)

Diagnostic Data

- Hemoglobin, 9.1 g/dl; hematocrit, 27.3%
- Beta-hCG level, 150 mIU/ml indicating pregnancy at approximately 1 month gestation
- Ultrasound: negative for fetal activity

Height/Weight/Vital Signs

- 160 cm, 77 kg; body mass index (BMI), 30.1

- Blood pressure, 140/90; heart rate, 92 beats per minute; respiratory rate, 18 breaths per minute; room air oxygen saturation, 97%; temperature, 37.1°C

PATHOPHYSIOLOGY

Abnormal uterine bleeding is often a result of benign fibroid tumors (myomas), polyps, hormonal imbalances of progesterone and estrogen, retention of the placenta post-childbirth, or early pregnancy failure. The uterus is a muscular, pear-shaped, hollow organ lined by the endometrium which thickens in response to estrogen and, once ovulation occurs, progesterone prepares the lining for implantation of an embryo as shown in Figure 34-1. The IVF process includes administering hormonal medications to the patient, harvesting several eggs after ovulation, egg retrieval and fertilization in a petri dish, incubation, and transfer of the embryo 2 to 5 days later into the uterus. Approximately one-third of all women have mild to moderate cramping or light bleeding during the first trimester of pregnancy; however, if the bleeding is followed by severe cramping, miscarriage is likely. Miscarriages occur most often during the first 3 months of pregnancy and result in 15–20% of all clinically recognized pregnancies. Ultrasound examinations and beta-hCG tests are done when vaginal bleeding is present and early termination of the pregnancy is suspected. The term "missed abortion" is used to define a nonviable pregnancy retained for a minimum of 8 weeks. An "incomplete abortion" is the term to define the passage of some fetal or placental tissue; however, some of the tissue is retained within the uterus. Anatomic representation of the uterus and cervix is shown in Figure 34-1.

SURGICAL PROCEDURE

The patient is positioned in lithotomy with her legs in stirrups. A tenaculum is inserted into the vagina to provide stability and expose the cervix. A uterine sound is inserted into the cervix to determine the safe depth that the cervical dilators and curettes can be inserted. When an incomplete abortion occurs, the cervix is frequently open. When the cervix is closed, it must be dilated. Metal dilators of increasing diameter are inserted into the cervix to dilate it approximately 1.5 cm. Once this opening is achieved, either a sharp curette is used to scrape the lining of the uterus or vacuum aspiration is used to evacuate the contents of the uterus. Suction aspiration can be done via electric vacuum or manual aspiration with a 60-ml syringe and a cannula. This process is illustrated in Figure 34-2.

ANESTHETIC MANAGEMENT AND CONSIDERATIONS

Preoperative Period

1. Discuss the common coexisting diseases of women who present for D&C.

Women of all ages and with varying medical conditions present for D&C. Women under the age of 40 may have unexplained bleeding due to hormonal imbalance and oftentimes coexisting endocrine pathology is present. Menstrual abnormalities have been linked to obesity in young women. Women over the age of 40 may have abnormal bleeding due to endometrial cancer. Cardiac disease is associated with the postmenopausal period and is often present. Anemia is often present in women who have experienced hemorrhage. Since this patient has experienced vaginal bleeding for the past 2 weeks, she is anemic. Physiologic compensation in response to mild to moderate degrees of anemia that develops gradually in a healthy female, frequently does not pose additional surgical and anesthetic risk.

Figure 34-1 *Anatomic representation of the uterus and cervix.*

A — Speculum

B — Clamp Speculum Dilator

C — Curette Speculum Clamp

Figure 34-2 *Instrumentation used for the D&C procedure.*

2. Discuss the impact of anemia on tissue oxygenation.

Each gram of hemoglobin binds with 1.39 ml of oxygen. A normal hemoglobin for women ranges from 12.1 to 15.1 g/dl. Excessive vaginal bleeding from any cause can result in decreases in hemoglobin and, as a consequence of that decrease, a lowering of arterial content of oxygen (CaO_2). The decrease in CaO_2 will impact delivery of oxygen to the tissues. Compensation occurs due to the production of 2,3-diphosphoglycerate as a result of anaerobic metabolism and result in a rightward shift of the oxygen-hemoglobin dissociation curve which facilitates release of oxygen from hemoglobin. Increased sympathetic nervous system tone stimulates the myocardium to increase cardiac output in order to provide more oxygen at a tissue level. The patient has a 9.1 g/dl hemoglobin and a hematocrit of 27.3% and a heart rate on the high end in compensation for the anemic state. It is critical that the anesthetist maximize the oxygenation to assure adequate tissue delivery. A higher fraction inspired oxygen delivery should be a consideration.

3. Describe the potential link between obesity and infertility.

The incidence of obesity has dramatically increased over the last decade and has reached epidemic proportions within the United States. The presence of obesity is associated with all age groups and its incidence is increasing rapidly in women in their childbearing years. Researchers have found that obese women of reproductive age have up to a 67% higher incidence of miscarriage as compared to women of normal weight. The risk of miscarriage further increases in obese women who receive infertility treatment. Obese women also have a higher incidence of polycystic ovaries, abnormal ovulation, and hormonal imbalances. These factors impact the ability of a woman to become pregnant and to sustain the pregnancy to full term.

4. Explain the implications of BMI and anesthetic risk.

BMI is a calculation of body fat based on height and weight. The formula to calculate BMI = (weight in pounds/[height in inches] × [height in inches]) × 703, or in the metric system BMI = (weight in kilograms/[height in meters] × [height in meters]). A normal BMI is between 18.5 and 24.9. Overweight individuals have a BMI between 25 and 29.9 and obese individuals a BMI greater than 30. Obesity increases the morbidity and mortality associated with anesthesia due to its impact on the various physiologic systems. Obese individuals have an increased metabolic demand, oxygen consumption, incidence of sleep apnea, abdominal pressure, the volume of distribution for lipid soluble drugs, cardiac output, and risk of developing arrhythmias due to myocardial hypertrophy. These patients have a decreased functional residual capacity and gastro-esophageal sphincter tone. There is an increased risk of gastric aspiration and preoperative prophylaxis accompanied with a rapid sequence induction is indicated. Preoperative data that should be assessed prior to surgical intervention include an electrocardiogram to identify any ischemia, arrhythmias, and hypertrophy and a chest x-ray to evaluate heart size and evidence of pulmonary hypertension. Consultation with a cardiologist to evaluate the patient's cardiovascular status is warranted if the patient has a history of cardiac related symptoms.

5. Discuss the physiologic and hormonal changes associated with pregnancy that may increase the risk of gastric aspiration.

During pregnancy, there is an increase in progesterone. Progesterone antagonizes the effects of motilin which is an amino acid peptide that is secreted into the mucosa of the proximal portion of the small intestine and results in the onset of uterine contractions. This substance facilitates gastric emptying. Thus, increased progesterone secretion delays gastric emptying. Furthermore, placental gastrin secretion results in increased gastric acidity, decreased lower esophageal tone, and increased intragastric pressure. Patients who present for anesthesia who are between 12 and 14 weeks pregnant should be considered to be a "full stomach" and are believed to be at increased risk of gastric aspiration.

Intraoperative Period

6. Discuss the airway management concerns for a patient who is obese.

The anesthetic technique that can be utilized for this procedure includes general anesthesia, spinal anesthesia, or sedation with paracervical block. If general anesthesia is indicated due to the specific patient situation, a mask technique or insertion of a laryngeal mask airway (LMA) is unsuitable for airway management for obese patients. Since the obese patient is at risk for aspiration, the potential for a difficult airway, and obstructive sleep apnea, placement of an endotracheal tube should be accomplished. The head-elevated laryngoscopy position (HELP) in which the head and neck are elevated above the chest and abdomen improves the view of laryngeal structures by aligning the airway axes during direct laryngoscopy. The reverse Trendelenburg position allows for increased diaphragmatic excursion and functional residual capacity. This maneuver allows for more effective preoxygenation prior to the induction of anesthesia.

7. Describe the anesthetic considerations associated with the lithotomy position.

Improper positioning may lead to nerve injuries in the lower extremities. The nerves that are predisposed to compression and damage include the femoral, sciatic, obturator, lateral femoral cutaneous, and common peroneal. Nerve injury in the lithotomy position has been reported to be 1:3608 patients. Of these injuries, 78% involve the common peroneal nerve, 15% the sciatic nerve, and 7% the femoral nerve. These nerve injuries are most common among patients who are thin, endure a prolonged surgical procedure, and smoke cigarettes. The common peroneal nerve is a branch of the sciatic nerve which is responsible for sensory and motor innervation to the lower leg, feet, and toes. It is anatomically positioned lateral to neck of fibula below the knee. Injury can occur with compression of lateral aspect of knee against stirrup can result in foot drop and paresthesias to the lower extremity. In order to avoid common peroneal nerve damage, it is essential to pad the stirrup and properly place the lower leg in order to avoid compression.

Injury to the hip joints can also occur when patients are placed in the lithotomy position.

Proper care while initiating the lithotomy position includes raising or lowering both legs simultaneously and avoiding external rotation and hip flexion beyond 110 degrees. Injury to the common peroneal nerve will result in foot drop, the inability to evert the foot, and the loss of dorsal extension of the toes. Sciatic nerve injury can result from excessive external rotation and pressure in the region of the sciatic notch. Sciatic nerve injury results in weakness or paralysis of muscles below knee, and numbness of the foot and lateral half of the calf. The anesthetist must be vigilant when raising the foot of the operating table in order to avoid injuries to the fingers and hands when the arms are tucked on the either side of the body.

8. Discuss the ventilatory and cardiovascular changes that are associated with the lithotomy position.

In a ventilated patient, peak inspiratory pressure and end-tidal carbon dioxide ($ETCO_2$) values will increase, and vital capacity and functional residual capacity decreases. Depending on the degree of hip flexion, abdominal contents are displaced upward on the diaphragm and impede lung excursion especially when patients are placed in the Trendelenburg position. These physiologic changes are amplified for patients who are obese and significant ventilation–perfusion mismatch resulting in hypoxemia and hypercarbia can occur. The risk of gastric aspiration increases during general anesthesia when patients are placed in the lithotomy position.

The estimated blood volume contained in both legs is between 250 to 500 ml. When placed in the lithotomy position, gravity increases the flow of blood from the legs increasing the central blood volume. Perfusion to the lower extremities is reduced and central venous pressure and pulmonary capillary wedge pressure is increased. This position also promotes venous stasis increasing the potential for deep vein thrombus formation. When the lithotomy position is combined Trendelenburg, cardiac output decreases.

9. Discuss the advantages and disadvantages of providing regional anesthesia for a D&C.

A major advantage of a spinal or epidural regional technique is that airway maintenance and artificial ventilation is frequently unnecessary. Other advantages include decreased anesthetic requirements for providing sedation, postoperative analgesia, decreased cardiopulmonary depression, and a lower incidence of postoperative nausea and vomiting (PONV).

A disadvantage for using neuraxial anesthesia for use during a D&C procedure is the duration of the anesthetic relative to the short length of the procedure. In obese patients, a regional technique may be technically challenging to perform due to difficulties identifying the iliac crests or the spinous processes, problems with depth of needle insertion, and epidural catheter migration associated with changes in position. Another issue may be an unexpected high block due to different dosing requirements in the obese. Researchers have found to be a direct positive correlation with increase in weight and the height of the block with any given dose. It is theorized that increased abdominal tissue mass exerts pressure on the abdominal vasculature which directly increases the blood volume within the epidural venous plexus. The engorged veins push inward on the dura mater decreasing the volume of cerebrospinal fluid within the subarachnoid space. Since the patient is awake when a regional technique is performed, premedication and continuous sedation with a benzodiazepine and/or an opioid should be considered as the patient is often anxious and may be emotionally distraught.

10. Discuss the advantages and disadvantages of providing general anesthesia for a D&C.

An advantage associated with general anesthesia is that the patient is unconscious and not aware of the sounds of the suction which can be bothersome for a woman who has endured a miscarriage. Furthermore, the pelvis is completely relaxed and the pelvic exam by the gynecologist can be accomplished most effectively.

Disadvantages associated with general anesthesia include an increased risk of aspiration and nerve injury, the potential for difficult airway management, and an increased incidence of PONV. If inhalation agents are administered, there is a dose-related increased risk for uterine atony or relaxation that may increase the incidence of bleeding. Anesthetic-related complications are considered greatest with general anesthesia for D&C.

11. Discuss the effects of inhalation agents on uterine smooth muscle.

All of the inhalation agents relax uterine smooth muscle by decreasing the availability of intracellular free calcium and inhibiting contraction. The degree of uterine relaxation is dependent on the dose that is administered. Uterine atony is associated with increased blood loss. Desflurane and sevoflurane cause a greater uterine relaxant effect as compared to isoflurane, at 1.5 MAC.

12. Explain the pharmacologic properties of oxytocin (Pitocin).

Oxytocin is a hormone that is produced in the paraventricular nuclei of the hypothalamus and is secreted from the posterior pituitary. The physiologic action associated with oxytocin includes stimulation of uterine contraction. A synthetic form is administered to increase the frequency and force of uterine contractions. When a spontaneous abortion is associated with uncontrolled bleeding, the surgeon will ask the anesthetist to administer 10 units of oxytocin to enhance uterine contraction.

13. Describe the technique that is used to correctly administer a paracervical block.

A paracervical block is considered a nerve block and is usually performed by the gynecologist. The technique for the block involves the use of a local anesthetic, usually 1% lidocaine, 1% lidocaine with 0.005 mg/ml epinephrine, or 3% chloroprocaine. To enhance the comfort of the patient and to decrease anxiety, sedation by using a benzodiazepine and small doses of propofol should be considered. Under sterile technique, in the lithotomy position, the cervicovaginal joint is identified with the index finger. A 10-ml syringe and 23-gauge needle with a needle extender are used to inject 1 to 3 ml volumes of local anesthetic at 0.5 cm depth, 1 cm depth, and 1.5 cm depth slowly in the cervicovaginal joint at the 4 or 5 o'clock and 7 or 8 o'clock positions (5 to 10 ml total at each location) to reach the sacrouterine ligaments. This intervention, as shown in Figure 34-3, anesthetizes Frankenhauser's ganglion which is the location for the visceral sensory never fibers to the upper vagina, cervix, and uterus. The anesthetist should be aware of volumes of local injected and vigilant for possible signs of local anesthetic toxicity when large volume of local anesthetic are used.

14. Discuss the possible complications associated with the D&C procedure.

As with any procedure, the anesthetic risks are determined by the patient's preoperative comorbid diseases and overall health status. The risks

Figure 34-3 *Location of the paracervical block.*

related to anesthesia for a D&C are usually related to airway management difficulties, light anesthesia, or nerve injury. The risk of surgical complications associated with the D&C procedure is relatively low. The surgical complications include uterine perforation, cervical tear, infection, and bleeding. The anesthetist must be prepared for periods of peak surgical stimulation. For example, when uterine dilators are inserted into the cervix, the anesthetic depth should be appropriate so that there is no patient movement which could increase the possibility of uterine perforation. The concentration of inhalation agent that is used should be decreased when possible to lessen the potential for uterine relaxation and bleeding.

Postoperative Period

15. Discuss postoperative nausea and vomiting management for patients having a D&C procedure.

The occurrence of PONV is associated with general anesthesia and gynecologic surgical procedures increase the risk. Certain factors have been associated with a higher incidence and unfortunately these factors apply to the patient scheduled for a D&C. They include female gender, outpatient, young adult, and gynecologic surgery. The patient presented also has an additional risk factor which is obesity. Adequate intravenous volume replacement is also essential to help reduce the possibility of PONV.

Most patients scheduled for a D&C are at high risk for PONV. In the past low-dose droperidol was considered a low cost-efficient agent to combat PONV. However, due to the black box warning issued in 2001 by the US Federal Drug Administration (FDA) related to cardiac QT prolongation and abnormal rhythms, it is no longer considered the drug of choice used for PONV prophylaxis. Dexamethasone has been found to be as effective as droperidol in preventing PONV. The exact mechanism of the antiemetic properties of steroids is unknown; however, it is postulated that decreasing prostaglandin synthesis or inhibiting neurokinin-1 receptors in the vomiting center has an antiemetic effect. The serotonin antagonist, ondansetron is effective in prevention and treatment of PONV.

Combination therapy using dexamethasone and a serotonin antagonist has been found to be of benefit for PONV prophylaxis as the emetogenic effects induced anesthetic agents involves a variety of receptors and neurologic pathways. By antagonizing these various receptors and pathways, decreasing PONV is frequently achieved.

16. Discuss the postoperative pain management for a patient who has had a D&C.

The character of the pain that is most frequently experienced after a D&C procedure is uterine cramps and duration extends for 24 hours. Oral acetaminophen with codeine is usually prescribed. Continuous administration of aspirin and ketorolac should be avoided to decrease the potential for uterine bleeding. Patients who experience persistent and severe pain should be evaluated for the possibility of a uterine perforation.

REVIEW QUESTIONS

1. The patient presenting for a D&C has a low hemoglobin value which shifts the oxyhemoglobin dissociation curve to right and:
   a. decreases the affinity between oxygen and hemoglobin.
   b. increases epinephrine release from the adrenal medulla.
   c. decreases the CO_2 production in peripheral tissues.
   d. increases baroreceptor stimulation in the carotid body and aortic arch.
2. The nerve that is most likely to be damaged from compression of the lateral aspect of the fibula immediately below the knee is the:
   a. sciatic nerve.
   b. obturator nerve.
   c. common peroneal nerve.
   d. femoral nerve.

3. The hormone that increases the risk of gastric aspiration during pregnancy is:
   a. estrogen.
   b. motilin.
   c. gastrin.
   d. progesterone.

4. A paracervical block anesthetizes the:
   a. uterus and cervix.
   b. cervix and vagina.
   c. uterus, cervix, and upper portion of the vagina.
   d. cervix, upper portion of vagina, and urethral orifice.

5. Which is true regarding the effect of inhalation agents on uterine tone?
   a. The degree of atony is dose dependent
   b. Causes uterine contraction
   c. Has minimal effects
   d. Increase intracellular calcium causing contraction

REVIEW ANSWERS

1. **Answer: a**
   A low hemoglobin value facilitates the production of 2,3-diphosphoglycerate caused by anaerobic metabolism. This situation decreases the affinity of hemoglobin and oxygen by causing a confirmation change in the hemoglobin molecule.

2. **Answer: c**
   The origin of the common peroneal nerve is on the outer surface of the fibula immediately below the knee. Damage to this nerve from pressure against the stirrup can result in foot drop and lower extremity parasthesia.

3. **Answer: d**
   Progesterone inhibits the effects of motilin thereby decreasing gastric motility.

4. **Answer: c**
   A paracervical block anesthetizes Frankenhauser's ganglion and provides anesthesia to the uterus, cervix, and upper portion of the vagina.

5. **Answer: a**
   Inhalation agents cause uterine atony that can increase blood loss. The degree of uterine atony is determined by the dose (concentration) of the inhalation agent that is administered. The greater the dose, the greater inhibition of uterine contraction.

SUGGESTED READINGS

Allen RH, Kumar D, Fitzmaurice G, et al. Pain management of first-trimester surgical abortion: effects of selection of local anesthesia with and without lorazepam or intravenous sedation. *Contraception* 2006;74:407–413.

Agostini A, Provansal M, Collette E, et al. Comparison of ropivacaine and lidocaine for paracervical block during surgical abortion. *Contraception* 2008;77(5):382–385.

Braimah FE, Arciaga P, Tekle E, et al. Evidence-based medicine: safety of moderate/heavy IV sedation (MHIVS) vs general endotracheal anesthesia (GETA) for d&c for spontaneous abortion. *Anesthesiology* 2004;101:A1203.

Brodsky JB, Lemmens HJ. Regional anesthesia and obesity. *Obes Surg* 2007;17:1146–1149.

Collins JS, Lemmons HJ, Brodsky JB, et al. Laryngoscopy and morbid obesity: a comparison of the "sniff" and "ramped" positions. *Obes Surg* 2004;14:1171–1175.

Glantz JC, Shomento S. Comparison of paracervical block techniques during first trimester pregnancy termination. *Int J Gynecol Obstetet* 2001;72:171–178.

Gomez PI, Gaitan H, Nova C, et al. Paracervical block in incomplete abortion using manual vacuum aspiration: randomized clinical trial. *Obstet Gynecol* 2004;103 (5 pt. 1):943–951.

Lopez JC, Vigil-de-Gracia P, Vega-Malek JC, et al. A randomized comparison of different methods of analgesia in abortion using manual vacuum aspiration. *Int J Gynecol Obstet* 2007;99(2):91–94.

Sinclair DR, Chung, F, Mezei G. Can postoperative nausea and vomiting be predicted? *Anesthesiology* 1999;91:1.

Swancutt DR, Luesley DM, Eastaugh JL, et al. Anaesthetic choice in the colposcopy clinic: a retrospective analysis of routinely collected data. *Int J Obstet Gynecol* 2008;115(5):646–652.

Yoo KY, Lee JC, Shin MH, et al. The effects of volatile anesthetics on spontaneous contractility of isolated human pregnant uterine muscle: a comparison among sevoflurane, desflurane, isoflurane, and halothane. *Anesth Analg* 2006;103:443–449.

Obstetric Surgery

XII

Cesarean Section

35

Greg Nezat

KEY POINTS

- Spinal anesthesia is considered an ideal choice for parturients undergoing cesarean section.
- Preeclampsia is a systemic disease process with multiple anesthetic considerations.
- A complete physical exam and history are critical when assessing the parturient with preeclampsia.
- The anesthetist must explain to the parturient in detail what to expect during a cesarean section.
- A plan of treatment for inadequate spinal analgesia must be outlined prior to cesarean section.
- Postoperative treatment of parturient with preeclampsia includes maintenance of adequate analgesia, hemodynamic control, maintenance of appropriate fluid and electrolyte balance, and seizure prophylaxis.

CASE SYNOPSIS

A 28-year-old parturient with an estimated fetal gestational age of 39 weeks presents to the labor and delivery unit where she is diagnosed as having preeclampsia. During an attempt at induction of labor, the fetus demonstrates a nonreassuring fetal heart rate. It is decided that a cesarean section will be performed.

PREOPERATIVE EVALUATION AND DEMOGRAPHIC DATA

Past Medical/Surgical History

- Previous cesarean section 22 months ago
- Tonsillectomy as a child—no anesthetic complications
- Gestational gastroesophageal reflux disease (GERD)
- Allergy to penicillin; develops rash

List of Medications

- Prenatal vitamins
- Magnesium sulfate
- Tums

Diagnostic Data

- Hemoglobin, 10 g/dl; hematocrit, 30%; platelet, 125 mm^3
- Glucose,139 mg/dl
- Blood urea nitrogen, 13 mg/dl; creatinine, 0.8 mg/dl
- Electrolytes: sodium, 140 mEq/l; potassium, 3.9 mEq/l; chloride, 104 mEq/l; carbon dioxide, 24 mEq/l
- 24-hour urine protein, 320 mg/l

Height/Weight/Vital Signs

- 163 cm, 100 kg
- Blood pressure,150/98; heart rate, 90 beats per minute; respiratory rate, 18 breaths per minute; room air oxygen saturation, 98%; temperature, 98.9°F
- Fetal heart rate, 130–140 beats per minute

PATHOPHYSIOLOGY

Preeclampsia is a systemic disease process which does not have a clearly defined pathogenesis. The exact etiology of preeclampsia is unknown but the condition affects 5–9% of all pregnancies with 85% of cases of preeclampsia affecting women in their first pregnancy. This condition is one of the most common comorbidities found in parturients. Risk factors that are associated with preeclampsia are included in Table 35-1. Multiple etiologic explanations exist for the development of preeclampsia including immunologic factors, genetic factors, a molecular variant of angiotensinogen, factor V Leiden mutation, excessive maternal inflammatory response to pregnancy, endothelial factors, abnormal increases of intracellular free calcium concentration, promotion of endothelial expression of procoagulants, and altered handling of fatty acids by the liver.

Table 35-1   Risk Factors for Preeclampsia
• History of preeclampsia
• Family history of preeclampsia
• Nulliparity
• Primipaternity
• Chronic hypertension and renal disease
• Obesity
• Insulin resistance
• Gestational diabetes
• Sickle cell disease
• Multiple pregnancies

Regardless of the exact etiology of preeclampsia, endothelial damage causes increased platelet aggregation, decreased production of vasodilatory substances, increased glomerular capillary permeability, and increased sensitivity to norepinephrine and angiotensin. The manifestations of these pathologic changes include thrombocytopenia, increased liver enzymes, increased systemic vascular resistance, and proteinuria and edema.

SURGICAL PROCEDURE

Delivery by cesarean section accounts for approximately one third of all births in the United States, at about 1 million cases per year; it is one of the most common surgical procedures in the United States. Cesarean section is indicated for maternal factors such as arrested labor, prior cesarean section, abnormalities of placentation, or deteriorating maternal health (as in severe preeclampsia). Fetal factors, for example, macrosomia, malpresentation, and nonreassuring fetal status, may lead to delivery by cesarean section. Cesarean section involves entry of the peritoneal cavity using a Pfannenstiel incision followed by incision of the lower uterine segment. After delivery of the fetus and placenta the uterus and abdomen are closed. Complications can include hemorrhage, infection, and laceration of the uterus or bladder.

ANESTHETIC MANAGEMENT AND CONSIDERATIONS

Preoperative Period

1. Define the diagnostic criteria of mild and severe preeclampsia.

Mild preeclampsia is diagnosed during pregnancy if the following criteria are met:

- *Blood pressure:* Sustained systolic pressure of 140 mm Hg or sustained diastolic blood pressure at least 90 mm Hg after the 20th week of pregnancy in a parturient who had previously normal blood pressure
- *Proteinuria:* Greater than 300 mg in a 24-hour period
- *Edema:* Not a reliable sign of preeclampsia as it is present in approximately 30% of all parturients

Severe preeclampsia is diagnosed during pregnancy if at least one of the following criteria is met:

- *Blood pressure:* Systolic pressure greater than 160–180 mm Hg or a diastolic pressure greater than 110 mm Hg.
- *Proteinuria:* > 5 g over a 24-hour period or a "dipstick" urine of +3 or +4
- *Oliguria:* Urine output of less than 500 ml in a 24-hour period
- *Neurologic symptoms:* Headache, visual disturbances, or other cerebral symptoms; the presence of grand mal seizures that are not related to other neurologic or metabolic conditions are diagnostic of eclampsia
- *Other associated symptoms:* Epigastric pain, pulmonary edema, liver dysfunction of unknown etiology, and thrombocytopenia.

2. Identify appropriate assessment interventions commonly used to evaluate the parturient with preeclampsia.

- Vital signs: blood pressure, heart rate, oxygen saturation, temperature, respiratory rate
- Physical exam/history: headache, epigastric pain, visual disturbances, seizures

- Laboratory assessment:
  - Hematocrit and hemoglobin should be assessed for hemoconcentration—a common finding in the hypertensive patient and one which supports the diagnosis of preeclampsia.
  - Platelet counts are obtained to assess for thrombocytopenia.
  - Renal function can be assessed with measures of serum uric acid and creatinine levels. Uric acid levels during pregnancy are typically lower than normal range and levels of 5 mg/dl are considered abnormal. Likewise, creatinine levels during pregnancy are approximately 0.5 mg/dl and levels of 0.9 mg/dl are considered abnormal during pregnancy. Urine protein is collected over a 24 hour period and serves as a marker for renal dysfunction.
  - Increasing serum transaminase levels can suggest progression of the disease. Decreased serum albumin levels suggest capillary leakage and can be used to help quantify the extent of the disease. Increasing levels of lactic acid dehydrogenase (LDH) are suggestive of hemolysis. Any patient with signs or symptoms of severe preeclampsia, clinical signs of coagulopathy, or right upper quadrant pain should have coagulation studies completed (PT/aPTT, fibrinogen, and D-dimer).

3. List the major teaching points the anesthetist should address with both the parturient and their significant other prior to cesarean section.

A thorough explanation of the sequence of events during the spinal anesthetic placement and the surgical procedure has a tremendous benefit to both the patient and the patient's significant other. When patients and their families know what to expect, they frequently experience less anxiety prior to the surgery. Additionally, a thorough explanation builds patient confidence in the anesthetist.

The parturient should inform the anesthetist of any symptoms of low blood pressure such as feelings of anxiety, diaphoresis, or nausea. The patient should be informed that they will feel pressure and movement during the cesarean section, especially during the period of time immediately before delivery. The patient should be made aware of the possibility of nausea and vomiting associated with the exteriorization of the uterus.

4. Discuss the preoperative medications that are commonly administered prior to cesarean section.

While experts have not reached a consensus on the use of premedications prior to cesarean section, the most recent report by the American Society of Anesthesiologists Task Force Obstetric Anesthesia (2006) recommends that the practitioner "consider the timely administration of nonparticulate antacids, H2 receptor antagonists, and/or metoclopramide for aspiration prophylaxis."

Intraoperative Period

5. Explain the clinical effects of spinal anesthesia in a patient with preeclampsia.

Spinal anesthesia can usually be safely administered in a patient with *mild* preeclampsia. A common side effect of the administration of spinal anesthesia is a hypotension. In patients who have intravascular volume depletion, such as those with preeclampsia, hypotension can rapidly ensue because of the abrupt onset of the sympathectomy from preganglionic B fiber blockade. In order to reduce the chance of rapidly developing and severe hypotension after the placement of a subarachnoid block (SAB), the rapid infusion of a balanced salt solution (typically 10 ml/kg) or 500 ml of colloid, should be started immediately prior to SAB. Due to the short intravascular half life of balanced salt solutions, if administration is accomplished more than 15 minutes prior to the SAB, then intravascular volume expansion may be inadequate.

Patients will typically have at least a T10 sensory nerve block 4 minutes after spinal placement and a T4 sensory nerve block 8 minutes after placement. As the spinal becomes established, the patient will feel warmth, tingling, numbness, and heaviness in their lower extremities and these sensations will move up their torso. Inactivation of proprioceptive nerves at the level of the T6 dermatome which innervates the intercostal muscles will cause some patients to feel as though they cannot breathe. This can provoke feelings of claustrophobia; however, informing the patient preoperatively that this sensation may occur can reduce the likelihood of anxiety.

In the event of a significant drop in blood pressure, typically 20% below the baseline values, the patient will often report feelings of restlessness and nausea before the blood pressure monitor will display a reading. This symptom is associated with central medullary hypoxia. In addition to the sympathectomy that results from the SAB, the gravid uterus can cause aortocaval compression especially if the mother is in the supine position. Sustained left uterine displacement (SLUD) decreases the degree of compression and can restore adequate preload and reduce afterload. Figure 35-1 depicts the aorta and inferior vena cava in relation to the uterus. It is reasonable to administer vasopressors to avoid severe hypotension. Intravenous (IV) fluids should be infused rapidly if hypotension occurs.

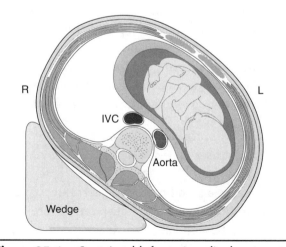

Figure 35-1 *Sustained left uterine displacement.*

6. Identify the dermatome level of sensory blockade needed if neuraxial anesthesia is used during cesarean section.

Typically, a T4 to T5 dermatome sensory blockade is desirable. Patients who have a sensory block as low as T6 (located at the tip of the xiphoid process) can usually tolerate the manipulation involved in cesarean section.

7. Construct a plan of treatment for a patient who experiences inadequate sensory blockade during cesarean section.

Multiple steps should be taken when assessing an inadequate spinal and deciding on an appropriate course of action. Some patients experience of fear and anxiety and any sensation (e.g., pressure, pulling) may be interpreted as pain. If the patient confirms that she feels pressure or pulling and not sharp pain, then reassure her that these sensations are normal. Also, encourage the patient's significant other to talk with the patient thereby providing a distraction from the sensations. If it is determined that the patient is having pain, determine the location of the pain. If it is near the incision site, the surgeon has the option of injecting low concentrations of local anesthetic medication at the incision site. If this intervention is ineffective, or if the pain is not located at the incision site, the anesthetist has a few options.

If the surgery has not started, an epidural may be placed and dosed slowly to achieve an appropriate sensory block. Another option is to postpone the case until the SAB completely recedes and administer a second SAB. The optimum time to wait for a second attempt has not been definitively determined and a second SAB can result in a high or complete spinal.

If the surgery has already commenced and the patient feels pain, the anesthetist can administer small doses of ketamine (10–40 mg IV). Ketamine is a potent analgesic; however, it should be used with caution because it can provoke a significant increase in blood pressure due to the drug's sympathomimetic activity. Administration of midazolam is prudent after the baby has been delivered to decrease the potential for emergence delirium. Rapid acting narcotics such as IV fentanyl in 25–50 mcg boluses and/or giving nitrous oxide, in a 50% mixture with oxygen can also be used, but only after delivery and clamping of the umbilical cord has occurred.

General anesthesia is the final and definitive option but is associated with a greater probability of airway difficulties, especially in the edematous, preeclamptic patient. General anesthesia can also provoke significant hemodynamic variability as well as neonatal respiratory depression.

8. Compare the advantages and disadvantages of spinal and epidural anesthesia in the parturient with preeclampsia.

The advantages associated with SAB include:

- Rapid onset
- Relative ease of placement
- Reliability

The disadvantages associated with SAB include:

- Rapid onset of a sympathetic blockade
- Hypotension
- Potential for a postdural puncture headache
- High SAB resulting in severe hypotension, loss of consciousness, and severe bradycardia
- Inadequacy of sensory blockade

The advantages associated with epidural anesthesia include:

- Gradual, controlled onset of sympathetic blockade
- Ability to titrate the volume of local anesthetic to the desired dermatome level
- Improved intervillous blood flow

The disadvantages associated with epidural anesthesia include:

- Possibility of sudden onset hypotension
- Potential for inadequacy, patchy, or unilateral blockade

- Potential for local anesthetic toxicity
- Potential for intravascular injection
- Increased level of technical difficulty during placement as compared to spinal anesthesia
- Increased risk of epidural hematoma in patients who develop coagulopathies

9. Describe the controversy related to the timing of antibiotic administration during cesarean section.

Historically, antibiotics (typically 1–2 g IV cefazolin or 900 mg IV clindamycin for patients who have a penicillin allergy) are administered after delivery of the neonate. Administering antibiotics prior to delivery was thought to possibly increase the potential for neonatal sepsis. Recent research has shown that administering cefazolin prior to skin incision is superior as compared to after the umbilical cord is clamped. This practice results in a decrease in total post-cesarean infectious morbidity and did not increase neonatal complications or sepsis. While some anesthetists have adopted administering antibiotics before skin incision, presently this practice is not universally accepted.

10. Compare the use of phenylephrine and ephedrine when treating hypotension after SAB.

Ephedrine has long been considered the drug of choice for treatment of neuraxial anesthesia induced hypotension. However, recommendations made by the American Society of Anesthesiologists Task Force on Obstetric Anesthesia (2006) state that administering phenylephrine may be preferable as compared to ephedrine for hypotension that ensues during routine pregnancies. It is thought that phenylephrine results in improved fetal acid-base balance when compared to ephedrine. The use of phenylephrine in patients with bradycardia, especially during the period in which the level of the SAB is still variable, profound bradycardia can occur. Blockade of sympathetic outflow at the level of the cardioaccelerator fibers (T1 through T5) combined with arterial constriction which initiates the baroreceptor response is the physiologic rationale

for this response. A reasonable approach may be to administer small doses of ephedrine (10–20 mg) prior to the administration of phenylephrine.

11. Describe the pharmacologic treatment for uterine atony.

After delivery of the fetus, an IV infusion of oxytocin, 20 U/l, is typically administered. In the setting of uterine atony an additional 20 U of oxytocin can be added to the existing oxytocin infusion. If this intervention fails to increase uterine tone, methylergonovine (methergine) (0.2 mg IM) can be administered. It must be used with caution in patients with hypertension, particularly when used concomitantly with ephedrine or phenylephrine. An additional pharmacologic agent, prostaglandin F2-alpha (250 mcg IM) can also be used to treat uterine atony. Like methylergonovine, prostaglandin F2-alpha can cause exaggerated hypertension. This medication can provoke bronchospasm in asthmatic patients. After the use of either methylergonovine or prostaglandin F2-alpha, the anesthetist should consider ordering antidiarrheal medications as these agents cause diarrhea.

12. Describe the therapeutic range and the side effects of increasing plasma levels of magnesium sulfate.

It is vitally important to maintain magnesium sulfate plasma levels within the therapeutic range. Subtherapeutic levels can result in seizures caused by inadequate treatment of preeclampsia and high levels can result in complete paralysis. Magnesium levels and the associated physiologic response are included in Table 35-3.

13. Examine the anesthetic implications associated with magnesium sulfate therapy.

Magnesium sulfate therapy can exacerbate the hypotension that is associated with neuraxial anesthesia. In the majority of preeclamptic patients, a decrease in blood pressure can be treated by fluid and vasopressors. Magnesium sulfate also prolongs the effects of nondepolarizing muscle

Table 35-3	Side Effects Associated with Increasing Plasma Levels of Magnesium Sulfate

- 1.5–2.0 mg/dl: Normal plasma concentration
- 4.0–8.0 mg/dl: Therapeutic range
- 5–10 mg/dl: ECG changes (widened QRS complex, PQ interval prolongation)
- 10 mg/dl: Loss of deep tendon reflexes
- 15 mg/dl: SA and AV block, respiratory paralysis
- 20–25 mg/dl: Cardiac arrest

relaxants (NDMR). If paralysis is necessary during general anesthesia, NDMRs should be carefully titrated to effect and assessment via nerve stimulation is prudent. While magnesium sulfate may prolong the duration of action of depolarizing muscle relaxants, the standard intubating dose of succinylcholine should not be reduced.

14. Explain the mechanism of action and the effects of magnesium sulfate in the patient with preeclampsia.

Treatment with magnesium sulfate is considered a first-line treatment for preeclampsia and it exerts anticonvulsant, vasodilator, and tocolytic properties. Magnesium sulfate likely exerts its anticonvulsant actions by reducing cerebral vasoconstriction and by centrally mediating cerebral N-methyl-D-aspartate receptors. Its peripheral vasodilatory effects are attributed to directly or indirectly competing with calcium, by increasing cyclic guanosine monophosphate, by decreasing angiotensin-converting enzyme levels, and by increasing endothelial cell production of PGI2.

15. Describe the unique communication aspects of the operating room environment during a cesarean section.

During cesarean section, the patient is not sedated and their significant other is present. The expectant parents likely have little to no experience in an operating room environment and are not accustomed to the sights, sounds, and smells that accompany surgery. The anesthetist must keep in mind these facts as they contribute to a situational disorientation on the part of the patient and their significant other. Additionally, the anesthetist will be communicating with the surgeon throughout the procedure.

Postoperative Period

16. Explain the importance of maintaining magnesium sulfate therapy in the postoperative period.

Magnesium sulfate therapy is typically continued for 24–48 hours after cesarean delivery. Postpartum convulsions are uncommon; however, continuation of magnesium sulfate reduces the risk of seizures.

17. Describe the goals of the postoperative management preeclamptic patients who have had a cesarean section.

- **Adequate analgesia**: Patients receiving spinal anesthesia for cesarean section may receive 0.1 to 0.2 mg of intrathecal preservative free morphine as well as nonsteroidal anti-inflammatory drugs such as ketorolac intravenously. The disadvantages associated with intrathecal narcotics include delayed respiratory depression, pruritus, and nausea and vomiting.
- **Maintenance of hemodynamic control**
- **Maintenance of intravascular volume**: Magnesium sulfate therapy is continued until the patient begins to recover from the signs and symptoms of preeclampsia such as hypertension, coagulopathy, or oliguria.
- **Assessment of electrolyte values**

REVIEW QUESTIONS

1. At which serum magnesium value(s) does the loss of deep tendon reflexes occur in parturients?
   a. 10 mEq/l
   b. 20–25 mEq/l

c. 15 mEq/l

d. 4–6 mEq/l

2. Which is not a reliable sign of preeclampsia?

   a. Proteinuria greater than 300 mg in a 24-hour period

   b. Systolic blood pressure greater than 140 mm Hg

   c. Edema

   d. Diastolic blood pressure of 90 mm Hg or higher

3. One possible site of action of the anticonvulsant effect of magnesium sulfate is:

   a. gamma-aminobutyric acid receptors.

   b. muscarinic receptors.

   c. cerebral N-methyl-D-aspartate receptors.

   d. oxytocin receptors.

4. Which agents are used to treat maternal hypotension and may provide improved fetal acid-base balance when compared to ephedrine?

   a. Epinephrine

   b. Vasopressin

   c. Oxytocin

   d. Phenylephrine

5. Which medication is associated with bronchospasm in patients with asthma?

   a. Magnesium sulfate

   b. Prostaglandin F2-alpha

   c. Methylergonovine

   d. Pitocin

REVIEW ANSWERS

1. **Answer: a**

   The loss of deep tendon reflexes in parturients undergoing magnesium therapy typically occurs at 10 mEq/l.

2. **Answer: c**

   Edema is not a reliable sign of preeclampsia as it is present in approximately 30% of all parturients.

3. **Answer: c**

   Cerebral N-methyl-D-aspartate receptors are thought to be the site of action of anticonvulsant properties associated with magnesium sulfate.

4. **Answer: d**

   Phenylephrine, when used to treat maternal hypotension, may provide improved fetal acid-base balance when compared to ephedrine.

5. **Answer: b**

   Prostaglandin F2-alpha is association with bronchospasm in asthmatic patients.

SUGGESTED READINGS

American Society of Anesthesiologists Task Force on Obstetric Anesthesia. Practice guidelines for obstetric anesthesia: an updated report by the American Society of Anesthesiologists Task Force on Obstetric Anesthesia. *Anesthesiology* 2007;106(4):843–863.

Aya AG, Vialles N, Tanoubi I, et al. Spinal anesthesia induced hypotension: a risk comparison between patients with severe preeclampsia and healthy women undergoing preterm Cesarean delivery. *Anesth Analg* 2005;101(3):869–875.

Lee A, Ngan K, Gin T. A quantitative systematic review of randomized controlled trials of ephedrine versus phenylephrine for the management of hypotension during spinal anesthesia for Cesarean delivery. *Anesth Analg* 2002;94:920–926.

Loughrey JP, Yao N, Datta S, et al. Hemodynamic effects of spinal anesthesia and simultaneous intravenous bolus of combined phenylephrine and ephedrine versus ephedrine for Cesarean delivery. *Int J Obstet Anesth* 2005;14(1):43–47.

Osbourne LA. Obstetric anesthesia. In: Nagelhout JJ, Plaus KL, eds. *Nurse Anesthesia*, 4th ed. St. Louis, MO: Elsevier Saunders, 2009.

Reed A, Lombard C, Leann K, et al. Hemodynamic changes associated with spinal anesthesia for cesarean delivery in severe preeclampsia. *Anesthesiology* 2008;108(5):802–811.

Reidy J, Douglas J. Vasopressors in obstetrics. *Anesth Clin* 2008;26:75–88.

Sullivan SA, Smith T, Chang E, et al. Administration of cefazolin prior to skin incision is superior to cefazolin at cord clamping in preventing postcesarean infectious morbidity: a randomized, controlled trial. *Am J Obstet Gynecol* 2007;197(3):455e1–455e5.

Thigpen BD, Hood AW, Chauhan S, et al. Timing of prophylactic antibiotic administration in the uninfected laboring gravida: a randomized clinical trial. *Am J Obstet Gynecol* 2005;192(6):1864–1869.

Visalyaputra S, Rodanant O, Somboonviboon W. Spinal versus epidural anesthesia for cesarean delivery in preeclampsia: a prospective randomized, multicenter study. *Obstet Gynecol Surv* 2006;61(2):84–85.

Williamson W, Burks D, Pipkin J, et al. Effect of timing of fluid bolus on reduction of spinal induced hypotension in patients undergoing elective Cesarean section. *AANA* 2009;77(2):130–136.

Disclaimer: The views expressed in this article are those of the author and do not necessarily reflect the official policy or position of the Department of the Navy, Department of Defense, or the United States government.

Cervical Cerclage

36

Lynn L. Lebeck

KEY POINTS

- Anesthetists need to minimize fetal drug exposure.
- Maintenance of placental perfusion by avoidance of maternal hypotension is critical.
- There are specific steps which help to avoid maternal complications: aspiration, aortocaval compression.
- Addressing maternal anxiety is imperative.

CASE SYNOPSIS

A 32-year-old woman, gravida 3 para 0, presents from the OB/GYN's office. She is now at 18 weeks' gestation and has evidence of cervical shortening and dilation to 1 cm and is scheduled to undergo an emergent cervical cerclage.

PREOPERATIVE EVALUATION AND DEMOGRAPHIC DATA

Past Medical/Surgical History

- Two prior second-trimester pregnancy losses at 19 and 21 weeks' gestation
- No previous medical or surgical history

List of Medications

- Prenatal vitamins

Diagnostic Data

- Hemoglobin, 12.2 g/dl; hematocrit, 33.4%
- Electolytes: sodium, 139 mEq/l; potassium, 4.1 mEq/l; chloride, 104 mEq/l; carbon dioxide, 21 mEq/l

Height/Weight/Vital Signs

- 165 cm, 78 kg
- Blood pressure, 112/64; heart rate, 71 beats per minute; respiratory rate, 16 breaths per minute; room air oxygen saturation, 98%

PATHOPHYSIOLOGY

Incompetent cervix can be the result of trauma or an inherent deficiency in structure or function of the cervix that leads to repeated second-trimester spontaneous abortions. These second-trimester losses often have three specific characteristics: painless cervical dilation, herniation then rupture of membranes, and short labor ending in delivery of live but extremely immature fetus.

The incidence of cervical incompetence ranges from 0.001 to 1.84%. Diagnosis of cervical incompetence is accomplished by observation of cervical shortening or dilation or protrusion of membranes through the cervical os. Diagnosis can also be made on the basis of past history, such as in this patient, if other causes of recurrent pregnancy loss have been ruled out. Serial examinations utilizing a variety of methods which include manual examination, ultrasound, or magnetic resonance imaging (MRI) may be used to evaluate cervical dilation and length and subsequent changes in order to determine if cervical cerclage is warranted.

SURGICAL PROCEDURE

The majority of pregnant women with an incompetent cervix will undergo a transvaginal placement of a cervical cerclage. The two types of cerclage procedures are McDonald and Shirodkar. The Shirodkar sutures are placed within the cervical mucosa following dissection of the bladder to the level of the internal cervical os, resulting slightly greater blood loss. The McDonald suture, which leaves the mucosa intact, is illustrated in Figure 36-1.

In rare instances, patients with a failed transvaginal cervical cerclage or those with little cervical structure, a transabdominal cerclage may be used. Transabdominal cervical cerclage (TAC) was first described in 1965 with an open laparotomy approach to insert a suture above the cardinal and uterosacral ligaments. There have been some reports of laparoscopic placement and the most recent case studies include the use of da Vinci robot and other robotic-assisted laparoscopic surgeries for placement of the suture. Prepregnancy TAC can be accomplished to avoid the complications of manipulation of the pregnant uterus and increased bleeding. The overall use of TAC is low being limited by the need for a clear diagnosis of cervical pathology and the technical challenges and learning curves associated with the surgery. A cervical cerclage needs to be removed prior to or at the onset of labor if a vaginal delivery is to occur; however, the usual mode of delivery following the transabdominal approach is via a cesarian section.

A   B

Figure 36-1   *Placement of sutures used for the McDonald cervical cerclage.*

There is a low incidence of cervical dystocia or failure of dilation secondary to cerclage.

ANESTHETIC MANAGEMENT AND CONSIDERATIONS

Preoperative Period

1. Describe the physiologic changes of pregnancy that impact anesthesia management of the parturient during the second trimester.

- **Cardiovascular:** Increases in heart rate (↑25%), stroke volume (↑25%), and cardiac output (↑50%), begin as early as 2–3 weeks' gestation and continue to rise into the second trimester. There are no further increases in cardiac performance that occur until labor and delivery process. Despite the increase in cardiac output, maternal blood pressure declines due to decreases in systemic vascular resistance, with the greatest decline occurring about the 20th week. Increased perfusion to the uterus, kidneys, skin, and skeletal muscle occurs throughout gestation. Aortocaval compression syndrome results in a 50% increase in femoral venous pressure, indicating decreased blood return to the heart (preload). This can be observed as early as 13–16 weeks' gestation and can result in severe hypotension and uteroplacental insufficiency.

- **Respiratory:** The increases in oxygen consumption, as a result of the increased metabolic demands of the fetus and placenta, result in changes within the respiratory system that occur when a woman is likely to undergo cervical cerclage. Approximately half of the 45% increase in tidal volume occurs in the first trimester with a corresponding rise in minute ventilation which results in a decrease in $PaCO_2$ and an increase in pH. Reduction in functional residual capacity begins in the fifth month of pregnancy and this change is not a primary determinant of decreased lung volume at the time of gestation that a cerclage would be performed.

- **Gastrointestinal:** The barrier pressure or difference between the lower esophageal high-pressure zone and the intragastric pressure decreases during pregnancy placing the parturient at increased risk for pyrosis (heartburn) and pulmonary aspiration if undergoing general anesthesia. The rotation and displacement of the gastroesophageal junction as pregnancy progresses is believed to contribute to the increasing incidence of gastroesophageal reflux. Therefore, the parturient should be treated as a full stomach with the appropriate precautions regardless of the method of anesthesia selected.

2. Differentiate between early and late pregnancy with respect to the need for:

- **Gastric aspiration precautions:** Early in pregnancy, the esophageal gastric junction has not been displaced so the risk of aspiration and pyrosis is lower as compared to late pregnancy. However, oral administration of a nonparticulate antacid is recommended for all parturients. In late pregnancy, additional treatment for gastric volume and acidity may be needed. Rapid sequence induction is used in pregnant women unless there is some rare contraindication.

- **Left uterine displacement (LUD):** Aortocaval compression can be detected as early as 13–16 weeks of gestation and, therefore, LUD should be initiated for all pregnant women. The anesthesia provider must be aware that, in late pregnancy, the vascular effects associated with aortocaval compression remain present even with LUD due to the increased weight of fetus, placenta, and amniotic fluid.

- **Fetal monitoring:** In early pregnancy confirmation of fetal heart rate (FHR) prior to a cerclage is sufficient. There is evidence to suggest that continuous FHR monitoring should be performed if the cerclage is performed after 16–20 weeks of gestation.

- **Avoidance of teratogenicity:** Although no current anesthesia drugs have been conclusively proven to be teratogenetic in humans when administered in therapeutic doses, there have been studies that suggest the existence of an association. It is prudent to minimize fetal exposure when possible.

3. Evaluate the advantages and disadvantages of regional/neuraxial and general anesthesia for surgical procedures in pregnancy.

When the surgical procedure permits, regional techniques offer the advantage of minimal exposure of anesthetic medications to the fetus and the ability of the patient to spontaneously breathe without the need for endotracheal intubation. Peripheral tissues, including those in the airway, become edematous due to increase in blood volume that occurs during pregnancy, which can make intubation more difficult to accomplish. Spinal anesthesia is most advantageous due to the low amount of drug that will be administered to provide and adequate sensory blockade and optimal surgical conditions. The primary disadvantage of regional anesthesia is caused by the sympathectomy that results from beta-preganglionic sympathetic fiber blockade. As a result, maternal hypotension can occur and decrease placental perfusion.

General anesthesia, when needed, provides superior uterine relaxation to facilitate replacement of bulging membranes prior to cervical cerclage when early cervical dilation has occurred. The uterine relaxation may decrease uterine irritability and premature uterine contraction. Disadvantages associated with general anesthesia include increased fetal drug exposure, the potential for difficult intubation, and increased risk of maternal aspiration. Postoperative vomiting may put undue strain on the suture.

4. Recognize the psychologic impact of prior pregnancy losses and anxiety over outcome of this pregnancy in the patient undergoing cervical cerclage.

Many women undergoing cervical cerclage have already suffered one or more miscarriages due to extreme prematurity at birth. Understandably,

they may be very anxious at the time of this procedure due to the uncertainty of being able to successfully carry this pregnancy to term. Anxiety may be heightened in cases where cervical dilation or bulging of membranes is already present. Establishing a rapport is important as little to no premedication for anxiolysis or intraoperative sedation is utilized in order to minimize fetal exposure.

5. Describe the selection of preoperative medications for the pregnant woman undergoing cervical cerclage.

Use of preoperative medications is usually minimal and frequently limited to a nonparticulate antacid (Bicitra) or other aspiration precautions (H_2 blocker, cimetidine; gastrokinetic, metoclopramide). Although no particular anesthetic agents or techniques have been proven teratogenic in humans, it is best to avoid unnecessary exposure during the time period of organogenesis (15–56 days' gestation). A cerclage is not frequently performed beyond this time period but emergency surgery may be required during pregnancy.

Intraoperative Period

6. Describe the physiologic changes that are associated with the lithotomy position.

Circulatory changes that occur as a result of lithotomy include an increase in the central blood volume and a decrease in perfusion pressure in the extremities. The higher the legs are placed above the heart the greater the effect. The reverse Trendelenburg position further amplifies the shifts in blood volume and perfusion.

Sympathectomy resulting from spinal or epidural anesthesia can contribute to the shift in blood volume. Hypotension may occur when the patient is returned to the supine position. Since placental perfusion is dependent on maternal blood pressure, avoiding hypotension is vitally important. Inappropriate positioning or pressure from leg holders can result in a nerve injury which necessitates proper padding and positioning. Care should be taken to return both legs to the center before replacing them in the supine position to avoid injuring the patient's hips.

7. Identify the level of sensory blockade needed if neuroaxial anesthesia is used during transvaginal placement of a cervical cerclage.

Cervical cerclage does not require neuroaxial blockade above T10 so a low spinal or "saddle block" is sufficient. A transabdominal approach to cerclage will require a higher dermatome level of blockade; however, it is less than a T4 block used for cesarian delivery.

8. Formulate a plan to maintain placental perfusion.

Uterine blood flow (UBF) is dependent on uterine arterial and venous pressure and uterine vascular resistance. The formula that is used to calculate UBF is shown in Equation 36-1. UBF is decreased if a decrease in uterine arterial pressure or an increase in uterine vascular resistance occurs. In order to avoid fetal hypoperfusion and maintain UBF, the anesthetist can support the maternal blood pressure by administering intravenous fluid. If vasopressors (ephedrine or phenylephrine) need to be administered for prolonged and severe hypotension, then these medications should be used judiciously since the sympathomimetic effects will increase uterine vascular resistance.

Postoperative Period

9. Discuss the potential adverse maternal and fetal outcomes following cervical cerclage.

The risks of aspiration, hypotension, and positioning injuries are all potential complications. Additional maternal risks include those related to anesthesia (nausea, vomiting) and those related to the procedure (infection, premature uterine con-

tractions, bleeding, tearing, or scarring with subsequent failure of the cervix to dilate in labor). There is the potential for amniotic membrane rupture, chorioamnionitis, and premature delivery. Cervical cerclage is not as effective in the prevention of preterm delivery as once believed, particularly in cases of shortened cervix. Although cervical cerclage does reduce the incidence of delivery prior to 34 weeks, neonatal mortality is unchanged and the risk of maternal postpartum fever is increased.

10. Describe a method for performing cerclage if advanced cervical dilation and or ballooning of membranes has occurred.

Emergency cerclage can be performed if advanced dilation or bulging of fetal membranes has occurred. This is accomplished by using a sterile inflatable balloon to gently push the fetal membranes into the cavity allowing placement of a cerclage over the balloon introducer. The balloon is deflated and the cerclage is tightened as the introducer is withdrawn. Use of balloons that can be inflated up to 10 cm and the protection provided by the introducer may result in greater use of the technique in the future. Risks that are associated with this procedure include maternal infection, chorioamnionitis, rupture of membranes, and premature delivery.

REVIEW QUESTIONS

1. An advantage of neuroaxial blockade for the patient having cervical cerclage placement is:
   a. minimizing the amount of drug that is administered.
   b. decreasing the blood loss during the procedure.
   c. distinguishing the signs and symptoms of bladder perforation.
   d. reducing postoperative pain.
2. Maternal blood pressure normally decreases during the first and second trimester of pregnancy due to:
   a. decrease in blood viscosity.
   b. increase in placental perfusion.

Equation 36-1   Formula Used to Determine Uterine Blood Flow

Uterine blood flow = Uterine arterial − Uterine venous pressure/Uterine vascular resistance

c. decrease in vascular resistance.

d. increase in heart rate.

3. Which intervention is recommended for all parturients to decrease the risk of gastric aspiration?

  a. Use of a high pressure cuff endotracheal tube

  b. Nasogastric suctioning prior to extubation

  c. Metoclopramide

  d. Nonparticulate antacid

4. Changes in barrier pressure at the gastroesophageal junction during pregnancy result from:

  a. increased acidity of gastric secretions.

  b. decreased gastric pressure.

  c. displacement of the junction.

  d. decreased progestin.

5. Which formula is most representative of UBF?

  a. Uterine arterial pressure $\times$ uterine venous pressure $-$ O_2 placental consumption.

  b. Uterine (arterial pressure $-$ venous pressure)/uterine vascular resistance

  c. CO $\times$ 0.04

  d. SV $\times$ HR/CO (uterine vascular resistance)

REVIEW ANSWERS

1. **Answer: a**

  Spinal anesthesia is the anesthetic technique of choice for cervical cerclage because it reduces the amount of intravenous medication administered and therefore, its impact on mother and fetus is minimal.

2. **Answer: c**

  The smooth muscle within vessel walls is relaxed by the hormones of pregnancy, resulting in a decrease in systemic vascular resistance allowing the maternal vasculature to accommodate for the increase in cardiac output without increasing blood pressure.

3. **Answer: d**

  Nonparticulate antacid should be given orally prior to any anesthesia administration to the parturient.

4. **Answer: c**

  As pregnancy progresses, the intragastric pressure increases but the rise in lower esophageal tone that would normally occur in response is prevented by the rotation and displacement of the gastroesophageal junction caused by the gravid uterus.

5. **Answer: b**

  The difference between uterine arterial pressure and uterine venous pressure divided by uterine vascular resistance is the equation that is used to calculate UBF.

SUGGESTED READINGS

Barmat L, Glaser G, Davis G, et al. Da Vinci-assisted abdominal cerclage. *Fertil Steril* 2007;88(5):1437e1-e3.

Bimbach DJ, Browne IM. Anesthesia for obstetrics. In: Miller RD, ed. *Millers Anesthesia*, 6th ed. Philadelphia: Elsevier Mosby, 2005:2337–2339.

Chantigian RC, Chantigian PDM. Problems of early pregnancy. In: Chestnut DH, ed. *Obstetric Anesthesia*, 4th ed. Philadelphia: Elsevier Mosby, 2009:319–337.

Gaiser R. Physiologic changes in pregnancy. In: Chestnut DH, ed. *Obstetric Anesthesia*, 4th ed. Philadelphia: Elsevier Mosby, 2009:15–35.

Levinson G. Anesthesia for surgery during pregnancy. In: Hughes SC, Levinson G, Rosen MA, eds. *Schnider and Levinson's Anesthesia for Obstetrics*, 4th ed. Philadelphia: Lippincott Williams & Wilkins, 2002:249–265.

Marenco JE, Santos AC. Anesthesia for nonobstetric surgery during pregnancy. In: Braveman FR, ed. *Obstetric and Gynecologic Anesthesia: The Requisites in Anesthesiology.* Philadelphia: Elsevier Mosby, 2006:18–24.

Simcox R, Shennan A. Cervical cerclage: a review. *Int J Surg* 2007;5:205–209.

Taslimi MM, El-Sayed Y, Carvalho B, et al. Obstetric surgery. In: Jaffe RA, Samuels SI, eds. *Anesthesiologist's Manual of Surgical Procedures*, 3rd ed. Philadelphia: Lippincott Williams & Wilkins, 2004:674–676.

Tsatsaris V, Senat MV, Gervaise A, et al. Balloon replacement of fetal membranes to facilitate emergency cervical cerclage. *Obstet Gynecol* 2004;98(2):243–246.

Wolfe L, DePasquale S, Adair CD, et al. Robotic-assisted laparoscopic placement of transabdominal cerclage during pregnancy. *Am J Perinatol* 2008;25:653–655.

Intraoperative Maternal Hemorrhage Caused by Uterine Rupture

37

Michael Rieker

KEY POINTS

- Uterine rupture is a potentially catastrophic complication of pregnancy.
- Uterine rupture may result from abnormalities of uterine anatomy, forceps delivery, external version procedure, connective tissue disease, or other causes; but the most widely recognized cause is a uterine scar from previous surgery.
- Cesarean delivery represents the most common nondiagnostic surgery in the United States, accounting for over 1 million births annually.
- To reduce the complications associated with cesarean delivery and to enjoy the benefits of a vaginal birth, approximately 10% of women who have had a cesarean delivery will deliver a subsequent child vaginally (~50,000 annually). This practice of "vaginal birth after cesarean" is abbreviated as VBAC.
- A woman attempting a VBAC may be at increased risk of uterine rupture or failed labor.
- Uterine rupture, although infrequent, calls for an immediate response by the anesthetist to assist with maternal and fetal rescue.
- Uterine rupture may likely be associated with severe hemorrhage, and the anesthetist will be responsible for a challenging fluid resuscitation in this situation.

CASE SYNOPSIS

A 30-year-old woman presents to the obstetric unit. The obstetrician reports that she is in early labor, but that the labor will be augmented with oxytocin. An order is written for the patient to be administered an epidural, upon her request.

PREOPERATIVE EVALUATION AND DEMOGRAPHIC DATA

Past Medical/Surgical History

- History of endometriosis with pelvic adhesions
- Five pack/year smoking history, but quit since becoming pregnant
- Heartburn with gastroesophageal reflux 1 time per week

- Noninsulin-dependent diabetes mellitus, well controlled by diet
- Obstetric history: gravida 3 para 2
- Cesarean delivery; epidural anesthesia
- Laparoscopy for endometriosis; general anesthesia without complications

The patient's obstetric history is present in Table 37-1.

List of Medications
- Prenatal vitamins daily
- Calcium carbonate as needed for heartburn/reflux

Diagnostic Data
- Hemoglobin, 12 g/dl; hematocrit, 36%; white blood count, 12,000/mm³; platelet count, 120,000/mm³
- Airway is assessed as Mallampati class III

Height/Weight/Vital Signs
- 163 cm, 84 kg
- Blood pressure, 110/64; heart rate, 82 beats per minute; respiratory rate, 16 breaths per minute

PATHOPHYSIOLOGY

Cesarean delivery is accomplished by making an incision in the uterus to allow delivery of the fetus. The most common approach is through the Pfannenstiel (bikini line) incision in the abdominal wall, followed by a transverse cut across the lower segment of the uterus, not far above the cervix. Previously common was the vertical, or classical incision as is depicted in Figure 37-1. In spite of the larger access provided for delivery of the baby by the vertical incision, this approach has become less popular due to the resulting increased potential for uterine rupture with subsequent pregnancies. The classical incision is associated with increased rupture risk because the myometrial fibers are separated longitudinally, and the incision extends upward toward the fundus of the uterus, where the strongest contractions occur during labor.

A number of physiologic changes occur during pregnancy to foster favorable maternal and fetal hemodynamics. Maternal blood volume rises, with a disproportionate rise in plasma volume, in relation to red blood cell mass. This change produces the "physiologic anemia of pregnancy" which serves to promote blood flow to the placenta and to also limit red cell loss during the inevitable bleeding that occurs with delivery. Another physiologic change which occurs in anticipation of this bleeding is an increase in blood coagulation factors.

SURGICAL PROCEDURE

During the prenatal period, uterine rupture is treated by emergency cesarean delivery in order to separate the fetus from the dysfunctional uterus, and to control maternal bleeding. A rupture that is diagnosed postnatally is treated by a laparotomy to repair or remove the damaged uterus. A wide retractor called a bladder blade is commonly used to prevent trauma to the bladder, which overrides the lower uterus. There is an increased incidence of bladder damage during cesarean surgery following uterine rupture, so the anesthetist must be vigilant for lack of urine output or for blood in the urine during

Table 37-1	Obstetric History		
PREGNANCY	**DATE**	**MODE OF DELIVERY**	**NOTES**
1	3.5 years ago	Vaginal	
2	22 months ago	Cesarean	Prolapsed cord
3	Current; 41 weeks gestational age		Macrosomia

Figure 37-1   *Classical uterine incision. (See Color Plate.)*

this procedure. An example of a classical uterine incision is present in Figure 37-1.

ANESTHETIC MANAGEMENT AND CONSIDERATIONS

Preoperative Period

1. Discuss the pertinent points in the preanesthetic evaluation and planning for a patient undergoing VBAC.

In addition to the typical assessment of the labor patient, some special factors should be considered when the patient planning vaginal delivery has had a previous cesarean (this process is referred to as a trial of labor [TOL]). The risk factors for failure of TOL or for uterine rupture should be assessed to determine the appropriate level of vigilance and monitoring due the patient. Uterine rupture can result in significant blood loss and it is imperative that blood products are available for infusion. Established policy and logistics of blood acquisition in the institution must be considered in determining whether the patient should be tested for blood type and antibody screen, or whether blood should be cross-matched. Staff availability is another crucial factor in the safe treatment of patients undergoing TOL. There are differing interpretations of guidelines by the American College of Obstetricians and Gynecologists which state that providers should be *immediately available* when a patient is undergoing a TOL. Institutional policy should dictate whether *immediate* availability implies that a surgical team is on the delivery unit, in the hospital, or available for call-back from outside.

2. Identify risk factors which may predict complications or failure of VBAC.

Certain factors increase the success of VBAC, including history of previous vaginal delivery (particularly if it was a VBAC), spontaneous onset of labor, cervical effacement > 75%, no more than one previous uterine incision, and clinically adequate pelvis. While models to predict uterine rupture in a given patient lack reliability, the following factors are associated with increased rates of uterine rupture or failure of vaginal delivery in patients undergoing TOL.

- Vertical (or *classical*) uterine incision
- Potentially recurring indication for previous cesarean
- Increasing number of uterine incisions
- Interval is less than 24 months since prior cesarean
- No history of a previous vaginal delivery
- Dystocia, or need for induction or augmentation of labor
- Macrosomia (> 4000 gm)
- Postterm or multiple gestations
- Obesity

The current patient has three favorable historical factors: she is in spontaneous labor; she has had a vaginal delivery previously; and her first cesarean delivery was for prolapsed umbilical cord. The previous vaginal delivery indicates a proven uterus, as opposed to the scenario where unsuitable pelvic dimensions were the cause of the prior cesarean. Likewise, prolapsed cord is a nonrecurring indication. Unlike cephalopelvic disproportion, it would not be expected that the underlying condition for the first cesarean would also complicate this pregnancy. However, this patient has a number of factors that detract from her chance of success including:

- She is obese, with a body mass index of 31.8 kg/m².
- Her baby is large (not uncommon among diabetic patients).
- It has been just less than 24 months since her cesarean surgery, which suggests less-than-optimal time for uterine scar strengthening.
- Although she is in spontaneous labor, her labor will be augmented by oxytocin. The need for augmentation, as well as the increased muscle tension it produces, confer negative risk factors.

3. Compare and contrast the advantages of different anesthetic techniques in managing VBAC.
As with a number of obstetric complications which forebode emergency cesarean delivery, it is valuable to have a functioning epidural in place in a VBAC patient. Catastrophic uterine rupture may not allow time, nor may it be appropriate for epidural anesthesia for the cesarean surgery, but in the case of a lesser uterine rupture, it is beneficial to have the option of using a functioning epidural. A combined spinal-epidural technique typically does not employ the epidural catheter during the initial period following subarachnoid injection. It may be favorable to utilize a traditional epidural technique, so that any deficiencies in epidural function may be identified and remedied immediately. In the present case, the patient has diabetes, which is associated with abnormal vascular development of the uteroplacental unit. This may make uteroplacental insufficiency more likely when her contractions increase in intensity. Her obesity also places her at higher risk for epidural catheter malfunction.

There is a theoretical concern that because abdominal pain is a sign of uterine rupture, epidural analgesia may mask this important sign and delay diagnosis of the complication. Experience shows that the visceral pain of uterine rupture, like that of bladder distention, is difficult to obliterate with moderate epidural analgesia. Therefore, concerns that providing epidural analgesia will prevent diagnosis of uterine rupture are unfounded.

4. Formulate a plan for management of a VBAC patient during labor.
Anesthetic management for VBAC needs not be significantly different from that of routine patients, other than assuring availability of a rapid response in case of emergency. The anesthetist should be assured of prompt availability of blood products because uterine rupture is frequently associated with significant blood loss. Depending on institutional logistics, this may warrant cross-matching type and screen only, or if emergency blood is rapidly available, no additional preparation. As with all obstetric patients, the preanesthetic evaluation includes an assessment of the airway, in anticipation of the possibility of emergency surgery. As noted previously, epidural analgesia is acceptable. While literature lends little objective information regarding the possibility of an epidural to mask signs of uterine rupture, prudence would suggest that the level of sensory blockade should allow for some awareness of abdominal sensation. The anesthetist should maintain lines of communication with the obstetric provider and labor nurse, and also maintain availability for a rapid response when caring for a VBAC patient.

5. Recognize the unique factors which should heighten the anesthetist's awareness and surveillance of a VBAC patient.
Any sign that natural labor is not progressing well may indicate a heightened level of awareness for complications of uterine rupture. Such signs include fetal heart rate abnormalities, dystocia or prolonged labor, and the need for high-dose oxytocin. Dystocia occurs in approximately one-half of uterine ruptures, and variable or late decelerations

occur as prodromal signs in the majority of cases of uterine rupture.

An epidural catheter is inserted and a T10 level of sensory block is achieved, with pain score of 0/10. The epidural infusion is 0.1% bupivacaine + fentanyl 2 mcg/ml, infusing at 10 ml/hr. The first stage of labor lasted 5 hours, and the patient is now pushing in the second stage. She begins to complain of breakthrough pain, and she is given a rest from pushing while you are called in to re-dose her epidural. As you arrive, she complains of increasingly severe pain.

6. Differentiate between various causes of pain which may exist in this patient.

- **Inadequate analgesia**: Epidural coverage of sacral dermatomes needed for second-stage analgesia may be lacking. Preservation of sacral motor function (plantar flexion via S1/superficial peroneal nerve) bolsters this supposition.
- **Placental abruption**: Vascular compromise from smoking history or diabetes in this patient increases her risk of placental abruption. Abnormally copious vaginal bleeding may be an accompanying sign.
- **Uterine rupture**: Pain is a less reliable sign of uterine rupture than is a change in the fetal heart rate. Uterine rupture typically manifests as diffuse, nonlocalized pain which may break through moderate epidural analgesia. A uterine hyperstimulation pattern or an abrupt cessation of contractions may be noted on the tocodynamometer. The fetal heart rate will likely show abnormalities such as repetitive late or variable decelerations progressing to a prolonged (terminal) deceleration and fetal bradycardia. Loss of fetal station may also occur.
- **Fetal malposition**: Dystocia and continuous back pain can result from a malpositioned fetus, such as being in the occiput posterior (OP) position. Similar to pathologic conditions, this pain may not subside between contractions. However, its recognition is suggested by

pain in the dermatomes of the lumbar plexus or sacrum, and a fetal head that is identified on vaginal examination to be in the OP position.
- **Other causes**: These include acute appendicitis, rupture of the abdominal rectus muscles, bladder rupture, hepatic rupture (right upper quadrant pain associated with severe HELLP syndrome), and vascular thrombosis (mesenteric, iliac, etc., due to the hypercoagulable state of pregnancy).

You evaluate the fetal heart rate and uterine monitor and observe the pattern is consistent with variable decelerations in Figure 37-2. The patient is complaining of severe abdominal pain. Uterine rupture is diagnosed.

Intraoperative Period

7. Describe the expected obstetric management of a patient with uterine rupture.

A patient with symptomatic uterine rupture, particularly if accompanied by fetal distress, will require an emergent cesarean delivery in order to provide the best opportunity for survival of the fetus. Many cases of uterine rupture are of a mild degree, often asymptomatic, and termed uterine dehiscence. These may not be recognized unless failure of vaginal delivery leads to a cesarean delivery, and the dehiscence is diagnosed upon visualizing the uterus. A uterine rupture that is severe may lead to cessation of placental perfusion, thus necessitating immediate cesarean delivery. If the uterus is severely damaged or if uncontrollable bleeding occurs, a hysterectomy may also be carried out following delivery of the infant.

While potentially catastrophic, the overall incidence of uterine rupture is close to only 1%, and better still, the incidence of fetal injury is only around 10% following uterine rupture. Nonetheless, a significant uterine rupture presents a true emergency, and maternal and neonatal well-being will be best served by a very expeditious delivery and resuscitation. In the routine cesarean delivery, uterine incision may disrupt the life-sustaining milieu of the fetus, so it is desirable for the surgeon

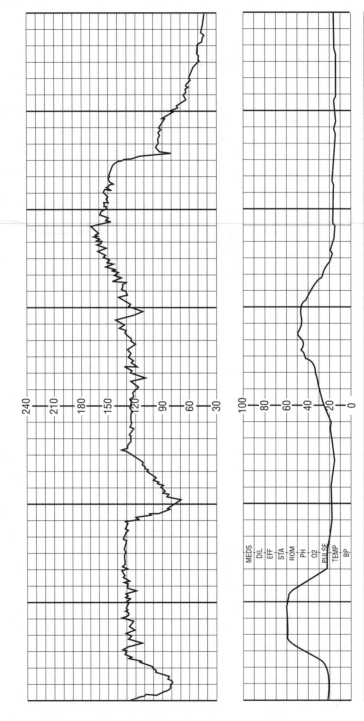

Figure 37-2   *Fetal heart rate tracing showing variable decelerations following uterine rupture.*

to expeditiously delivery of the infant within 2 minutes following uterine incision. This time frame is supported by animal models which demonstrate physiologic compromise in this interval, following umbilical cord occlusion. Also carrying the potential to disrupt placental perfusion (particularly if the placenta has implanted anteriorly on the site of the eventual rupture), a uterine rupture should likewise demand extreme haste in delivering the infant.

The American College of Obstetricians and Gynecologists recommends that in the case of urgent or emergent cesarean delivery, the delivery should be accomplished within 30 minutes of the decision to do so ("decision-to-incision" time). However, in the case of uterine rupture, 30 minutes may be too long to ensure survival for a fetus with severely compromised perfusion. Therefore, effective management of a uterine rupture requires availability of the obstetric, anesthesia, and surgical nursing team in order to affect delivery within a time frame closer to 15 minutes. Retrospective data predict a reasonably low incidence of significant neonatal injury or death if delivery is affected within this time frame. Institutional practice and logistics will influence the feasible response time, but when possible, the anesthetist managing a patient undergoing VBAC should not be required to become involved in other anesthetics, lest they lose the ability to respond rapidly in the case of a uterine rupture. Staff availability for rapid response is the most important asset to ensure effective management of a catastrophic uterine rupture.

8. Order the steps in the anesthetic management of a patient with uterine rupture.
As indicated previously, rapid delivery of the fetus is paramount in the case of uterine rupture. Anesthesia intervention should begin as soon as rupture is identified, and may include intensifying the epidural anesthesia prior to transport to the operating room, preparation for possible or planned general anesthesia, and procurement of blood products. Uterine rupture is associated with significant bleeding and may lead to rapidly developing disseminated intravascular coagulation (DIC). For these reasons, anesthesia care should prepare for an emergent hysterectomy following the delivery, and assess the need for red blood cell and clotting factor administration. The anesthetist must estimate the anticipated blood loss to decide whether epidural anesthesia will be sufficient, or if general anesthesia will facilitate better control of physiologic parameters. Having a history of gastroesophageal reflux and obesity, the present patient has additional risk factors for aspiration pneumonitis. It would be worthwhile to utilize a regional technique for her, as long as it is appropriate. Table 37-2 summarizes the anesthetic management for a patient who has experienced a uterine rupture.

Table 37-2 Anesthetic Management of Uterine Rupture

1. Assess severity of maternal and fetal compromise to determine the type of anesthesia indicated.
2. Assist with transport to the operating room as quickly as possible.
3. If epidural anesthesia is appropriate and a catheter is in place, begin dosing immediately with 3% chloroprocaine or 2% carbonated lidocaine.
4. Obtain 2–4 units of packed red blood cells and plasma.
5. Ensure, through general or regional anesthesia, that surgery can proceed in the shortest amount of time after entering the operating room.
6. Anticipate the need for aggressive fluid and blood replacement due to uterine bleeding and the likelihood of disseminated intravascular coagulation.

9. Formulate a plan to manage blood replacement.

While vaginal delivery is typically associated with approximately 500 ml of blood loss, and cesarean delivery is associated with 1000 ml, a uterine rupture can be expected to typically lead to 1500 to 2000 ml loss. Approximately 25–50% of women who experience uterine rupture will require blood products. Shock occurs in a similar incidence. In the patient in this case, her history of endometriosis and previous laparoscopy suggests that the cesarean delivery may be associated with even more surgical challenges and resultant bleeding.

Although obstetric patients are generally of good health, the physiologic anemia of pregnancy may prompt practitioners to treat with blood products earlier. Packed red cells will provide oxygen carrying capacity. In an ideal situation, blood would be type- and cross-matched; however, in the absence thereof, uncrossed type-specific or O-negative blood may need to be administered if the patient's condition does not allow time for preparation of other products.

There is a large margin of safety in the amount of clotting factor that can be lost without clinical significance. At the same time, uterine rupture may lead to massive transfusion, and red cells may also need to be supplemented with plasma. Ligation of the uterine arteries may be used by the surgeon to control massive hemorrhage, but at times hemorrhage becomes uncontrollable. The possibility of requiring unconventional approaches, such as administration of recombinant factor VIIA, should be considered. A fluid and blood warmer should be used to maintain body temperature and avoid further compromise of clotting factor function.

10. Distinguish the anesthetist's responsibility to the mother and to the neonate.

Being involved in a case where neonatal outcomes are poor is a heart-wrenching experience. In a smaller hospital, staff resources for neonatal resuscitation may not be as ample as in larger institutions. The scenario of a significant uterine rupture may present a quandary for the anesthetist when a hemorrhaging mother and an asphyxiated neonate can both benefit from the anesthetist's intervention. The anesthetist's primary duty is to their original patient, the mother. If the mother is stable, and lack of personnel or expertise calls for the anesthetist to become involved with care of the neonate, the decision to divert attention from the primary patient must be made by the anesthetist after weighing the risks and benefits. The guiding principle should be, however, that the primary responsibility is to the mother, even when the health of the neonate is compromised.

11. Debate the advantages and disadvantages of using salvaged blood in obstetric emergencies.

Uterine rupture may result in significant amounts of blood loss. Massive transfusions alone, and particularly when involving commingling of maternal and fetal blood, frequently lead to development of DIC. Historically, there has been reluctance to use salvaged blood in obstetrics due to concerns about causing amniotic fluid embolism and alloimmunization of the mother from exposure to fetal antigens which would be included in the salvaged blood. A mounting body of case report evidence indicates that these fears are largely unfounded, provided that the cell salvage system utilizes a leukocyte filter and a washing process. With these factors in place, the amount of fetal tissue, hemoglobin, and amniotic fluid to be infused into the mother have not demonstrated appreciable increases in hematologic complications. However, many practitioners will limit the amount of blood that is collected for salvage during the period of amniotomy until the placenta is delivered. The American College of Obstetricians and Gynecologists has even recommended blood salvage as a means of managing hemorrhage for placenta accreta. In cases of religious preferences against the receipt of banked blood, cell salvage is an alternative option for managing hemorrhage.

Postoperative Period

The baby was delivered with Apgar scores of 5 (1 minute) and 7 (5 minute). The neonatal intensive care unit team handled infant resuscitation. The anesthetist administered 6 l of lactated Ringer's solution and 3 units of packed red blood cells. The epidural was left in place for postoperative analgesia.

12. Describe the potential for uterine rupture postpartum following VBAC.

The risk of uterine rupture does not exist exclusively during active labor. There have been case reports of uterine rupture antepartum in patients who are not in labor. Likewise, a patient may successfully deliver a VBAC, and then experience a uterine rupture postpartum. The anesthetist may be called upon to provide anesthesia for emergency hysterectomy, even following successful VBAC. Hemorrhage is the second most common cause of obstetric complications, and hemorrhage may result from a variety of factors, both anatomic and hematologic. Postpartum bleeding should alert the anesthetist of the possibility of an emergent procedure such as curettage for removal of retained placenta, hysterotomy, for placenta accreta, or possibly hysterectomy for uterine rupture.

REVIEW QUESTIONS

1. Which is the greatest risk factor for uterine rupture in a patient undergoing VBAC?
   a. Classical uterine incision.
   b. History of three previous vaginal deliveries.
   c. Oxytocin augmentation of labor.
   d. Transmural myomectomy 15 months prior to VBAC

2. Uterine rupture would most likely be characterized by which signs and symptoms?
   a. Painless vaginal bleeding.
   b. Early decelerations of the fetal heart rate.
   c. Fetal tachycardia with loss of variability.
   d. Variable decelerations and abdominal pain.

3. Which is the optimal decision to incision response time for initiating a cesarean delivery for uterine rupture?
   a. 15 minutes
   b. 30 minutes
   c. 45 minutes
   d. 60 minutes

4. What is the most important asset to ensure safe management of a patient for VBAC?
   a. Intrauterine pressure monitoring
   b. Epidural in place immediately upon onset of labor
   c. Staff availability to initiate a cesarean delivery rapidly
   d. Type- and cross-matched blood available on the labor ward

5. In the case of a bleeding mother and a compromised neonate, the professional *duty* of the anesthetist is to the:
   a. neonate primarily, if intubation of the neonate is indicated.
   b. mother primarily, but may incorporate the neonate if required and if the mother is stable.
   c. mother only, even if stable and the infant is in cardiac arrest.
   d. whichever patient has a greater chance of survival.

REVIEW ANSWERS

1. **Answer: a**
   A classical (longitudinal) uterine incision presents the greatest risk factor for uterine rupture in a patient undergoing VBAC because the orientation of the cut between muscle fibers does not lead to development of a strong scar. It also implies that the scar extends toward the fundus of the uterus, where the greatest tension is formed during contractions.

2. **Answer: d**
   Uterine rupture would most likely be characterized by variable decelerations of the fetal heart rate and abdominal pain.

3. **Answer: a**

   In contrast to other indications for emergency cesarean delivery, the optimal time for initiating a cesarean delivery for uterine rupture is within 15 minutes.

4. **Answer: c**

   Staff availability to initiate a cesarean delivery rapidly is the most important asset to ensure safe management of a patient for VBAC. Rapid delivery is absolutely crucial to best ensure fetal survival following a catastrophic uterine rupture.

5. **Answer: b**

   In the case of a bleeding mother and a compromised neonate, the professional *duty* of the anesthetist is to the mother primarily, but may incorporate the neonate if required and if the mother is stable.

SUGGESTED READINGS

Allam J, Cox M, Yentis SM. Cell salvage in obstetrics. *Int J Obstet Anesth* 2008;17(1):37–45.

American College of Obstetricians and Gynecologists. Placenta accrete. ACOG committee opinion no. 266. *Obstet Gynecol* 2002;99(1):169–170.

Kaneko M, White S, Homan J, et al. Cerebral blood flow and metabolism in relation to electrocortical activity with severe umbilical cord occlusion in the near-term ovine fetus. *Am J Obstet Gynecol* 2003; 188:961–972.

Leung AS, Leung EK, Paul RH. Uterine rupture after previous cesarean delivery: maternal and fetal consequences. *Am J Obstet Gynecol* 1993;169(4): 945–950.

Levit K, Stranges E, Ryan K, et al. *HCUP Facts and Figures, 2006: Statistics on Hospital-based Care in the United States*. Rockville, MD: Agency for Healthcare Research and Quality, 2008. Available online at http://www.hcup-us.ahrq.gov/reports.jsp. Accessed September 14, 2009.

Macones GA, Peipert J, Nelson DB, et al. Maternal complications with vaginal birth after cesarean delivery: a multicenter study. *Am J Obstet Gynecol* 2005;193(5): 1656–1662.

Martin JA, Hamilton BE, Sutton PD, et al. Births: final data for 2004. *Natl Vital Stat Rep* 2006;55(1):1–104.

Martinez-Biarge M, Garcia-Alix A, Garcia-Benasach F, et al. Neonatal neurological morbidity associated with uterine rupture. *J Perinat Med* 2008;36(6):536–542.

Smith JG, Mertz HL, Merrill DC. Identifying risk factors for uterine rupture. *Clin Perinatol* 2008;35(1):85–99.

Spong CY, Landon MB, Gilbert S, et al. Risk of uterine rupture and adverse perinatal outcome at term after cesarean delivery. *Obstet Gynecol* 2007;110(4): 801–807.

Labor Epidural

38

Michael Rieker

KEY POINTS

- Approximately two thirds of labor patients in the United States receive epidural analgesia.
- Despite the potential for systemic effects, epidural analgesia can provide more complete pain relief with less maternal somnolence or neonatal respiratory depression than that resulting from parenteral analgesics.
- In the absence of a patient history suggesting otherwise, laboratory evaluation is not required prior to initiating epidural analgesia.
- The most common risks associated with epidural analgesia include backache, epidural failure, postdural puncture headache (PDPH), and transient neurologic symptoms.
- Testing for improper placement is paramount to safe epidural administration; however, the traditional test dose for intravascular placement may be difficult to interpret and may cause side effects in the laboring patient.
- Inadequate pain relief or total failure of epidural analgesia may occur in 6–10% of patients.
- Epidural analgesia for labor should ideally eliminate pain while allowing the maximal amount of motor strength possible and preserving maternal awareness of uterine contractions.

CASE SYNOPSIS

A 27-year-old woman presents in early labor. She states that she requests an epidural analgesia for labor.

PREOPERATIVE EVALUATION AND DEMOGRAPHIC DATA

Past Medical/Surgical History

- Protein C deficiency
- History of tobacco use
- Table 38-1 provides the patients obstetric history

Table 38-1 Obstetric History			
PREGNANCY	DATE	MODE OF DELIVERY	NOTES
1	4 years ago	N/A	Spontaneous abortion
2	3 years ago	Vaginal	Blood clot in leg, postpartum
3	15 months ago	N/A	Spontaneous abortion
4	Current		39 weeks' gestational age

List of Medications

- Prenatal vitamins daily
- Heparin 5000 units subcutaneously, twice daily

Diagnostic Data

- Hemoglobin, 11 gm/dl; hematocrit, 34%; white blood count, 11,500/mm³; platelet count, 125,000/mm³
- Airway is assessed as Mallampati class III

Height/Weight/Vital Signs

- 157 cm, 110 kg
- Blood pressure, 130/84; heart rate, 85 beats per minute; respiratory rate, 14 breaths per minute

PATHOPHYSIOLOGY

During gestation, multiple physiologic changes occur in order to create a favorable environment for embryologic and fetal growth and also to prepare for the birthing event. These changes include an increase in blood volume, wherein the plasma volume increase is greater than the red blood cell increase, creating an apparent anemia. The minute ventilation is increased almost 50% above normal, but this is in response to an increase in oxygen consumption, so the pH is only slightly elevated, within the normal range. Increases in heart rate and stroke volume coupled with a reduction in peripheral vascular resistance

lead to an increase in cardiac output of 40–50%. This increase can be detrimental to patients with cardiac valvular dysfunction, especially considering that cardiac output may rise to nearly 80% above normal immediately following delivery. Hypercoagulability in pregnancy results from increased levels of most coagulation factors, except for factors XI and XIII, which are slightly decreased. Hormonal changes contribute to sensitivity to general and local anesthetic agents. Gastric function is not significantly altered during pregnancy; however, gastric emptying is delayed during labor. Considering also the presence of reduced lower esophageal sphincter tone and gastric compression from the gravid uterus, the laboring patient should be considered at risk for regurgitation and aspiration.

A term pregnancy is one in which the gestational age of the fetus is 37–42 weeks. While occasional uterine contractions may be experienced during the latter stage of pregnancy, onset of labor (including both contractions and cervical effacement) prior to 37 weeks gestational age is considered preterm labor. The triggering factor for normal labor onset is not clearly understood, but it may be related to oxytocin released from the posterior pituitary gland, or to changes in prostaglandin activity. Labor progresses through distinctive stages, as delineated in Table 38-2. Cervical effacement and dilation as well as uterine contractions are responsible for pain in the first stage of labor. Synthetic oxytocin is commonly administered to either induce labor or to augment natural labor contractions. Oxytocin may also be combined with prostaglandin administration for the purpose of encouraging cervical effacement and/or uterine contractions.

ANESTHETIC MANAGEMENT AND CONSIDERATIONS

Preoperative Period

1. List the indications for epidural analgesia for labor.

Historically, there existed concern that epidural analgesia impeded the progress of labor, even to

Table 38-2	Stages of Labor		
STAGE	CHARACTERISTIC	CLINICAL ENDPOINTS	PAIN PATTERN
I		Onset of regular contractions until full cervical dilation (10 cm)	T10–L1
(I latent)	Cervix effaces; slow change in dilation	~4 cm cervical dilation, rate of dilation increases rapidly to signify transition to active stage I	T10–L1
(I active)	Rapid dilation of cervix	Full dilation of cervix	T10–L1
II		From full cervical dilation until delivery of the fetus	S2–S4
III		From delivery of the fetus until expulsion of the placenta	

the extent of increasing the incidence of forceps or cesarean delivery. Over time, and perhaps due to changing patterns of obstetric anesthesia care, research to describe the relationship between epidural analgesia and instrumented delivery has been equivocal. While epidural anesthesia may prolong the second stage of labor in some patients, it does so to a degree that is overcome by the benefit of analgesia. By contrast, in some cases (particularly primiparous patients) epidural analgesia with a combined subarachnoid dose may speed the progress of labor. Contemporary practice, supported by the American College of Obstetricians and Gynecologists, utilizes a more liberal indication for epidural analgesia. Epidural analgesia is indicated if the patient is:

- in active labor.
- committed to delivery (i.e., there is not a chance that the patient will be discharged to return to the hospital later).
- in pain.
- desiring epidural analgesia.

2. Consider contraindications to epidural analgesia for labor.

You evaluate the fetal heart rate and uterine monitor and observe the patterns as shown in Figure 38-1.

Patient refusal is the absolute contraindication to epidural analgesia. Unlike anesthesia service for surgery, labor epidurals are purely optional. Therefore, the anesthetist must take meticulous care to obtain a thorough informed consent from the patient. General contraindications to regional techniques apply to the labor patient, as well. Thus, serious coagulopathies, active infection at the site of insertion, increased intracranial pressure, and physiologic factors such as severe aortic stenosis would likely preclude epidural placement. Patients on anticoagulants such as in the present case should be evaluated for the risk of epidural hematoma prior to deciding on a neuraxial technique. "Mini-dose" heparin, such as 5000 units subcutaneously twice daily, or use of nonsteroidal anti-inflammatory medications should not contraindicate a regional technique, unless other confounding factors exist. For patients on larger doses of heparin or fractionated heparin, accepted guidelines should be followed regarding timing of a neuraxial block in relation to medication administration as set forth by the most current recommendation made by the American Society of Regional Anesthesia.

With regard to obstetric factors, neuraxial blockade carries the side effect of sympathetic block and the resulting potential for hypotension.

Figure 38-1 *Late decelerations.*

Placental perfusion is directly related to maternal blood pressure and initiation of regional anesthesia should be weighed carefully in the presence of a nonreassuring fetal heart rate. Late decelerations, as pictured in Figure 38-1, are indicative of uteroplacental insufficiency, and hypotension from a regional block may be detrimental to the fetus in that scenario.

3. Discuss the necessary laboratory evaluation prior to initiating a labor epidural.

The physiologic anemia of pregnancy and benign leukocytosis can be anticipated in every parturient patient, and unless specific factors in the patient history dictate, there are no laboratory studies that must be carried out on a routine basis. In the case of preeclampsia, thrombocytopenic disease, and even possibly pregnancy-induced hypertension, a platelet count would be indicated. Frequently, as

in the case presented, pregnant patients present with idiopathic thrombocytopenia. Up to 10% of patients may be found with a platelet count below normal, and in a small number, the count may be less than 100,000/mm^3. There is much discussion and controversy regarding the lowest platelet count which allows for safe spinal or epidural block placement. A threshold of 100,000/mm^3 is a fairly conservative cut-off point. In the case of preeclampsia, the rate of drop of the platelet count should be considered as important as the absolute level, in determining the best course of action with regard to epidural placement. That is to say that a dropping platelet count may indicate epidural placement before the level reaches an anticipated point which would preclude placement. Likewise, a rapidly dropping level may give cause for concern that even though the absolute level is adequate, an anticipated significantly low nadir may predispose to bleeding complications after placement or upon removal of the catheter.

4. Describe the implications of a patient history which includes multiple miscarriages.

Multiple miscarriages such as noted in this case may stem from a variety of causes, commonly including hematologic and anatomic derangements. Abnormal uterine anatomy may prevent normal embryonic implantation or fetal growth. Coagulation abnormalities, specifically, thrombophilias, often lead to miscarriage. Examples of these thrombophilias include deficiencies of protein C or protein S, antiphospholipid (anticardiolipin antibody) syndrome, and factor V Leiden. The main anesthetic concerns of these conditions results from the associated anticoagulation used to suppress the process, and the resulting implications for regional anesthesia.

5. Outline the material risks and the potential benefits of epidural analgesia.

Risks:
- Failure or incomplete analgesia (6–10% of epidurals)
- PDPH (around 1% incidence)
- Persistent backache or sensory-motor impairment for up to a few months after discharge
- Infection at the insertion site, or in the central nervous system (CNS) (rare)
- Epidural hematoma
- Permanent nerve damage, total spinal/high spinal, and other complications; however, these are sufficiently rare that they may not be considered material risks.

Benefits:
- Potential for complete pain relief
- More complete analgesia than that provided by parenteral agents
- Less CNS depression than experienced with equipotent parenteral agents
- Ability to convert to surgical anesthesia, and avoid the dangers of general anesthesia in the case of cesarean delivery

6. Discuss implications of initiating epidural analgesia either early or later in labor.

As stated previously, a patient in active labor who is committed to delivery during the present admission may be given epidural analgesia upon request, provided that this plan fits with the obstetric management. The potential for an epidural placed early in labor to cause significant prolongation of labor or dystocia is not a material consideration in timing of delivery of the technique. Instead, practical considerations prevail; in most hospitals, initiation of epidural analgesia automatically relegates the patient to bed rest, unless a "walking epidural" program is in place. The patient considering an epidural early in labor should weigh her desire for pain relief against her desire to walk or even to ambulate only to the lavatory.

On the other end of the spectrum, healthcare workers frequently inform patients that they may not request an epidural after a particular point of cervical dilation. Similar to the concern surrounding early epidural placement, there is no absolute rule which precludes epidural placement based upon the stage of labor. However, practical considerations again prevail. In a patient in advanced labor, it may be very difficult to have her remain adequately motionless and cooperative for placement. The sitting position may cause discomfort to the mother and may cause fetal heart rate decelerations due to head compression at the perineum. Finally, there may not be adequate time for establishment of the block before delivery occurs. In this case, a subarachnoid technique seems particularly indicated to provide almost instantaneous pain relief.

The patient is positioned sitting for epidural insertion. A loss of resistance technique is used with saline, which is then injected into the epidural space prior to catheter insertion. The catheter is inserted 6 cm, but blood backflow on passive drainage occurs. The catheter is withdrawn 1 cm and flushed with saline. No further blood is aspirated. A test dose is administered, consisting of 3 ml of 1.5% lidocaine with epinephrine 1:200,000. No change in motor function or heart rate are observed. After the test dose, the epidural is loaded with 10 ml of 1% lidocaine in divided doses. The patient initially demonstrates a T10 sensory level. An infusion 0.1% bupivacaine + fentanyl 2 mcg/ml is initiated at 10 ml/hr. The patient remains comfortable for 3 hours, but then begins to complain of pain.

7. Compare the use of air vs saline in the loss of resistance syringe.

The choice between using air or saline for the loss of resistance (LOR) is often based on the clinician's preference and may be based on their tactile familiarity with one or the other substances as resistance is tested during the procedure. Provided that the volume of air injected is minimized, there are data supporting equivalence of efficacy and side effects between the two materials. However, air in the epidural space can ascend to produce the headache pain of pneumocephalus, and the severity of a PDPH can be increased by ascended epidural air, although the presence of air does not contribute to development of the PDPH initially. There is reasonable conjecture that an air bubble in the epidural space may dwell in space better occupied by local anesthetic solution, and some trials have found greater incidence of inadequate or patchy analgesia when air was used instead of saline for the LOR. Considering numerous factors disfavoring air, and that injection of saline reduces paresthesias and vein cannulations from the subsequent catheter insertion, it would be preferable for clinicians to use saline for the LOR technique.

8. Describe indications that give cues to needle location and appropriate responses to them.

The anesthetist should rely on more information than just the loss of pressure resistance to determine needle tip location in identifying the epidural space. A change in resistance accompanied by a gritty feel or sound during needle advancement can serve to indicate passage through the ligamentum flavum and should indicate more conservative advancements of the needle. Blood return into the needle or catheter obviously indicates penetration of an epidural vein, but more subtly suggests a needle tip position lateral to the midline, as the epidural veins tend not to be situated directly in the midline. In response to initial bloody return via the needle, the needle should be withdrawn and redirected with another LOR technique, with attention to assuring midline placement. In response to blood return via the catheter, the catheter may be withdrawn slightly and flushed with saline. If this maneuver withdraws the catheter from the vein, as evidenced by a lack of blood return and a negative intravenous (IV) test dose, the catheter may be dosed with anesthetic. The incidence of venous cannulation may be decreased by performing the epidural insertion with the patient in a lateral position, as opposed to the sitting position, wherein the epidural veins are more engorged. It is notable that the epidural veins are easily collapsible, and the inability to aspirate blood has little sensitivity for indicating vein cannulation. Passive gravity-assisted flow is a more sensitive indicator of a catheter situated in a blood vessel. Like bloody cannulations, paresthesias may indicate needle tip placement in a lateral epidural space. Paresthesias may indicate direct needle contact with or inside a nerve and injection should not take place. The needle should be withdrawn if any but the most fleeting paresthesia is encountered. Finally, while the epidural space is occupied by adipose tissue and a venous network, the epidural catheter should be expected to slide easily into the space through the epidural needle. Resistance to catheter advancement, particularly in the first 5 cm of insertion depth, may indicate placement outside of the epidural space. In this case, withdrawal of the entire needle–catheter unit and reinsertion of the needle may be preferable to continuing to secure and attempting to dose the catheter.

9. Debate the benefits of a shallow or deep catheter insertion depth.

There is a compromise between inserting the catheter adequately deep to buffer against movement causing withdrawal from the epidural space, and not inserting the catheter to a depth that promotes coiling or moving to a very lateral situation. The dividing line between these competing intentions is very thin, around the insertion depth of 5 cm. With a multiple-orifice catheter, the most proximate hole is usually situated 2 cm from the catheter tip. This would suggest that 2–3 cm is the absolute least depth a catheter may be inserted into the epidural space in order to have all orifices delivering medication into that space. On the other hand, the cause of many epidural failures is internal withdrawal of the catheter from the epidural space. A deeper insertion depth can provide some buffer against internal mobility of the catheter (in the space between the skin, where secured, and the epidural space). However, insertion depth beyond 4 cm increases the incidence of catheter coiling. This can lead to the catheter moving to one side or out the lateral vertebral foramen, causing a unilateral block, or it may even lead to catheter knotting. Insertion to a depth of 5–6 cm is a good compromise between the competing needs for adequate, but not excessive depth.

Intraoperative Period

10. Describe the level of anesthesia required for stage I and stage II of labor.

During stage I, pain is carried primarily via afferent nerves entering the spinal cord at T10 through L1. Therefore, adequate sensory block should be reflected in these dermatomes. During stage II, or the pelvic stage, pain is transmitted via the pudendal nerve to S2-S4 roots. As labor progresses, the extent of epidural blockade may need to be widened to assure coverage of the sacral dermatomes. In the absence of perineal pain to assess epidural coverage of sacral dermatomes, absence of plantar flexion of the foot indicates blockade of the S2 myotome, and provides a useful indication of caudal coverage of the epidural block.

11. Contrast the benefits of different anesthetic medications for a labor epidural infusion.

A wide variety of anesthetic mixtures may be used to provide epidural analgesia. Optimal epidural analgesia for labor manages the differential block that results from varying sensitivities of different nerves to local anesthetic effects. Differential block refers to blockade, but not all levels of nerve function in affected dermatomes. Ideally, the epidural will block all pain transmission, while leaving as much motor function preserved as possible, so as to not interfere with patient positioning, and "pushing" during stage II of labor. Lighter concentrations of anesthetic help preserve motor function, but may be more prone to breakthrough pain. Table 38-3 provides some representative epidural solutions, along with potential advantages and disadvantages associated with each of the various mixtures.

12. Discuss controversies and options related to performing the epidural test dose.

The epidural test dose is not used to verify optimal positioning of the catheter, but rather to rule out a catheter position that could lead to patient injury: in the intrathecal space, or in a blood vessel. The traditional test dose consists of a local anesthetic in a dose that would produce a definitive motor block if administered intrathecally, and epinephrine in a dose that would produce a heart rate rise if administered intravascularly. In the laboring patient, the heart rate can be very dynamic, and a rise in heart rate is not specific for epinephrine administration. Furthermore, if the epinephrine is injected intravascularly, it would be expected to cause a brief reduction in placental perfusion, and it could worsen any existing hypertension or pre-eclampsia. For these reasons, some variants on the test dose are sometimes preferred in the obstetric population.

Table 38-3   Examples of Medication Solutions Used to Administer Epidural Analgesia

SOLUTION	ADVANTAGES	DISADVANTAGES	REPRESENTATIVE USE
0.06% bupivacaine + epinephrine 1:800,000	Little to no motor block	Lighter sensory block; may be prone to break-through pain	Walking epidural
2 mcg/ml fentanyl	No motor block	Incomplete analgesia; increased opioid side effects apparent	Walking epidural; patient with allergy to all local anesthetics
0.125% bupivacaine + fentanyl 2 mcg/ml	Reliable analgesia; conservative compromise between analgesia and motor block		Typical continuous epidural solution
0.2% ropivacaine + fentanyl 2 mcg/ml	Possibly better analgesia with comparable motor block to 0.125% bupivacaine		Typical continuous epidural solution
0.08% ropivacaine + fentanyl 2 mcg/ml	Reliable analgesia; less toxicity potential than equipotent bupivacaine		Typical continuous epidural solution
0.25% bupivacaine ± opioids or epinephrine	Profound sensory block; resistant to breakthrough pain	Unnecessary motor block; increase in minor transient neurobehavioral deficits of neonate	Malpositioned fetus; "back labor"; opioid allergy

Following an intrathecal dose of anesthetic (when high-volume loading of the epidural is not needed), the IV test dose can be foregone, and a subarachnoid test can be used alone to assure that the infusion will not be administered into the intrathecal space. Other variants on the test dose include low, then high volume local anesthetic administration to determine intrathecal, and then IV placement. In this case, 2 ml of 2% lidocaine can be given first, with signs of lower extremity weakness after 5 minutes indicating intrathecal administration. Once the intrathecal position is ruled out, 5 ml of 2% lidocaine can be given, with signs of dizziness or other CNS symptoms indicating intravenous placement. Other drugs suitable for neuraxial administration but with characteristic IV responses may be substituted for epinephrine in the IV test dose, under particular circumstances. Fentanyl and isoproterenol are examples of agents that have been used in this way.

13. Discuss the procedural variants of the traditional labor epidural.

When the patient is in need of rapid analgesia without long-term effects or with minimal chance of late complications, à "single-shot spinal" may be used. This approach is useful when the patient is in very advanced labor and will deliver during the 60–90 minute duration of effects of the initial injection. With very small needles (27- or 29-gauge), the risk of PDPH may not be appreciably increased if the injection needs to be repeated. The single-shot injection is faster and easier to implement than an indwelling epidural, but it eliminates the benefit of an adaptable technique that can be extended for instrumented or surgical delivery, should either of those become necessary.

The combined spinal-epidural (CSE) technique is beneficial in the case of advanced or rapidly progressing labor, intense pain, a history of epidural failure, or the desire to avoid a heavy epidural loading dose (such as in the "walking" epidural). Medications useful for the intrathecal dose include fentanyl 10–20 mcg, sufentanil 5–10 mcg, bupivacaine 1.5–2.5 mg, ropivacaine 2–4 mg, or a combination of local anesthetic and opioid, including morphine. Following the intrathecal dose, the patient may be started on an epidural infusion, or epidural dosing may be deferred until the effects of the intrathecal dose subside. An intrathecal dose which does not contain morphine will typically provide a significant degree of analgesia for 60–90 minutes. If it is anticipated that an epidural infusion will be started eventually, it may be initiated immediately after CSE administration. In this way, the epidural space will be "loaded" by way of the slow infusion over the period during which the intrathecal dose is in effect. The epidural test dose may be used following a CSE, with the understanding that a high-volume test dose procedure may extend the height of spinal blockade and theoretically promote more local anesthetic diffusion through the dural puncture. Some providers omit the IV test dose following a CSE, in lieu of initiating the low-concentration infusion. This approach assumes that the low concentration of infusion (e.g., ≤ 0.125% bupivacaine) does not threaten systemic toxicity even if it is administered into a vein, while complete recession of the analgesia in the meanwhile would inform the practitioner that the medication is being delivered somewhere other than the epidural space.

The CSE technique derives analgesia from the intrathecal dose for the first 60–90 minutes; therefore, a nonfunctional epidural catheter is not discovered until after that period. As a result, while the CSE technique may aid in correct identification of the epidural space, it may also be disadvantageous in patients at risk for surgical delivery, as the anesthetist's ability to recognize catheter malfunctions is delayed. These competing considerations may create a conundrum when caring for an obese patient, such as the one that was presented. In this case, the selection of the CSE approach may be based largely on provider preference.

14. Discuss the side effects and treatment options for complications of epidural insertion.
A number of complications may occur during placement as outlined in Table 38-4.

Table 38-4 Epidural Complications and Management

COMPLICATION	MANAGEMENT
Blood in epidural needle	Withdraw needle and redirect
Blood in epidural catheter	Withdraw catheter (not while still in needle) to extent possible, flush, and use if clear. If continued blood, remove catheter and replace.
Cerebrospinal fluid via epidural needle or catheter	a. Remove needle and/or catheter and reinsert at different level b. Use catheter intrathecally, adjusting dosage accordingly
Paresthesia	Withdraw needle or catheter (not while still in needle) for all but the most transient paresthesias
Resistance on insertion of catheter	Remove catheter and needle as a unit (do not withdraw catheter through needle) and reinsert

Epidural catheter dislodgement may occur internally, if the catheter is secured to the relatively mobile soft tissue of the patient's back when seated, before moving the patient to a recumbent position in bed. This effect is minimal with a thin patient, but can be very pronounced with an obese patient. If inserting the catheter with the patient seated, it is advisable to instruct the patient to move to a lateral lying position before securing the catheter to the skin. A similar effect may result from edema formation which increases the distance from the epidural space to the skin, where the catheter is secured. See Figure 38-2.

15. Differentiate potential causes of breakthrough pain and their treatment.

- **Epidural misplacement:** block receding bilaterally, perhaps (but not always) visible disconnection of dislodgement at the site of insertion.
- **Malpositioned fetus:** fetus is positioned occiput posterior, causing pressure on parturient's sciatic nerve or others. The obstetric team can evaluate fetal position through palpation of the fontanelles.
- **Labor progression:** pain from T10 to L1 dermatomes in first stage, transitions to S2-S4 during second stage. Analgesia that does not reach sacral dermatomes may become unmasked as labor progresses to stage II.
- **Visceral pain:** bladder distention from sacral anesthesia may not be recognized by the patient and may present as diffuse abdominal pain.

Figure 38-2 *Internal dislodgement of the epidural catheter.*

- **Pathology,** such as placental abruption: smoking history or vascular compromise from diabetes or thrombophilia in this patient increase her risk of placental abruption. Vaginal bleeding may be an accompanying sign.

The patient pushed in stage II labor for 3 hours. The obstetrician plans to employ a vacuum extraction and calls for additional epidural dosing.

16. Formulate a plan for providing anesthesia for an instrumented vaginal delivery (ISV).

The use of vacuum extraction, and less commonly forceps delivery, may call for anesthetist intervention to intensify the level of a preexisting epidural block and to stand by for possible complications or conversion to cesarean delivery. With an existing epidural, elevating the patient's head to at least 30 degrees will reduce the incidence of "sacral sparing" or inadequate sacral blockade, as an additional bolus is given. The perineal dose typically consists of 5–10 ml of a rapidly-acting anesthetic such as 2–3% chloroprocaine or 2% lidocaine. If requested to provide anesthesia for ISV without an epidural in situ, an intrathecal dose of 2–3 mg bupivacaine followed by elevating the patient's upper body will provide rapid effects, with less sacral sparing than an epidural. However, considering the risk of operative intervention, providing this intrathecal dose as part of a CSE technique provides a useful back up, providing that there is time to perform this procedure.

Postoperative Period

17. Describe potential removal complications of the epidural catheter.

Complications associated with the removal of an epidural catheter are very rare. In a patient with coagulopathy, bleeding may be incited by catheter removal. For this reason, catheter removal should be delayed during an interval of significant coagulopathy, or therapeutic levels of low molecular weight heparin and similar medications. The other class of removal complications involves mechanical problems related to the catheter becoming fixed in place. This can result from a variety of causes and has been reported as occurring even immediately after initial insertion. A soft polyurethane catheter shows a greater propensity for becoming stuck in place, although these catheters perform more favorably in terms of ease of insertion and incidence of vein cannulations. The soft catheter also has a lower breaking strength than the polyamide nylon type, and so forceful removal attempts may more likely lead to catheter breakage. In the case of the inability to remove a catheter, methods to facilitate removal include changing the patient's position, applying steady gentle traction to the catheter, allowing hours to days of rest time before reattempting removal, and general anesthesia with muscle relaxation.

REVIEW QUESTIONS

1. Which is absolutely required prior to insertion of a labor epidural?
   a. Platelet count $> 140,000/mm^3$
   b. Cervical dilation > 4 cm
   c. Maternal desire for an epidural
   d. Ruptured amniotic sac
2. Which epidural medication would provide the greatest degree of motor block?
   a. Lidocaine 1%
   b. Bupivacaine 0.25%
   c. Fentanyl 2 mcg/ml
   d. Ropivacaine 0.1%
3. Pain from stage I of labor is transmitted through which spinal nerve distribution?
   a. C5–C8
   b. T4–T8
   c. T10–L1
   d. S2–S4
4. Which condition is least associated with pain?
   a. Malpositioned fetus
   b. Placenta previa
   c. Bladder distention
   d. Placental abruption

5. Which complication associated with epidural analgesia occurs with an incidence of approximately 1%?
   a. Inadequate analgesia
   b. Postdural puncture headache
   c. Backache
   d. Nerve damage

REVIEW ANSWERS

1. **Answer: c**
   Maternal desire for an epidural. Traditional approaches required that epidural analgesia not be initiated until the parturient had achieved a cervical dilation of at least 4 cm. This approach was borne of concern that epidural effects would inhibit labor. While some studies have demonstrated a prolongation of labor in patients with epidural, the degree of prolongation is not detrimental.
2. **Answer: b**
   Bupivacaine 0.25%, although this strength also provides reliable analgesia
3. **Answer: c**
   T10–L1. Pain during the second stage is transmitted via S2-S4.
4. **Answer: b**
   Placenta previa is characteristically not painful. The other choices should be considered in cases of breakthrough pain.
5. **Answer: b**
   Postdural puncture headache. Backache and inadequate analgesia occur much more frequently. Nerve damage is a very rare event.

SUGGESTED READINGS

Abrao KC, Francisco RP, Miyadahira S, et al. Elevation of uterine basal tone and fetal heart rate abnormalities after labor analgesia: a randomized controlled trial. *Obstet Gynecol* 2009;113(1):41–47.

Asai T, Yamamoto K, Hirose T, et al. Breakage of epidural catheters: a comparison of an arrow reinforced catheter and other nonreinforced catheters. *Anesth Analg* 2001;92:246–248.

Goodman SR, Smiley RM, Negron MA, et al. A randomized trial of breakthrough pain during combined spinal-epidural versus epidural labor analgesia in parous women. *Anesth Analg* 2009;108(1): 246–251.

Girard T, Kern C, Hösli I, et al. Ropivacaine versus Bupivacaine 0.125% with fentanyl 1mcg/ml for epidural labour analgesia: is daily practice more important than pharmaceutical choice? *Acta Anaes Belg* 2006;57: 45–49.

Halpern SH, Carvalho B. Patient-controlled epidural analgesia for labor. *Anesth Analg* 2009;108(3):921–928.

Hamilton CL, Riley ET, Cohen SE. Changes in the position of epidural catheters associated with patient movement. *Anesthesiology* 1997;86(4):778–784; discussion 29A.

Orbach-Zinger S, Friedman L, Avramovich A, et al. Risk factors for failure to extend labor epidural analgesia to epidural anesthesia for cesarean section. *Acta Anaesthesiol Scand* 2006;50(7):793–797.

Sakala C, Declercq ER, Corry MP. Listening to mothers: The first national U.S. survey of women's childbearing experiences. *JOGN Nurs* 2006;31(6):633–634.

Sia AT, Lim Y, Ocampo C. A comparison of a basal infusion with automated mandatory boluses in parturient-controlled epidural analgesia during labor. *Anesth Analg* 2007;104(3):673–678.

Van de Velde M, Dreelinck R, Dubois J, et. al. Determination of the full dose-response relation of intrathecal bupivacaine, levobupivacaine, and ropivacaine, combined with sufentanil, for labor analgesia. *Anesthesiology* 2007;106:149–156.

Laparoscopy for Adnexal Mass During Pregnancy

39

Edward Waters

KEY POINTS

- Approximately 2% of pregnant women will require nonobstetric surgery during pregnancy; these are often abdominal surgeries involving laparoscopy.
- If conditions permit, surgery during pregnancy should be accomplished during the second trimester.
- Numerous anesthetic agents can be used safely during pregnancy.
- Maintenance of maternal oxygen saturation and blood pressure during the intraoperative period is critical to avoiding fetal hypoxia from inadequate uteroplacental perfusion.
- Perioperative monitoring of fetal heart rate and uterine tone is prudent.

CASE SYNOPSIS

A 26-year-old woman who is at 29 weeks of gestation is evaluated in the anesthesia clinic for a diagnostic laparoscopy for an adnexal mass detected on routine ultrasound.

PREOPERATIVE EVALUATION AND DEMOGRAPHIC DATA

Past Medical/Surgical History

- Tonsillectomy, without anesthetic complications at 9 years of age

List of Medications

- Prenatal vitamins (folic acid, calcium, iron)

Diagnostic data

- Hemoglobin, 12.5 g/dl; hematocrit, 37.5%
- Sodium, 139 mEq/l; potassium, 4.1 mEq/l; chloride, 105 mEq/l; carbon dioxide (CO_2), 24 mEq/l
- Blood urea nitrogen, 8 g/dl; creatinine, 0.4 g/dl

Height/Weight/Vital Signs

- 175 cm, 73 kg
- Blood pressure, 110/60; heart rate, 78 beats per minute; respiratory rate, 22 breaths per minute; oxygen saturation on room air, 99%; temperature, 36.9°C

PATHOPHYSIOLOGY

Adnexal masses are diagnosed in 2% of pregnancies and can include ovarian cysts and benign or malignant tumors. Ovarian cysts are often incidental findings noted during routine ultrasonography for pregnant patients. Diagnostic workup for ovarian cysts includes ultrasound and computed tomography (CT) or magnetic resonance imaging (MRI). Ovarian cysts can cause pelvic pain, infertility, nausea, and vomiting. If large enough, cystic masses can obstruct normal labor. If the cyst is small, management involves observation because the majority of cysts will resolve spontaneously. If the cyst is large (> 5–10 cm), suspicious for malignancy, or persists for a prolonged time surgery is indicated.

SURGICAL PROCEDURE

The need for nonobstetric surgery in the pregnant patient is not a rare occurrence. Approximately 1 in 50 pregnant women will require surgery at some point during their pregnancy. Conditions most likely to lead to surgery in this population include trauma, appendicitis, cholecystitis, adnexal masses, breast masses, trauma, and cervical incompetence. While surgery during pregnancy is usually performed to treat maternal pathology, the well-being of maternal–fetal unit as a whole must be taken into account when planning anesthetic care. Important goals in the care of the pregnant patient for nonobstetric surgery include:

- Mitigating increased maternal risk arising from the physiologic changes of pregnancy.
- Minimizing fetal exposure to potentially teratogenic agents.

- Prevention of preterm labor.
- Avoidance of fetal asphyxia secondary to uterine hypoperfusion or maternal hypoxia.

ANESTHETIC MANAGEMENT AND CONSIDERATIONS

Preoperative Period

1. Discuss how the physiologic changes of pregnancy affect surgical risk.

The dramatic anatomic and physiologic adaptations that occur during pregnancy preserve the pregnancy and facilitate labor and delivery. Changes in the majority of maternal organ systems are seen during pregnancy; most important to anesthetic management are changes in the central nervous, pulmonary, cardiovascular, and gastrointestinal systems. The physiologic changes associated with pregnancy are summarized in Table 39-1.

Due largely to the effect of progesterone on the central nervous system (CNS), the pregnant patient experiences increased sensitivity to inhaled, intravenous, and local anesthetics. Furthermore, the subarachnoid and epidural spaces are reduced in volume due to the anatomic changes of pregnancy resulting in increased rostral spread of anesthetic agents injected into these spaces.

Oxygen consumption during pregnancy is dramatically increased, whereas functional residual capacity is diminished; this leads to a potential for significant hypoxia in poorly ventilated patients. An increased minute volume is normally seen in the pregnant woman as a result of an increase in both tidal volume and respiratory rate. The alveolar hyperventilation that occurs during pregnancy leads to a state of chronic compensated respiratory alkalosis. Difficult endotracheal (ET) intubation and epistaxis (in the case of nasal intubation) can result due to capillary engorgement of the mucosa of the upper airways as early as the first trimester of pregnancy.

The maternal cardiovascular system is dramatically changed by pregnancy. An increase in

Table 39-1	Physiologic Changes Associated with Pregnancy	
RESPIRATORY SYSTEM		
Minute ventilation	Increased 50%	
Tidal volume	Increased 40%	
Respiratory rate	Increased 15%	
Functional residual capacity	Decreased 20%	
$PaCO_2$ 32 to 35 mm Hg	Decreased	
Oxygen consumption	Increased 20%	
$PaCO_2$-$ETCO_2$ −1 to +1 mm Hg	Decreased	
CARDIOVASCULAR SYSTEM		
Cardiac output	Increased 40%	
Stroke volume	Increased 25%	
Heart rate	Increased 25%	
Systemic vascular resistance	Decreased	
Systolic blood pressure	Unchanged	
Diastolic blood pressure	Decreased	
HEMATOLOGIC SYSTEM		
Plasma volume	Increased 40–50%	
Hematocrit ~35%	Decreased	
CENTRAL NERVOUS SYSTEM		
Minimum alveolar concentration	Decreased	
GASTROINTESTINAL SYSTEM		
Lower esophageal sphincter tone	Decreased	
Barrier pressure	Decreased	
METABOLIC		
Free drug availability	Increased	
Plasma cholinesterase activity	Decreased	

cardiac output is the product of an increase in heart rate, intravascular volume, and stroke volume. The increased cardiac output, like the increased minute volume, helps the pregnant woman meet the metabolic needs of the fetoplacental unit. The generalized vasodilatation typical during healthy pregnancies leads to decreased systemic vascular resistance during pregnancy and increases sensitivity to the vasodilating effects of anesthetics.

The effect of pregnancy on gastric motility and acid secretion remain subjects of debate among experts related to gastrointestinal physiology. What is not in question is the fact that lower esophageal sphincter tone and gastric barrier pressure are decreased in pregnancy, placing pregnant women at increased risk of pulmonary aspiration.

2. Select the optimal time for surgery in the pregnant patient.

In the pregnant patient, elective surgery should be delayed until after delivery. If the need for surgery is pressing, it is preferably performed during the second trimester. If possible, surgery is best avoided during the first trimester due to the fact that fetal organogenesis occurs during this period. Third-trimester surgery is associated with increased risk of preterm labor and the possibility that the surgeon will experience increased technical difficulty due to the presence of the gravid uterus.

3. Explain the evaluation and preparation of a pregnant patient for anesthesia and surgery.

The preanesthetic assessment of a pregnant patient includes an evaluation of organ systems taking into account the changes expected in pregnancy. Obstetric consultation should be obtained regarding perioperative monitoring of fetal heart rate and uterine tone. The patient's obstetrician may also be consulted regarding the possible need for tocolysis. In addition to the above, preparation of a pregnant patient for anesthesia and surgery should include aspiration prophylaxis and pneumatic compression devices.

Pneumatic compression devices are indicated in pregnant patients due to the increased risk of deep vein thrombosis (DVT) resulting from the hypercoagulable state normal in pregnancy which is exacerbated by surgical trauma. Anxiolytics may be warranted due to the fact that increased catecholamine levels can cause vasoconstriction leading to decreased uteroplacental perfusion.

Intraoperative Period

4. Analyze which anesthetic technique is optimal for this surgery.

Research fails to demonstrate improved fetal outcomes associated with any particular anesthetic technique. A common, prudent practice is to employ regional techniques whenever possible due to the fact that fetal exposure to anesthetic agents is minimized and maternal risk for pulmonary aspiration is reduced. Most surgery during pregnancy is performed for intra-abdominal pathology that commonly requires general anesthesia. Increased maternal sensitivity to anesthetic agents necessitates reducing the amount of medication that is administered by approximately 30% to prevent accidental overdosage. Regardless of the technique employed, maintenance of adequate uteroplacental perfusion and maternal oxygenation is essential. Table 39-2 summarizes the most important anesthetic considerations in the pregnant patient undergoing nonobstetric surgery.

5. Examine the advantages and disadvantages of laparoscopic surgery during pregnancy.

A pregnant woman who presents with abdominal discomfort poses a diagnostic challenge for the clinician

Table 39-2   Anesthetic Considerations in Pregnant Patients Undergoing Laparoscopic Surgery

PREOPERATIVE

- Defer elective surgery until after delivery.
- Urgent surgery should be scheduled during the second trimester, if possible.
- If possible, use of a regional anesthetic technique may be prudent.
- Obstetric consultation should be obtained for recommendations regarding fetal heart rate monitoring and the use of tocolytics in the perioperative period.

INTRAOPERATIVE

- Patient should be placed in the left lateral decubitus position to minimize hypotension.
- Recognize and address the increased risk for difficult airway and pulmonary aspiration.
- Reduce dose of anesthetic agents due to increased maternal sensitivity.
- If mechanical ventilation is used, minute volume should be adjusted to maintain $ETCO_2$ at preoperative level.
- Maintain adequate maternal blood pressure and oxygenation to assure uteroplacental perfusion.
- Intra-abdominal pressure should not exceed 15 mm Hg.
- Continuous fetal heart rate monitoring in the intraoperative period should be considered.
- Intraoperative pneumatic compression devices should be employed to minimize venous thrombus.

POSTOPERATIVE

- Intraoperative pneumatic compression devices should be continued in the postoperative period to minimize risk of venous thrombus.
- Early ambulation should be encouraged to minimize risk of venous thrombus.
- Uterine tone should be monitored and tocolysis instituted if signs of preterm labor noted.
- Continuous fetal heart rate monitoring should be continued in the postoperative period.

who must distinguish between common pregnancy related symptoms and symptoms resulting from a potential pathology. This process is further complicated by the anatomic changes that are associated with pregnancy. Laparoscopy is valuable in this circumstance, providing a useful tool for both diagnosis and definitive treatment. Other beneficial effects of laparoscopic surgery include decreased intraoperative blood loss, reduced postoperative analgesic requirements, and the fact that the technique tends to facilitate early ambulation which is important for reducing the risk of thromboembolic complications.

Some clinicians have expressed concern regarding the use of laparoscopy in pregnant patients and this concern focuses principally on two issues: establishment of the pneumoperitoneum (PnP) and the physiologic effects of the PnP. Establishment of a PnP involves insufflation of CO_2 into the peritoneal space via either blind placement of a verres needle or open placement of a trocar, either of which has the potential to traumatize organs in the abdomen. Both techniques, when proper precautions are followed, are considered acceptable practice.

The physiologic effects of the CO_2 PnP have the potential to exacerbate preexisting cardiovascular and pulmonary pathophysiology. The physiologic effects associated with PnP are listed in Table 39-3. Anesthetic considerations for management of the pregnant woman undergoing laparoscopic surgery must take these changes into account and will be discussed in more detail later.

The Society of American Gastrointestinal and Endoscopic Surgeons has published well-developed guidelines for laparoscopic surgery during pregnancy. Careful anesthetic and surgical management allows pregnant patients to benefit from laparoscopic surgical techniques.

6. Describe airway and respiratory management of the pregnant woman undergoing nonobstetric laparoscopic surgery.

General anesthesia should be preceded by denitrogenation. Induction and ET intubation, using an

Table 39-3	Physiologic Effects Associated with Pneumoperitoneum	
RESPIRATORY SYSTEM		
Peak inspiratory pressure	Increased	
Pulmonary compliance	Decreased	
Vital capacity	Decreased	
Functional residual capacity	Decreased	
CO_2 delivery to lungs·	Increased by 30%	
Intrathoracic pressure	Increased	
CARDIOVASCULAR SYSTEM		
Cardiac output	Decreased	
Mean arterial pressure	Increased	
Systemic vascular resistance	Increased	
GASTROINTESTINAL SYSTEM		
Postoperative emesis	40–60%	

ET tube one size smaller than customarily used in nonpregnant women, should be accomplished expeditiously by the rapid sequence induction with cricoid pressure. Due to decreased functional residual capacity (FRC) and increased oxygen (O_2) demand, pregnant women experience rapid desaturation during even short periods of apnea.

Carbon dioxide homeostasis deserves special consideration. Absorption of CO_2 from the PnP increases the delivery of CO_2 to the lungs. End tidal carbon dioxide ($ETCO_2$) monitoring reliably reflects the partial pressure of arterial CO_2 ($PaCO_2$) in the patient and should be monitored closely. In the pregnant patient undergoing general anesthesia, minute ventilation will need to be adjusted to maintain an $ETCO_2$ in the low normal range typically seen during pregnancy (32 to 36 mm Hg). Providing adequate minute ventilation can be challenging due to the fact that a gravid uterus and the presence of the PnP can compromise diaphragmatic excursion leading to decreased lung compliance. Inadequate ventilation increases the potential risk of fetal and maternal acidosis. Hyperventilation can lead to alkalosis, resulting in a left shift of the oxyhemoglobin disassociation curve and impaired exchange of oxygen between the maternal and fetal circulation.

7. Review some of the cardiovascular issues seen in this population and appropriate anesthetic management.

Pregnant women can experience aortocaval compression as early as 20 weeks' gestation; because of this fact, patients undergoing surgery should be positioned in such a manner that the uterus is displaced to the left optimizing maternal preload and placental perfusion. In addition to the risk of decreased preload caused by aortocaval compression, insufflation of the abdomen to establish a PnP decreases venous return. Intravascular volume should be optimized prior to induction of anesthesia. Generalized vasodilation occurs during normal pregnancy, putting the woman receiving anesthesia at risk for sudden decreases in blood pressure. The development of hypotension may be mitigated by the effects of the PnP which causes increased systemic vascular resistance. The risk of hypotension can be reduced by avoiding high doses of inhaled agents. If the patient experiences a significant drop in blood pressure (systolic blood pressure below 100 mm Hg or a decrease exceeding 20%), the hypotension should be treated aggressively to ensure adequate uteroplacental perfusion since the uterus lacks the ability to autoregulate. Both phenylephrine and ephedrine have been used successfully to support the maternal blood pressure and preserve uteroplacental perfusion.

8. Identify the teratogenic risks of surgery and anesthesia in the pregnant patient.

Teratogenicity refers to significant structural or functional changes in a newborn resulting from prenatal treatment. This complex phenomenon involves the susceptibility of the species as well as the dose, duration of exposure, and timing of exposure to the agent during gestation. The risk of fetal harm resulting from anesthetics has been the subject of much concern on the part of the general public and clinicians.

Most anesthetic drugs (with the exception of neuromuscular blocking medications) are highly lipid soluble and therefore cross the placenta and enter the fetal circulation. In spite of the potential risk of fetal injury, very few drugs are thoroughly studied to determine whether their use is safe in pregnancy. This is largely due to the multiple scientific and ethical challenges that drug testing in pregnancy presents. A list of widely recognized teratogenic drugs is found in Table 39-4.

Despite many years of clinical experience and several studies, no anesthetic agent has been definitively identified as having teratogenic effects. The ability to conclusively affirm the safety of an anesthetic agent in pregnant women (or, for that matter, most drugs) is constrained by the limited number of studies in this population.

Table 39-4 Drugs Reported to Have Human Teratogenic Effects
Angiotensin-converting enzyme inhibitors
Aminoglycosides
Androgens
Antithyroid medications
Carbamazepine
Cocaine
Corticosteroids
Cytotoxic agents
Diethylstilbestrol
Estrogens
Ethanol
Lithium
Penicillamine
Phenytoin
Retinoids
Tetracycline
Thalidomide
Valproic acid
Warfarin

Two anesthetic agents have been implicated as having teratogenic effects. An association between maternal benzodiazepine use and increased risk of cleft lip and palate in newborns was suggested following case reports. This association was not supported by later case-controlled and prospective studies. In lab studies involving rodents, exposure to very high levels of nitrous oxide (N_2O) use led to abortion and congenital malformations. Observational studies examining human exposure to N_2O in normal concentrations fails to establish an association between N_2O and abortion or congenital malformation.

9. Explain the role of fetal heart rate monitoring in the management of patients undergoing nonobstetric surgery.

Whether or not to use fetal heart rate monitoring is a decision which is best made considering the specific circumstances surrounding the patient and surgery in question and after consultation between obstetric, surgical, and anesthetic practitioners. If a decision is made to employ fetal monitoring in the perioperative period, it is essential to have qualified personnel present to operate and interpret the monitor(s).

Fetal heart rate monitoring can be easily accomplished after 22 to 24 weeks' gestation using surface transducers. Intraoperative monitoring may be problematic due to the fact that transabdominal monitor placement can interfere with the surgical field. In these cases, options include omitting monitoring during the intraoperative period or the use of a vaginal probe.

Fetal exposure to anesthetic agents has the effect of eliminating beat-to-beat variability, and is not of concern. Persistent fetal bradycardia (Fig. 39-1) at any point in the perioperative period indicates fetal compromise and should trigger actions directed toward improving delivery of oxygen to the fetus. Depending on the circumstances, actions to improve fetal oxygenation may include left uterine displacement, tocolysis, release of surgical retraction, as well as support of maternal blood pressure and oxygenation.

Figure 39-1 *Fetal heart rate monitoring involves monitoring and correlating the fetal heart rate (upper graph) and uterine contractions (lower graph). Normal fetal heart rate is 110 to 160 beats per minute. Note the repeated episodes of fetal bradycardia in the upper tracing.*

Postoperative Period

10. Plan the postoperative care of a pregnant patient following nonobstetric surgery.

Postoperative care of surgical patients should devote considerable attention to managing pain and nausea. These priorities are of even greater significance in the population under consideration due to the fact that pregnancy and laparoscopic surgery put the patient at especially high risk for nausea and vomiting and the risk that increased levels of catecholamines accompanying pain can cause decreased uteroplacental blood flow.

Special considerations in the postoperative care of pregnant women undergoing nonobstetric surgery include prophylaxis against venous thrombosis and monitoring of the fetal heart rate and uterine tone. Measures to reduce the risk of venous thromboembolism include sequential compression hose, anticoagulation (avoiding the teratogenic agent warfarin), and early ambulation.

Preterm labor presents significant risk to the well-being of the fetus and accounts for 70% of perinatal morbidity and mortality. Monitoring of the fetal heart rate and uterine activity for 12 to 24 hours after surgery may be warranted with timely intervention for fetal bradycardia or preterm labor indicated if these conditions are detected.

REVIEW QUESTIONS

1. Low maternal blood pressure can lead to poor perfusion of the placenta due to the:
   a. increased maternal circulating volume.
   b. lack of uterine vascular autoregulation.
   c. left shift of the oxyhemoglobin curve.
   d. presence of fetal hemoglobin.
2. Maternal hyperventilation can lead to:
   a. altered uterine tone.
   b. decreased cardiac inotropy.
   c. increased risk of persistent fetal circulation.
   d. left shift of the oxyhemoglobin disassociation curve.

3. Absence of fetal beat-to-beat variability during administration of general anesthesia to the mother is considered:
   a. a normal fetal response.
   b. a sign of damage to the fetal nervous system.
   c. an indication for emergent delivery.
   d. an indication for tocolysis.
4. Which technique used for prophylaxis of thromboemboli is contraindicated during pregnancy?
   a. Early ambulation
   b. Low–molecular weight heparin
   c. Sequential compression hose
   d. Warfarin
5. In the setting of nonobstetric surgery during pregnancy, the greatest cause of fetal morbidity and mortality is:
   a. congenital defects.
   b. maternal death.
   c. postoperative infection.
   d. preterm labor.

REVIEW ANSWERS

1. **Answer: b**
   Because the uterine vasculature is not autoregulated, placental blood flow is directly dependent on the dynamic between perfusion pressure and vascular resistance.
2. **Answer: d**
   Hyperventilation causes a left shift of the oxyhemoglobin disassociation curve which inhibits the off loading of oxygen from maternal to fetal hemoglobin.
3. **Answer: a**
   The absence of beat-to-beat variability is common when the fetus is exposed to general anesthetic agents and will resolve with cessation of the precipitating agent.
4. **Answer: d**
   Warfarin is a known human teratogen.
5. **Answer: d**
   Preterm labor accounts for 70% of perinatal morbidity and mortality.

SUGGESTED READINGS

ACOG Committee on Obstetric Practice. ACOG Committee Opinion Number 284, Nonobstetric surgery in pregnancy. *Obstet Gynecol* 2003;102(2):431.

Andrade SE, Gurwitz JH, Davis RL, et al. Prescription drug use in pregnancy. *Am J Obstet Gynecol* 2004;191(2): 398–407.

Hawkins JL. Nonobstetric surgery during pregnancy. In: Atlee JL, ed. *Complications in Anesthesia,* 2nd ed. Philadelphia: Saunders, 2007:799–801.

Hepner D, Kodali B, Segal S. Pregnancy and complications of pregnancy. In: Fleisher L, ed. *Anesthesia and Uncommon Diseases,* 5th ed. Philadelphia: Saunders, 2006:547–577.

Hong JY. Adnexal mass surgery and anesthesia during pregnancy: a 10-year retrospective review. *Int J Obstet Anesth* 2006;15(3):212–216.

Penning DH. Does anesthesia increase the risk of the parturient undergoing nonobstetric surgery? In: Fleisher L, ed. *Evidence Based Practice of Anesthesiology*. Philadelphia: Saunders, 2004: 407–411.

Reynolds JD, Booth JV, de la Fuente S, et al. A review of laparoscopy for nonobstetric-related surgery during pregnancy. *Curr Surg* 2003;60(2):164–173.

Rosenberg L, Mitchell AA, Parsells JL, et al. Lack of relation of oral clefts to diazepam use during pregnancy. *N Engl J Med* 1983;309(21):1282–1285.

Society of American Gastrointestinal and Endoscopic Surgeons. Guidelines for diagnosis, treatment and use of laparoscopy for surgical problems during pregnancy. Society of American Gastrointestinal and Endoscopic Surgeons Web site. Available online at: http://www.sages.org/Publication/id/23/. Accessed January 28, 2009.

Steinbrook RA. Anaesthesia, minimally invasive surgery and pregnancy. *Best Pract Res Clin Anaesthesiol* 2002;16(1):131–143.

Urologic Surgery

XIII

Radical Prostatectomy

40

Jessica Bair

KEY POINTS

- Since the average age of men who develop prostate cancer is greater than 50 years, patients presenting for radical prostatectomy frequently have at least one comorbidity.
- The most common intraoperative complications associated with radical prostatectomy are acute hemorrhage and positioning injuries.
- Presently, there are several surgical options and anesthetic choices for patients with prostate cancer.
- Accurate monitoring of blood loss as well as plan for fluid and blood replacement is imperative.

CASE SYNOPSIS

A 69-year-old man presents to his urologist with increased urinary frequency and urgency. He undergoes a thorough urologic workup that reveals his prostate-specific antigen (PSA) is elevated. His doctor performs a digital rectal exam and palpates several irregular nodules. The results from a prostate biopsy definitively reveal that the patient has prostate cancer. His urologist recommends a radical prostatectomy and explains the risks and benefits of the various surgical options which include traditional open approach, laparoscopic, and robot-assisted laparoscopic technique. The patient chooses the robot-assisted laparoscopic approach.

PREOPERATIVE EVALUATION AND DEMOGRAPHIC DATA

Past Medical/Surgical History

- Hypertension
- Coronary artery bypass graft (CABG) performed 2 years ago
- Well-controlled asthma
- Osteoarthritis
- 12 pack/year smoker, stopped smoking 2 weeks ago

List of Medications

- Atenolol
- Hydrochlorothiazide
- Singulair inhaler
- Aspirin
- Sildenafil (Viagra)

Diagnostic Data

- Hemoglobin, 14.1 g/dl; hematocrit, 40.9%
- Blood urea nitrogen (BUN), 17 mg/dl; creatinine, 1.0 mg/dl
- Electrolytes: sodium, 141 mEq/l; potassium, 3.4 mEq/l; chloride, 101 mEq/l; carbon dioxide (CO_2), 25 mEq/l
- Glucose, 144 mg/dl
- PSA, 11 ng/ml (reference range 0–4.5 ng/ml for age 61–70 years)

Height/Weight/Vital Signs

- 185 cm, 86 kg
- Blood pressure, 161/96; heart rate, 78 beats per minute; respiratory rate, 14 breaths per minute; room air oxygen saturation, 99%; temperature, 37.4°C
- 12-Lead electrocardiogram (ECG): normal sinus rhythm with a right bundle branch block, heart rate, 72 beats per minute
- Exercise stress test: no evidence of ischemia
- Cardiac Doppler ultrasound: estimated ejection fraction, 55%

PATHOPHYSIOLOGY

It is estimated that up to one third of men develop cellular dysplasia consistent with prostate cancer by 50 years of age. The incidence of prostate cancer increases with age and, at 75 years of age, the possibility rises to approximately 75%. Prostate cancer is the second leading cause of mortality due to cancer-related deaths. Prostate cancer generally occurs in men over the age of 50. Therefore, it is reasonable to expect a high incidence of comorbidities such as hypertension and diabetes in this patient population. Prostate cancer is considered a slow progressing cancer. Early detection and prompt treatment significantly increase the probability of survival.

The initial routine screening for prostate cancer is achieved by assessing PSA blood test results. It is theorized that if every man lived long enough, he would develop prostate cancer. The information provided by PSA testing has limitations which include the sensitivity and specificity of the results. There are many factors that can cause falsely elevated PSA results such as a urinary tract infection. More recently, the upper limits in the reference range of the PSA is indexed in relation to patient age. A digital rectal exam provided by a urologist and a prostate biopsy are necessary to definitively diagnose the presence of prostate cancer.

Approximately 95% of prostate cancer is caused by adenocarcinoma. Androgens and estrogens affect prostate epithelial proliferation, thereby supporting carcinogenesis. However, not all patients who develop prostate cancer have elevated androgen levels. The incidence of prostate cancer differs according to various ethnic groups. African American men are 60% more likely to develop the disease as compared to Caucasian men.

Once a patient is diagnosed with prostate cancer and a prostate sample is obtained, the tumor is staged using the TNM Classification System (T = tumor, N = nodes, M = metastasis) and the Gleason grading scale both, of which are included in Tables 40-1 and 40-2. It is believed that several predisposing factors for developing prostate cancer include increased age, race, family history, and a high-fat diet. The exact mechanism that triggers prostate cancer remains unknown. Patient symptomatology varies significantly and ranges from no symptoms to those that are associated with benign prostatic hypertrophy (BPH) which include urinary hesitancy, frequency, retention, urgency, and incontinence. If these symptoms are present, it is likely the tumor has

Table 40-1 TNM Staging of Prostate Cancer	
PRIMARY TUMOR	
STAGE	**DESCRIPTION**
Tx	Primary tumor cannot be assessed
T0	No evidence of primary tumor
	Clinically unapparent tumor not palpable or visible by imaging
T1	T1a – Tumor incidental, found in 5% or less resected tissue
	T1b – Tumor incidental, found in more than 5% resected tissue
	T1c – Tumor identified by needle biopsy (because of elevated PSA)
	Tumor is confined within the prostate gland
T2	T2a – Tumor involves one lobe
	T2b – Tumor involves both lobes
	Tumor extends through the prostatic capsule
T3	T3a – Extracapsular extensions (unilateral or bilateral)
	T3b – Tumor invades the seminal vesicles
T4	Tumor is fixed or invades adjacent structures other than seminal vesicles: bladder neck, external sphincter, rectum, levator muscles, and/or pelvic wall
REGIONAL LYMPH NODES	
STAGE	**DESCRIPTION**
Nx	Regional lymph nodes have not been assessed
N0	No regional lymph node metastasis
N1	Regional lymph node metastasis
DISTANT METASTASIS	
STAGE	**DESCRIPTION**
Mx	Distant metastasis has not been assessed
M0	No distant metastasis
M1	M1a – Nonregional lymph nodes
	M1b – Bone
	M1c – Other sites

grown large enough to partially occlude the urethra and surgical intervention is necessary.

SURGICAL PROCEDURE

The traditional approach for radical prostatectomy occurs through a lower abdominal midline extraperitoneal incision extending from the umbilicus to the symphysis pubis. Presently, laparoscopic and robotic-assisted surgical approaches are rapidly becoming increasingly popular.

The procedure involves removing the entire prostate gland, the seminal vesicles, the ejaculatory ducts, and a portion of the bladder neck. Sometimes the surrounding lymph nodes are

Table 40-2	Gleason Grading of Prostate Cancer
GRADE	**DESCRIPTION**
Grade 1	Small, uniform glands with minimal nuclear changes
Grade 2	Medium-sized acini, still separated by stroma but more closely arranged
Grade 3	The most common finding in prostate cancer biopsies, show marked variation in glandular size and organization with infiltration of stromal and neighboring tissues
Grade 4	Markedly atypical cells with extensive infiltration into the surrounding tissues
Grade 5	Sheets of undifferentiated cancer cells

removed and examined for pathologic staging. There are bilateral neurovascular bundles adjacent to the prostatic capsule. This neural tissue allows a man to achieve a penile erection. Surgeons may try to preserve sexual function by preserving the nerve bundles. The procedure is called a nerve-sparing prostatectomy. In patients with a history of impotence, these nerve bundles are removed (non–nerve-sparing prostatectomy). Once the prostate gland is removed, the bladder neck and urethra are reanastomosed over an indwelling urinary catheter. The catheter helps surgeons visualize and align the two edges of the urethra as they are rejoined. This reestablishes a path for urine flow.

Radical prostatectomy procedures are increasingly being done by the laparoscopic approach. A subset of the laparoscopic approach is the robot-assisted laparoscopic prostatectomy, in which the da Vinci surgical robot is employed. The robot offers the surgeon more precise motor movements as well as the ability to obtain a magnified view of the surgical field during dissection. These attributes are particularly beneficial for the intracorporeal anastomoses, which is technically challenging. Three to six trochars are placed in the abdominal wall as a pathway for the camera and instruments. Through these ports, the retroperitoneal space is insufflated with CO_2 gas. Steep Trendelenburg (30–45%) is required for the laparoscopic approach as gravity mobilizes the abdominal contents toward the diaphragm providing a clear view of the surgical field and ample space to safely dissect the prostate gland.

ANESTHETIC MANAGEMENT AND CONSIDERATIONS

Preoperative Period

1. Describe the comorbidities that are likely found in this patient population.

Due to the advancing age of this patient population, these men frequently present with at least one or more coexisting disease process such as hypertension, diabetes mellitus, renal dysfunction, myocardial infarction, arrhythmias, and emphysema. Renal impairment is probable in cases that have had chronic urinary obstruction. It is estimated that patients 65 years and older have at least one comorbid factor. The incidence of commonly occurring pathophysiologic disease states associated with patients who have prostate cancer is listed in Table 40-3.

Table 40-3	Incidence of Comorbidities in Patients with Prostate Cancer
Chronic obstructive pulmonary disease	10%
Coronary artery disease	10%
Hypertension	10%
Diabetes	5%
Renal failure	1%

2. Determine a comprehensive plan to ensure this patient's health is optimized preoperatively.

Cardiovascular System Due to the physiologic stress induced by anesthesia and laparoscopic surgery, a comprehensive cardiac evaluation is necessary prior to the surgical procedure. A degree of cardiac pathology must be suspected since this patient is nearly 70 years of age, has a history of essential hypertension, CABG 2 years prior, and diabetes mellitus. A thorough preoperative work-up would include a 12-lead ECG, a treadmill cardiac stress test, and clearance from a cardiologist. Hemodynamic control will be an essential aspect of the anesthetic management for this patient.

The patient should be instructed to continue taking all of his daily medications, except for the aspirin and Viagra until the day of surgery. Aspirin should be stopped 2 weeks prior to surgery to decrease prolonged bleeding. A discussion of the medication Viagra will occur later in this chapter.

Respiratory System His bronchial asthma is well controlled and, as a result, pulmonary function tests are not required. This patient also smokes cigarettes which, along with asthma, further increases the possibility of hyperreactive airway and chronic obstructive pulmonary disease (COPD).

Renal System Patients with chronic urinary obstruction may develop renal insufficiency. The BUN and creatinine values for this patient are within limits.

Antibiotic Prophylaxis The primary infecting microorganism that results in postoperative infection after radical prostatectomies are coliforms. A quinolone antibiotic (Ciprofloxin) or an aminoglycoside antibiotic (Gentamicin) should be administered immediately prior to surgical incision.

Preoperative Laboratory Assessment Hemoglobin and hematocrit values will be obtained to compare these results to those performed intraoperatively after surgical blood loss and hemodilution have occurred. Due to the potential for severe blood loss, type and screen for packed red blood cells is prudent. However, a type and cross-match is required for an open radical prostatectomy due to the increased blood loss that occurs.

The patient is regularly taking hydrochlorothiazide, a diuretic used to treat hypertension. His electrolytes should be checked to make certain the results are within normal limits. Lastly, his blood sugar should be checked prior to surgery. His blood glucose value is 144 mg/dl. If this result is elevated as compared to his baseline values, the cause is most probably the result of the stress response and no treatment is warranted at this time. Serial glucose values will be assessed intraoperatively.

3. Discuss the pharmacology of sildenafil (Viagra) and any physiologic concerns regarding its use within the perioperative period.

During sexual arousal, there is an influx of blood into the corpus cavernosum due to the relaxation of smooth muscle causing an erection. This response is mediated by the production of nitric oxide (NO). Cyclic-guanosine monophosphate (cGMP) is responsible for smooth muscle relaxation and is produced from GTP when NO activates guanylyl cyclase. Phosphodiesterase controls the length of time the cGMP works. Phosphodiesterase 5 (PDE 5) is the phosphodiesterase isoenzyme that terminates the action of cGMP on the corpus cavernosum. Viagra inhibits PDE 5 thereby allowing the accumulation of cyclic-GMP, which sustains penile erection. The use of Viagra is contraindicated with concurrent organic nitrates, such as nitroglycerin, because it potentiates the actions of NO. The synergistic effects of this drug combination could cause a precipitous drop in the patient's blood pressure that is minimally responsive to adrenergic agonists. Considering this patient's history of a CABG, the use of nitroglycerin is a sound pharmacologic choice if hypertension ensues. If the patient has taken Viagra in the 24 hours before surgery, the use of nitroglycerin would be absolutely contraindicated and the safest course of action is to postpone surgery.

Intraoperative Period

4. State the advantages and disadvantages of administering various antihypertensive medications to this patient.

Beta-adrenergic antagonists, commonly referred to as beta-blockers, can be cardioselective, only antagonizing β1 receptors, or nonselective, antagonizing both β1 and β2 receptors. Beta-blocking drugs have negative inotropic (contractility), negative chronotropic (rate), and negative dromotropic (speed of cardiac conduction) effects on the myocardium and result in decreased cardiac output (CO), a component of blood pressure. By increasing oxygen supply and decreasing myocardial oxygen demand, beta-blocking medications are cardioprotective.

It is important to note that β2 receptor blockade in the lungs results in bronchiolar smooth muscle constriction, which can result in bronchospasm. This patient is already predisposed to developing bronchospasm due to his smoking history, COPD, and asthma. Therefore, beta-blocking medications must be used with extreme caution in patients with these disease states. Since beta blockers can cause acute congestive heart failure (CHF), the anesthetist should consider the patient's ejection fraction prior to administration. This patient's ejection fraction is estimated to be 55% which is nearly a normal value.

Since anesthesia and surgery are both extremely physiologically stimulating events, such as tachycardia and hypertension, can occur. Patients receiving beta-blockers preoperatively should not abruptly discontinue taking medications because hypertension, arrhythmias, angina, and myocardial infarction can occur. Beta-blocking medications that can be administered intravenously during the perioperative period include:

- ***Propranolol (Inderal)*** is a nonselective β1 and β2 receptor antagonist. Propranolol has a long duration of action and, for this reason, the oral form is frequently prescribed for chronic therapy.

- ***Metoprolol (Lopressor)*** is a nonselective β1 and β2 receptor antagonist. However, due to the intrinsic sympathomimetic effects of metoprolol, patients with decreased ejection fraction may benefit.

- ***Labetalol (Trandate)*** is a nonselective β1, β2, and alpha 1 receptor antagonist. Alpha 1 receptor antagonism results in vascular dilation which results in decreased systemic vascular resistance (SVR). The beta-blocking effects associated with Labetalol are significantly more potent that the alpha 1 blocking effects at a ratio of 7 to 1, respectively.

- ***Esmolol (Brevibloc)*** is a short-acting selective β1 antagonist. It is metabolized in the plasma by nonselective red blood cell esterases and, as a result, this drug's elimination half-life is only 10 minutes. The degree of β1 selectivity may be compromised and β2 receptor blockade can occur when the medication is administered as an intravenous bolus.

5. Compare the anesthetic options for open radical prostatectomy and laparoscopic prostatectomy.

The prostate is innervated by sympathetic nerve fibers that originate in the T10-12 and L1-2 segments of the spinal cord and by parasympathetic nerve fibers originating from S2-4. The innervation of the prostate and bladder neck makes neuraxial anesthesia an option for open radical prostatectomy. Spinal and epidural anesthesia have been administered with success and the benefits of regional anesthesia include decreased blood loss, reduced postoperative pain, and a shorter postanesthesia recovery when compared to general anesthesia. Disadvantages associated with neuroaxial anesthesia include prolonged surgical length, extremes in positioning (i.e., exaggerated lithotomy for the perineal approach), and the possibility of massive blood loss. A combined epidural and general anesthetic is associated with less blood loss and allows for postoperative pain management.

Neuraxial anesthesia is an anesthetic option for laparoscopic prostatectomy. However, the pressure exerted by the pneumoperitoneum on the diaphragm and the need for steep Trendelenburg positioning make breathing difficult. There is also the potential for bowel injury secondary to patient movement. Therefore, general anesthesia is considered the gold standard for open and laparoscopic radical prostatectomy.

6. Describe the potential nerve injuries that are associated with positioning for radical prostatectomy.

Most anesthetic-related nerve injuries are the result of overstretching and compression of a nerve, or from hypoperfusion. During an open prostatectomy, the patient is positioned supine. The table is flexed at the level of the anterior superior iliac spine and the patient's legs are placed in a low lithotomy position.

The two most often reported anesthetic-related nerve injuries are ulnar nerve neuropathy and brachial plexus injury; both of which can result from improper positioning of the upper extremities. The upper extremities are placed on armrests and must not be abducted greater than 90 degrees from the body or stretching of the brachial plexus can occur. The entire length of each arm must be padded and secured, including the ulnar groove. Pressure points should be reassessed every 15 minutes during the intraoperative period.

Injuries that occur most often to the nerves of the lower extremities during lithotomy positioning are the common peroneal, sciatic, obturator, and femoral. The length of the legs as well as the popliteal space should be padded and supported. Lateral placement of the knees can stretch the obturator nerves. Lifting and lowering the lower extremities simultaneously can avoid lumbar sacral nerve injuries. In the lithotomy position, damage to the common peroneal nerve results from direct pressure on the posterior and inferior surface of the head of the fibula against the leg support. This is an example of a compression injury. Femoral nerve damage can occur from the lithotomy position when the thigh is hyperextended. This is an example of a stretch injury.

Sensory injuries occur more frequently than motor injuries. If the injury results in numbness or tingling, these symptoms usually resolve within 1 week. Any neurologic injury that is sustained should be evaluated by a neurologist. This patient has osteoarthritis and proper positioning is imperative to help avoid nerve injury. The prolonged length of the procedure and extreme Trendelenburg may further predispose him to positioning-related injuries.

7. Explain the physiologic changes that occur with steep Trendelenburg, lithotomy, and laparoscopic surgery.

The physiologic stress that is experienced during laparoscopic prostatectomy is a dynamic process. The individual's compensatory response for the physiologic changes varies. The most significant changes occur to the cardiovascular system and respiratory system.

Cardiovascular System   The cardiovascular system is affected by laparoscopic surgery and specifically the pneumoperitoneum in the following ways:

1. *Increased SVR (increased afterload)*
2. *Increased pulmonary vascular resistance (PVR)*
3. *Decreased venous return (decrease preload)*
4. *Increased mean arterial pressure (MAP)*
5. *Decreased CO*

Increasing the patient's circulating volume by administering intravenous fluid helps offset decreases in CO and venous return. Instrumentation of the airway and surgical trauma increases sympathetic nervous system predominance. Increases in afterload causes increased myocardial oxygen consumption, which is of great concern in patients with preexisting cardiac pathology. Additionally, when the legs are placed in lithotomy, there is approximately 300–400 ml of blood that passively increased central blood volume. Lastly, the Trendelenburg position further exacerbated this situation. These factors support the need for a comprehensive preoperative cardiac evaluation.

Inhalation agents, narcotics, and adrenergic antagonists directly or indirectly cause a decrease in SVR, PVR, and sympathetic nervous system tone resulting in decreased myocardial oxygen consumption. Insufflation during creation of the pneumoperitoneum may initiate the celiac reflex caused by stretching of the abdominal cavity. The response causes increased vagal tone which can manifest as arrhythmias, hypotension, bradycardia, and possibly asystole. Treatment of the celiac reflex that causes hemodynamic instability includes immediate evacuation of the pneumoperitoneum and then administration of an anticholinergic (atropine) if necessary.

Respiratory System The pneumoperitoneum increases intra-abdominal pressure and the Trendelenburg position allows the abdominal contents to move cephalad and impinge on the diaphragm. The result is both a decrease in functional residual capacity (FRC) and a decrease in thoracolumbar compliance which support ventilation perfusion mismatch. Also, insufflation is accomplished using CO_2 gas. Systemic absorption of CO_2 occurs over time and can result in acidosis. Increasing minute ventilation is imperative to maintain normocapnia and provide oxygenation. Since peak airway pressures (PAP) will be elevated, increasing the tidal volume will further increase PAP. This patient has COPD and dramatically increasing PAP could result in barotrauma. Ventilation using a set pressure as compared to a set volume may help to decrease PAP. Therefore, increasing the respiratory rate while maintaining PAP to achieve normocapnia and adequate arterial oxygenation is recommended.

8. Identify potential intraoperative complications that can occur during robot-assisted laparoscopic prostatectomy.
Robot-assisted laparoscopic prostatectomy is associated with unique complications. A list of potential complications is listed in Table 40-4.

9. Review the benefits of this patient's choice of laparoscopy over laparotomy.
It has been demonstrated that the inflammatory response associated with tissue trauma is decreased with laparoscopic surgical procedures. Measurement of two mediators of inflammation, C-reactive protein and interleukin-6 are decreased during laparoscopic surgery when compared to a traditional open approach. Robot-assisted laparoscopic radical prostatectomy results in less intraoperative blood loss, less postoperative pain, greater nerve sparing success, and decreased time until ambulation

Table 40-4   Potential Complications Associated with Robot-Assisted Laparoscopic Prostatectomy

Extraperitoneal insufflation resulting in subcutaneous emphysema

Potential for hypercarbia resulting in acidosis

CO_2 gas embolism

Arterial hypoxemia

Endotracheal tube migration

Barotrauma resulting in a pneumothorax

Stimulation of the celiac reflex resulting in hemodynamic instability

Increased cardiac workload resulting in myocardial ischemia

Retinopathy, airway and cerebral edema resulting from prolonged steep Trendelenburg positioning

Acute and massive hemorrhage

Unintentional surgical trauma to the bowel, bladder, abdominal organs, and vascular structures postoperatively. Together, these factors result in shorter length of hospitalization and a higher rate of patient satisfaction.

10. Evaluate a fluid management plan for patients having laparoscopic prostatectomy.

Hypotension can occur after the induction of anesthesia due to the relative intravascular volume depletion due to "nothing-by-mouth" (NPO) guidelines and the myocardial depression and vasodilation that occurs with anesthetic agents. Fluid replacement must account for the following factors:

- Hourly maintenance rate
- NPO deficit
- Insensible or surgical loss

Administration of isotonic crystalloid solutions such as lactated Ringers or normal saline should be used. Hespan, a colloid solution can also be used; however, coagulopathy can occur if a total volume of greater than 20 ml/kg is administered.

The anesthetist must continuously assess the amount of blood loss that occurs. Physiologic signs of intraoperative hemorrhage include tachycardia and hypotension. In response to blood loss, both SVR and stroke volume increase to compensate for decreased intravascular volume. The degree of hypovolemia may be moderate to severe when signs of hemorrhage ensue. The estimated blood loss during radical prostatectomy is 200–700 ml but is frequently between 50–100 ml after a laparoscopic approach. Figure 40-1 is used to calculate allowable blood loss for this patient.

$$\frac{EBV \times (Hi-Hf)}{Hi} = ABL$$

ABL, allowable blood loss; Hi, initial hematocrit; Hf, final lowest acceptable hematocrit; EBV, estimated blood volume = weight in kilograms multiplied by the average blood volume (65–70 ml/kg).

Figure 40-1 *Formula used to calculate allowable blood loss.*

The actual blood loss may be difficult to accurately determine because, after the bladder neck is severed, urine flows directly into the surgical field mixing with blood. Serial assessment of the patient's hematocrit is imperative to most objectively quantify the degree of blood loss. There is no single hematocrit value that necessitates the need for blood transfusion. This decision should be based on the patient's preoperative level of functioning, assessment of hemodynamic factors, and the progress of the surgery. Hemoglobin and hematocrit values should be rechecked in the recovery room and during the patient's hospital stay.

11. Discuss the importance of maintaining normothermia throughout the procedure.

Even during laparoscopic surgery, a dramatic and rapid decrease in core temperature can occur. The negative effects associated with hypothermia can adversely affect the patient's surgical and anesthetic outcome. Coagulopathy leading to increased surgical bleeding and altered hemostasis, decreased drug metabolism resulting in prolonged emergence from anesthesia, and postoperative shivering which greatly increases myocardial oxygen demands can result from hypothermia.

The primary mode of heat loss that patients experience during surgery is by radiation. Core temperature monitoring should be assessed using an esophageal probe. An esophageal stethoscope also allows for continuous assessment of high quality breath sounds. Maintaining body temperature can be accomplished by using:

- Heated air warming blanket
- Fluid warming system
- Covering the patient's head
- Avoiding the use of high liter fresh gas flow
- Using warmed irrigation in the surgical field

12. Describe the reason that indigo carmine or methylene blue is administered during laparoscopic prostatectomy.

As with other laparoscopic surgical procedures, injury to the ureters is a known complication. A tear or inadvertent damage is difficult to identify during laparoscopic visualization, so it is common for the surgeons to ask the anesthetist to administer indigo carmine or methylene blue to determine ureteral integrity. Hepatic metabolism is minimal and both dyes are primarily excreted by the kidneys within approximately 10 minutes after intravenous administration. If ureteral damage has occurred or ureteral reanastomosis in necessary, the surgeon can detect the blue colored urine and then repair the defect.

The choice of which dye to use is dependent on the hospital drug formulary and the surgeon's preference. These medications can produce an increased blood pressure; however, the degree of hypertension is frequently mild and the duration is short. It is proposed that the hypertension occurs due to the inhibition of NO which is a potent vasodilator. Additionally, the oxygen saturation displayed by the pulse oximeter will artificially decrease due to the blue color of the dyes. The physiologic effects associated with methylene blue and indigo carmine includes:

Methylene blue
- Methemoglobinemia if large doses are administered
- Hypertension
- Dysrhythmias
- Hyperthermia
- Anaphylaxis

Indigo carmine
- Bradycardia
- Hypertension
- Methemoglobinemia if large doses are administered

Postoperative Period

13. Create a postoperative plan for this patient.
If venous congestion of the airway is suspected, it is appropriate to take the patient to the recovery room intubated. Deflating the endotracheal tube cuff and verifying the presence of an air leak can help confirm the presence of swelling. Administration of sedative and analgesic medications is warranted.

The patient's vital signs should be closely monitored throughout the postoperative period and, as previously mentioned, serum hemoglobin and hematocrit values should be obtained. The urine collection system should be monitored for bleeding.

The CO_2 gas used during laparoscopic surgery is converted to carbonic acid. Carbonic acid has been implicated with causing peritoneal irritation. It has been reported that as many as 80% of patients report neck or shoulder pain in the 24-hour postoperative period. The diaphragmatic peritoneal pain is referred to the shoulder via the phrenic nerve. This pain can be difficult to distinguish from cardiac pain and is effectively treated by administering ketorolac.

REVIEW QUESTIONS

1. Which medication decreases heart rate, decreases myocardial contractility, and causes a decrease in SVR?
   a. Esmolol
   b. Labetalol
   c. Metoprolol
   d. Atenolol
2. Elevating the patient's legs into the lithotomy position causes:
   a. an decrease in afterload.
   b. a decrease in SVR.
   c. an increase in myocardial oxygen consumption.
   d. an increase in CO_2 production.
3. Which is an advantage of robotic laparoscopic surgery for prostatectomy as compared to a traditional open abdominal approach?
   a. Increased blood loss
   b. Decreased risk of infection
   c. Decreased inflammatory mediator response
   d. Decreased ability to maintain normothermia
4. Which physiologic phenomena can occur with both indigo carmine and methylene blue?
   a. Anaphylaxis
   b. Hypotension
   c. Bradycardia
   d. Methemoglobinemia

5. Which is associated with perioperative hypothermia?
   a. Decreased drug metabolism
   b. Hypercoagulation
   c. Hypotension
   d. Decreased myocardial oxygen consumption

REVIEW ANSWERS

1. **Answer: b**
   Labetalol is a nonspecific β1, β2 antagonist which decreases myocardial contractility and heart rate. This medication is also an alpha-1 antagonist which decreases SVR and blood pressure.

2. **Answer: c**
   Raising the patient's legs into the lithotomy position causes an increase in central blood volume. The predominant cardiovascular effect is increased preload which causes an increase in myocardial oxygen consumption.

3. **Answer: c**
   Robotic-assisted laparoscopic surgery for radical prostatectomy is associated with a decreased inflammatory mediator response, decreased blood loss, and slower heat loss as compared to an open approach. The rate of infection is comparable for both procedures.

4. **Answer: a**
   Both methylene blue and indigo carmine can produce allergic reactions that can result in anaphylaxis.

5. **Answer: a**
   Hypothermia is associated with a decrease in metabolic rate resulting in decreased hepatic metabolism of medications. Postoperative shivering resulting from hypothermia dramatically increases myocardial oxygen consumption.

SUGGESTED READINGS

Atallah F, Khedis M, Seguin P, et al. Postoperative analgesia and recovery after open and laparoscopic prostatectomy. *Anesth Analg* 2004;99:1878–1879.

Cherian VT. Anesthetic implication of urology surgery. *Indian J Urol* 2006;22:194–200.

Cucchiara RF, Faust RJ. Patient positioning. In: Miller RD, ed. *Anesthesia*, 5th ed. Philadelphia: Churchill Livingstone, 2000:1017–1031.

Gerges FJ, Kanazi GE, Jabbour-Khoury SI. Anesthesia for laparoscopy: a review. *J Clin Anesth* 2006;18(1):67–78.

Joris JL. Anesthesia for laparoscopic surgery. In: Miller RD, ed. *Anesthesia*, 5th ed. Philadelphia: Churchill Livingstone, 2000:2003–2019.

Malhorta V. Anesthesia considerations radical prostatectomy. *Rev Esp Anestesiol* 2006;29(1):S89–S91.

Monk TG, Weldon BC. The renal system and anesthesia for urologic surgery. In: Barash P, Cullen BF, Stoelting RK, eds. *Clinical Anesthesia*, 4th ed. Philadelphia: Lippincott Williams and Wilkins, 2001:1026–1027.

Mycek MJ, Harvey RA, Champe PC. Drugs for erectile dysfunction. In: Harvey RA, Champe PC, eds. *Pharmacology*, 2nd ed. Philadelphia: Lippincott Williams and Wilkins, 2000:477–478.

Mycek MJ, Harvey RA, Champe PC. Adrenergic antagonists. In: Harvey RA, Champe PC, eds. *Pharmacology*, 2nd ed. Philadelphia: Lippincott Williams and Wilkins, 2000:71–80.

Salonia A, Crescenti A, Suardi N, et al. General versus spinal anesthesia in patients undergoing radical retropubic prostatectomy: results of a prospective, randomized study. *J Urol* 2004;64(1):95–100.

Stoelting RK, Dierdorf SF. Cancer. *Anesthesia and Co-Existing Disease*, 4th ed. Philadelphia: Churchill Livingstone, 2002:597–598.

Sass Elisha

KEY POINTS

- It is estimated that approximately 77% of patients who present for transurethral resection of the prostate (TURP) have one or more preexisting medical conditions.
- Systemic absorption of irrigation fluid used during TURP can result in fluid volume overload, dilutional hyponatremia, and metabolic acidosis.
- Factors that most significantly influence the volume of irrigating fluid absorbed during TURP include the hydrostatic pressure of the irrigating solution, the number and size of open venous sinuses during resection, the peripheral venous pressure, and the duration of resection.
- Depending on the severity of dilutional hyponatremia, severe neurologic and cardiac compromise can occur rapidly.
- Perioperative complications that are associated with TURP include TURP syndrome, hemorrhage, hypothermia, sepsis, bladder perforation, and myocardial dysfunction.

CASE SYNOPSIS

A 75-year-old man has developed urinary obstruction caused by benign prostatic hypertrophy (BPH). He is scheduled by his urologist to have a TURP procedure.

PREOPERATIVE EVALUATION AND DEMOGRAPHIC DATA

Past Medical/Surgical History

- Noninsulin-dependent diabetes, hypertension

List of Medications

- Hydrochlorothiazide, terazosin hydrochloride (hytrin), finasteride (propecia)

Diagnostic Data

- Hemoglobin, 13.2 g/dl; hematocrit, 39.4%; glucose, 139 mg/dl; blood urea nitrogen, 15 mg/dl; creatinine, 1.1 mg/dl
- Electrolytes: sodium, 139 mEq/l; potassium, 3.9 mEq/l; chloride, 104 mEq/l; carbon dioxide, 24 mEq/l

Height/Weight/Vital Signs

- 180 cm, 78 kg
- Blood pressure, 152/84; heart rate, 61 beats per minute; respiratory rate, 16 breaths per minute; room air oxygen saturation, 98%; temperature, 36.8°C
- Electrocardiogram (ECG): normal sinus rhythm; heart rate, 66; left ventricular hypertrophy; ejection fraction, 50%

PATHOPHYSIOLOGY

Benign prostatic hypertrophy (BPH) is a nonmalignant and progressive condition that will occur in approximately 90% of men during their lifetimes. Transurethral resection of the prostate is the second most common surgical procedure performed in men older than 65 years of age.

Urethral obstruction is caused by both a static and a dynamic component. Due to the effect of testicular hormones, the median and lateral lobes of the prostate become enlarged and cause a mechanical (static) obstruction that narrows the urethral lumen resulting in urinary retention (Fig. 41-1). The dynamic aspect of urinary obstruction is the result of smooth muscle tension of the prostate and bladder neck that further inhibits urine flow. Depending on the degree of obstruction, the inability to urinate can cause mild to severe discomfort and hydronephrosis.

There is a complex venous network that surrounds the prostatic capsule. This anatomic feature is significant because veins within this complex will be ligated during surgical resection. This will allow irrigating solution to enter systemic circulation. Depending on the amount and rapidity of bleeding and the amount and rapidity of absorption of irrigating fluid, the patient can develop severe anemia, dilutional hyponatremia and hypervolemia, and metabolic acidosis (see Fig. 41-1).

SURGICAL PROCEDURE

Removal of the hypertrophic prostatic tissue is accomplished via a resectoscope that is placed in the urethra. Irrigating solution is continuously infused during the procedure while the surgeon applies either a cutting current to resect small pieces of the prostate or a coagulating current to control bleeding. This process is accomplished by using an energized wire loop that is inserted through the resectoscope as depicted in Figure 41-2.

ANESTHETIC MANAGEMENT AND CONSIDERATIONS

Preoperative Period

1. Discuss the type and frequency of various coexisting diseases that are associated with patients presenting for TURP.

The speed at which BPH develops is dependent on the individual and is progressive. The average age of male patient with BPH that causes significant urinary obstruction is approximately 70 years. Therefore, patients presenting for TURP often have significant systemic coexisting disease. The type and frequency of pathophysiology associated with patients presenting for TURP are listed in Table 41-1. It is estimated that approximately 77% of these patients have one or more preexisting medical conditions.

2. Describe the potential link between cardiovascular dysfunction and BPH.

In addition to testicular hormones, BPH is thought to be enhanced by metabolic syndrome. The components of metabolic syndrome include hypertension, diabetes, obesity, insulin resistance, and dyslipidemia. These factors are thought to be a predisposition for developing prostate cancer. Men with evidence of increased inflammatory mediator values such as C-reactive protein are also more likely to develop BPH. Another proposed mechanism for BPH is impaired blood flow caused by vascular insufficiency. There is evidence to support an association between hypertension and BPH which may be caused by sympathetic nervous system hyperactivity. Of those that develop symptoms of urinary obstruction, a higher mean arterial pressure is associated with increased prostate size. Additionally, it is believed that intraprostatic inflammation plays a significant role in the development and progression of BPH.

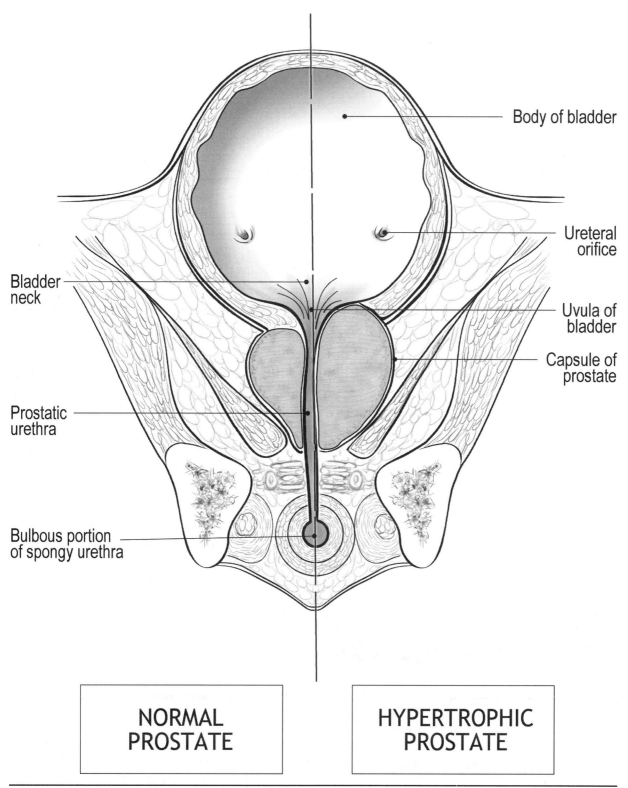

Body of bladder

Ureteral orifice

Bladder neck

Uvula of bladder

Capsule of prostate

Prostatic urethra

Bulbous portion of spongy urethra

NORMAL PROSTATE

HYPERTROPHIC PROSTATE

Figure 41-1 *Anatomic representation of normal and hypertrophic prostate. Note the urethral obstruction caused by benign prostatic hypertrophy.*

Figure 41-2   *Components of a resectoscope that is used to perform TURP.*

3. Examine the autonomic and sensory innervation to the prostate gland.
Autonomic nervous system responses are initiated via adrenergic, cholinergic, neuromodulators (adenosine), and nonadrenergic noncholinergic (nitric oxide) mechanisms. Sympathetic innervation arises from the superior hypogastric plexus and extends from T10-L2. The autonomic nervous system modulates the growth and secretory function to the prostate gland. These effects are the result of alpha-1 adrenergic stimulation. Beta-2 adrenergic stimulation aids in maintaining normal cellular integrity.

Table 41-1	Medical History and Frequency of Disease Associated with Patients Having TURP

- Hypertension, 31.6%
- Ischemic heart disease, 18.2%
- Myocardial infarction, 12.3%
- Arrhythmia, 12.4%
- Chronic obstructive pulmonary disease, 11.6%
- Diabetes, 11.2%
- Renal insufficiency, 9.8%

The inferior hypogastric plexus (pelvic nerves) are formed from the division of the splanchnic, hypogastric, pudendal, and sacral nerves. Parasympathetic innervation originates from S2-S4 via muscarinic receptors. It has been postulated that alpha-1 adrenergic overstimulation can lead to prostatic hyperplasia. A combination of other chemical substances such as nitric oxide, adenosine, and vasoactive intestinal polypeptides may influence smooth muscle tone and blood flow.

The exact spinal cord location of the sensory ganglia from the prostate gland is unknown. Sensory information is relayed at two different spinal cord segments. It appears that the majority of sensory innervation originates from the T12-L2 and L5-L6 levels. An illustration that diagrams the autonomic nervous systems innervation to the genitourinary is included in Figure 41-3.

4. Explain the mechanism of action and physiologic effects of medications used to treat BPH.
Terazosin hydrochloride, an alpha-adrenergic antagonist, is predominantly alpha-1 receptor specific and produces minimal alpha 2 blockade. The

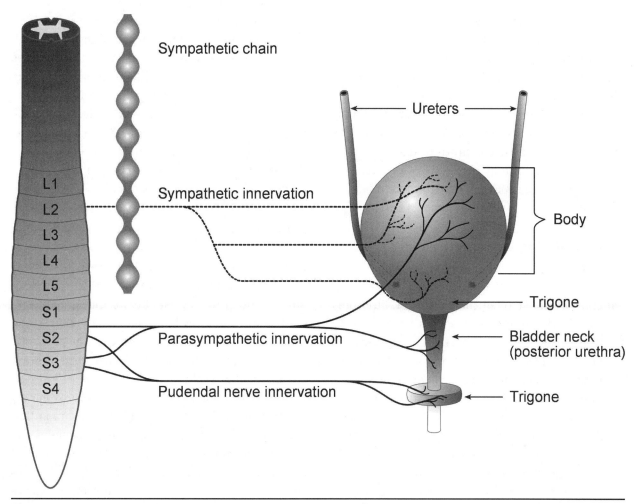

Figure 41-3   *Autonomic nervous system innervation to the genitourinary system.*

physiologic effect of this medication on the prostate gland is a decrease in smooth muscle contraction within the prostatic capsule and the bladder neck, thereby decreasing the symptoms associated with urinary obstruction. However, terazosin hydrochloride does not decrease or slow the progression of BPH. Terazosin hydrochloride is also used as an antihypertensive medication resulting in decreased arterial tone.

A metabolic byproduct of testosterone, dihydrotestosterone (DHT) is synthesized by 5 alpha reductase (5AR). DHT binds to androgen receptors on the prostate gland and accelerates cellular proliferation. Finastride is a 5AR inhibitor (5ARI) decreases the formation of DHT. Finasteride and

other 5ARIs help to decrease symptoms of urinary obstruction and decrease prostatic hyperplasia.

5. Describe the importance of administering antibiotic prophylaxis for TURP.

The incidence of bacteriuria and urinary tract infections (UTI) following TURP surgery is approximately 6%. Most of these cases resolve spontaneously after the urethral catheter is removed. For this reason, prescribing antibiotics to all patients having TURP is a controversial practice. However, it is estimated that the incidence of septicemia ranges from 1 to 4%. The mortality rate for patients older than 65 years of age who develop septicemia is 20%.

The cause of UTI after TURP is multifactorial. Sources of infections include inflamed tissue within the prostatic capsule, urethral flora, contamination during surgery, and urethral catheter colonization. The most effective antibiotic regimen has not been determined. Cephalosporins are most commonly administered preoperatively. The use of preoperative antibiotics has been shown to decrease postoperative bacteriuria by nearly twofold. The signs and symptoms of septicemia are discussed later in this chapter.

Intraoperative Period

6. Describe the anatomic and physiologic changes associated with lithotomy position.

Patients are most often placed in low lithotomy for TURP. The lithotomy position is associated with a decrease in functional residual capacity and patients who have a history of chronic obstructive pulmonary disease may have difficulty breathing. When the legs are raised, the central venous blood volume is increased by approximately 500 ml. As a result, myocardial workload is increased. Venous stasis and peripheral ischemia occur most often in patients with preexisting vascular insufficiency.

Ligaments in the lower legs and lumbar region are stretched. The lumbar curve is decreased

which can cause the level of spinal anesthesia to spread cephalad potentially resulting in a high spinal. This is most likely to occur within minutes after the spinal anesthetic has been administered. It is imperative to pad areas of the lower leg to avoid injury. The nerves at risk for injury include the common peroneal (lateral knee) and saphenous (inner knee). The obturator, femoral, and lateral femoral cutaneous nerves can be injured if hyperflexion of the thighs occurs.

7. Examine the differences between various irrigating solutions used during TURP.

Continuous irrigation through the resectoscope is necessary during TURP in order to dilate the prostatic urethra, provide visibility for the surgeon, and dilute and wash away blood and resected prostatic tissue. The advantages and disadvantages related to various irrigating solutions used for TURP are summarized in Table 41-2.

Normal physiologic osmolarity is approximately 280 mOsm/l. Absorption of irrigating solution that is significantly hyperosmolar or hypo-osmolar can have severe physiologic effects. The definition of osmolarity is the movement of water from a higher concentration to a lower concentration across a semipermeable membrane. Therefore, creating

Table 41-2 Characteristics of Irrigating Solutions Used for TURP			
SOLUTION	**OSMOLARITY (mOsm/l)**	**ADVANTAGES**	**DISADVANTAGES**
Glycine 1.5%	200	• Decreased TURP syndrome	• Hyperglycinemia • Hyperammonemia
Cytal: 2.7% sorbitol 0.54% mannitol	167	• Decreased TURP syndrome	• Hyperglycemia • Lactic acidosis
Distilled water	0	• Superior visibility	• Hemolysis • Hyponatremia
Normal saline 0.9%	308	• Minimal effects with absorption	• Current dispersion
Lactated Ringers	274	• Minimal effects with absorption	• Current dispersion

extracellular fluid hypotonicity in relation to the intracellular fluid will cause cellular swelling and lysis. If the extracellular fluid is hypertonic in relation to the intracellular fluid, cells crenate (shrink).

- Glycine 1.5%: Glycine is the most common irrigating solution used in North America. It is an essential amino acid and inhibitory neurotransmitter that is naturally present in the body. The metabolic byproduct of glycine is ammonia, a potent cerebral and myocardial depressant which can cause decreased level of consciousness and decreased cardiac output. Glycine is cardiotoxic and has been associated with cardiac hypokinesis and elevated troponin I levels. Ammonia decreases the production and release of norepinephrine from postsynaptic nerve terminals resulting in hypotension. Hyperglycinemia can cause transient visual disturbances ranging from blurred vision to blindness and may last from 24 to 48 hours. It is theorized that the inhibitory effects of glycine interrupt retinal synaptic transmission. Vision improves as glycine is metabolized and excreted.
- Cytal (2.7% sorbitol/0.54% mannitol): Mannitol, a sugar alcohol compound, is not metabolized and is rapidly excreted by the kidneys. However, sorbitol is metabolized to fructose which can result in hyperglycemia. It is theorized that during glycolysis, fructose metabolism occurs preferentially over glucose metabolism. Therefore, pyruvate and lactate are liberated resulting in lactic acidosis.
- Distilled water: This solution is rarely used in the United States because of the hypo-osmolarity and the concern over causing cell lysis.
- Normal saline/lactated Ringers: It would seem that these solutions would be ideal for TURP due to their relative iso-osmolarity and lack of metabolic byproducts. However, due to the electrolytes in these solutions (cations), current dispersion occurs making it difficult for the urologist to accurately focus on the electrical current.

8. Cite factors that affect the volume of irrigating fluid absorbed systemically during TURP.

The four factors that have the most significant influence on the volume of irrigating fluid absorbed during TURP include:

- The hydrostatic pressure of the irrigating solution. The pressure is determined by the height of the irrigating solution container. The ideal height of the irrigation bag to maintain adequate surgical visibility is 60 cm.
- The number and size of open venous sinuses during resection. A larger prostate gland has a greater surface area and during resection, a greater number of venous sinuses are exposed to irrigant. Also, intermittent coagulation of the bleeding vessels will decrease absorption.
- The peripheral venous pressure. Absorption is greatest when the venous pressure is lowest.
- The duration of resection. Approximately 10 to 50 ml of irrigant can be absorbed into systemic circulation per minute of resection. Ideally, TURP procedures should last no longer than 60 minutes.

9. Explain the physiologic alterations associated with the absorption of irrigating fluid.

Absorption of irrigating fluid increases vascular volume and dilutes plasma proteins, which cause a decrease in protein oncotic pressure. This effect results in the movement of fluid from the intravascular to the interstitial compartment. For each 100 ml of fluid diffusing into the interstitial space, 10 to 15 mEq of sodium is lost to the intravascular space resulting in dilutional hyponatremia. Hypocalemia can also occur. Serum potassium values can increase by 15–25% due to intravascular hemolysis. These cellular changes can result in severe metabolic acidosis known as TURP acidosis. Additionally, hypervolemia can ensue causing cerebral edema, myocardial ischemia, and congestive heart failure. The cardiac effects are dependent on the amount of fluid absorbed, the rate of fluid absorption, the size of the patient, and the patient's cardiac reserve. Factors that increase the likelihood of TURP syndrome include resection time greater than 60 minutes, prostatic weight greater than 30 g, inexperienced surgeon, and total irrigant volume of greater than 30 l.

10. Correlate the signs and symptoms associated with TURP syndrome with various serum sodium values.

It is vital to realize that a specific serum sodium value may result in loss of consciousness and cardiovascular collapse in one patient, whereas another patient that has the identical serum sodium will not exhibit signs and symptoms of TURP syndrome. The best method of avoiding the consequences of TURP syndrome is preventing the situation from occurring. The neurologic and cardiac manifestations associated with acute hyponatremia are listed in Tables 41-3 and 41-4.

11. Construct a plan of treatment for a patient who develops TURP syndrome.

The signs and symptoms associated with TURP syndrome vary dramatically and will determine the

Table 41-3   Neurologic Manifestations Associated with Acute Hyponatremia

SERUM SODIUM (mEq/l)	
120	Mild Signs/Symptoms
	• Dizziness
	• Headache
	• Nausea
115	Moderate Signs/Symptoms
	• Retching
	• Restlessness
	• Confusion
110	Severe Signs/Symptoms
	• Loss of consciousness
	• Seizures
	• Respiratory arrest

Table 41-4   Cardiac Manifestations Associated with Acute Hyponatremia

SERUM SODIUM (mEq/l)	
120	• Hypotension
	• Decreased myocardial contractility
	• Initial widening of QRS complex
115	• Bradycardia
	• Widening QRS complex
	• Possible ventricular ectopy
110	• Ventricular tachycardia
	• Ventricular fibrillation
	• Cardiac arrest

plan of treatment. Interventions used to treat TURP syndrome are listed in Table 41-5.

12. Explain the advantages and disadvantages of neural blockade for TURP.

The individual patient's preoperative profile is most important when determining an anesthetic technique for any surgical procedure. The ideal level of sensory blockade resulting from neural blockade is the T10 dermatome. The advantages and disadvantages of neuraxial blockade are listed in Table 41-6.

Table 41-5   Treatment Plan for TURP Syndrome

- Stop surgery
- ACLS/BLS protocol as needed
- Check electrolytes, specifically serum sodium values every 20 minutes
- Administer diuretics (furosemide)
- Treat seizure activity (benzodiazepine, barbiturate, propofol, airway management)
- Hypertonic saline (3% or 5%), not to exceed 100 ml/h infusion rate
- Invasive hemodynamic monitoring

Table 41-6 Advantages and Disadvantages of Neuraxial Blockade for TURP	
ADVANTAGES	**DISADVANTAGES**
• The major advantage is the ability to assess the patient's level of consciousness as an early monitor to detect TURP syndrome. This is the reason that neural blockade is considered the technique of choice by many practitioners. • The ability to assess chest pain and/or shortness of breath cause by myocardial ischemia and/or volume overload. • The ability to assess abdominal pain caused by a bladder perforation. • Decreased vascular resistance will lessen the possibility of hypervolemia. • It is controversial if neuroaxial blockade decreases blood loss during TURP.	• Moderate to severe hypotension can occur as a result of peripheral vascular dilation. This effect will be potentiated in patients taking alpha-adrenergic antagonists for BPH. • Due to arthritic changes associated with aging, placement can be difficult. • Decreasing venous resistance can increase the amount of irrigation absorption that occurs through open venous sinuses. • Dysphoria that can result in patient movement when benzodiazepine, narcotics, and other central nervous system depressants are administered.

13. Compare and contrast between signs and symptoms of an extraperitoneal bladder perforation and an intraperitoneal bladder perforation.

Bladder perforation can occur as a result of increased pressure from the irrigating solution or from the cutting current of the energized wire loop. Urologists should be aware that the amount of fluid output should be similar to the amount of fluid introduced into the bladder. Bladder perforation can occur in two different regions within the bladder, either intraperitoneal or extraperitoneal. The signs and symptoms associated with bladder perforation and are listed in Table 41-7.

The only sign that may be indicative of an intraperitoneal bladder perforation during general anesthesia is bradycardia caused by the leakage of irrigation into the peritoneal cavity which initiates the celiac reflex. Most small extraperitoneal bladder perforations resolve spontaneously, but urethral catheter placement is used to minimize bladder pressure. The majority of large extraperitoneal perforations or intraperitoneal perforations are treated by direct surgical closure.

14. Discuss factors that affect the estimated blood loss during TURP.

The average estimated blood loss during TURP is 300 to 400 ml. The total blood loss is highly variable but is most closely related to the size of the prostate and duration of resection. Blood loss is increased

Table 41-7 Comparison Signs and Symptoms Associated with Extraperitoneal and Intraperitoneal Bladder Perforation	
EXTRAPERITONEAL PERFORATION	**INTRAPERITONEAL PERFORATION**

• Discomfort
  1. Periumbilical
  2. Inguinal
  3. Suprapubic
• Periumbilical/ inguinal tissue distention
	• Discomfort
	  1. Chest
	  2. Upper abdomen
	  3. Shoulder tip (diaphragmatic irritation)
	• Nausea and vomiting
	• Abdominal rigidity
	• Shortness of breath
	• Diaphoresis
	• Hiccups

Equation 41-1

Blood loss = (Hct % of irrigant × total volume of irrigant)/preoperative Hct %

---

with prostatic size of greater than 45 g and resection time greater than 90 minutes. The average blood loss is estimated to be 10 to 15 ml/gram of resected prostate. Having blood available to transfuse is dependent on size of the prostate and the patient's current hemoglobin value and physiologic condition. Dilution of the blood by the irrigation makes estimating blood loss difficult. Equation 41-1 can be used to calculate the estimated blood loss.

Intraoperative blood loss can be decreased if the surgical technique includes frequent application of a coagulating current. Newer resectoscopes use bipolar current instead of unipolar current which is associated with less bleeding and decreased fluid absorption.

A postoperative subclinical disseminated intravascular coagulation (DIC) syndrome occurs in less than 1% of patients. The exact mechanism is unknown; however, the cause may be related to resected prostate tissue that enters central circulation during resection. Treatment for DIC includes administering fibrinogen, platelets, and cryoprecipitate.

Postoperative Period

The total resection time for this surgery was 105 minutes. In the postanesthesia care unit, the patient exhibits the following acute symptoms: restlessness, confusion, shivering, blood pressure of 80/46, respiratory rate of 32, sinus tachycardia with intermittent unifocal premature ventricular contractions (PVCs) rate of 102, room air oxygen saturation of 93%, and temperature of 35.4°C.

15. List potential postoperative complications and frequency that can occur following TURP.

If the bladder irrigation is not warmed, then average temperature loss after TURP is 1° to 1.5°C. Hypothermia can inhibit coagulation and increase myocardial

---

Table 41-8 Frequency of Postoperative Complications Associated with TURP

- Mortality: < 1%
- TURP syndrome: mild 2%, severe 0.5%
- Hemorrhage requiring transfusion: 4%
- Hypothermia: unknown
- Sepsis: 1%
- Bladder perforation: 1%
- Postoperative hemorrhage: 5%
- Subclinical disseminated intravascular coagulation: 1%
- Myocardial infarction: 0.5%
- Transient myocardial ischemia: as high as 20%

---

oxygen demand. Other postoperative complications associated with TURP are listed in Table 41-8.

16. Discuss potential causes and diagnostic criteria that could cause this clinical scenario.

Potential postoperative complications that can occur after TURP surgery include:

- Bladder perforation: discomfort in the abdominal and/or the inguinal region, no urine output from the urethral catheter. A urology consultation is necessary.
- Hyponatremia: obtain a serum sodium value, treat hyponatremia as discussed previously.
- Hypervolemia: listen to bilateral lung fields, obtain chest x-ray, consider diuretics.
- Hemorrhage: obtain hemoglobin/hematocrit value. Administer blood if necessary.
- Hypothermia: confirm temperature value of 35.4°C, forced air warming, consider meperidine to decrease shivering when oxygen saturation improves.
- Myocardial ischemia/infarction: obtain chest x-ray, obtain 12-lead ECG, administer volume if no signs of congestive heart failure, administer phenylephrine, check calcium levels as a potential cause of hypotension, consult a cardiologist.

Treatment for this patient would include providing high-flow oxygen, warming measures, and diagnosing the specific cause(s) of this scenario prior to definitive treatment.

REVIEW QUESTIONS

1. An advantage of neuraxial blockade for monitoring patient's having TURP surgery includes:
   a. assessing neurologic function.
   b. determining the speed of irrigation absorption.
   c. distinguishing signs and symptoms of bladder perforation.
   d. estimating blood loss.
2. Which intervention is indicated for treatment of TURP syndrome?
   a. Administering 3% sodium chloride at a rate of 200 ml/h.
   b. Administering etomidate to decrease the seizure threshold.
   c. Administering furosemide.
   d. Assessing hemoglobin value every 20 minutes.
3. Abdominal rigidity, shoulder tip pain, and shortness of breath are associated with:
   a. common peroneal nerve compression.
   b. extraperitoneal bladder perforation.
   c. intraperitoneal bladder perforation.
   d. myocardial ischemia.
4. A serum sodium value of _____ mEq/l is associated with confusion, widening QRS complex, and bradycardia.
   a. 110
   b. 115
   c. 120
   d. 125
5. Which irrigation fluid is associated with direct myocardial depression?
   a. Cytal
   b. Glycine
   c. Isotonic crystalloids
   d. Distilled water

REVIEW ANSWERS

1. **Answer: a**
   Spinal anesthesia is the anesthetic technique of choice for TURP surgery because it allows the anesthetist to monitor the patient's neurologic function. Altered mental status may be indicative of dilutional hyponatremia.
2. **Answer: c**
   TURP syndrome is associated dilutional hyponatremia. Administering lasix promotes diuresis which decreases intravascular volume restoring protein oncotic pressure. As a result, sodium returns from the interstitial space restoring intravascular sodium concentration.
3. **Answer: c**
   These signs and symptoms are associated with an intraperitoneal bladder perforation
4. **Answer: b**
   Although no one serum sodium value ensures specific signs and symptoms, a sodium value of 115 mEq/l is associated with confusion, widening QRS complex, and bradycardia.
5. **Answer: b**
   Glycine is metabolized to ammonia which is a direct myocardial depressant.

SUGGESTED READINGS

Berger AP, Bartsch G, Deibl M, et al. Atherosclerosis as a risk factor for benign prostatic hyperplasia. *BJU Int* 2006;98(5):1038–1042.

Collins JW, Macdermott S, Bradbrook RA, et al. The effect of the choice of irrigation fluid on cardiac stress during transurethral resection of the prostate: a comparison between 1.5% glycine and 5% glucose. *J Urol* 2007;177(4):1369–1373.

Gibbons EP, Cohen J, Nelson JB, et al. Correlation between risk factors for vascular disease and the American Urological Association Symptom Score. *BJU Int* 2007;99(1):97–100.

Hahn RG. Fluid absorption in endoscopic surgery. *Br J Anaesth* 2006;96:8–20.

Mebust WK, Holtgrewe HL, Cockett AT, et al. Transurethral prostatectomy: immediate and postoperative complications. Cooperative study of 13 participating institutions evaluating 3,885 patients. *J Urol* 2002; 167(1):5–9.

Mishra VC, Allen DJ, Nicolau C, et al. Does intraprostatic inflammation have a role in the pathogenesis and progression of benign prostatic hyperplasia. *BJU Int* 2007;100:327–331.

O'Hara JF, Cywinski JB, Monk TG. The renal system and anesthesia for urologic surgery. In: Barash P, Cullen BF, Stoelting RK, eds. *Clinical Anesthesia*, 5th ed. Philadelphia: Lippincott Williams and Wilkins, 2006:1026–1029.

Okeke LI. Effect of warm intravenous and irrigating fluids on the body temperature during transurethral resection of the prostate. *BMC Urol* 2007;18:7–15.

Oulette SM, Owens S. Renal anatomy, physiology and pathophysiology. In: Nagelhout JJ, Zaglaniczy KL, eds. *Nurse Anesthesia*, 3rd ed. St. Louis, MO: Elsevier Saunders, 2005:658–659.

Qiang W, Jianchen WU, MacDonald R, et al. Antibiotic prophylaxis for transurethral prostatic resection in men with preoperative urine containing less than 100,000 bacteria per ml: a systematic review. *J Urol* 2005;173(4):1175–1181.

Extracorporeal Shock Wave Lithotripsy

42

Pamela Binns-Turner

KEY POINTS

- Careful monitoring of the electrocardiogram (ECG) for dysrhythmias, such as ventricular tachycardia, is necessary due to the timing of extracorporeal shock waves.
- The shock waves, which are aimed toward the patient's flank region, are painful.
- Location for anesthesia is often outside of the operating room which may involve poor lighting, small spaces, high noise level, and a safety risk (e.g., radiation exposure).
- Extracorporeal shock wave lithotripsy (ESWL) is noninvasive but may cause bacteremia in susceptible patients.

CASE SYNOPSIS

A 57-year-old man has complained of right flank pain and hematuria for 4 days. An x-ray shows evidence of a renal calculus located in the right upper calyx. He is scheduled to have ESWL to the right kidney by his urologist.

PREOPERATIVE EVALUATION AND DEMOGRAPHIC DATA

Past Medical/Surgical History

- Hypercholesterolemia
- Hypertension
- Insulin-dependent diabetes mellitus
- Three-vessel coronary artery bypass graft (CABG) 5 years ago; no anesthetic complications

List of Medications

- Zocor (simvastatin)
- Lopressor (metoprolol)
- Aspirin
- Multivitamin
- NPH and Lantus insulin

Diagnostic Data

- White blood cell count, $4.7 \times 10^9/l$
- Hemoglobin, 13.7 g/dl; hematocrit, 41%
- Platelets, $215 \times 10^9/l$
- Sodium, 136 mEq/l; potassium, 4.8 mEq/l; chloride, 102 mmol/l
- Blood urea nitrogen (BUN), 21 mg/dl; creatinine, 1.5 mg/dl
- Glucose, 133 mg/dl
- Partial thromboplastin time, 30 s; prothrombin time, 12.3 s; international normalized ratio, 1.1 s
- Kidneys, ureters, bladder x-ray: right renal calculi

Height/Weight/Vital Signs

- 183 cm, 104 kg; body mass index, 31 kg/m^2
- Blood pressure, 136/65; heart rate, 71 beats per minute; respiratory rate, 18 breaths per minute; room air oxygen saturation, 97%; temperature, 98.1°F
- 12-Lead ECG: NSR with 1-degree AV block and left axis deviation

PATHOPHYSIOLOGY

Renal calculi are hardened crystalline masses often referred to as a "kidney stones." They can exist within the kidney, as shown in Figure 42-1, or the ureter and cause hydronephrosis. Nephrolithiasis, a condition where calculi are present in the kidneys or urinary tract, is more common in men than women (3:1 ratio) and less common in Asian and African Americans. It is estimated that between 10 and 15% of adults in the United States will develop kidney stones. People who live in the southeastern region of the country have the highest incidence of nephrolithiasis. The potential causes for the development of kidney stones include diet and mineral content and fluoride concentration in drinking water. Frequent episodes of nephrolithiasis may occur in association with a host of metabolic disorders such as renal tubular acidosis, Dent disease, hyperparathyroidism, and medullary sponge kidney. The rate of calcium

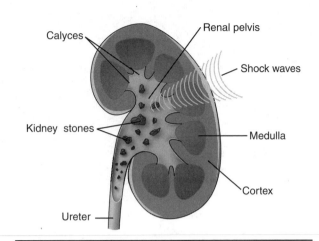

Figure 42-1 *Kidney stones present in the renal calyces.*

excretion as well as pH of the urine plays a factor in the composition of the calculus formation. These stones are formed of calcium oxalate (80%), uric acid, calcium phosphate, cystine, and struvite. Compositional analysis of stones can be used as an integral component in prevention of future stone formation. The signs and symptoms associated with nephrolithiasis are listed in Table 42-1.

Diagnosis of kidney stones is accomplished by assessing signs and symptoms that are commonly associated with nephrolithiasis; kidney, ureter, bladder (KUB) abdominal x-ray; intravenous pyelogram; computed tomography (CT) scan; blood tests (increased white blood cells hypercalcemia,

Table 42-1 Signs and Symptoms Associated with Kidney Stones
• Severe flank/back/groin pain
• Dysuria
• Hematuria
• Pyuria
• Nausea and vomiting
• Hydronephrosis
• Urinary frequency
• Fever and chills

elevated BUN/creatinine); urinalysis presence of red blood cells; bacteria; protein; casts; crystalline formations; and urine culture. Most kidney stones that are less than 4 mm in diameter will spontaneously pass out of the kidney through the ureter and into the bladder. However, if the diameter of the stone is greater than 6 mm in diameter, the need for surgical intervention may be necessary.

SURGICAL PROCEDURE

Lithotripsy is a therapeutic medical procedure used to disintegrate stones in the urinary tract and renal pelvis. ESWL is a noninvasive technique using a focused, high intensity acoustic pulse emitted from a water-filled device (shock wave generator) which is in contact with the patient's skin at the level of the kidney (approximately L2 vertebrae) as shown in Figure 42-2. With older ESWL devices, it was necessary to submerge the patient's entire body in a warm water bath while the procedure occurred. Due to advances in the technologic construction of ESWL units, this process is no longer necessary. If the treatment is to occur outside of the anesthetizing area such as in a mobile trailer, all of the necessary anesthesia and emergency equipment must be present. Since the shock waves have the same acoustic density as water, the energy passes through tissue planes and shears the stone instead of damaging tissue. Thousands of pulsatile

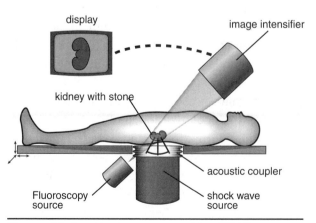

Figure 42-2 *Equipment used for ESWL.*

Table 42-2 Side Effects Associated with ESWL
• Dysrhythmias
• Nausea and vomiting
• Pleural injury
• Renal parenchymal or subcapsular hemorrhage
• Impaired skin integrity
• Hypertension

shock waves of energy are focused on the calculi. The kidney stone is visualized by fluoroscopy or ultrasound. The fragments of stone are then able to pass into the bladder and be eliminated from the body. Care must be used when positioning and securing the patient to the ESWL table. As the table and lithotripter move in response to the stone's position, padding of extremities and frequent visual inspection are warranted to prevent nerve injury. The shock wave generator produces noise, and the patient's ears are covered to avoid acoustic trauma. A temporary ureteral stent is frequently placed at the end of this procedure to maintain urinary flow and ureteral patency. The overall complication rate associated with ESWL is approximately 5–15%. The side effects caused by the treatment can be mild or severe and a list of the potential complications is listed in Table 42-2.

ANESTHETIC MANAGEMENT AND CONSIDERATIONS

Preoperative Period

1. Discuss the anesthetic options available for ESWL.

A number of anesthetic techniques are available for an ESWL procedure. General anesthesia can be utilized as well as intravenous sedation under monitored anesthesia care using a propofol or remifentanil infusion, subcutaneous infiltration of local anesthesia, or the application of topical anesthesic such as dimethyl sulfoxide (DMSO) or eutectic mixture of local anesthesic (EMLA) cream.

If neuraxial anesthesia is chosen (spinal or epidural), a T6 dermatome sensory blockade is desirable because renal innervation by sympathetic fibers is located between T10 and L1. A spinal block can be performed by using local anesthesia and/or sufentanil.

2. Identify the anesthetic concerns related to this patient's medical history and ESWL.

Hypertension, Hyperlipidemia, and CABG   Although ESWL is a noninvasive surgical procedure, the patient can experience a significant amount of pain which has been described by patients as being snapped by a rubber band in the flank region. The number of shock wave pulses that are needed to obliterate the stone varies depending on its composition. However, a typical ESWL treatment results in hundreds of pulses.

A painful experience activates the sympathetic nervous system, and the cardiovascular response includes tachycardia, increased myocardial contractility, increased rate of cardiac conduction, and vasoconstriction. Since this patient has risk factors that are associated with cardiac dysfunction, increased myocardial oxygen demand without the ability to increase supply can result in ischemia and infarction. His medication regimen also includes metoprolol (Lopressor) which he should continue taking throughout the perioperative phase.

Obesity   This patient is considered obese as per body mass index. Obesity will increase the difficulty of positioning the patient's kidney area directly over the shock wave generator. Also, due to the association between obesity and the presence of redundant airway tissue, obstruction of the airway during intravenous sedation can occur. Since the patient cannot move during the procedure, dysphoria and agitation are best avoided.

Aspiring Therapy   Intraoperative and postoperative bleeding can occur after an ESWL treatment. It is prudent to discontinue his aspirin for 10 days before surgery.

Table 42-3   Contraindications to ESWL

Obstruction distal to the kidney stone
Anticoagulation
Bleeding disorders
Abdominal aortic aneurysm > 5 cm
Automated internal cardiac defibrillator
Pacemaker
Renal artery aneurysm
Acute urinary tract infection
Pregnancy
Morbid obesity

3. List the contraindications to having an ESWL procedure.
Contraindications to ESWL are included in Table 42-3.

Intraoperative Period

4. Evaluate the potential for cardiac dysrhythmias in relation to a patient's cardiac morbidity.
Since the shock waves can result in cardiac dysrhythmias, the timing of the pulses are linked to the ECG. Referred to as a gaited ESWL, the energy is discharged 20 ms after the R wave in the cardiac cycle. The R wave is the electrical event that coincides with ventricular depolarization and stimulation that occurs prior to the R wave, can result in severe dysrhythmias such as ventricular tachycardia. The event immediately proceeding the R wave when the shock wave is emitted correlates with the absolute refractory period. A supramaximal stimulus that is applied to the cardiac myocyte during this period will not result in depolarization, and the potential for dysrhythmia formation is decreased.

Patients with a cardiac pacemaker or automatic internal cardiac defibrillator (AICD) should be carefully monitored for heart rate and rhythm abnormalities. Although rarely needed, a magnet should be readily available to reprogram the pacemaker if necessary. Prior to ESWL therapy, placement of a magnet over most types of AICD will temporarily inhibit the detection of tachyarrhythmias. The focal point of the shock wave generator should be greater than 15 cm away from the cardiac device.

5. Compare the impact of positive pressure ventilation and spontaneous ventilation on the ESWL procedure.

Stone movement is more profound with spontaneous ventilation due to the involvement of structures within the abdomen during diaphragmatic contraction and relaxation to achieve tidal volume respirations. With positive pressure ventilation, stone movement can be decreased and controlled by changing the tidal volume, respiratory rate, and peak inspiratory pressures. Even small changes in location of the calculus as a result of ventilation can prolong the ESWL treatment and increase the number of shocks necessary to effectively eliminate the stone. This predisposes the patient to a greater risk of complications (e.g., bruising, bleeding).

Postoperative Period

6. Summarize the mechanism for hematuria following ESWL.

Although shock waves are focused on the calculus, some tissue damage within the urinary tract and/or renal parenchyma may occur as a result of time and intensity of shock waves. A small amount of hematuria may occur after ESWL but it is usually limited to approximately 24–48 hours after treatment.

REVIEW QUESTIONS

1. Which cardiovascular response is most likely to occur during extracorporeal shock wave lithotripsy?
   a. Cardiac dysrhythmias
   b. Hypotension
   c. Hypertension
   d. Congestive heart failure

2. Which is not a contraindication for having an ESWL procedure?
   a. 6-cm abdominal aortic aneurysm
   b. Ureteral obstruction distal to the calculus
   c. History of myocardial infarction 2 years prior
   d. von Willebrand disease

3. Anesthetic techniques that can be used for ESWL include all of the following except:
   a. general anesthesia.
   b. spinal anesthesia.
   c. local anesthetic infiltration.
   d. peripheral blockade.

4. The shock wave is timed to discharge 20 ms after the _____ wave during gaited ESWL to avoid cardiac dysrhythmias.
   a. P wave
   b. R wave
   c. Q wave
   d. T wave

5. Blockade at which dermatome level is necessary to perform an ESWL under spinal anesthesia?
   a. T4
   b. T5
   c. T6
   d. T7

REVIEW ANSWERS

1. **Answer: a**
   Cardiac dysrhythmias may occur due to the mechanical stress exerted by the shock waves on the cardiac conduction system. Patients with a history of dysrhythmias or a cardiac pacemaker are at increased risk.

2. **Answer: c**
   A patient who has had a myocardial infarction 2 years ago but is medically optimized and has been evaluated by a cardiologist can have ESWL. The other patient conditions are contraindications to this procedure.

3. **Answer: d**
   A peripheral nerve block will not provide adequate analgesia during ESWL.

4. **Answer: b**

Shock waves in a gaited ESWL should be timed to discharge 20 ms after the R wave on the patient's ECG. This period corresponds with the absolute refractory period minimizing the risk of cardiac dysrhythmias.

5. **Answer: c**

A T6 dermatome sensory block is necessary because the innervation to the kidney is from sympathetic nerves that arise from the T10-L1 spinal nerve distribution.

SUGGESTED READINGS

Coe FL, Evan A, Worcester E. Kidney stone disease. *J Clin Invest* 2005;115:2598–2608.

Cormack JR, Hui R, Olive D, et al. Comparison of two ventilation techniques during general anesthesia for ESWL: high-frequency jet ventilation versus spontaneous ventilation with a laryngeal mask airway. *Urology* 2007;70:7–10.

Juknevicius I, Hruska KA. Renal calculi (nephrolithiasis). In: Goldman L, Ausiello D, eds. *Textbook of Medicine*, 22nd ed. Philadelphia: Saunders, 2004:761–767.

Lee C, Weiland D, Ryndin I, et al. Impact of type of anesthesia on efficacy of medstone STS lithotripter. *J Endourol* 2007;21:957–960.

Medina HJ, Glavin EM, Dirckx M, et al. Remifentanil as a single drug for extracorporeal shock wave lithotripsy: a comparison of infusion doses in terms of analgesic potency and side effects. *Anesth Analg* 2005;101(2):365–370.

Oulette SM. Renal anatomy, physiology, pathophysiology, and anesthesia management. In: Nagelhout JJ, Plaus K, eds. *Nurse Anesthesia*, 4th ed. Philadelphia: Elsevier, 2009:718–719.

Sorenson C, Chandhoke P, Moore M, et al. Comparison of intravenous sedation versus general anesthesia on the efficacy of the Doli 50 lithotriptor. *J Urol* 2002;168(1):35–37.

Terlecki RP, Triest JA. A contemporary evaluation of the auditory hazard of extracorporeal shock wave lithotripsy. *Urology* 2007;70(5):898–899.

Yilmaz E, Batislam E, Basar M, et al. Can prilocaine infiltration alone be the most minimally invasive approach in terms of anesthesia during ESWL? *Urology* 2007;68:24–27.

Zimhony O, Goland S, Malnick DH, et al. Enterococcal endocarditis after extracorporeal shock wave lithotripsy for nephrolithiasis. *Postgrad Med J* 1996;72:52–58.

Plastic and Reconstructive Surgery

XIV

Breast Reconstructive Surgery

43

Tatiana Bevans

KEY POINTS

- Preoperative identification of the patient's chemotherapeutic agent regimen is essential. An anesthetic plan must account for the potential physiologic and pharmacologic effects associated with these medications.
- Anesthetic considerations vary related to the type of breast reconstruction performed. The specific surgical technique employed is individualized to patient's needs and preferences.
- Patients who have comorbidities presenting for breast reconstructive surgery are at increased risk for complications throughout the perioperative period. These comorbidities most typically include hypertension, diabetes mellitus, dyslipidemia, active smoking, and obesity.
- Postoperative complications may require reoperation for debridement and drainage and include hematoma, seroma, infection, skin flap necrosis, and implant exposure.

CASE SYNOPSIS

A 59-year-old woman with diagnosed breast cancer is scheduled for modified radical mastectomy with immediate transverse rectus abdominus myocutaneous (TRAM) flap reconstruction.

PREOPERATIVE EVALUATION AND DEMOGRAPHIC DATA

Past Medical/Surgical History

- Lumpectomy and biopsy for breast mass
- Hypothyroidism
- Chemotherapy as a treatment for breast cancer

List of Medications

- Doxorubicin hydrochloride (Adriamycin)
- Hydrochlorothiazide
- Synthroid
- Phenergan

Diagnostic Data

- Hemoglobin, 12.3 g/dl; hematocrit, 36.6%; platelets, 219/mm³; glucose, 93 mg/dl; blood urea nitrogen, 21 mg/dl; creatinine, 0.9 mg/dl
- Electrolytes: sodium, 137 mEq/l; potassium, 3.9 mEq/l; chloride, 105 mEq/l; carbon dioxide, 24 mEq/l

Vital Statistics

- 170 cm, 79 kg; body mass index, 27.2 kg/m² (overweight)
- Blood pressure, 121/79; heart rate, 78 beats per minute; respiratory rate, 16 breaths per minute; room air oxygen saturation, 99%; temperature, 36.9°C
- Electrocardiogram (ECG): normal sinus rhythm; heart rate, 72 beats per minute
- Echocardiogram: Ejection fraction (EF) = 68% and there are no associated wall motion abnormalities. In her history and physical exam, it is noted that she has occasional shortness of breath and fatigue during exertion.

PATHOPHYSIOLOGY

Each year over 211,000 women and 1700 men are diagnosed with breast cancer. Adenocarcinoma is the most common cause of breast cancer and the process of cellular dysplasia begins in the cells' lining the ducts and lobules of the breast. Risk factors for breast cancer include family history, nulliparity, early menarche, advanced age, obesity, and personal history of breast cancer. Women who have the genetic mutation BRCA 1 or BRCA 2 have a 40 to 85% increased risk of developing breast cancer over their lifetimes. Some women with this gene mutation undergo prophylactic mastectomies. Breast cancer is commonly treated with a combination of surgery, radiation therapy, chemotherapy, and hormone therapy. Breast reconstruction may be immediate or scheduled during a subsequent surgery for patients who choose to undergo mastectomies. There are two

different types of postmastectomy reconstruction: prosthetic implant-based reconstruction and autologous tissue-based reconstruction. Many factors influence the choice of reconstruction technique including the type and location of the cancer, the extent of resection necessary, medical and surgical risk factors of the patient, desired size and shape of the reconstructed breast, and patient preference.

SURGICAL PROCEDURE

Implant-Based Reconstruction

Current prosthetic reconstruction may involve a single-stage implant reconstruction with either a standard or an adjustable implant, a two-stage tissue implant reconstruction, or a combined implant with autologous tissue reconstruction. Immediate single-stage reconstruction is best suited for women with small breasts and women who qualify for skin-sparing techniques. Advantages of skin-sparing techniques include improved symmetry after reconstruction due to preservation of a breast envelope. In some patients, superior results are obtained with a two-stage reconstruction.

With a two-stage reconstruction, a tissue expander is placed in the submuscular pocket during the primary procedure. The deflated expander exerts minimal tension on the mastectomy flap. Complete muscular coverage minimizes the risk of expander exposure in the event of flap necrosis. Postoperatively, the expander can be slowly filled through an internal port until the desired volume is achieved. During the second stage procedure, the temporary expander is exchanged for a permanent implant. A partial or complete capsulotomy is performed at this time to maximize breast projection and ptosis as shown in Figure 43-1.

Combined Implant and Autologous Tissue Reconstruction

A combined implant with autologous or donor tissue reconstruction can allow for complete wound closure

Figure 43-1 *Capsulotomy before placement of the permanent breast implants. (See Color Plate.)*

as shown in Figure 43-2. Tissue is most commonly retrieved from the latissimus dorsi myocutaneous flap. The tissue is rotated from the back to the anterior chest to create the breast. This type of flap may not be ample, and the implant is placed between the latissimus and pectoralis muscle to increase the volume of the reconstruction. The duration of implant-based breast reconstructive surgery ranges from 2 to 9 hours (mean 4 hours).

Autologous Tissue Reconstruction

The distinct advantage of autologous tissue breast reconstruction is that the reconstructed breast looks and feels more natural. Results from autologous tissue reconstruction are more consistent over the woman's lifetime. One of the disadvantages of autologous reconstruction is that it is a more complex procedure, requiring a longer surgical procedure and a greater period of convalescence. Three different types of flaps are most commonly used for these procedures: latissimus flaps (see previous text), TRAM flaps, and deep inferior epigastric perforator (DIEP) flaps.

A TRAM flap procedure is performed to replace the breast tissue with an ellipse of tissue from the rectus abdominus muscle. The pedicle TRAM

Figure 43-2 *The beginning of surgical closure of the wound. Note that the muscle layer is sutured over the breast implant to prevent implant exposure. (See Color Plate.)*

flap maintains the original blood supply through the superior epigastric artery. The donor tissue is rotated into position, contoured, and then secured in place. A free TRAM flap involves microvascular anastomoses of the inferior epigastric artery to either the thoracodorsal or internal mammary vessels. The blood supply to the flap is temporarily suspended until this reanastomoses occurs. This method allows for transfer of larger amounts of tissue than the pedicle TRAM flap. If TRAM flap hypoperfusion and failure occurs, then surgical flap debridement or hematoma evacuation will be instituted. Increased body mass index, smoking, and radiation treatment all increase the potential

for TRAM flap failure. The duration for a TRAM flap varies greatly from 5 to 12 hours (mean 7.5 hours).

The DIEP flap has been used recently to minimize donor site morbidities seen with other autologous options such as abdominal wall deformities and muscle weakness. The DIEP flap uses the inferior epigastric artery as the vascular supply that can be dissected without sacrificing any muscle tissue or fascia. Deep inferior epigastric perforator flaps have been shown to improve perfusion to the reconstructed breast and survival. This technique does not require surgical microvascular expertise, longer operative times, and the need for intense postoperative flap monitoring.

ANESTHETIC MANAGEMENT AND CONSIDERATIONS

Preoperative Period

1. Identify the comorbidities that increase mortality from breast cancer.

Mortality from breast cancer significantly increases when it is associated with systemic disease states including diabetes, renal failure, stroke, liver disease, and previous cancer. Mortality also increases with increased age. Women who are older than 65 years of age account for approximately 45% of all new breast cancer cases. Smoking and obesity increase flap failure and decrease wound healing associated with reconstruction.

2. Describe reasons that obesity complicates the anesthetic and surgical management of patients with breast cancer.

Obese women are more likely to develop breast cancer due to increased production of estrogen. These patients have a higher incidence of flap complications, flap failure, and impaired wound healing. Obesity causes numerous pathophysiologic processes that affect multiple organ systems including:

- *Cardiovascular system:* There is an interrelationship between obesity and cardiovascular disease. Hypertension and dyslipidemia can result in the development of concentric hypertrophy and coronary artery disease. As a result, myocardial performance is decreased. There is increased myocardial oxygen demand and, during periods of physiologic stress, myocardial ischemia, myocardial infarction, and congestive heart failure can occur.
- *Respiratory system:* Chest wall compliance is decreased in obese patients resulting in restrictive lung disease. Total lung capacity and functional residual capacity are also decreased. These effects contribute to the rapid development of arterial hypoxemia from premature airway closure and ventilation–perfusion mismatch.

Obesity is associated with the presence of redundant airway tissue which can make ventilation and intubation difficult or impossible. Obstructive sleep apnea and chronic hypercarbia are associated with obesity. Optimal alignment of the laryngeal, pharyngeal, and oral axes by ramping the patient and achieving a sniffing position is warranted. Thorough preoxygenation prior to the induction of anesthesia is vital to decrease the possibility of hypoxemia.

- *Endocrine system:* People who are obese are at increased risk of developing noninsulin-dependent diabetes. The incidence increases as body mass index increases and results in altered glucose metabolism and impaired insulin receptor sensitivity. Perioperative assessment of blood glucose is warranted.
- *Gastrointestinal system:* Obesity has been associated with decreased gastric emptying time and gastroesophageal reflux disease. Preoperative gastrointestinal prophylaxis with a gastrokinetic agent, histamine receptor type 2 antagonist, and nonparticulate antacid is indicated for obese patients who are at increased risk of gastric aspiration.
- *Hepatic system:* Due to the infiltration of hepatocytes with triglycerides, morbid obesity is associated with nonalcoholic fatty liver disease. The degree of hepatic compromise can be assessed by results from liver function tests. Hepatic dysfunction is associated with coagulopathy and decreased metabolism of anesthetic medications.

3. Identify commonly used chemotherapeutic agents and discuss the anesthetic implications.

Chemotherapeutic agents such as bleomycin, adriamycin, methotrexate, and tamoxifen affect the anesthetic plan and intraoperative care. This patient has taken adriamycin which has the potential to cause cardiotoxicity. Even small doses of adriamycin can cause cardiotoxicity.

Myocardial dysfunction can be acute or chronic. Manifestations associated with the acute form which are reversible include arrhythmias, ST-T wave abnormalities, and decreased EF. The severity of the effects associated with chronic treatment with adriamycin is dose dependent and can result in congestive heart failure. The frequency of significant cardiomyopathy is estimated to be between 1 to 10% if the total dose of Adriamycin is less than 450 mg/m². The proposed mechanism of action by which adriamycin decreases cardiac performance results from myofibril degeneration and myocardial mitochondrial dysfunction.

Due to the synergy between the cardiotoxic effects produced by adriamycin, myocardial depression caused by the inhalation anesthetic agents and physiologic stress produced by surgery and anesthesia, a comprehensive preoperative cardiac evaluation is essential. A list of commonly used chemotherapeutic agents, the physiologic changes, and the associated anesthetic considerations are present in Table 43-1.

Table 43-1 Common Chemotherapeutic Agents Used to Treat Breast Cancer: Physiologic Effects and Anesthetic Considerations

	BLEOMYCIN	DOXORUBICIN HYDROCHLORIDE (ADRIAMYCIN)	METHOTREXATE (TREXALL, AMETHOPTERIN)	TAMOXIFEN (NOLVADEX)
Physiologic effects	• Pulmonary toxicity	• Cardiac toxicity: transient dysrhythmias, ECG changes, irreversible cardiomyopathy, and congestive heart failure • Cardiac risk is increased with increasing dose, prior radiotherapy, and female gender • Myelosuppression resulting in thrombocytopenia, anemia, and leukopenia	• Renal dysfunction • Hepatic dysfunction • Anemia	• Nausea and vomiting • Dehydration
Anesthetic considerations	• Avoid FiO₂ > 30% to prevent pulmonary fibrosis and edema • Chest x-ray • Arterial blood gas as indicated by history and physical • Pulmonary function testing as indicated by history and physical	• ECG • Echocardiography to evaluate for cardiomyopathy • Complete blood count to evaluate for myelosuppression	• Complete blood count • Blood urea nitrogen • Creatinine • Liver function tests	• Intravenous hydration • Antiemetic medication

4. Discuss the anesthetic considerations regarding intravenous (IV) placement.

It is best to avoid placing IV catheters or taking serial blood pressure measurements on the mastectomy side to avoid the development of lymph edema. If bilateral mastectomies were performed, the anesthetist should place the IV on the side opposite from where the lymph node dissection occurred. If bilateral lymph edema exists, or if bilateral lymph node dissection was performed, external jugular or internal jugular cannulation should be considered. An option for patients without diabetes is to place the IV in a lower extremity.

5. Discuss the anesthetic considerations for blood pressure assessment including arterial line placement.

Patients with heart disease, anemia, bilateral lymph edema, or other comorbid factors may benefit from the placement of an arterial line. An arterial line will allow for easy access for blood sampling, and provide real-time and reliable blood pressure measurements. Placing the blood pressure cuff on the leg is also an option in select patients when upper extremity blood pressure monitoring is contraindicated.

6. Discuss the anesthetic considerations for preoperative sedation.

Because the surgeon routinely marks the chest wall while the patient is standing during the preoperative phase, caution against providing heavy sedation must be exercised during this time. An example of preoperative chest wall markings is shown in Figure 43-3. Due to the possibility of redundant airway tissue and the reduction of functional residual capacity, oversedation can result in airway obstruction and hypoxemia.

Intraoperative Period

7. Explain how blood pressure control affects flap perfusion.

One of the complications of the TRAM flap procedure is postoperative necrosis of the newly constructed breast. Therefore, maintenance of mean arterial pressure within 20% of preoperative values allows for adequate perfusion pressure to the flap tissue. Extremes in blood pressure should be avoided. Hypertension frequently causes excessive bleeding and hypotension can result in hypoperfusion to the graft. It is important to avoid the use of vasopressors to treat hypotension, as vasoconstriction of the arterial vasculature will restrict blood flow to the flap. The blood pressure is most effectively supported by administering fluids.

8. Identify how volume replacement affects hemostasis.

Synthetic colloids such as hespan and hetastarch are useful for volume expansion. Administration of these products is associated with decreased hemostasis and, as a result, their application for breast reconstruction surgery is limited. In order to avoid infusing a large volume of crystalloid, patients may benefit from use of albumin. Intraoperative assessment of serial hemoglobin values is necessary to ensure adequate oxygen-carrying capacity. The decision to administer blood, fresh frozen plasma, and platelets should be based on the patient's preoperative physical status, hemodynamic stability, laboratory values, and surgical hemostasis.

9. Discuss the anesthetic considerations for autologous blood donation and transfusion.

Autologous blood donation is the collection of the patient's own blood prior to elective surgery. This blood can be autotransfused if necessary during the intraoperative or postoperative periods. It has not been proven that the risk of transmission of communicable bloodborne diseases is less with autologous blood as compared to banked blood. Autologous donation is associated with a higher rate of postoperative transfusion. This phenomena is most likely due to relative preoperative anemia caused by autologous donation. It has been determined that fewer than half of patients who donate autologous blood receive their own

Figure 43-3   *Preoperative marking prior to stage 2 breast reconstructive surgery. (See Color Plate.)*

blood. Risks associated with autologous blood transfusion include the potential for posttransfusion anemia, bacterial contamination, and human error resulting in blood typing incompatibilities. Transfusions are not routinely required for breast reconstructive surgery and, as a result, autologous blood donation is infrequently performed for reconstructive breast surgery.

10. Discuss the anesthetic implications of administering nitrous oxide for TRAM flap reconstruction.
During TRAM flap reconstruction, the abdominal donor site is often closed as though the patient has undergone an abdominoplasty. Since nitrous oxide is highly diffusible, its use should be avoided to prevent abdominal distention. Avoiding the use of nitrous oxide will allow for optimal cosmetic results.

11. Explain the rationale for maintaining normothermia during breast reconstructive surgery.
Normothermia should be maintained during breast reconstructive surgery, particularly during flap reconstruction. Hypothermia causes vasoconstriction thus restricting blood supply to the flap and, therefore, maintenance of normothermia is important to optimize flap perfusion. Hypothermia can

also result in decreased hemostasis causing hematoma formation, postoperative shivering which significantly increases myocardial oxygen demand, and decreased hepatic metabolism and renal excretion of drugs leading to delayed emergence from anesthesia.

12. Explain the advantages and disadvantages for using dextran during breast reconstructive surgery.

Pharmacologic antithrombotic prophylaxis that occurs with the use of dextran can be used during flap reconstructive surgery to minimize the risk of TRAM flap hypoperfusion and necrosis caused by microvascular thrombus formation. However, risks associated with dextan administration include coagulopathy and anaphylaxis. Breast reconstruction is an elective surgery. High-risk patients are frequently offered reconstructive surgery using breast implants rather than flap reconstruction to minimize the risk of microvascular thrombosis. As a result, dextran is not routinely administered intraoperatively.

13. Identify changes in patient positioning that is required during intraoperative breast reconstructive surgery.

Mastectomies and breast reconstructive surgeries are usually performed in a supine position with mild flexion. In order to gain access for the latissimus dorsi flap harvest, the patient will be placed in the lateral decubitus position. After placement of the implant or flap construction, the patient may be moved to a sitting position to assess the overall appearance and symmetry of the breast reconstruction. Hypotension can occur when the patient is moved abruptly into a sitting position. It is important to secure both arms in order to keep them from falling forward and to avoid brachial plexus and ulnar nerve injury. Lastly, holding the endotracheal tube is important to decrease the potential for accidental extubation or right mainstem intubation.

Postoperative Period

14. Discuss methods for postoperative pain control.

There are numerous pain management modalities that can be used to decrease postoperative pain. These strategies include patient-controlled analgesia, thoracic epidural, intercostal nerve block, thoracic paravertebral nerve block, IV administration of narcotics, and oral pain medication. Decreasing postoperative pain is important because it inhibits sympathetic nervous system hyperactivity and allows patients to breathe deeply in order to prevent atelectasis.

15. Discuss the long-term postoperative care necessary after breast reconstructive surgery.

Many patients will undergo subsequent surgical procedures because breast implants are not considered permanent devices. The implants may need to be replaced over a period of years due to the development of contractures, migration, leakage, or rupture. Reintervention for scar revision and nipple reconstruction is also common. Advancements in surgical techniques for nipple reconstruction can be accomplished using monitored anesthesia care. Breast tissue is reconfigured into a nipple. Tattooing techniques are used and the new nipple is colored to match the color of the areola.

REVIEW QUESTIONS

1. Maintenance of intraoperative blood pressure during breast reconstructive surgery is best controlled by administering:
   a. ephedrine to maintain preoperative mean arterial pressure.
   b. hespan and lactated Ringers.
   c. a crystalloid solution and blood.
   d. a phenylephrine (Neo-Synephrine) bolus.
2. Which preoperative evaluation(s) are indicated for a patient receiving bleomycin?
   a. ECG and echocardiography obtained to determine potential cardiac toxicity

b. Liver function tests obtained to determine potential hepatic impairment

c. Blood urea nitrogen and creatinine obtained to determine potential renal impairment

d. Arterial blood gas and chest x-ray obtained to determine potential pulmonary impairment

3. A diabetic patient is scheduled for a right mastectomy with lymph node dissection. Which is the best area to place an IV?
   a. Left hand
   b. Right hand
   c. Left leg
   d. Right leg

4. Which patient is the highest risk for developing breast cancer?
   a. A patient with a negative BRCA 1 and 2 gene
   b. A positive BRCA 2 gene and history of ovarian cancer
   c. A morbidly obese 30-year-old woman
   d. A woman with a 20 pack/year smoking history

5. Which perioperative intervention(s) will help to ensure TRAM flap perfusion?
   a. Controlled hypothermia and normotension
   b. Normothermia, normotension, normocarbia
   c. Intraoperative dextran infusion
   d. Controlled hypotension to prevent bleeding

REVIEW ANSWERS

1. **Answer: c**

   Administration of adequate crystalloid is necessary in order to minimize intraoperative hemodynamic variability. Administration of hespan should be limited due to decreased hemostasis. Blood products should be administered judiciously as anemia decreases oxygen carrying capacity and patients can develop a coagulopathy.

2. **Answer: d**

   Bleomycin is an antitumor agent with known pulmonary toxic properties. Bleomycin

pulmonary toxicity occurs in 10% of patients and the signs and symptoms manifest as a dry, hacking cough, dyspnea, tachypnea, and fever. Changes in pulmonary function tests occur in 20% of patients who receive bleomycin. Pulmonary complications include pulmonary fibrosis and interstitial pneumonitis. Arterial blood gas and chest x-ray analysis are important preoperative tests used to evaluate for potential pulmonary toxicity.

3. **Answer: a**

   IV line placement should be avoided on the side of lymph node dissection to help prevent the development of lymphedema. It is best to avoid placement of the IV line in the foot of a diabetic patient due to the potential for compromised wound healing and diabetic ulcers.

4. **Answer: b**

   Women with the gene mutation BRCA 1 or 2 are considered very high risk for developing breast cancer.

5. **Answer: b**

   Adequate blood supply to the flap is necessary for TRAM flap survival. Normothermia is important to prevent vasoconstriction associated with hypothermia. Normotension allows for adequate perfusion of the flap, preventing ischemia and flap death associated with hypotension. Normocarbia helps prevent vasoconstriction associated with hypocarbia.

SUGGESTED READINGS

Andrades P, Fix RJ, Danilla S, et al. Ischemic complications in pedicle, free, and muscle sparing transverse rectus abdominis myocutaneous flaps for breast reconstruction. *Ann Plast Surg* 2008;60(5):562–567.

Arellano R, Gan BS, Salpeter MJ, et al. A triple-blinded randomized trial comparing the hemostatic effect of large-dose 10% hydrosyethyl starch 264/0.45 versus 5% albumin during major reconstructive surgery. *Anesth Analg* 2005;100(6):1846–1853.

Carlson GW, Page AL, Peters K, et al. Effects of radiation therapy on pedicled transverse rectus abdominis myocutaneous flap breast reconstruction. *Ann Plast Surg* 2008;60(5):568–572.

Kahn DM, Karanas YL, Pardun J. Breast surgery. In: Jaffe RJ, Samuels SI, eds. *Anesthesiologist's Manual of Surgical Procedures*. Philadelphia: Lippincott Williams and Wilkins, 2004:916–922.

Moller JF, Nikolajsen L, Rodt SA, et al. Thoracic paravertebral block for breast cancer surgery: a randomized double-blinded study. *Anesth Analg* 2007; 105(6):1848–1851.

Reavey P, McCarthy C. Update on breast reconstruction in breast cancer. *Curr Opin Obstet Gynecol* 2008; 20(1):61–67.

Spear SL, Newman MK, Bradford MS, et al. A retrospective analysis of outcomes using three common methods for immediate breast reconstruction. *Plast Reconstr Surg* 2008;122(2):340–347.

Spear SL, Mardini S, Ganz JC. Resource cost comparison of implant based breast reconstruction versus TRAM flap breast reconstruction. *Plast Reconstr Surg* 2003;112(1):101–105.

Vega SJ, Nguyen VT, Forsberg C, et al. Efficacy of preoperative autologous blood donation in free TRAM flap breast reconstruction. *Plast Reconstr Surg* 2008;121(5):241–246.

Warren AG, Morris DJ, Houlihan MJ, et al. Breast reconstruction in a changing breast cancer treatment paradigm. *Plast Reconstr Surg* 2008;121(4):1116–1126.

Liposuction

44

Vickie S. Jordan

KEY POINTS

- Many patients undergoing liposuction have acute and chronic coexisting disorders related to obesity or massive weight loss (MWL).
- The systemic absorption of wetting solution can potentially result in fluid volume overload, lidocaine toxicity, and epinephrine toxicity.
- Estimating blood loss is dependent on the liposuction technique employed as well as total aspirate obtained.
- Compliance with fluid resuscitation guidelines coupled with urinary output monitoring aids in the prevention of hypovolemia and hypervolemia in the patient undergoing liposuction.
- Perioperative complications associated with liposuction include bacterial infection, pulmonary and fat embolism, lidocaine toxicity, perforation, fluid volume overload, and hypothermia.

CASE SYNOPSIS

A 43-year-old woman presents for elective liposuction for body contouring of the flanks, back, inner and outer thighs, and abdomen utilizing the tumescent technique. Intraoperatively, the patient will be placed in the prone position to obtain access to the back and flank area. The planned amount of aspirate is 4000 ml.

PREOPERATIVE EVALUATION AND DEMOGRAPHIC DATA

Past Medical/Surgical History

- Smoking
- Hypertension
- MWL of 58 kg; status postbariatric surgery
- Anxiety
- Bilateral tubal ligation and cholecystectomy; no anesthetic complications

List of Medications

- Avalide
- Fexofenadine
- Lexapro
- Hormone replacement therapy
- Multivitamin

Diagnostic Data

- Hemoglobin, 12.7 g/dl; hematocrit, 36.8%
- Electrolytes: sodium, 137 mEq; potassium, 3.7 mEq/l; carbon dioxide, 25 mEq/l; glucose, 97 mg/dl

Height/Weight/Vital Signs

- 165 cm, 117 kg
- Blood pressure, 142/87; heart rate, 72 beats per minute; respiratory rate, 18 breaths per minute; room air oxygen saturation, 97%; temperature, 36.2°C.
- Electrocardiogram (ECG): normal sinus rhythm with occasional premature atrial contractions; nonspecific T-wave abnormalities
- Chest x-ray (CXR): no acute disease process, heart normal in size

PATHOPHYSIOLOGY

Obesity/Lipodystrophy

Body mass index (BMI) is a calculation derived from a patient's height and weight expressed in kilograms per meter squared (kg/m^2). Persons with a BMI greater than 20% are by definition, obese, while those with a BMI greater than 30% are classified as morbidly obese. A multitude of pathophysiologic changes are associated with obesity as summarized in Table 44-1.

SURGICAL PROCEDURE

Suction-assisted lipoplasty is the most common elective cosmetic procedure performed in the United States. Liposuction involves removing subcutaneous adipose tissue through a cannula with the aid of an external source of suction. Various liposuction techniques are included in Table 44-2. The wetting

Table 44-1	Pathologic Conditions Associated with Obesity
CARDIOVASCULAR	
Hyperlipidemia	
Hypertension	
Venous insufficiency	
Peripheral vascular disease	
Coronary artery disease	
Ventricular hypertrophy	
RESPIRATORY	
Restrictive lung disease	
Obstructive sleep apnea	
Redundant airway tissue	
Hypoventilation syndrome	
OTHER PATHOLOGY	
Diabetes	
Gastroesophageal reflux disease	
Cerebrovascular disease	
Cirrhosis	
Cholecystitis	
Impaired wound healing	

solution used for liposuction may or may not contain additives such lidocaine with epinephrine and their significance is discussed further in this chapter. Additionally, the subsequent use of laser-assisted liposuction may be used in conjunction with the wetting solution to facilitate greater volumes of aspirate. MWL secondary to bariatric surgery has resulted in nearly 56,000 body contouring procedures being performed in the United States.

ANESTHETIC MANAGEMENT AND CONSIDERATIONS

Preoperative Period

1. Discuss medications that could potentially interact with the tumescent fluid.

- Antidepressants, monoamine oxidase (MAO) inhibitors, and beta-blockers. Potential side

Table 44-2   Commonly Performed Liposuction Techniques

TECHNIQUE	WETTING SOLUTION (WS)	WS: ASPIRATE	BLOOD LOSS
Dry technique	No wetting solution is utilized	N/A	20–45% of total aspirate
Tumescent technique	0.025–0.1% lidocaine and epinephrine 1:100,000 in normal saline or lactated Ringer's solution	3:1	1% of total aspirate
Superwet technique	Normal saline or lactated Ringer's solution with epinephrine and sometimes lidocaine	1:1	1% or less of total aspirate
Ultrasound-assisted technique	Used in conjunction with tumescent or superwet technique	Dependent on technique used in conjunction with ultrasound	1% of total aspirate

effects of beta-blockers are bradycardia, claudication, and sedation.

- MAO inhibitors result in an increased availability of norepinephrine which affects the central nervous system (brain) as well as the sympathetic nervous system. A potential side effect of the MAO inhibitor phenelzine is sedation.
- Tricyclic antidepressants may result in seizure-like activity on the electroencephalogram.
- The anticholinergic effects of tricyclic antidepressant increase the likelihood of central anticholinergic syndrome if atropine or scopolamine are administered.
- Oral contraceptives and hormone replacement therapy increases the risk for deep vein thrombosis.
- Oral estrogen increases the risk of venous thromboembolism in postmenopausal women.
- Venous thrombosis and pulmonary embolism has been associated with the use of third-generation progestins in low estrogen.

2. Discuss obesity and related coexisting diseases associated with patients having elective liposuction.

Obesity is present in 50% of the population in America. Patients with a BMI > 20% are at increased risk for perioperative complications related to acute and chronic medical conditions such as type 2 diabetes, hypertension, and coronary artery disease. Cardiac manifestations related to obesity included an increased myocardial workload, hypertension, and ventricular hypertrophy. Obstructive sleep apnea (OSA) frequently occurs in obese patients and, when coupled with deep sedation, there is an increase in respiratory risk factors. Increases in pulmonary blood flow and pulmonary vasoconstriction due to chronic hypoxia can result in pulmonary hypertension and cor pulmonale in the obese patient with OSA.

Although liposuction is commonly performed with the utilization of local block or tumescent anesthesia, many anesthetists administer sedation to help the patient better tolerate the brief periods of discomfort experienced during the punctures necessary to instill the subdermal infiltration of the local anesthetic. Of particular concern in the postoperative period is the increased risk of postoperative apnea associated with the use of opioids and sedatives. Gastrointestinal concerns associated with obesity include factors that predispose the patient to aspiration pneumonitis which includes hiatal hernia, gastroesophageal reflux, decreased gastric emptying, and increased acidity of gastric.

Fatty liver infiltrates which may lead to cirrhosis, can decrease metabolism of medications increasing the likelihood of local anesthetic toxicity. Strict diets and strenuous exercise resulting in weight loss could cause hypoalbuminemia, electrolyte imbalances, or fluid/electrolyte deficiencies.

3. Discuss the importance of administering prophylactic antibiotics for the patient undergoing liposuction.
- Necrotizing fasciitis with overwhelming infection and toxic shock syndrome is a known fatal complication associated with liposuction.
- Causative organisms have been identified as *Streptococcus pyogenes* and *Staphylococcus aureus*.
- Autopsy reports have shown bacterial invasion from the perineal area.
- The most common class of antibiotic administered preoperatively for anesthetic procedures is a cephalosporin.
- Current evidence-based practice recommends that prophylactic antibiotic treatment be instituted within 60 minutes of surgical incision.
- Subsequent doses of antibiotics are determined based on the antibiotics half-life and duration of the surgery.

Factors that Contribute to Infection
- Patient factors: Extremes of age, malnutrition, obesity, diabetes, hypoxemia, remote infection, corticosteroid therapy, recent operation, chronic inflammation, and prior irradiation
- Perioperative factors: Long preoperative hospitalization, no preoperative shower, hair removal, and prior antibiotic therapy
- Intraoperative factors: Intraoperative contamination, lengthy operation, excessive electrocautery, foreign material, wound drainage, epinephrine wound injection, intraoperative hypotension, and massive transfusion

Intraoperative Period

4. Describe the physiologic alterations and potential complications associated with the prone position.
The prone position is associated with cardiac, respiratory, and cerebral complications.

Decreased preload, cardiac output, and blood pressure are associated with venous compression from tension of the abdominal muscles which causes blood to pool in the lower extremities.

Increased work of breathing results from compression of the abdomen and thorax and decreased lung compliance. In cases of head rotation in the prone position, cerebral venous drainage and cerebral blood flow is also diminished.

5. Examine the differences for various liposuction techniques.
Dry Technique
- Performed without the use of infiltration of subcutaneous solutions before suctioning.
- Disadvantages of the dry technique are swelling and discoloration.
- Blood loss is 20–45% of the aspirate obtained.
- Transfusion is usually required when large volumes of fat are removed.
- Avoid aspirate volumes greater than 1000 ml because of the risk of large blood loss volumes.
- Never performed in conjunction with ultrasound-assisted liposuction because of the possibility of thermal injuries from the ultrasound.

Wet Technique
- Infiltration of 200–300 ml of wetting solution into the operative site before suctioning begins.
- The solution may or may not contain additives such as lidocaine, epinephrine, and/or bicarbonate.
- Epinephrine added to the solution results in a significant decrease in the volume of blood loss to 4–30% of the aspirate.

Tumescent Technique

- Tumescent fluid is composed of a liter of lactated Ringer's solution containing 40 ml of lidocaine, 1 ml 1:1000 epinephrine, and 20 ml 8.4% sodium bicarbonate.
- The segmental injection of tumescent fluid prior to suctioning.
- Doses of 35 mg/kg of patient weight have reportedly been safely infiltrated although the FDA recommends the maximum dose of 7 mg/kg of lidocaine with epinephrine in the adult.
- Variations of the tumescent formula consist of a liter of lactated Ringer's solution or normal saline with 0.05–1.0% lidocaine and 0.5 to 1:1,000,000 epinephrine and sodium bicarbonate 2.5 to 12.5 mEq/l.
- The tumescent technique employs the practice of infiltrating 3–4 ml of infiltrate for each 1 ml of aspirate.
- An advantage of this technique is epinephrine induced hemostasis caused by vasoconstriction which reduces blood loss to 1% of the volume of aspirate.

Superwet Technique

- Major difference between the superwet technique and the tumescent technique is the amount of aspirate infiltrated.
- Utilizes a 1:1 ration of aspirate to infiltrate.
- Composition of the infiltrate is either saline or Ringer's lactate with epinephrine and sometimes lidocaine.
- Blood loss with this technique has been found to be comparable to blood loss in the tumescent technique at 1% of the aspirate.

Ultrasound-Assisted Liposuction

- Cannula or probe that delivers fat-liquefying ultrasonic energy to adipose tissue in fibrous areas.
- Adipocytes go through a series of expansion and compression cycles, resulting in implosion of the cell.

- Wetting solution used in conjunction with the ultrasound probe emulsifies fat and aids in cooling the heat generated.
- Blood loss is consistent with the superwet technique at 1% of the aspirate which is comparable to the tumescent technique.

Comparisons of the different techniques utilized to perform liposuction are described in Table 44-2.

6. Explain the physiologic alterations that manifest with intravascular absorption of lidocaine and epinephrine in the tumescent fluid used during liposuction.

Local anesthetics have the potential to cause systemic toxicity because these medications cause blockade of cellular sodium channels through the entire body. Untoward effects that occur to the neurologic and cardiovascular systems are dependent on the plasma concentration of the local anesthetic. When a patient begins to develop local anesthetic toxicity, the first signs and symptoms are associated with the neurologic system and include ringing sound in the ears, numbness around the lips, dizziness, and tinnitus. Higher plasma concentrations associated with local anesthetic toxicity manifest as altered level of consciousness, seizures, respiratory arrest, and finally cardiac compromise.

The greatest determining factor of the lidocaine plasma level during tumescent liposuction is due to hepatic degradation. The liver's maximum clearance capacity is approximately 250 mg of lidocaine per hour. Hepatic enzymes and blood flow are the predominant factors affecting lidocaine metabolism. The plasma half-life of lidocaine is 1.8 hours but hepatic disease can increase it to 4.9 hours. Decreased hepatic blood flow as found in congestive heart failure drastically reduces the rate of elimination of lidocaine. Cardiac and cerebral events occur if the peak metabolic capacity of lidocaine is impaired by drug interactions or hepatic dysfunction. Depression of the intracardiac conduction system and ventricular contractility resulting in asystole can occur. Treatment for cardiac arrest resulting from local anesthetic toxicity includes, but is not limited to, the infusion of intralipids. The addition of epinephrine- to lidocaine-containing solutions reduces the absorption of the local anesthetic by approximately one third. To date there have been no documented cases of epinephrine toxicity because very little of the diluted epinephrine is minimally absorbed. However, the anesthetist should be alert to the potential sympathomimetic effects caused by epinephrine. Lidocaine can potentiate the effects of nondepolarizing neuromuscular-blocking drugs.

7. Explain the process of estimating blood loss during liposuction.

- Two major determinants of blood loss in liposuction are the amount of blood in each milliliter of aspirate which can be determined by the technique used and the total aspirate obtained.
- Total blood loss can be calculated by multiplying the percent of blood in the aspirate by the total amount suctioned.
- Blood loss in the tumescent technique is approximately 1% of the aspirate.

8. Explain the fluid resuscitation guidelines for the patient undergoing liposuction.

- There are currently no definitive guidelines that exist for fluid management during liposuction.
- Factors that guide perioperative fluid homeostasis include close monitoring of intravenous (IV) fluid administered, wetting solution infiltrated, amount of aspirate, estimated blood loss, and urinary output.
- Aspirate is defined as the total volume of fat and fluid obtained during liposuction.
- Approximately 60–70% of wetting solution remains and is absorbed as hypodermoclysis.
- The volume of fluids to be infused should be guided by the patient's vital signs and urinary output.
- Patients with less than 5 l of aspirate removed should receive maintenance fluid only.

- Patients with greater than 5 l removed should receive maintenance + 0.25 ml of IV fluid for each milliliter of aspirate over 5000 ml.
- Guidelines for fluid resuscitation are listed in Table 44-2.

Postoperative Period

The total time required to perform the liposuction was 130 minutes. The amount of wetting solution infiltrated was 4300 ml and the total amount of aspirate obtained was 3800 ml. Fluid resuscitation with crystalloid was 3400 ml and the urinary output was 625 ml. The dressings and compression garment were applied and the patient was extubated once she was completely awake after the application. Vital signs in the postanesthesia care unit were blood pressure, 167/92; heart rate, 119 beats per minute; respiratory rate, 26 breaths per minute; and temperature, 35.1°C.

9. Discuss the following potential complications associated with liposuction.

Embolism

- Pulmonary embolus is the largest single cause of mortality in patients undergoing liposuction, 4.6 per 100,000 patients.
- Embolism may result from fat or venous thrombosis.
- Pulmonary embolism presents as shortness of breath, pleuritic pain, cough, hemoptysis, palpitations, wheezing, and angina-like pain.
- Deep venous thrombosis (DVT) signs and symptoms include: leg pain, Hohmann's sign, swelling and erythema, tachycardia, and warmth of the extremity.
- Intermittent pneumatic leg compression devices are recommended for the prophylactic prevention of pulmonary thromboembolism.
- Some of the risk factors for DVT and pulmonary embolism include thrombophlebitis, smoking, obesity, previous DVT, hormone replacement therapy/oral contraceptives.
- Treatment for pulmonary embolism/ DVT includes heparin, thrombolytics,

low–molecular weight heparin, hemodynamic support.

Pulmonary Edema

- Hyperhydration that results from the infusion of IV fluid for the treatment of hypotension.
- Hypodermoclysis that results from the wetting solution being rapidly absorbed.

Intestinal or Organ Perforation

Organ perforation has been reported in the presence of an existing abdominal scar on rare occasions. Susceptible areas for major damage from perforation include the abdomen, thorax, retroperitoneum, major vessels, and the kidney. The signs and symptoms of organ perforation may not manifest for several days thus, the patient presents with an acute abdomen or sepsis requiring an emergency laparotomy to repair the injury.

Hypothermia

Hypothermia is defined as body temperature < 36.5°C. The primary mechanism by which patients lose heat within the operating room is by radiation which occurs rapidly in the operating room. Wetting solutions injected into patients, even if prewarmed, are frequently less than body temperature. Infused IV fluids are also a source of heat loss by way of convection. Perioperative hypothermia can result in increased discomfort, infection, bleeding, decreased metabolism of medications, and shivering which can prolong discharge. Methods that can reduce the risk of hypothermia are present in Table 44-3.

REVIEW QUESTIONS

1. What is the approximate blood loss for the patient who has undergone tumescent liposuction with 4500 ml of total aspirate obtained?
   a. 450 ml
   b. 1500 ml
   c. 2250 ml
   d. 45 ml

2. Which is an initial sign associated with local anesthetic toxicity?
   a. Seizures
   b. Dizziness
   c. Respiratory arrest
   d. Bradycardia

3. What is the calculated fluid volume replacement *in addition to the maintenance* that the patient undergoing large volume liposuction should receive? The patient weighs 117 kg, 5900 of wetting solution has been infiltrated, and 5500 ml of total aspirate obtained.
   a. Wetting solution + 500 ml
   b. Wetting solution + 125 ml
   c. Wetting solution + 250 ml
   d. Wetting solution + 6000 ml

4. Which complication causes the highest mortality for a patient having liposuction?
   a. Hypothermia
   b. Pulmonary embolism
   c. Organ perforation
   d. Necrotizing fasciitis

Table 44-3   Methods Used to Prevent Intraoperative Hypothermia
Warming the skin preparation solution, intravenous, and infiltrative fluids
Applying forced-air warming blanket
Increasing the operating room temperature
Warming the infiltration solution to 37°C at the time of injection
Cover the patient's head and appendages to help minimize the exposed surface area

5. Which class of anesthetic medications can be potentiated by lidocaine?
   a. Inhalation anesthetics
   b. Nitrous oxide
   c. Nondepolarizing muscle relaxants
   d. Benzodiazepines

REVIEW ANSWERS

1. **Answer: d**
   The tumescent technique reduces blood loss to 1% of the volume of aspirate.

2. **Answer: b**
   An initial sign that is associated with local anesthetic toxicity is dizziness.

3. **Answer: b**
   500 ml $\times$ 0.25 = 125 ml, patients with greater than 5 l of aspirate removed should receive maintenance + wetting solution + 0.25 ml of IV fluid/cc of aspirate greater than 5000 ml.

4. **Answer: b**
   Pulmonary embolus is the greatest single cause of mortality in patients undergoing liposuction, 4.6 per 100,000 patients.

5. **Answer: c**
   Lidocaine can potentiate nondepolarizing neuromuscular-blocking medications.

SUGGESTED READINGS

Agency for Healthcare Quality and Research. Composite measure: adult Medicare patients having surgery who had prophylactic antibiotics begun at the right time and ended at the right time. Available online at: http://www.ahrq.gov/qual/nhdr06/measurespec/patient_safety.htm. Accessed September 1, 2008.

Caballini M, Preis F, Casati A. Effects of mild hypothermia on blood coagulation in patients undergoing elective plastic surgery. *Plast Reconstr Surg* 2005;116:316–321.

Canonico M, Oger E, Plu-Bureau G, et al. Hormone therapy and venous thromboembolism among postmenopausal women: impact of the route of estrogen administration and progestogens: the ESTHER Study. *Circulation* 2007;115:840–845.

DeJong R, Grazer F. Perioperative management of cosmetic liposuction. *Plast Reconstr Surg* 2000;107:1039–1044.

Karmo F, Milan M, Silbergleit A. Blood loss in major liposuction procedures: a comparison study using suction-assisted versus ultrasonically assisted lipoplasty. *Plast Reconstr Surg* 2001;108:241–247.

Kenkel J. Practice advisory on liposuction. *Plast Reconstr Surg* 2004;113:1494–1496.

Kenkel J, Lipschitz A, Luby M, et al. Hemodynamic physiology and thermoregulation in liposuction. *Plast Reconstr Surg* 2004;114:503–513.

Middeldorp S. Oral contraceptives and the risk of venous thromboembolism. *Gend Med* 2005; 2 Suppl A:S3–S9

Most D, Kozlow B, Heller J, et al. Thromboembolism in plastic surgery. *Plast Reconstr Surg* 2005;115:20e–30e.

Robles-Cervantes J, Martinez-Molina R, Cardenas-Camarena L. Heating infiltration solutions used in tumescent liposuction: minimizing surgical risk. *Plast Reconstr Surg* 2005;115:1077–1081.

Mandibular Osteotomy

45

Joseph A. Joyce

KEY POINTS

- Maxillofacial surgery is performed for the following pathologic reasons: musculoskeletal and craniofacial abnormalities, dental osseous misalignment, soft tissue deformities, maxillofacial trauma, maxillofacial infection, or tumor growth.
- Airway management for patients having maxillofacial surgery is dependent on the type of surgery that is being performed and the patients' comorbidities. Nasal intubation with a specialized Ring-Adair-Elwyn (RAE) endotracheal tube provides optimal surgical access and visualization.
- Strategies to control postoperative nausea and vomiting (PONV) are extremely important because of the increased potential for aspiration of gastric contents and decreased access to the airway caused by the surgical intervention.
- Blood loss during maxillofacial surgery may be as large as 1500 ml as a result of the complexity and extensive nature of the surgical procedure.

CASE SYNOPSIS

A 15-year-old girl with maxillary insufficiency and prognathia is scheduled to have a LeFort 1 and bilateral sagittal split osteotomies.

PREOPERATIVE EVALUATION AND DEMOGRAPHIC DATA

Past Medical/Surgical History

- No past surgical history

Medication List

- None

Diagnostic Data

- Hemoglobin, 12.7 g/dl; hematocrit, 37.4%

Height/Weight/Vital Signs

- 173 cm, 86 kg
- Blood pressure, 115/78; heart rate, 82 beats per minute; respiratory rate, 18 breaths per minute; Temperature, 37°C; room air oxygen saturation, 99%
- Airway classification Mallampati 1; 7-cm thyromental distance; full range of motion cervical spine without discomfort; both nares appear normal size without any narrowing or obstruction to airflow.

PATHOPHYSIOLOGY

Maxillofacial surgery represents a large variety of procedures that range from simple (extraction of teeth) to complex (facial reconstruction after a trauma). There are many indications for tooth extractions which include severe caries, pulpal necrosis, odontalgia, aiding orthodontic corrections, removal of impacted molars, and for cosmetic improvement. Orthognathic procedures are carried out on both maxillae and mandible and are indicated for psychological and/or aesthetic reasons, medical concerns, or functional/developmental abnormalities.

Maxillofacial trauma can be the result of a blunt force, such as a motor vehicle accident, penetrating trauma or result from a thermal injury. Blunt and/or penetrating trauma may produce extensive injury due to production of secondary projectile—teeth or bone fragments—that damage surrounding soft tissues. Other indications for maxillofacial surgery include maxillary insufficiency, prognathia, macrognathia, retrognathia, maxillomandibular complex asymmetry, temporomandibular joint/facial pain, and obstructive sleep apnea. This patient presented with maxillary insufficiency and prognathia for surgical correction/resculpting to improve appearance and dentition alignment.

RELEVANT ANATOMY

Twenty-two bones form the head and facial skeleton. The skull is divided into two regions: the *calvaria* and *facial* skeleton. The calvaria is comprised of 8 bones: frontal, occipital, temporal (2), parietal (2), sphenoid, and ethmoid—all of which form the rigid structure for the brain. The remaining 14 bones form the face—that part of the skeleton is most closely associated with visual appearance. These bones are nasal (2), lacrimal (2), superior maxillary (2), zygomatic (2), palate (2), inferior turbinate (2), vomer, and mandible. The teeth lend structure and composition and contribute significantly to the facial skeleton. Figures 45-1 and 45-2 illustrate the complexity of the craniofacial skeleton.

The face is divided into three areas: the upper, middle, and lower face. The upper face is comprised of the frontal bone and is bound by the frontozygomatic and frontonasal sutures/articulations. The middle of the face begins with the orbits and extends downward to, and includes, the upper teeth. The lower face is comprised of the lower teeth and mandible.

SURGICAL PROCEDURE

There are three distinct facial fractures and the anatomic description is classified into one of three LeFort categories. Figure 45-3 depicts the region of the craniofacial skeleton that is characteristic of each type of fracture.

LeFort 1 Fracture/Osteotomy

The LeFort 1 fracture occurs along the maxillary alveolar rim. This fracture arises from the nasal septum toward the lateral pyriform rims and traverses above the apices of the teeth. The fracture occurs below the zygomaticomaxillary junction and interrupts the pterygoid plates by crossing the pterygomaxillary junction. The LeFort 1 osteotomy closely follows the fracture lines and produces separation of the maxilla and the palate.

The surgical incisions are made inside the mouth at the junction of the upper lip and the gum. The bony separation is accomplished with an oscillating saw. The maxilla may be mobilized as a whole or in two or more segments, depending on the anatomic indications, and may be adjusted anteriorly, posteriorly, inferiorly, or any variable combination of these directions, dictated by the presenting anatomic inadequacy. The maxilla is repositioned by several millimeters then secured with titanium plates and screws. Typically, the duration of surgery is approximately 2.5 to 3.5 hours, but may be longer depending on the number of maxillary segments created for the procedure. The patient's age may also contribute to the length of the procedure because of the density of bone that must be transected. This procedure advances the midface to achieve a more aesthetically pleasing facial construction as well as more

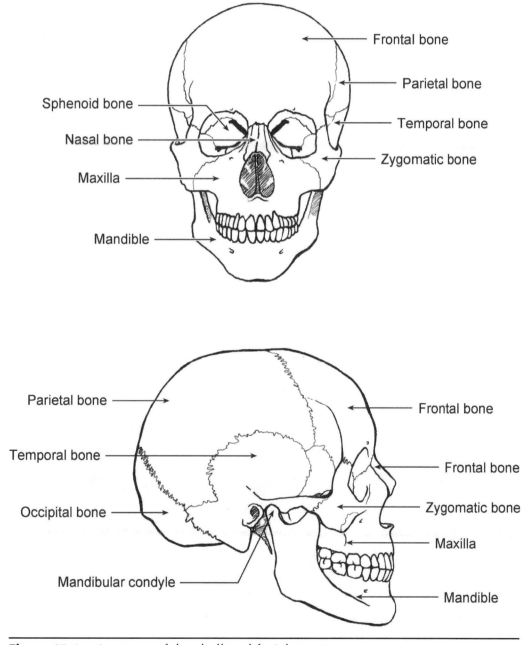

Figure 45-1 *Anatomy of the skull and facial structures.*

Figure 45-2   *Craniofacial skeleton.*

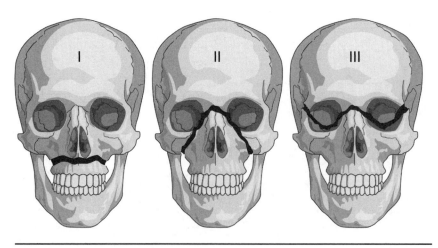

Figure 45-3   *LeFort classification system.*

efficient functionality of a number of facial structures including dental occlusive alignment and nasal passages/airway. Frequently, this procedure may be completed in an office setting and/or an outpatient/ambulatory care setting.

LeFort 2 Fracture/Osteotomy

The LeFort 2 fracture forms a pyramidal shape that traverses the nasal bridge via the nasofrontal suture. The bone disruption crosses the maxillae via the frontal process, through the lacrimal bones, inferior orbital floor/rim, frequently through the orbital foramen, and finally through the anterior wall of the maxillary sinus. The base of the pyramid is formed as the fracture lines travel beneath the zygoma, traverses the pterygomaxillary fissure, and extends through the pterygoid plates.

The LeFort 2 osteotomy is not commonly performed. Because of the nature of this surgical undertaking, it is reserved for patients in whom growth of the center of the face has been greatly deficient. The target patient is one in whom the facial redesign requires movement of the facial center, maxillae, and nose simultaneously. The LeFort 2 is a major surgical undertaking requiring surgical incisions in three locations: the junction of the upper lip and gum, a bicoronal incision (from ear to ear across the crown of the head), and either transconjunctival or blepharoplasty incisions. Scalp reflection and accessing the nose and face center along with the results in significant blood loss. Blood transfusions may be required intra- and/or postoperatively. Due to the extensive nature of the surgery, the degree of bruising and edema that is likely to occur, compounded by the high level of postoperative pain and potential for nausea and vomiting, it is prudent for this patient to remain intubated and sedated and receive assisted or controlled mechanical ventilations for the first 24 hours or more.

LeFort 3 Fracture/Osteotomy

The LeFort 3 fracture produces separation of the face from the calvaria. As a result of the LeFort 3 fracture, the skull has three "mobile" components—the calvaria, face, and mandible—rather than the normal two segments, the mandible and the skull. The LeFort 3 fracture is also called craniofacial dysjunction. The LeFort 3 begins in a fashion similar to the LeFort 2 fracture: the nasofrontal and frontomaxillary sutures are separated and the fracture traverses the medial orbit walls through the nasolacrimal groove and the ethmoid bone. Extension of the fracture line into the optical canals is generally prevented by the thick sphenoid bone resulting in fracture lines instead traversing the orbit floor and across the lateral orbital wall via the zygomaticofrontal junction and zygomatic arch. The fracture lines are completed via the base of the ethmoid bone's perpendicular plate, through the vomer, and the sphenoid bone's pterygoid plates.

The LeFort 3 procedure is reserved for patients with extremely deficient midfacial growth and development. This procedure is accomplished via incisional approaches described in the LeFort 2 procedure. Other procedural aspects that are similar to the LeFort 2 procedure include the extensive dissection required, the lengthy duration of the procedure, the high degree of bruising and edema, and the large blood loss that is frequently associated with potential for blood transfusions. As with the LeFort 2, this patient should remain intubated and sedated with controlled ventilations for at least the first 24 hours postoperatively. The potential complications that are associated with LeFort osteotomies are listed in Table 45-1.

Mandibular Sagittal Split Osteotomy

In terms of complexity, the mandibular sagittal split osteotomy (MSSO) may be one of the more "simple" orthognathic procedures. This procedure involves incisions, usually two, at or near the third molars. These molars are frequently extracted about 6 months prior to this surgical procedure. The mandible is split bilaterally. The splits are the locations where a few millimeters of bone may be removed or added to produce the desired correction in

Table 45-1	Potential Complications Associated with LeFort Osteotomies

- Arteriovenous fistulas
- Fractures to pterygoid plate, sphenoid bone, middle cranial fossa
- Infraorbital nerve traction injury
- Lacrimal duct injury
- Stensen duct injury
- Velopharyngeal insufficiency
- Avascular necrosis
- Maxillary sinusitis
- Nasal–septal buckling
- Nasal–septal deviation
- Ophthalmic duct injury

Table 45-2	Potential Complications Associated with Mandibular Sagittal Split Osteotomy

- Avascular necrosis
- Inferior alveolar artery bleeding
- Mental nerve injury
- Proximal segment malposition
- Condylar resorption
- Gingival recession
- Unanticipated fractures
- Inferior mandibular border contour irregularity
- Masseteric artery bleeding
- Unfavorable sagittal split

Table 45-3	Potential Complications Associated with Maxillofacial Surgery

- Bleeding
- Devitalization of teeth
- Gingival recession
- Hardware exposure
- Malocclusion
- Malunion/nonunion of bone
- Postoperative infection
- Respiratory decompensation
- Dental injury
- Unanticipated fractures

mandible length. The splits are stabilized in their new position using titanium plates and screws. The MSSO is the least time-consuming orthognathic procedure, usually requiring about 1.5 to 2.5 hours. Frequently the MSSO is combined with various forms of the LeFort 1 procedures to correct various facial growth disparities. Potential complications that are associated with an MSSO procedure and maxillofacial procedures are listed in Tables 45-2 and 45-3.

ANESTHETIC MANAGEMENT AND CONSIDERATIONS

Preoperative Period

1. Identify the structural components that comprise the airway.

The airway begins within the face/facial skeleton. The airway originates at the external nares and vestibulum oris (mouth) through the nasal and oral cavities continuing to the nasopharynx and oropharynx then on to the larynx and glottis to enter the trachea. From the trachea, the airway divides into numerous subdivisions of the bronchial tree to culminate in the alveoli. There are three concha or turbinates that are present on the lateral walls of the nasal cavity opposite of the nasal septum: superior, middle, and inferior. The superior and middle turbinates are formed from the ethmoid bone, while the inferior turbinate is an osseous formation that articulates with the ethmoid, lachrymal, maxillae, and palatine bones. These bony formations disrupt airflow and redirect air into the various sinuses within the facial skeleton. The turbulence that is created prolongs the time the air is in contact with the mucosa of the turbinates. As a result, there is increased moisture and heat as air moves into the lungs.

2. List the important factors necessary to determine the airway management technique to be used for patients having maxillofacial surgery.
Airway management for patients having maxillofacial surgery is dependent on the type of surgical procedure that will be performed. A discussion with the surgeon regarding the surgical requirements is imperative. Orthognathic procedures—those producing reshaping/resculpting of the bony structures of the face—require general anesthesia. Due to the nature and complexity of orthognathic procedures, airway management will require a nasal intubation.

3. Describe the preparation process for nasotracheal intubation.
Tracheal intubation via the nasal approach differs from the oral approach in that the anesthetist must prepare both nares prior to intubation. Factors that need to be assessed during the preoperative evaluation include:

- The amount of airflow via the nares/nasal passages
- Is one nare narrower than the other?
- Is the nasal septum deviated significantly in one direction?
- Does the patient perceive a restriction to inspiration or extubation via the nasal passages?
- Does this patient have unilateral choanal atresia?

Despite the assessment to determine the degree of patency of the nasal passages, both nares should be prepared for endotracheal tube placement. Medications applied directly to the nasal mucosa produce vasoconstriction which reduces the thickness of the mucosal tissue and decreases the potential for bleeding during intubation. This can be accomplished by using a decongestant nasal spray such as dilute phenylephrine, oxymetazoline nasal, a 4% cocaine solution, azelastine, ipratropium, or cromolyn nasal sprays. Utilizing a 4% cocaine solution offers the added action of anesthetizing the mucosal surfaces and local vasoconstriction.

Prior to nasotracheal intubation, the right or left nare that the anesthetist determines to be most patent should be further dilated using nasal airways. To help facilitate nasal intubation, it is reasonable to insert a nasal airway that is equal to or slightly larger than the endotracheal tube that will be placed. Nasal passage dilation can be done prior to entering the operating room, but insertion of the nasal airways may produce significant discomfort despite the use of the lidocaine jelly. Typically, dilation of the nasal passage is undertaken immediately after induction of anesthesia. Any of the three turbinates may be dislodged or injured during dilation or intubation which will result in significant bleeding. The blood can obscure visualization during direct laryngoscopy process and increase the risk of aspiration.

4. Explain the importance of the "golden triangle" in relation to intubation for maxillofacial surgery.
The "golden triangle" is the facial region outlined by the nose and a portion of the maxilla. The apex of the triangle originates at the frontonasal sutures with the base angles at or near the corners of the mouth. This area is nicknamed the "golden triangle" because it is a highly vascular region. The nose is central to this triangular area. As such, relatively mild trauma in this area can produce a seemingly disproportionate amount of bleeding. The anesthetist must be as gentle as possible during the insertion of nasal airways and the endotracheal tube to minimize the degree of trauma produced during endotracheal tube placement.

Intraoperative Period
5. Identify the potential complications associated with nasal intubation.
The most common complications associated with nasal intubation include epistaxis, turbinectomy, and dental trauma. If an unintended turbinectomy occurs during nasal dilation or intubation, blood will pool in the oropharynx and may obstructing the anesthetist's view of the epiglottis and glottis.

The endotracheal tube may tamponade the nasal bleeding. However, after extubation, the bleeding can resume. This blood causes aspiration and may initiate a laryngospasm at the end of surgery.

One potential injury that may occur is a pressure injury to the forehead due to constant contact of the endotracheal tube connector. For this reason, during the process of securing the endotracheal tube, padding should be placed between the forehead and the universal connector. If a specialized nasal RAE tube is not used, the placement of a standard endotracheal tube can cause pressure on the nare and surrounding tissues causing necrosis. The surgical repair for maxillofacial fracture is shown in Figure 45-4.

Cerebral injury is another rare but potential complication associated with nasal intubation for patients who have sustained a LeFort 2 or LeFort 3 fracture as a result of a traumatic injury. The cribriform plate separates the superior portion of the nasal cavity from the cranial vault. If it is damaged, placement of a nasogastric tube or endotracheal tube can result in direct neurotrauma. Nasal intubation is absolutely contraindicated for patients who have sustained these fractures.

6. *Discuss interventions that can be used to decrease blood loss during maxillofacial surgery.*
Due to the intricacy, complexity, and anatomic region associated with maxillofacial surgery, the amount of blood loss can range from 250 and 1500 ml. If the surgery requires bone grafting and the graft(s) are taken from the patient, then the iliac crest or ribs are frequently the preferential sites. The amount of blood loss may be increased as the result of the additional incisions and bone harvesting. Currently, there is no absolute hemoglobin value at which the patient should receive a transfusion. The decision to initiate a transfusion should be based on the patient's comorbid factors and anesthetic course. Blood should be made available for patients having moderate and major craniofacial surgical procedures. Methods that the anesthetist can employ to help decrease blood loss includes:

- *Reverse Trendelenburg* positioning to facilitate venous drainage from the head.

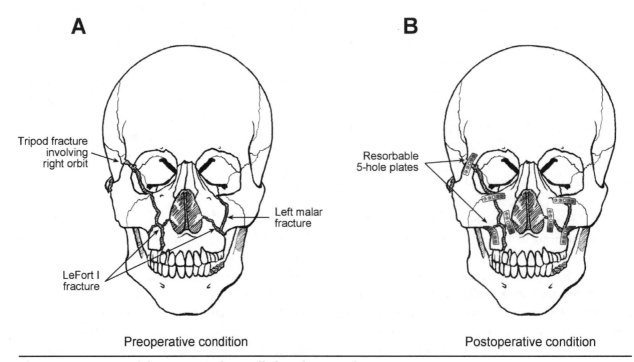

Figure 45-4 *Facial fractures and maxillofacial surgical repair.*

- Maintain *normothermia* to preserve adequate platelet function
- *Deliberate hypotension* can be employed to maintain the patient's mean arterial pressure (MAP) between 50 and 65 mm Hg. In patients who have cardiovascular or neurovascular insufficiency, coronary and cerebral perfusion as determined by autoregulation is increased. Therefore, decreasing MAP to this degree may result in myocardial and/or cerebral ischemia/infarction.

Deliberate hypotension can be achieved by administering increased doses of anesthetic agents (narcotics, inhalation agents, propofol infusion), Beta blockers or vasodilators (nitroprusside infusion). A combination of medications is most frequently used.

Postoperative Period

7. Identify strategies to reduce/eliminate/prevent PONV for patient having maxillofacial surgery.

Retching, with or without vomiting, can disrupt the alignment of the jaw and increase bleeding. The patient's jaws may be secured together using either rubber bands or, less frequently, wires. The limited access increases the potential for aspiration of gastric contents. The anesthetist must balance the

Table 45-4   Extubation Considerations
• Respiratory function
• Return/presence of protective airway reflexes
• Soft tissue edema
• Surgical time
• The presence of pathology
• Hemodynamic stability
• Intermaxillary fixation
• Level of consciousness
• Pain management requirements
• Potential for postoperative bleeding

need to influence operative blood loss with efforts to reduce or eliminate PONV.

Hypotension, hypovolemia, and narcotic administration are all factors that contribute to the development of PONV. Interventions that can be used to prevent PONV may entail administration of any of several different classes of medications such as gastrokinetic medications (metoclopramide), steroids (dexamethasone), 5-HT3-receptor antagonists (odansetron or dolasetron), or combination of these medications. Other factors that should be assessed include the degree of hypovolemia that can be treated by administrating intravenous fluids and the presence of pain.

8. Relate crucial factors to consider for extubation after maxillofacial surgery.

A significant amount of facial and tracheal edema develops during extensive maxillofacial procedures due to fluids that have entered the interstitial space and from surgical trauma. Careful assessment of the degree of tracheal edema can be achieved by deflating the endotracheal tube cuff immediately prior to extubation to determine if a leak occurs during a positive pressure breath. If tracheal edema is present or ventilation and intubation were difficult during the induction, it is prudent to keep the patient intubated. Airway management will almost certainly be more difficult or impossible post surgical repair. Table 45-4 lists factors that should be considered prior to tracheal extubation.

REVIEW QUESTIONS

1. Which is not a valid indication to perform an orthognathic procedure?
   a. Improved aesthetics
   b. Alleviation of obstructive sleep apnea
   c. Myofascial pain relief
   d. Temporal arteritis
2. Which description is indicative of a LeFort 2 fracture?
   a. Disarticulation of the mandible at the temporomandibular joints

b. Nasofrontal and frontomaxillary sutures are separated and the fracture traverses the medial orbit walls through the nasolacrimal groove

c. Fracture forming a pyramidal shape that extends from above the nose and traverses the zygomatic arches

d. Separation of the midfacial skeleton from the maxilla associated with sphenoid sinus disruption

3. Which intervention may reduce blood loss during maxillofacial surgery?

a. Elevating the patient's head 15 degrees

b. Maintaining hypothermia

c. Maintaining normotension

d. Decreasing the depth of anesthesia

4. Which complication is not associated with a nasal intubation?

a. Turbinectomy

b. Esophageal intubation

c. Epistaxis

d. Cranial intubation

5. Which is the most crucial reason to administer PONV prophylaxis for patients having maxillofacial surgery?

a. Decreased/limited access to the patient's airway

b. Excess blood loss

c. Increased postoperative sedation

d. Facial numbness

REVIEW ANSWERS

1. **Answer: d**

Each of the goals listed are among the indication for maxillofacial/orthognathic surgical procedures with the exception of temporal arteritis.

2. **Answer: c**

A triangular fracture that extends above the bridge of the nose to below the zygomatic arches is consistent with a LeFort 2 fracture.

3. **Answer: a**

Elevating the patients head will facilitate venous drainage and decrease venous pressure. This will lead to decreased blood

loss. The other intervention listed may increase bleeding from the surgical site.

4. **Answer: b**

Epistaxis and turbinectomy are the most common complications associated with a nasal intubation. Cranial intubation can occur if extreme pressure is exerted on the endotracheal tube if a sphenoid sinus fracture is present such as with a LeFort 2 or 3 fracture. An esophageal intubation is not considered to be a complication during nasal intubation.

5. **Answer: a**

The relative restrictive nature of the surgical intervention, edema formation and bandages may impede the ability of the anesthetist to control the patient's airway.

SUGGESTED READINGS

Choi WS, Samman N. Risks and benefits of deliberate hypotension in anaesthesia: a systematic review. *Int J Oral Maxillofac Surgery* 2008;37(8):687–703.

Clark S, Stone J. Anesthesia for ear, nose, throat, and maxillofacial surgery. In: Nagelhout JJ, Plaus K, eds. *Nurse Anesthesia*. 4th ed. Philadelphia: WB Saunders, 2009:937–939.

Dale RA. Dentoalveloar trauma. *Emerg Med Clin North Am* 2000;18:521–538.

Elsalanty ME, Genecov DG, Genecov JS. Functional and aesthetic endpoints in orthognathic surgery. *J Craniofac Surg* 2007;18(4):725–733.

Kim SG, Park SS. Incidence of complications and problems related to orthognathic surgery. *J Oral Maxillofac Surg* 2007;65(12):2438–2444.

Krohner RG. Anesthetic considerations for oral and maxillofacial surgery. *Int Anesthesiol Clin* 2003;41(3):67–89.

Mayhew JF. Airway management for oral and maxillofacial surgery. *Int Anesthesiol Clin* 2003;41(3):57–65.

Org TK, Banks RJ, Hildreth AJ. Surgical accuracy in LeFort 1 maxillary osteotomies. *Br J Oral Maxillofac Surg* 2001;39:96–102.

Silva AC, O'Ryan F, Poor DB. Postoperative nausea and vomiting (PONV) after orthognathic surgery: a retrospective study and literature review. *J Oral Maxillofac Surg* 2006;64(9):1385–1397.

Ueki K, Marukawa K, Shimada M. The assessment of blood loss in orthognathic surgery for prognathia. *J Oral Maxillofac Surg* 2005;63(3):350–354.

Orthopedic Surgery

XV

Anterior Cervical Discectomy/Fusion

46

Gary D. Clark and Nicholas C. Curdt

KEY POINTS

- Patients who require anesthesia for anterior cervical discectomy/fusion (ACDF) may be difficult or impossible to intubate due to the inability to place them in a "sniffing position" and properly align the oral, laryngeal, and pharyngeal axes.
- A comprehensive preoperative neurologic evaluation of the patient's sensory and motor function is imperative.
- There is the potential for damage to critical structures within the neck resulting from surgical trauma.
- Postoperative respiratory distress can occur due to unilateral recurrent laryngeal nerve injury, airway edema, hematoma, tracheal laceration, and pneumothorax.

CASE SYNOPSIS

A 45-year-old woman has paresthesias and numbness in the left shoulder, arm, and finger tips. Her electrocardiogram (ECG) and cardiac stress test are normal. The paresthesias and numbness are caused by cervical nerve compression as shown on magnetic resonance imaging (MRI). She is scheduled for an ACDF by the neurosurgeon.

PREOPERATIVE EVALUATION AND DEMOGRAPHIC DATA

Past Medical/Surgical History

- Hypertension
- Hysterectomy

List of Medications

- Atenolol

Diagnostic Data

- Hemoglobin, 13.2 g/dl; hematocrit, 39.4%
- Electrolytes: sodium, 139 mEq/l; potassium, 3.9 mEq/l; chloride, 104 mEq/l; carbon dioxide, 24 mEq/l

Height/Weight/Vital Signs

- 168 cm, 65 kg
- Blood pressure, 135/70; heart rate, 61 beats per minute; respiratory rate, 18 breaths per minute; room air oxygen saturation, 98%; temperature, 36.8°C
- ECG: Normal sinus rhythm; heart rate, 64 beats per minute
- Cardiac stress test (treadmill): within normal limits; no evidence of ischemia, infarction, or syncope during exertion

PATHOPHYSIOLOGY

Adult men and women between the ages of 40 and 55 are most commonly affected by cervical degeneration as part of the aging process. However, degenerative changes are readily documented in many adults with radiography and MRI beginning about 30 years of age. Instability of the cervical disc can result from traumatic or destructive (neoplastic, degenerative, congenital) disruption of stabilizing elements (anterior and posterior longitudinal ligaments, pedicles, and articulations). It still remains unclear why some patients have an increased risk of experiencing cervical spine deterioration and nerve compression.

Pain, weakness, paresthesias, and numbness of the neck, shoulder, arms, and hands is the result of a rupture or herniation of the annulus fibrosus of the disc. The annulus tears on the cervical disc compressing the nerve root or spinal cord at the cervical level. The bulging of the disc allows the softer inner nucleus to compress the nerve root or spinal cord. Narrowing and compression of the nerves in the cervical region can also result from the formation of osteophytes (spondylosis) or congenital narrowing of the space (stenosis) and symptoms associated with disc degeneration will not occur until later in life, as shown in Figure 46-1. A rupture or tear can be the result of age, degeneration, or traumatic injury. The cervical vertebrae are more susceptible to injury because of a greater range of motion, the small distance between the vertebrae, and the complexity of the anatomy in this region.

While it is inexplicable why some patients are affected more than others, degenerative cervical disc disease is thought to be the result of fibrous changes to the gelatinous disc resulting in less pliability. Degeneration occurs most commonly at the vertebral segments extending from C5 through C7. The resulting cervical compression can hinder blood flow and result in a cervical canal

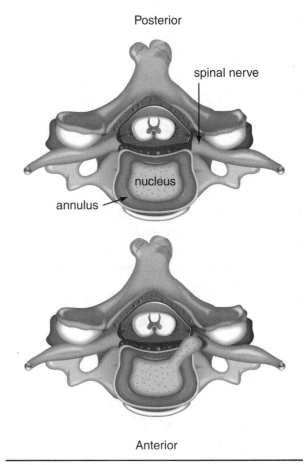

Figure 46-1 *Superior view of left herniation of cervical disc.*

narrowing. The diminished blood flow can produce myelopathy and neural injury which can be progressive and can result in permanent spinal cord damage if left untreated. Patients who have cervical degeneration can have further numbness, pain, or irritation by flexion, extension, or rotation of the head and neck. Therefore, even minimal manipulation of the head and neck could produce serious and/or permanent injury.

CONSERVATIVE TREATMENT OPTIONS

Treatment options range from conservative and palliative to emergency surgical intervention. The conservative treatments include rest, use of nonsteroidal medications, cervical traction, physical therapy, pain medication, and instructional exercises used to strengthen the muscles of the neck, upper back, and shoulders. Some patients benefit from conservative treatment; however, patients who continue to experience pain and functional limitations are candidates for ACDF.

SURGICAL PROCEDURE

The anterior approach is the most common surgical technique used for ACDF. A skin incision is made on the anterior aspect of the neck and then tissue is retracted to expose the anterior cervical spine. The surgical approach occurs between the esophagus and trachea medially, and the sternocleidomastoid muscle and carotid sheath laterally. The omohyoid muscle and recurrent laryngeal nerve are retracted inferiorly. Hand-held retractors or self-retaining retractors are utilized to provide initial exposure of the anterior vertebral column and the adjacent longus colli muscles. Tissue is removed from the disc to relieve the pressure that is exerted on the nerve root. Following the discectomy, the vertebra is fused to the superior or inferior vertebra with bone, mechanical plates, and/or screws in order to prevent dislocation. The anatomy and muscles surrounding the cervical spine are included in Figure 46-2.

Once removal of the disc occurs, there are several methods by which surgeons use in order to

fill or secure the intervertebral space with instruments called pituitaries, curettes, and/or kerrisons. These techniques use either an autograft (patient's bone) or allograft (cadaver bone) and are placed between the vertebral bodies. One such surgical method for ACDF is the Smith-Robinson technique. The bone graft is inserted into the disc space in order to maintain a neutral position, as shown in Figure 46-3. Vertebral fusion results over time as the bone graft heals. However, the implantation of plates and screws provides additional vertebral stabilization, as shown in Figure 46-4.

SURGICAL COMPLICATIONS

The most common complications resulting from ACDF surgery includes:

- Thrombophlebitis
- Infection
- Nerve damage
- Graft inadequacy (migration, erosion, degradation)
- Nonunion of the cervical vertebrae
- Chronic pain

ANESTHETIC MANAGEMENT AND CONSIDERATIONS

Preoperative Period

1. Discuss the coexisting diseases that are associated with patients presenting for ACDF.
A thorough preoperative evaluation is a standard of care and it is one of the most important components of providing anesthesia for any patient. Specific information and documentation of symptoms should include the following: sensory and motor function and factors that causes an exacerbation of the symptoms. There is also the potential for gastric immobility caused by parasympathetic and sympathetic dysfunction that occurs at the level of the cervical vertebra.

The type and amount of medications that are used to treat pain should be investigated to determine the extent of the patient's perceived discomfort

Figure 46-2 *Anterior view of anatomy and muscles of the neck covering the cervical spine.*

Figure 46-3 *Placement of the graft between vertebra.*

and the potential for increased anesthetic requirements due to the development of functional and or dispositional tolerance. Patients should remain on their current pain medication regimen until the morning of surgery. Abrupt withdrawal of narcotics for patients with severe pain will increase sympathetic nervous system innervation leading to tachycardia, hypertension, and seizure activity.

2. Describe the importance of a thorough assessment of the patient's cardiovascular function prior ACDF surgery.

Anesthesia and surgery can cause significant hemodynamic variability throughout the perioperative period. Optimizing the patient's cardiac status prior to the day of surgery is necessary to decrease the possibility of cardiovascular dysfunction which includes labile blood pressure, dysrhythmias, myocardial ischemia, myocardial infarction, and heart failure.

Figure 46-4 *Anterior cervical discectomy with plate fixator.*

This patient has a history of hypertension which is being treated with atenolol. She states that she takes her medication every day and she was instructed to take her atenolol the day of surgery. The ECG that was obtained during exertion showed that by increasing heart rate and myocardial oxygen demand that coronary artery reserve (supply) was sufficient and there was no evidence of ischemia, infarction, or syncope.

3. Explain the anesthetic concerns related to airway management and ACDF surgery.

Airway assessment is vitally important for all patients having anesthesia; however, there are added concerns for patient's having ACDF surgery. If the patient has sustained a traumatic injury or if it is determined that the cervical spine is unstable, the patient may be placed in an external fixation device. Prophylactic neck immobilization and/or traction using in-line manual axial stabilization technique may be necessary during airway management. In this circumstance, elevating the patient's head to achieve a "sniffing" position is absolutely contraindicated. In a nonacute situation, certain movements of the neck may cause an exacerbation of the existing symptoms or cervical nerve root and/or spinal cord damage. Positioning the patient's head prior to the anesthetic induction allows the anesthetist to ensure that the position does not cause pain in the neck or in the arms, which is indicative or pressure on the brachial plexus. Care must be taken not to move the neck or head far from the position that was comfortable. The less extension and manipulation of the neck, the less likely injury to the cervical spine during airway management and surgery will occur. The anesthetist must be cautious with neck mobility and airway management with all patients who have had previous ACDF surgery. Alternative plans for ventilation and intubation must be available for patients who have either acute or nonacute cervical spine injuries.

A meticulous preoperative examination assessing the mobility of the neck, ability to open the mouth, and feasibility of intubation should be considered prior to the anesthetic induction. The application of cricoid pressure is controversial and should be initiated with caution as downward pressure of the cricoid ring in order to occlude the esophagus against the cervical vertebrae can cause neurologic damage. Administration of succinylcholine is contraindicated for patients with chronic myopathies that result in muscle wasting. Proliferation of extrajunctional acetylcholine receptors occurs and, due to the depolarizing effects of succinylcholine, this response may result in severe hyperkalemia that is life threatening.

Regional anesthesia can be used to supplement anesthesia for ACDF but the use of this technique does not provide adequate anesthetic and surgical conditions. Retraction of the trachea and the esophagus is extremely stimulating and, therefore, general anesthesia is the technique of choice for ACDF. A superficial and deep cervical plexus block provides analgesia during the intraoperative and postoperative period.

Intraoperative Period

4. Describe the importance of proper positioning for patient's having ACDF.

The patient's arms are most frequently tucked at their sides to allow for adequate surgical access. Proper patient positioning and padding must occur prior to the surgical incision because it will be more difficult to assess pressure on the bony prominence during the surgical procedure. Ensuring that the arms are abducted less than 90 degrees and that all pressure points are padded decreases the potential for nerve injury.

A gel roll is frequently placed under the shoulders by the surgeon to hyperextend the neck and to maximize the surgical exposure. The patient's head should be properly supported to decrease the pressure exerted on the cervical vertebrae and the patient occiput. Careful positioning of the endotracheal tube, which should be shifted to the corner of the mouth contralateral to the incision and free from traction is suggested.

5. Describe the monitoring considerations and techniques used for the ACDF patient.

Neurologic monitoring may be used during the ACDF, but these techniques are not commonly employed during anterior approach in the neck because nerve roots are more readily identifiable as compared to the posterior approach. If neurologic monitoring is to be used, the anesthetist should discuss the anesthetic plan with the surgeon and the neurophysiologist so that the anesthetic management and interdisciplinary communication can be optimized.

Somatosensory evoked potentials (SSEPs) are sensitive to the neurologic depressant effects of the inhalation agents at a concentration of greater than 0.5 volume percent of the minimal alveolar concentration (MAC). Typically, 0.5 MAC of any volatile agent with the addition of 50% nitrous oxide decreases the amplitude and increases the latency of the SSEP waveforms which can produce unreliable results. Intravenous anesthetic medications such as narcotics do not affect the evoked potential waveform to the extent associated with the inhalation agents. Thus, total intravenous anesthesia (TIVA) can be used as an alternative anesthetic technique. Since SSEP monitoring is used to assess the dorsal or posterior sensory component of spinal cord transmission, paralytics will not adversely affect the evoked potential.

Motor evoked potentials (MEPs) can be used to assess the integrity of the ventral or anterior portion of the spinal cord during ACDF. MEPs are not affected by the inhalation or intravenous anesthetic agents; however, MEPs are affected by neuromuscular blocking agents. Incomplete paralysis as assessed by the neuromuscular blocking monitor, train of four ratio of 3 out of 4, can allow for adequate monitoring of MEPs. Occasionally, both MEP and SSEP monitoring are used simultaneously

for patients who are at increased risk of spinal cord injury due to the severity of their disease process.

6. Examine the fluid requirements necessary for patients having ACDF.

The estimated blood loss that is most often associated with ACDF is less than 50 ml. However, due to the close proximity of major arterial and venous structures to the surgical site, there is the potential for significant bleeding. If a large amount of blood loss is anticipated, then autologous blood infusion, cell saver blood salvage, and normovolemic hemodilution are all methods that can be employed.

Intraoperative and postoperative tissue swelling surrounding the surgical site is always a concern during ACDF procedures. Excessive administration of fluid should be avoided because it will increase edema formation and increase the possibility of developing superior vena cava syndrome. For procedures that exceed 2 hours, a urinary catheter is indicated to assess urine output and to avoid bladder distention. Intravenous fluids that contain glucose should be avoided because if periods of neurologic ischemia occur, increased lactic acid is produced during anaerobic metabolism.

7. Describe the anesthetic and surgical complications associated with ACDF.

Acute spinal cord injury can occur during ACDF as a result of inadvertent pressure, edema formation, or partial or complete disruption. The most severe circumstance that can occur is rapidly developing spinal shock. Efferent sympathetic nervous system impulse transmission will not occur to organ systems below the level of the cervical spinal cord trauma. This will result in parasympathetic nervous system predominance and manifest as bradycardia, and vasodilation causing hypotension and heat loss. The treatment for acute neurogenic shock includes administration of intravenous fluids, vasopressors, and forced air warming. Invasive monitoring such as an arterial line and central venous pressure catheter should be used to guide fluid therapy.

Major vascular injury can occur as a result of surgical trauma to major vasculature in the neck region including the internal and external jugular veins, superior and inferior thyroid artery, or carotid artery. Blood loss can be rapid and extensive. If the carotid artery is damaged, the potential of acute dissection and emboli formation increase the potential for a stroke. The anesthetist should be acutely aware of the potential for postoperative hematoma formation and airway compromise if vascular injury has occurred.

Airway compromise can result from unilateral recurrent laryngeal nerve damage and hematoma formation which impinges on the trachea, airway edema, and tracheal laceration. The degree of airway and tracheal edema can be directly assessed via fiberoptic examination or indirectly by performing a leak test. The endotracheal tube cuff is deflated, and positive pressure breaths are administered to determine if an air leak occurs. This should be accomplished before the endotracheal tube is removed. If an air leak does not exist, then the patient should not be extubated. If intubation is initially difficult, then extubation can be performed over an Eschmann stylet or a tube exchanger so that immediate reintubation is possible. Lastly, if the surgical procedure was prolonged and associated with excessive traction, it may be most prudent for the patient to remain intubated. A complete list of complications that can occur during the perioperative management of patients having ACDF is included in Table 46-1.

Postoperative Period

Two hours after the surgical procedure is complete, the surgeon calls you from the intensive care units and she states that this patient is having difficulty swallowing. He also has a hematoma at the surgical site. The patient is scheduled for an emergent neck exploration.

Table 46-1   Complications Associated with ACDF
• Acute spinal cord injury
• Spinal nerve injury
• Dural tear
• Anterior spinal artery syndrome
• Hematoma
• Venous air embolism
• Airway edema
• Unilateral recurrent laryngeal nerve injury
• Pneumothorax
• Superior vena cava syndrome
• Hemorrhage
• Vascular injury
• Tracheal laceration

8. Discuss the various airway management techniques that can be safely used in this situation.

The major focus of this scenario revolves around the potential for the patient to rapidly develop respiratory distress and respiratory arrest due to compression of the trachea by the hematoma. A hematoma can occur rapidly after the neck incision is closed or slowly over a period of hours as blood is sequestered into the tissues. Since there is very little room for blood to exist within tissue planes adjacent to the neck, a small amount of blood can cause severe tracheal impingement. Additionally, tracheal deviation can occur without the presence of a large hematoma that is assessed externally. The definitive and initial intervention to resolve this situation is to have the surgeon remove the sutures and evacuate the hematoma.

There is no single airway management technique that is absolutely contraindicated in this scenario. It is possible that even if a complete view of the glottic opening was visualized during induction that the hematoma has dramatically shifted the anatomic airway structures so that visualization is difficult or impossible. An extraglottic device such as a laryngeal mask airway or mask ventilation may not be an effective method to maintain a patent airway. A fiberoptic intubation may prove challenging if edema and blood are present. Additionally, anesthetizing the airway with nebulized lidocaine can cause complete airway collapse, and maintaining spontaneous respirations are important. Lastly, tracheotomy placement as the initial method for establishing the airway is also an option. Having the supplies and ability to perform and emergency tracheotomy is vital.

REVIEW QUESTIONS

1. A symptom that is associated with cervical disc herniation includes:
   a. dilated pupils.
   b. paresthesias occurring in the shoulder and neck.
   c. lower back pain.
   d. frequent headaches.
2. Which of the following interventions is not appropriate for a patient who has sustained an acute cervical spine injury?
   a. Fiberoptic intubation
   b. "Sniffing" position
   c. Awake intubation
   d. In-line manual axial stabilization
3. Which sign is associated with acute neurogenic shock?
   a. Hypertension
   b. Hyperthermia
   c. Bradycardia
   d. Hypocarbia
4. Which regional anesthetic technique can be administered to decrease postoperative pain after ACDF?
   a. Cervical plexus block
   b. Transtracheal block
   c. Intercostal nerve block
   d. Superior laryngeal nerve block

5. There is an increased risk of stroke from emboli entering the brain associated with damage to the:
   a. internal jugular vein.
   b. inferior thyroid artery.
   c. external jugular vein.
   d. carotid artery.

REVIEW ANSWERS

1. **Answer: b**
   Paresthesias of the neck, shoulders, arms, and sometimes the fingers are frequent symptoms of nerve root compression in the cervical vertebra. Irreversible paresthesias and/or paralysis may follow if allowed to persist. Conservative treatment can be initiated with medications, cervical injections, or traction. However, more severe symptoms are more aggressively treated with surgery.
2. **Answer: b**
   Elevating and extending the head which is necessary in order to achieve optimal alignment of the oral, laryngeal, and pharyngeal axes ("sniffing position"), is absolutely contraindicated in patients with suspected or actual cervical spine injuries and acute spinal cord trauma can occur as a result of this maneuver.
3. **Answer: c**
   Sympathetic nervous system denervation is caused by cervical spinal cord damage. The result is parasympathetic nervous system predominance which includes bradycardia, hypotension, and hypothermia.
4. **Answer: a**
   Providing a deep and superficial cervical plexus block can be used to decrease the postoperative pain associated with ACDF.
5. **Answer: d**
   Damage to the carotid artery can cause acute dissection and damage to the intima of the vessel. Microemboli formation can occur and lodge in a cerebral vessel, resulting in decreased blood flow and an ischemic stroke.

SUGGESTED READINGS

Ahn Y, Lee SH, Chung SE, et al. Percutaneous endoscopic cervical discectomy for discogenic cervical headache due to soft disc herniation. *Neuroradiology* 2005;47(12):924–930.

Aker J. Neuroanatomy, neurophysiology, and neuroanesthesia. In: Nagelhout JJ, Zaglaniczy KL, eds. *Nurse anesthesia*. 3rd ed. St. Louis, MO: Elsevier Saunders, 2005:591–631.

Anderson PA, Subach BR, Riew KD. Predictors of outcome after anterior cervical discectomy and fusion: a multivariate analysis. *Spine* 2009;34(2):161–166.

Banoub M. Pharmacologic and physiologic influences affecting sensory evoked potentials: implications for perioperative monitoring. *Anesthesiology* 2003;99(3):716–737.

Imani F, Jafarian A, Hassani V, et al. Propofol-alfentanil vs propofol-remifentanil for posterior spinal fusion including wake-up test. *Br J Anaesth* 2006;96(5):583–586.

Drummond JC, Englander RN, Gallo CJ. Cerebral ischemia as an apparent complication of anterior cervical discectomy in a patient with an incomplete circle of Willis. *Anesth Analg* 2006;102:896–899.

Moshour GA, Stallmer ML, Kheterphal S, et al. Predictors in intubation in patients with cervical spine limitations. *J Neurosurg Anesthesiol* 2008;20:110–115.

Pajewski TN, Arlet V, Phillips LH. Current approach on spinal cord monitoring: the point of view of the neurologist, the anesthesiologist and the spine surgeon. *Eur Spine J* 2007;16:S115–S129.

Sagi HC, Beutler W, Carroll E, et al. Airway complications associated with surgery on the anterior cervical spine. *Spine* 2002;27(9):949–953.

Smith PN, Balzer JR, Khan MH, et al. Intraoperative somatosensory evoked potential monitoring during anterior cervical discectomy and fusion in nonmyelopathic patients—a review of 1,039 cases. *Spine J* 2007;7(1):83–87.

Posterior Spinal Reconstructive Surgery

47

Sass Elisha

KEY POINTS

- A comprehensive preoperative examination is vital in order to determine an individualized plan of care prior to posterior spinal reconstructive surgery.
- Correct prone positioning can decrease the possibility of nerve injury, decrease intraoperative blood loss, and decrease the possibility of postoperative visual impairment.
- Due to the potential for severe hemorrhage, serial hemoglobin and hematocrit values should be obtained and various techniques for intraoperative blood salvage should be available.
- Cerebral and coronary artery autoregulation must be considered when providing deliberate hypotensive technique.
- A venous air embolism (VAE) can occur during posterior spinal reconstructive surgery as air is entrained into the complex venous network surrounding the spinal cord.
- The integrity of the sensory or dorsal aspect of the spinal cord can be continuously assessed using somatosensory evoked potentials (SSEP).
- Anesthetic agents used for maintenance of general anesthesia increase latency and decrease amplitude during SSEP monitoring.

CASE SYNOPSIS

A 14-year-old girl has adolescent idiopathic scoliosis (AIS) which limits her functional ability and is also physiologically compromising. She is scheduled by her orthopedic surgeon to have posterior spinal reconstructive surgery.

PREOPERATIVE EVALUATION AND DEMOGRAPHIC DATA

Past Medical/Surgical History

- Scoliosis with decreased functional limitations
- Asthma

List of Medications

- Albuterol as needed
- Prednisone

Diagnostic Data

- Hemoglobin, 17.8 g/dl; hematocrit, 53%
- Glucose: 88 mg/dl; blood urea nitrogen (BUN), 15 mg/dl; creatinine, 1.0 mg/dl
- Electrolytes: sodium, 139 mEq/l; potassium, 4.0 mEq/l; chloride, 104 mEq/l; bicarbonate, 20 mEq/l
- Cobb angle of 80 degrees from T9 to L3; the curvature is convex toward the patient's right side
- Arterial blood gas: pH, 7.36; PCO_2, 33 mm Hg; PaO_2, 76 mm Hg; HCO_3, 21 mEq/l; base excess, 1.8; room air oxygen saturation, 94%
- Pulmonary function test: Forced expiratory volume (FEV_1), 60% of predicted; FEV_1/FVC, 90% of predicted
- Chest x-ray: There is significant overcrowding of the left ribs and a mechanical decrease in lung span of the right lung. A gross estimate of the bone density is normal without evidence of obvious cortical thickness to medullary cavity disproportion. There is no cardiac hypertrophy, masses, air, or fluid collections.
- Electrocardiogram (ECG): normal sinus rhythm; heart rate, 92 beats per minute; ejection fraction, 55%

Height/Weight/Vital Signs

- 163 cm, 58 kg
- Blood pressure, 122/78; heart rate, 94 beats per minutes; respiratory rate, 22 breaths per minute; room air oxygen saturation, 96%; temperature, 36.9°C

PATHOPHYSIOLOGY

Spinal reconstructive surgery is performed to correct a curvature that occurs to the spinal column. There are gradations of spinal column deformation which range from minor to severe. Minor deformations may be improved by the use of an external bracing device. Moderate to severe curvatures are frequently treated utilizing surgical interventions and can limit functions of activities of daily living, normal lung development, and alter cardiac and respiratory status. Identifying scoliosis prior to adolescent growth is vital since the primary vertebral curvature can become more severe. In most instances, scoliosis is idiopathic and it occurs approximately six times more frequently in women than in men. However, there may be a familial genetic predisposition for scoliosis. Other causes of scoliosis include neuromuscular pathology, myopathy, congenital, and spinal column instability. Pathologic conditions associated with scoliosis are included in Table 47-1.

Scoliosis, a lateral curvature of the spine, can be present in both the lumbar and thoracic vertebrae. In addition to the lateral curvature, the vertebrae are malrotated and thus the ribs can cause impingement on the lung pleura, resulting in inadequate lung development, restrictive lung disease, pulmonary hypertension, and respiratory insufficiency. The alterations that occur to respiratory dynamics include ventilation–perfusion mismatch, decreased vital capacity, decreased expiratory reserve volume, decreased total lung capacity, decreased functional residual capacity, and increased residual volume. Figure 47-1 depicts scoliosis with thoracic cage involvement.

Table 47-1   Pathophysiologic Conditions Associated with Patients Presenting for Spinal Reconstructive Surgery
• Muscular dystrophy
• Cerebral palsy
• Spina bifida
• Congenital heart disease
• Gastroesophageal reflux
• Dwarfism
• Myasthenia gravis

Figure 47-1   *Spinal column deformity with associated rib cage abnormality associated with severe scoliosis.*

The severity of scoliosis and degree of functional limitation is routinely quantified by assessing the Cobb angle from an x-ray. Since an x-ray only shows an anterior and posterior view, there are limitations when diagnosing the degree of lateral rotation of individual vertebrae. A Cobb angle of 10 to 15 degrees indicates a minor deformity and, frequently, there is no functional limitation. An angle measuring between 20 and 40 degrees is initially treated using an external bracing device. Treatment for a curvature between 40 and 50 degrees is controversial; however, experts agree that a Cobb angle of ≥ 50 degrees warrants surgical correction. Respiratory function and vital capacity is significantly decreased for patients who have a

Cobb angle greater than 90 degrees which results in hypoxemia and hypercarbia. Patients with a Cobb angle ≥ 30 degrees are at risk for postoperative respiratory insufficiency.

In patients with congenital scoliosis, the malformation of the thoracic cage can inhibit normal lung development. As a result of hypoxemia, hypoxic pulmonary vasoconstriction increases pulmonary vascular resistance which causes increased right ventricular workload. Concentric hypertrophy can occur from pressure overload that, if untreated, will result in right ventricular dysfunction and eventual failure. Additionally, hypoxemia and hypercarbia increase sympathetic nervous system activation, thereby increasing systemic vascular resistance, central catecholamine release, and myocardial work-load. If the vertebral curvature is angled toward the patient's left side, the heart and mediastinal structures can be shifted caudad which can cause cardiomegaly if pulmonary hypertension or a right ventricular outflow tract obstruction is present.

There are numerous physiologic syndromes that are associated with patients who have scoliosis, including muscular dystrophy, cerebral palsy, spina bifida, congenital heart disease, gastroesophageal reflux, dwarfing syndrome, and myasthenia gravis. A thorough review of the patient's medical history and comprehensive preoperative examination are necessary to develop an individualized anesthetic plan of care.

SURGICAL PROCEDURE

The goal of spinal reconstruction surgery is to straighten the spine, achieve improved balance between the torso and pelvis, and maintain surgical correction. However, disadvantages to traditional surgical correction include vertebral fusion resulting in decreased mobility, inhibition of the normal growth process which can lead to truncal deformity and decreased pulmonary maturation, and chronic pain. For this reason, surgical correction of scoliosis is best attempted prior to complete skeletal development.

The type of surgical correction performed is dependent on the patient's pathophysiology and the surgeon's experience and preference. The instrumentation that is implanted will cause vertebral fusion within 1-year postprocedure. The hardware can be removed after this time if the patient develops chronic back pain. If a posterior surgical approach is chosen, then a midline incision is made from the midthoracic to lower lumbar vertebrae. Once the vertebrae are exposed, pedicle hooks or screws are secured to the lateral aspects of the vertebrae. Pedicle screws are associated with improved surgical correction and improved postoperative pulmonary function. The pedicle hooks or screws anchor the rods that are placed

on both sides of the vertebral column. The rods are inserted and then manipulated to cause tension or distract the vertebrae. Distraction causes stimulation and expansion of the growth plate, a phenomena named the Hueter–Volkmann principle. In the past, the gold standard for spinal instrumentation was Harrington rods. Presently, there are numerous other manufacturers of hardware used for posterior spinal instrumentation.

Anterior spinal fusion involves a transthoracic and possibly retroperitoneal approach to the spinal column. Removal of the vertebral discs and implantation of instrumentation occurs. Since this approach involves a flank incision, rib resection, and major body cavity intrusion, there is a potential for rapidly occurring massive hemorrhage. There is a need for preferential ventilation of one lung and, therefore, a double-lumen endotracheal tube (ETT) is necessary. It has not been definitively determined that anterior spinal fusion yields improved results as compared to posterior spinal fusion for adolescents with idiopathic scoliosis.

With the development of minimally invasive surgical procedures, emerging technology and improved techniques result in decreased surgical trauma, decreased blood loss, and equivalent or superior outcomes. Using an anterior vertebral approach using video-assisted thoracoscopic instruments to place large nitinol staples, inserting vertebral bone anchors with flexible ligament tethers, and implanting "growing rods" (which can be elongated and distracted using an external remote control device) are all being investigated as potential future treatment modalities used to treat scoliosis.

ANESTHETIC MANAGEMENT AND CONSIDERATIONS
Preoperative Period

1. Define the pertinent preoperative assessment data for posterior spinal reconstructive surgery.
Neurologic A thorough neurologic examination of both motor and sensory functioning of the upper

and lower extremities is imperative in order to be able to accurately assess limitations that can occur as a result of the surgical procedure and prone positioning. This patient does not have upper or lower body motor or sensory deficits.

Respiratory Pulmonary function testing (PFT) was completed and her results are indicative of restrictive lung disease. Restrictive lung disease can be divided into two categories: intrinsic, which involves lung parenchyma, or extrinsic, caused by thoracic cage deformation, inadequate respiratory muscle function, or pleural disease. The results of the PFT testing are estimated by comparing a patient's performance to the performance of healthy subjects who are the same age, weight, and gender. In patients with restrictive lung disease, all measured lung volumes are decreased. FEV_1 is the volume of gas that is forcibly exhaled in 1 second. A normal FEV_1 is 80% of predicted; however, this patient's FEV_1 is only 60%. Forced vital capacity (FVC) is the total volume of gas that is forcibly exhaled in one breath. A normal FEV_1/FVC ratio is 80% and this patient's ratio is 90% indicating similar small volumes for both FEV_1 and FVC. A low FEV_1 and a normal or increased FEV_1/FVC ratio is indicative of restrictive lung disease. Decreased FRC and ventilation–perfusion mismatch increase the risk for rapid intraoperative desaturation. Due to the loss of elastic properties of the lungs, vigilant monitoring of peak airway pressures is essential to avoid barotrauma during mechanical ventilation. Furthermore, lung function does not improve dramatically during the postoperative period. The anesthetist and postanesthesia recovery unit staff must be aware of the potential for respiratory distress and failure.

Her ABG results are indicative of compensated respiratory alkalosis. Her Cobb angle is severe causing an extrinsic restrictive respiratory defect. Due to the inadequacy of ventilation as evidenced by low PO_2, there is a compensatory increase in minute ventilation primarily caused by increasing respiratory rate. This results in a low PCO_2. Notice that the low HCO_3 and negative base excess are indicative of compensated respiratory alkalosis.

Cardiovascular The patient's ECG shows normal sinus rhythm and near normal ejection fraction as measured by echocardiography. There is no evidence of cardiac hypertrophy or cardiomegaly on the chest x-ray.

Hematologic Her hemoglobin and hematocrit levels indicate polycythemia related to chronic hypoxia.

Endocrine The patient is taking prednisone on a regular basis to decrease symptoms associated with bronchial asthma. Knowing that this surgical procedure will cause severe physiologic stress, it is prudent to administer hydrocortisone 100 mg intravenously prior to surgery to avoid the possibility of acute adrenal crises. The anesthetist should be aware of the possibility of hyperreactive airway during the perioperative period. Her lungs should be auscultated preoperatively and bronchodilators should be used as needed.

Musculoskeletal This patient does not have musculoskeletal pathology. Scoliosis is associated with Duchenne muscular dystrophy and spina bifida. Duchenne muscular dystrophy is associated with malignant hyperthermia. In patients with spinal bifida who self-catheterize, there is the potential for the patient to develop a latex allergy.

Intraoperative Period

2. Summarize the importance of proper prone positioning relative to anatomic and physiologic implications.

Cardiovascular During prone positioning, it is important to minimize pressure on the abdomen because pressure on the vena cava and other venous structure will contribute to venous stasis in the lower body and could result in thrombus formation. Also, venous compression will decrease venous return to the heart and cause engorgement of the epidural venous plexus that increases intra-operative blood loss. Due to the long duration of spinal reconstructive surgery, patients frequently develop periorbital, facial, and airway edema.

Respiratory Chest excursion is decreased which can result in increased peak inspiratory pressure, decreased FRC, atelectasis, and increased ventilation–perfusion mismatch which can result in decreased oxygen saturation. For this reason, chest rolls must be positioned properly to minimize pressure on the anterior thoracic cage. Abdominal compression displaces the diaphragm cephalad further decreasing FRC and thoracic cage expansion. The anesthetist should recheck for equal bilateral and clear breath sounds after the prone position is achieved.

Prior to extubation, assessment of the degree of airway edema can be accomplished by direct visualization with a fiberoptic scope and the patient can be extubated over an ETT exchanger in the event that emergent reintubation is necessary. The decision to extubate the patient upon termination of the surgical procedure must be individualized to the patient. However, if the patient has compromised lung function prior to surgery, the duration of the procedure is prolonged, an anterior approach is performed, or an extreme volume of crystalloid, colloid, and blood is administered, the patient should remain intubated postoperatively and weaned from artificial ventilation over a 12-hour period.

Thoracic Outlet Syndrome Impingement on the nerves that comprise the brachial plexus and the subclavian artery between the first rib and the clavicle can cause permanent nerve damage and decreased perfusion to the arm. Preoperative assessment for the presence of thoracic outlet syndrome is accomplished by having the patient extend their arms above their head. If patients develop paresthesias in their hands or decreased quality of their radial pulses, their arms should be placed at their side throughout the intraoperative period.

Intraoperative Blindness Postoperative visual loss (POVL) can range from partial visual loss to permanent and complete blindness. POVL results from ischemic optic neuropathy (ION). The exact mechanism by which ION occurs has not been conclusively determined. However, possible reasons include ocular compression, decreased ocular nerve perfusion from microemboli, anemia, and edema formation. Methods to decrease the possibility of POVL include:

1. Ensuring that there is no pressure on both eyes throughout the procedure as well as maintenance of the head in a neutral position.
2. Maintenance of adequate mean arterial blood pressure (MAP). There is no one specific MAP that will ensure adequate cerebral perfusion pressure. Also, coronary and cerebral autoregulatory pressures are increased in patients with cardiovascular pathology.
3. An adequate amount of hemoglobin is necessary to facilitate oxygen delivery to peripheral tissues. There is no single minimum hemoglobin value that has been implicated with POVL.
4. Crystalloids are frequently administered as a component of volume replacement therapy. With judicious use of crystalloids, edema formation can cause ION. It is possible that anemia coupled with edema of the optic nerve can result in a higher incidence of ION.
5. Peripheral vasoconstriction associated with the use of phenylephrine can further decrease optic nerve perfusion.

Miscellaneous Concerns All joints including the fingers, hands, elbows, knees, ankles, and toes as well as genitalia must be padded and free of continual pressure. Axillary rolls must not impinge on the axillary arteries and bilateral radial pulses should be palpable. The patient's arms must not be abducted greater than 90 degrees in order to avoid a brachial plexus injury. Specialty positioning devices such as Relton or Wilson frames are used to keep the patient's thorax off of the operating table. Carefully securing the endotracheal tube is essential since saliva can decrease the adhesiveness of tape over time. Using a reinforced endotracheal tube will decrease the chance of kinking during intraoperative management.

3. List monitoring equipment that is used during spinal reconstructive surgery.

Application of standard monitoring equipment such as pulse oximetry, blood pressure, end-tidal carbon dioxide ($ETCO_2$) analysis, and five-lead ECG are used. An esophageal stethoscope will allow for continuous auscultation of breath sounds as well as a core temperature monitor. A urinary catheter is inserted to drain the bladder and to assess volume status. A urine output of 1–2 ml/kg/h is considered ideal. An arterial line is necessary in order to continuously assess blood pressure variability as a result of changes in anesthetic depth, deliberate hypotensive technique, and loss of intravascular volume. Additionally, serial ABG samples can be drawn. The choice to use central venous pressure monitoring should be determined by the patient's physical status. Pulmonary artery catheter placement and monitoring is not indicated for routine use.

4. Explain various strategies used to maintain adequate hemoglobin levels.

The estimated blood loss during spinal reconstructive surgery is highly variable and it is dependent on a number of factors, including preoperative coagulation status, type of surgical correction, experience of the surgeon, and amount of volume replacement. However, the anesthetist must be prepared to treat rapid and severe hemorrhage. A minimum of two large bore intravenous lines must be available. Fluid, blood, and blood products are infused through a fluid warming system. Strategies that can be used to preserve hemoglobin include:

- Deliberate hypotension (refer to question 7).
- Normovolemic hemodilution is accomplished by drawing blood prior to surgical blood loss.

The patient's hematocrit is decreased from 24–28%. Hypovolemia is treated by administering isotonic crystalloids or colloids at a ratio of 3 ml to each 1 ml of blood lost. The patient is transfused with their own blood after major surgical loss has transpired. Patients must be able to tolerate the physiologic stress associated with acute anemia and therefore this technique should not be employed in patients with severe cardiovascular or neurovascular pathology.

- Intraoperative blood salvage obtained from the surgical field using a cell saver system allows for transfusion of the patient's own red blood cells. Approximately 60–80% of blood loss can be replaced using this technique.
- Autologous or directed donor blood can be collected 2 to 3 weeks prior to surgery to be transfused as needed during the surgical procedure. For preoperative blood collection to occur, the patient's hemoglobin value should be greater than 11 mg/dl.

Despite the use of preoperative hematologic preparation or intraoperative blood salvage techniques, the patient should be typed and crossed and have a minimum of two units of available for infusion.

5. Discuss the pathophysiologic mechanism of venous air embolism (VAE) during posterior spinal reconstructive surgery.

A VAE, although rare, can occur during spinal reconstructive surgery as air is entrained into the complex venous network that surrounds the dura mater and spinal cord. During a posterior surgical approach, surgeons position patients prone with slight flexion in order to improve their vision and access to the operative field. As a result, the venous network is above the level of the heart and therefore air can be entrained into the traumatized veins.

The air that reaches the right atrium creates an air lock which decreases blood flow into the right heart. As a result, forward blood flow from the right atrium, right ventricle, and then to the pulmonary arteries

Table 47-2   Monitors Used for Detecting a Venous Air Embolism Listed in Order from Most Sensitive to Least Sensitive

- Transesophageal echocardiography
- Precordial Doppler positioned on the right sternal border between the 3rd and 6th ribs
- Increased pulmonary artery pressures
- Decreased $ETCO_2$
- Increased end-tidal nitrogen

Table 47-4   Treatment of a Venous Air Embolism

- Notify the surgeon to flood the surgical field with normal saline to decrease air intrusion
- 100% oxygen
- Fluid bolus
- Aspirate from central venous catheter
- Vasopressor administration
- Left lateral decubitus position

is impaired. Left ventricular preload is decreased resulting in hypotension. This explains the reason that hypotension and decreased $ETCO_2$ are signs that occur during VAE.

6. List monitoring modalities, signs, and symptoms and treatment for VAE.

The physiologic effects of VAE are dependent on the speed and amount of air that is entrained into the venous system. Signs and symptoms of VAE will be more severe the more air that is introduced to the venous system over a short period of time. The monitoring modalities, signs and symptoms and treatment for VAE are listed in Tables 47-2, 47-3, and 47-4, respectively.

7. Describe methods that can be used to induce deliberate hypotension.

Deliberate hypotension is frequently employed during spinal reconstructive surgery to decrease

Table 47-3   Signs and Symptoms of a Venous Air Embolism

- Hypotension
- Millwheel murmur
- Decreased oxygen saturation
- Decreased $ETCO_2$
- Increased end-tidal nitrogen
- Dysrhythmias

blood loss. By decreasing the patient's blood pressure, there is less blood loss from the vascular system resulting from surgical trauma. A variety of pharmacologic agents can be used to accomplish continuous hypotension. Anesthetic medications such as inhalation agents and narcotics are used initially to provide an adequate anesthetic depth and inhibit sympathetic nervous system hyperactivity. A variety of other pharmacologic adjuncts can be used such as vascular dilators, nitroglycerin or nitroprusside, calcium channel blockers, or beta blockers. It is imperative to use medications that can be titrated and that have a short duration of action for optimum control in the event that hypotension occurs from volume depletion.

Careful consideration must be taken to identify patients who are appropriate candidates for prolonged hypotension. Cerebral autoregulation occurs at MAP between 50 and 150 mm Hg and coronary artery autoregulation occurs at MAPs between 50 and 120 mm Hg. When the MAP decreases below 50 mm Hg, blood flow to the heart and the brain becomes pressure dependent. For patients with cardiac pathology, the vascular autoregulation curve is shifted to the right, necessitating higher MAP to ensure adequate perfusion. The disadvantages associated with hypotensive technique for spinal reconstructive surgery include cerebral and cardiac ischemia, spinal cord ischemia, optic nerve ischemia, and decreased renal perfusion.

8. Discuss the advantages and limitations of somatosensory evoked potential (SSEP) monitoring.
SSEP monitoring is used to detect spinal cord ischemia. If spinal cord ischemia is recognized and treated expeditiously, then spinal cord ischemia and paralysis can potentially be avoided. The risk of iatrogenic paraplegia is approximately 1%.

The major disadvantage associated with SSEP monitoring is the failure to detect ischemia that occurs to the ventral or anterior portion of the spinal cord which mediates motor function. SSEP monitoring allows assessment of the integrity of the sensory or dorsal or posterior aspect of the cord. Although a rare event, it is possible that adequate SSEP waveforms exist and the patient can still develop postoperative motor paralysis. There is conflicting evidence to support the routine use of SSEP monitoring during spinal reconstructive surgery since it has not been emphatically determined that this monitoring technique decreases morbidity and mortality.

Monitoring SSEP and motor evoked potentials (MEP) can be accomplished simultaneously. When both modalities are used, the SSEP monitoring electrode must be placed in the epidural space. This technique improves ability to safely monitor patients.

9. What are the advantages and disadvantages of performing an intraoperative "wake-up" test?
The intraoperative "wake-up" test is performed to assess movement to determine that the anterior or ventral portion of the spinal cord is intact. Preoperatively informing the patient that they will wake up momentarily and be instructed to move their feet is essential.

Communication with the surgical team is important so that the patient will regain consciousness at the appropriate time and in a controlled manner. Inhalation agents and neuromuscular blockade will be discontinued. Reassuring the patient as they awake and asking them to move their legs and feet is necessary. After bilateral motor function has been assessed, the patient is reanesthetized. The advantage of the "wake-up" test is confirmation of movement assures that the motor aspect of the spinal cord is undamaged. Disadvantages associated with a "wake-up" test include recall, dislodgement of spinal reconstruction hardware, potential of extubation, and VAE. Additionally, it is possible that permanent and untreatable paraplegia had already occurred prior to assessing for movement of the lower extremities.

10. Examine the component parts of an SSEP waveform.
- Wave latency is defined as the *time* between the application of a stimulus and the appearance of a neurologic response.
- Wave amplitude is defined as the *size* or *intensity* of the neurologic response that results from peripheral nerve stimulation.
- Wave morphology is defined as the general *appearance* of the electrical tracing as seen in Figure 47-2.

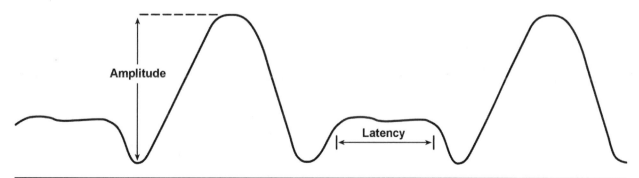

Figure 47-2 *Components of a normal SSEP waveform.*

Figure 47-3 *The influence of blood pressure on SSEP monitoring for spinal.*

Increased waveform latency and decreased waveform amplitude may be indicative of impending spinal cord impairment.

11. Describe causative factors that can result in increased SSEP waveform latency and decreased SSEP waveform amplitude.

- Stretching, torsion, or retraction of the spinal cord
- Decreased blood flow to the spinal cord
- Hypoxia
- Hypercarbia
- Anemia
- Anesthetic medications
- Dislodgement of SSEP monitoring probes
- Electrical interference (electrocautery)
- Extreme hypothermia

12. Cite interventions that should be employed if pathologic SSEP waveforms occur.

- Notify the surgeon
- Increase oxygen concentration
- Decrease anesthetic depth
- Ensure adequate blood pressure (as depicted in Fig. 47-3)
- Assess for anemia

13. Identify anesthetic medications that have an effect of SSEP waveform monitoring.

In order to maintain the integrity of the SSEP waveform during anesthesia, it is desirable to titrate

Table 47-5

MEDICATION	LATENCY	AMPLITUDE
Inhaled anesthetic agents	↑	↓
Nitrous oxide	0	↓
Propofol	↑	↓
Etomidate	↑	↑
Ketamine	0	↑
Barbiturates	↑	↓
Sufentanil/fentanyl/ remifentanil	↑	↓

Figure 47-4 *The effect of inhalation agent and nitrous oxide on SSEP monitoring.*

inhalation agents to < 1 MAC, since neurologic inhibition occurs in a dose-dependent fashion. Nitrous oxide potentiates the cerebral depressant effects of inhalation agents and will further increase latency and decrease amplitude during SSEP monitoring as seen in Figure 47-4. In addition, nitrous oxide is highly diffusible and will increase the size of a potential VAE. Lastly, if a transthoracic approach is performed, the use of nitrous oxide is not routinely used during one lung ventilation. Communication between the anesthetist, neurophysiologist, and surgeon is essential.

Postoperative Period

14. Describe postoperative pain control strategies for patients having posterior spinal reconstructive surgery.

The degree of postoperative pain is intense following postoperative spinal reconstructive surgery. Postoperative pain control is essential in order to facilitate adequate respiratory exchange. Methods that can be used to decrease postoperative pain include neuraxial opiates or intravenous opioids delivered by a patient-controlled analgesic

infusion. If a transthoracic approach is used, intercostal nerve blocks can be performed.

15. Review the potential postoperative complications that can occur following posterior spinal reconstructive surgery.

The potential postoperative complications associated with spinal reconstruction surgery include:

- Respiratory insufficiency
- Pneumothorax
- Hematoma formation
- Massive hemorrhage
- VAE
- Spinal cord injury
- Dislodgement of surgical instrumentation

REVIEW QUESTIONS

1. Which nerve(s) can be injured if the patient's arms are abducted greater than 90 degrees during prone positioning?
   a. Ulnar
   b. Brachial plexus
   c. Radial
   d. Intercostal

2. The changes in lung volume that are associated with moderate to severe scoliosis include:
   a. decreased vital capacity.
   b. decreased residual volume.
   c. increased total lung volume.
   d. increased expiratory reserve volume.

3. Which monitoring modality is most sensitive for detecting a venous air embolus?
   a. Increased pulmonary artery pressures
   b. Decreased $ETCO_2$
   c. Increased end-tidal nitrogen
   d. Precordial Doppler

4. The portion of the spinal cord that relays efferent motor responses is the:
   a. anterior.
   b. posterior.
   c. dorsal.
   d. lateral.

5. Inhaled anesthetic agents affect SSEP monitoring by:
   a. increasing amplitude and decreasing latency.
   b. decreasing amplitude and increasing latency.
   c. decreasing amplitude and decreasing latency.
   d. increasing amplitude and increasing latency.

REVIEW ANSWERS

1. **Answer: b**
   The brachial plexus originates from the 5th cervical vertebrae and extends through the 1st thoracic vertebrae. Motor or sensory deficits may be temporary or permanent if the patients are abducted greater than 90 degrees.

2. **Answer: a**
   Due to the physical impingement of the thoracic cage on the lungs and the potential for impaired lung development, vital capacity measure during inspiration is decreased. Residual volume is increased while both total lung volume and expiratory reserve volume are decreased.

3. **Answer: d**
   While the most sensitive monitor for detecting a VAE is transesophageal echocardiography, the next most sensitive monitor choice is a precordial Doppler.

4. **Answer: a**
   The anterior or ventral portion of the spinal cord transmits motor information from the brain to the periphery.

5. **Answer: b**
   The neurologic inhibitory effects of the inhaled agents decrease SSEP wave amplitude and increases latency in a dose-dependent manner.

SUGGESTED READINGS

Cheh G, Lenke L, Padberg AM, et al. Loss of spinal cord monitoring signals in children during thoracic kyphosis correction with spinal osteotomy: why does it occur and what should you do? *Spine* 2008;3(10):1093–1099.

Elisha S. Cardiovascular anatomy, physiology and pathophysiology. In: Nagelhout JJ, Zaglaniczny KL, eds. *Nurse anesthesia*, 3rd ed. St. Louis, Missouri: Elsevier Saunders, 2005:425–460.

Epstein NE. Bloodless spinal surgery: a review of the normovolemic hemodilution technique. *Spine* 2006;31(19):2227–2230.

Fehlings MG, Kelleher MO. Intraoperative monitoring during spinal surgery for neuromuscular scoliosis. *Nat Clin Prac Neurol* 2007;3(6):318–319.

Gambrall MA. Anesthetic implications for surgical correction of scoliosis. *AANA Journal* 2007;75(4):277–284.

Grottke O. Intraoperative wake up test and postoperative emergence in patient's undergoing spinal surgery. *Anesth Analg* 2004;99(5):1521–1527.

Kim YK, Lenke LG, Cho SK, et al. Comparative analysis of pedicle screw versus hook instrumentation in posterior spinal fusion of adolescent idiopathic scoliosis. *Spine* 2004;29(18):2040–2048.

Lee LA, Roth S, Posner KL, et al. The American Society of Anesthesiologists Postoperative Visual Loss Registry: Analysis of 93 spine surgery cases with postoperative visual loss. *Anesthesiology* 2006;105:652–659.

Othman Z. Hypotension-induced loss of intraoperative monitoring data during surgical correction of Scheuermann kyphosis. *Spine* 2004;29(12):258–265.

Park C. The effect of patient positioning on intraabdominal pressure and blood loss in spinal surgery. *Anesth Analg* 2000;91(3):552–557.

Redding G, Song K, Inscore S, et al. Lung function asymmetry in children with congenital and infantile scoliosis. *Spine J* 2008;8(4):639–644.

Wang Y, Fei Q, Qui G, et al. Anterior spinal fusion versus posterior spinal fusion for moderate lumbar/thoracolumbar adolescent scoliosis: a prospective study. *Spine* 2008;33(20):2166–2172.

Anesthesia for Shoulder Arthroscopy

48

Molly Wright

KEY POINTS

- An important aspect of the anesthetic course is intraoperative and postoperative pain relief provided by an interscalene block.
- Injuries that occur to the brachial plexus are reduced when patients are positioned in the beach chair position as compared to the lateral decubitus position.
- In the beach chair position, when the blood pressure (BP) is taken on the arm, mean arterial pressure (MAP) is not reflective of the MAP in the brain.
- Patients in the beach chair position are at risk for an intraoperative stroke if low MAPs that are measured in the arm are assumed to be reflective of adequate cerebral and coronary perfusion due to the effect of gravity.

CASE SYNOPSIS

A 57-year-old man has been diagnosed with torn right rotator cuff caused by a work-related injury. He is scheduled to have a shoulder arthroscopy and repair of his right rotator cuff.

PREOPERATIVE EVALUATION AND DEMOGRAPHIC DATA

Past Medical/Surgical History

- Smoker with a chronic cough
- Gastroesophageal reflux disease

List of Medications

- Celecoxib (Celebrex)
- Omeprazole (Prilosec)

Diagnostic Data

- Hemoglobin, 15 g/dl; hematocrit, 46%
- Glucose, 109 mg/dl; blood urea nitrogen, 18 mg/dl; creatinine, 1.3 mg/dl
- Electrolytes: sodium, 139 mEq/l; potassium, 4.2 mEq/l; chloride, 106 mEq/l; carbon dioxide, 26 mEq/l

Height/Weight/Vital Signs

- 180 cm, 113 kg
- BP, 114/73; heart rate, 61 beats per minute; respiratory rate, 21 breaths per minute; room air oxygen saturation, 97%; temperature, 36.6°C
- Electrocardiogram: normal sinus rhythm

PATHOPHYSIOLOGY

Many advances have been made in orthopedic surgery in the last 30 years. Procedures that initially required hospitalization for several days are now performed via an arthroscopic approach which is less invasive and patients are routinely discharged from the hospital within 24 hours. The introduction of fiberoptics for visualization, smaller surgical instrumentation, and superior orthopedic techniques have led to the increasing popularity of less invasive arthroscopic shoulder surgery.

A rotator cuff injury involves one or more of the four muscles in the shoulder, as shown in Figure 48-1. This may be an acute injury, such as from a fall or trauma. The trauma may lead to hemorrhage and inflammation of the bursa. The swelling that occurs with this process decreases the space available under the acromion. This may then lead to impingement with abduction of the shoulder. A vicious cycle begins as inflammation progresses.

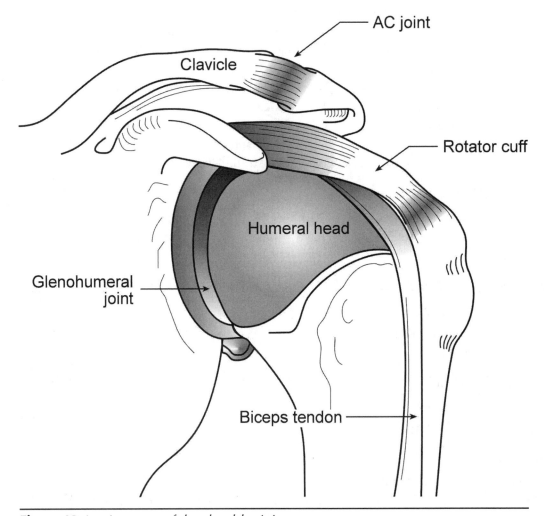

Figure 48-1 *Anatomy of the shoulder joint.*

The upper arm is connected to the shoulder joint by three bones: the clavicle, scapula, and humerus. Ligamentous support helps to stabilize the joint. Muscles of the rotator cuff (supraspinatus, infraspinatus, teres minor, and subscapularis) help keep the head of the humerus in place against the scapula allowing it to lift and rotate. This network of muscles and tendons form a covering around the top of the humerus. The actual rotator cuff tear exists within the supraspinatus muscle and is the cause of pain for many adults as is shown in Figure 48-2.

SURGICAL PROCEDURE

The type of surgery that is performed is dependent on the size and location of the tear. If the tendon is torn, it may require repair with suture via the arthroscope or by using an open technique. Sometimes the tendon may be torn away from the bone and the intervention may require a direct repair of the tendon to the bone. The surgeon may also remove part of the acromion (connected to the scapula), due to impingement on the tendon which could lead to a tear.

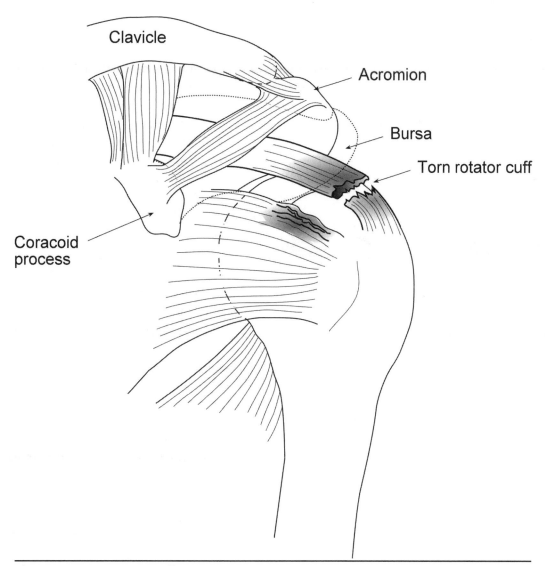

Figure 48-2   *Rotator cuff tear.*

In the beach chair position, traction on the operative arm is frequently applied in order to improve the operating conditions. The eyes must be protected from direct pressure and the head is secured with a Velcro strap or tape. The ears of the patient must be checked to ensure they are not pinched by the strap. The anesthetist should periodically visualize the head and neck, due to manipulation of the shoulder by the surgeon, assuring continuous alignment.

ANESTHETIC MANAGEMENT AND CONSIDERATIONS

Preoperative Period

1. Discuss the consent process for interscalene block for anesthetic management.

To gain an informed consent from the patient, explanation of the available anesthetic option of an interscalene block should be discussed. The patient needs to be informed of risks and possible complications as well as expectations of the anesthetic procedure. Table 48-1 lists the complications and benefits associated with an interscalene

| Table 48-1 | Complications and Benefits Related to Interscalene Blockade |

COMPLICATIONS

- Horner syndrome
- Brachial plexus injury
- Phrenic nerve injury
- Recurrent laryngeal nerve trauma
- Total spinal anesthetic
- Intravascular injection
- Intraneural injection
- Infection

BENEFITS

- Postoperative analgesia
- Shorter recovery time
- Rapid discharge time
- Unanticipated admission to the hospital for pain is reduced

block. A thorough history and a complete list of medications that the patient is taking should also be provided.

2. Explain the nervous system innervation to the rotator cuff.

Innervation to the rotator cuff originates from the cervical plexus dividing into roots, trunks, divisions, cords, and branches. The supraspinatus and infraspinatus muscles of the rotator cuff are innervated by the suprascapular nerve, the teres minor muscle by the axillary nerve, and the subscapularis muscle innervations is by the subscapular nerve.

3. Describe the method for placement of an interscalene block.

Before beginning a regional anesthetic of any type, check to see that emergency airway and resuscitation equipment is available and in working order. Also, observation of aseptic technique is essential.

To perform an interscalene block, the patient is positioned supine with the head facing away from the shoulder that is being anesthetized. The patient is asked to elevate the head slightly to bring the clavicular head of the sternocleidomastoid muscle into prominent view. The anesthetist's palpating finger is placed behind the sternocleidomastoid muscle and the patient is informed to relax the head lift. The palpable interscalene groove between the anterior and middle scalene muscle is palpated. The injection site in the interscalene groove lies at the level of the cricoid (C6). Local anesthetic is injected with a 25-g needle, followed by a 35–50 mm 21-g insulated needle. The needle which is connected to a plastic catheter is directed inward (toward the cervical plexus) and caudad 30–50 degrees. The stimulating current is set at 1.0 mA, 2Hz, and 0.1 msec. The insulated needle is advanced slowly until the nerve is stimulated and muscle contraction occurs. The intended response should include movement of the acromion as well as the deltoid muscle. Posterior extremity movement can occur from posterior needle placement, or diaphragm movement may be seen with stimulation of the phrenic nerve.

After securing the proper muscle movement of the affected shoulder, current of the nerve stimulator is then decreased slowly and continuously to approximately 0.35 mA, or to the lowest mA setting where muscle response continues to be slightly visible. Incremental local anesthetic injection, while intermittently aspirating to be sure that intravascular injection is not occurring, is accomplished.

Intraoperative Period

4. Describe the anatomic and physiologic changes that are associated with the beach chair position.

In comparison to the lateral position, surgeons often prefer the beach chair position for rotator cuff repair which improves visualization, decreases distortion of the intra-articular anatomy, and minimizes the potential for brachial plexus injury. Significant physiologic changes occur when patients are in the upright position as gravity pulls blood downward away from the thorax. MAP stroke volume (SV), cardiac output (CO), and PaO_2 all decrease. The alveolar–arterial oxygen gradient and pulmonary and vascular resistance all increase. When a patient is awake, these effects are compensated for by an increase in systemic vascular resistance (SVR) by up to 50–80%. However, this autonomic response is inhibited by general anesthetic medications, causing vasodilation and decreased CO.

Cerebral perfusion pressure (CPP) decreases by approximately 15% when a patient is in a sitting position and this value is calculated as shown in Equation 48-1. General anesthetic agents cause vasodilation, myocardial depression, and impaired

Equation 48-1
CPP = MAP − ICP (or CVP) ***CPP***, cerebral perfusion pressure; ***CVP***, central venous pressure; ***ICP***, intracranial pressure; ***MAP***, mean arterial pressure

venous return which can further impair cerebral blood flow. Inspiratory subatmospheric pressure during spontaneous ventilation increases venous return from the cerebral circulation, but this effect does not occur when positive pressure ventilation is initiated. Flexion of the head may obstruct the internal jugular veins and cause cerebral venous engorgement. Extension of the head may impair cerebral blood flow (CBF) resulting in cerebral ischemia.

The cerebral vasculature dilates and constricts to maintain constant blood flow to the brain. This concept, cerebral autoregulation, occurs when the patients MAP is between 50 and 150 mm Hg. When the MAP is above or below these values, the degree of CBF becomes pressure dependent. However, with poorly controlled hypertensive patients, autoregulation of CBF is shifted to the right, requiring a higher MAP to ensure adequate cerebral perfusion. In recent years, Drummond and others have emphasized that the lower limit of autoregulation should be increased to reflect a range of values from 70–93 mm Hg with a mean value of 80 ± 8 mm Hg. Some orthopedic surgeons request deliberate hypotension for shoulder arthroscopy, specifically rotator cuff repair. Decreasing the MAP to 50–60 mm Hg during deliberate hypotensive technique jeopardizes adequate CBF, especially in patients with chronic hypertension.

5. Examine the correct location for a blood pressure cuff and state the physiologic significance.

When placed in the supine position, the BP measured on the arm is similar to CPP in the absence of ICP. However, in the beach chair position, BP and MAP readings taken from the arm are *higher than the CPP* because blood flow from the heart must overcome the force of gravity. The difference in MAP when comparing the heart/arm and the brain will be equal to the hydrostatic pressure gradient. The mean brachial artery pressure obtained from a BP cuff may be 7–22 mm Hg lower than what is present in the brain.

If the BP at the heart/arm is 130/65 (MAP, 85 mm Hg) and the height of the external auditory meatus (representing the base of the brain) is 20 cm above the heart, the difference in BP at the heart compared to the brain will be 15 mm Hg. Thus, the MAP at the base of the brain will be 70 mm Hg. There will be a greater disparity in BP and MAP if the cuff is placed on the patient's leg. During this surgery, placement of an arterial line is unnecessary.

In a series of patients having shoulder surgery in the beach chair position, BP decreases ranged from 28–42% of control values, and hypotension was a likely cause of ischemic brain injury. It is recommended that MAP should be maintained at a minimum of 60 mm Hg in healthy patients that are assumed to have normal cerebral vasculature. For elderly patients with hypertension and/or known cerebral vascular disease, the cerebral autoregulation curve is shifted to the right and a higher MAP should be maintained.

Hypotension that occurs during arthroscopic surgery in the beach chair position should be aggressively treated. Treatment includes vigilant monitoring and titration of anesthetic gases, gradual position changes instead of abrupt changes, administration of IV fluid, and treatment with vasopressors as needed.

6. Explain the rationale for why the external auditory meatus is utilized as the landmark for the circle of Willis.

The auditory meatus is easily identifiable and it is relatively constant as an indicator of the location of the base of the brain and the circle of Willis. Measurements or estimates of the MAP can be made once the patient is in the beach chair position. The critical variable is the vertical distance from the circle of Willis to the BP cuff.

7. Discuss the importance of maintaining normocarbia for patients who are placed in the beach chair position.

Hypocapnia significantly reduces internal carotid artery and CBF. This change will be exacerbated when the patient is placed in the sitting position. Hence, significant hypocapnia should be avoided whenever possible to decreases the potential for cerebral hypoperfusion.

Postoperative Period

Surgery time for this procedure was 52 minutes. In PACU, the patient's vital signs were BP of 134/72, heart rate of 83 beats per minute, respiratory rate of 20 breaths per minute, oxygen saturation of 95–97%, and a temperature of 96.4°F. The patient required no additional pain medication.

8. List potential postoperative complications that can occur following arthroscopic rotator cuff repair under general anesthesia with an interscalene block.

Respiratory depression can occur in the postoperative period due to increased opioids administered during the surgical procedure. The anesthetist must be aware of the possibility of postoperative respiratory depression because analgesia provided by interscalene block the results in decreased postoperative pain.

REVIEW QUESTIONS

1. If a patient's CPP at the circle of Willis is 60 mm Hg, which is the corresponding CPP at the highest point in the brain?
   a. 69 mm Hg
   b. 60 mm Hg
   c. 51 mm Hg
   d. 55 mm Hg
2. The external auditory meatus is a landmark that:
   a. estimates the position of the most cephalad position of the brain.
   b. estimates the position of the base of the brain.
   c. estimates the MAP of the brain.
   d. estimates intracranial pressure.
3. Physical injury to the patient in the beach chair position for rotator cuff surgery:
   a. can result and somatosensory evoked potential monitoring is recommended.
   b. is a rare occurrence.

c. is most often associated with peroneal nerve injury.

d. can be prevented by assuring normal anatomic alignment throughout the procedure.

4. The brachial plexus originates as the cervical plexus at the spinal cord level of:

a. C8-T1.

b. C5-T1.

c. C2-C8.

d. C6-C8.

5. Hypocapnia that is associated with the sitting position:

a. causes minimal change in carotid blood flow.

b. causes increased cerebral blood flow.

c. causes a synergistic decrease in carotid blood flow.

d. causes increased blood flow velocity in the middle cerebral artery.

REVIEW ANSWERS

1. **Answer: c**

The cerebral perfusion pressure at the circle of Willis, or base of the brain, is 9 mm Hg lower gradient than the cephalad portion of the brain.

2. **Answer: b**

The external auditory meatus is easily recognized and represents the location of the base of the brain and the circle of Willis.

3. **Answer: d**

It is vital for the anesthetist to periodically assess the patient for normal anatomic alignment to prevent hyperextension of the neck, facial compression by surgical team, etc.

4. **Answer: b**

The brachial plexus stems from the ventral rami of C5 to T1 nerve roots in the majority of patients.

5. **Answer: c**

General anesthesia with hypocapnia alone can decrease internal carotid artery flow. Combined with the sitting position, this can decrease blood flow by an additional 18%.

SUGGESTED READINGS

Barret J, Harmon D, Loughnane F, et al. *Peripheral Nerve Blocks and Perioperative Pain relief.* Philadelphia: Elsevier Limited, 2005:63–71.

Bhatti M, Enneking T, Kayser F. Visual loss and ophthalmoplegia after shoulder surgery. *Anesth Analg* 2003; 96:899–902.

Bhatti MT, Enneking FK. Hypotensive technique and sitting position in shoulder surgery. *Anesth Analg* 2003; 97:1199.

Cullen DJ, Kirby RR. Beach chair position may decrease cerebral perfusion: catastrophic outcomes have occurred. *Anesthesia Patient Safety Foundation Newsletter* 2007;22:25–27.

Drummond JC. The lower limits of autoregulation: time to revise our thinking? *Anesthesiology* 1997;86: 1431–1433.

Jaffe R, Samuels SI. Shoulder/arm surgery. In: *Anesthesiologist's Manual of Surgical Procedures*, 3rd ed. Philadelphia: Lippincott Williams & Wilkins, 2004: 760–764.

Kirby RR, Cullen DJ. Complications of the beach chair position. In: Lobato E, Gravenstein N, Kirby RR, eds. *Complications in Anesthesiology*. Philadelphia: Lippincott Williams and Wilkins, 2007:844–853.

Miller RD. et al. Patient positioning and anesthesia for orthopedic surgery. In: *Miller's Anesthesia,* 6th ed. Philadelphia: Elsevier Churchill Livingstone, 2005:1162– 1164, 2421.

Nagelhout JJ, Plaus KL. Outpatient anesthesia. In: *Nurse Anesthesia,* 4th ed. St. Louis, MO: Saunders Elsevier, 2010:433–437, 902–913.

Pohl A, Cullen DJ. Cerebral ischemia during shoulder surgery in the upright position: a case series. *J Clin Anesth* 2005;17:463–469.

Hip Arthroplasty

49

Henry Talley

KEY POINTS

- Postoperative venous thromboembolism can be a devastating complication associated with total hip replacement. Interventions can be instituted to decrease the potential of thromboembolism.
- Advantages to providing regional anesthesia include decreased intraoperative blood loss, decreased perioperative deep vein thrombosis (DVT), and minimal need for airway manipulation or control.
- Since infection after total hip arthroplasty (THA) can be life threatening, confirmation and administration of antibiotics within 1 hour of incision is imperative.
- Respiratory compromise can occur in patients that are placed in the lateral decubitus position.
- Postoperative pain control will decrease sympathetic nervous system stimulation and allow for early ambulation.

CASE SYNOPSIS

An 86-year-old woman complained of right hip joint pain which resulted in pain and difficulty walking. As a result of the x-ray, she was diagnosed as a right hip fracture, and THA was scheduled.

PREOPERATIVE EVALUATION AND DEMOGRAPHIC DATA

Past Medical/Surgical History

- Rheumatoid arthritis
- Shortness of breath
- Hypertension
- Obesity (body mass index [BMI] = 32 kg/m^2)

List of Medications

- Celecoxib (Celebrex)
- Nifedipine (Adalat CC)
- Lipitor

Height/Weight/Vital Signs

- 170 cm, 96 kg
- Blood pressure, 150/88; heart rate, 72 beats per minute; respiratory rate, 16 breaths per minute; room air oxygen saturation, 97%; temperature, 36.7°C
- Electrocardiogram (ECG): normal sinus rhythm (occasional premature ventricular contraction), left ventricular hypertrophy
- Cardiac Doppler: ejection fraction (EF) 55%

Diagnostic Data

Hematology Report

- Hemoglobin, 10.9 g/dl; hematocrit, 32.7%
- Platelets: 62/mm^3
- White blood cells: 3.2/mm^3
- Lactate dehydrogenase, 224 U; erythrocyte sedimentation rate, 24 mm/hr
- Alkaline phosphatase, 14 U/dl

Pulmonary Function Test

- FVC, 67% (predicted, 6 l; measured, 4 l)
- FEV$_1$, 40% (predicted, 5 l; measured, 2 l)
- FEV$_1$/FVC, 60% (predicted, 83%; measured, 50%)

Dobutamine Stress Echo

- Left ventricle (LV) is normal in size and systolic function. EF = 55 ± 5%. The LV appears normal in size. LV systolic function is normal. Baseline LV diastolic function is consistent with abnormal relaxation (stage 1).
- Right ventricle (RV) is normal in size and systolic function.
- Left atrium (LA)/pulmonary veins: the LA is normal; the LA cavity is mildly dilated.
- Right atrium (RA)/inferior vena cava/superior vena cava: the RA is normal.
- Mitral valve: there is trivial mitral regurgitation
- Tricuspid valve (TV) is normal with trivial regurgitation; regurgitant velocity is 243.0 cm/s and estimated RV systolic pressure is 28 mm Hg.

- Aortic valve/left ventricular outflow tract: the peak gradient is 14.0 mm Hg; the mean gradient is 8 mm Hg; there is mild aortic regurgitation.

PATHOPHYSIOLOGY

There are more than 200,000 total hip replacements performed annually in North America. Progressively, severe arthritis of the hip joint, as seen in osteoarthritis (degenerative disease), is associated with aging and "wear and tear" of the joint over time. Patients scheduled for THA are usually older and often have preexisting medical conditions that may affect perioperative outcome. Osteoarthritis is the most common indication for hip arthroplasty, usually occurring after age 50 and often in individuals with a familiar history of arthritis. The hip joint, which contains the spheroid femoral head and acetabular cavity, degenerates over time and prevents the smooth movement of these surfaces causing pain. This process inhibits the ability of the patient to bear weight on the affected hip, and ambulation is frequently impaired. A comparison of the normal and abnormal hip joint is shown in Figure 49-1. Other factors that lead to degenerative joint disease include congenital hip joint abnormalities, traumatic injuries, and rheumatoid arthritis.

Rheumatoid arthritis is an autoimmune disease which causes inflammation of the synovial membrane producing greater amounts of synovial fluid than normal and damage to the articular cartilage, leading to pain and severe joint immobility. Inflammation associated with rheumatoid arthritis progression causes the formation of a mass known as a "pannus," causing the invasion and destruction of soft tissue, cartilage, and bone. Traumatic arthritis can result from a severe injury to the hip, causing a condition known as avascular necrosis, which can further cause hip bone necrosis and death of the bone (aseptic necrosis). Patients with any one of these conditions might

Figure 49-1   *Normal and abnormal right hip joint.*

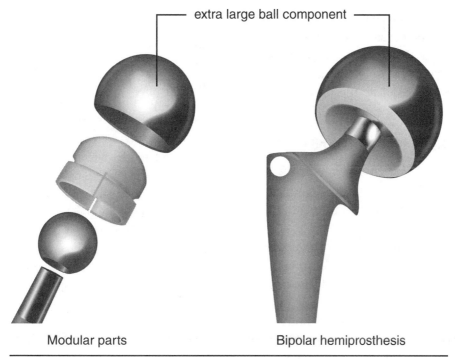

extra large ball component

Modular parts   Bipolar hemiprosthesis

Figure 49-2 *Bipolar hip joint prosthesis.*

benefit from a THA to relieve chronic pain and improve functional status.

SURGICAL PROCEDURE

The hip joint is a simple ball and socket joint formed by the femoral head and part of the pelvis called the acetabulum. When the cartilage is damaged and smooth movement is impeded, the joints become stiff and painful. THA, one of the most successful procedures in orthopedic surgery, is performed to improve mobility and relieve pain. Numerous hardware designs and materials are used for THA depending on surgeon preference. This procedure involves the dislocation of the femoral head from the acetabulum with excision of the arthritic femoral head and a portion of the femoral neck. The acetabulum is reamed to accept a cemented or cementless prosthetic metallic or plastic cup and this process is repeated to the femur so that the modular femoral stem and head component (metal or ceramic) can be inserted. Patients who have a BMI of greater than 50 kg/m^2 are at increased risk for developing postoperative complications. Table 49-1 lists the most common complications that are associated with THA.

ANESTHETIC MANAGEMENT AND CONSIDERATIONS

Preoperative Period

1. Describe the preoperative preparation for a patient having a THA.

Since THA is frequently an elective procedure, preparation of the patient should include a complete and comprehensive health and physical examination to assess the health of the patient and to identify any comorbid conditions that would potentially interfere with the perioperative period. Laboratory tests will be ordered as indicated by the findings in the history and physical. Anti-inflammatory medications will need to be discontinued at least 1 week prior to surgery to decrease the risks associated with platelet function and clotting. Additionally, preoperative radiographic examinations of the

Table 49-1	Most Common Complications Associated with a Total Hip Arthroplasty
• Infection
• Thromboembolism
• Nerve injury (femoral, obturator, lateral femoral cutaneous)
• Dislocation
• Implant failure
• Limb length discrepancy
• Periprosthetic fracture

hip joint and cervical spine x-rays are taken to assess flexion and extension in patients known to have rheumatoid arthritis if general anesthesia is a possibility. Flexion and extension of the cervical region and temporomandibular joint mobility is a major concern in patients with severe arthritis, which can make airway management difficult or impossible. A thorough dental evaluation is necessary for all patients and especially for those with poor dentition. While infection is uncommon with this procedure, bacteria accompanying dental disease can pose a major postoperative concern in these patients. Preoperative care or extraction of diseased teeth may be necessary before proceeding to surgery. Typing and cross-matching for the possibility of allogenic blood transfusion or preparation of autologous blood should be assured prior to the administration of anesthesia. If the procedure is urgent, a cell-saver system should be readily available. Any coexisting disease factors should be medically controlled to ensure optimization before surgery.

2. Discuss the preoperative concerns regarding this patient.

While the concern regarding the patient's rheumatoid arthritis is addressed during the preoperative preparation of the THA patient, the anesthetist must also remember that the systemic inflammatory disease arthritis can potentially affect every organ system in this patient. Preoperative evaluation for pericardial effusion and rhythm disturbances may require preoperative pacemaker (external) assistance. In addition to the routine, preoperative history and physical, this patient needs to be queried more as to the etiology and severity of her hypertension, the current therapy, and to determine if end-organ damage that accompanies chronic hypertension has occurred. Hypertension commonly affects a considerable proportion of the world population. Preoperative antihypertensive therapy is indicated; however, there is a lack of consensus concerning the preoperative evaluation and perioperative care of hypertension for patients having noncardiac surgery.

This patient might also benefit from a thorough renal examination. Urinalysis, serum creatinine, and blood urea nitrogen (BUN) may be necessary to obtain information about the presence and extent of renal parenchymal disease. Oftentimes, THA is indicated in the treatment of osteonecrosis; a condition often seen in patients with chronic renal failure (CRF) and believed to be associated with steroid use.

Lastly, while age alone is not an indication of cognitive dysfunction, the patient presenting with THA may also be prone to dementia of unknown etiology (sometimes called "multi-infarct dementia"). This is a concern to the anesthetist because failure to assess cognitive integrity during the preoperative period may lead to complication during the postoperative period. Additionally, if there is any concern regarding the cognitive status of this patient, there should also be concerns regarding the importance of the "informed consent."

3. Identify patient characteristics that increase the susceptibility to hip fracture.

Depending on etiology, the sex of the patient may be a factor increasing the susceptibility to hip fracture. Likewise, advanced age and obesity have been suggested as positive risk factors. Increased BMI was found to be a risk factor for total hip replacement caused by osteoarthritis. The variables related to the surgeon's decision to suggest the need for THA were the presence or absence of severe cardiovascular disease, physical subscale score, and amount of joint space narrowing. More recently, younger patients and patients with severe anatomic deformities are receiving THA procedures to improve activities of daily living.

4. Discuss the options for the anesthetic technique for THA.

For patients scheduled for THA, the choice of a neuraxial anesthetic, general anesthesia, or a combination of techniques can be offered. For some patients, the mention of regional anesthesia provokes fear of the needle stick and anxiety associated with being "awake" during the procedure. A thorough explanation of the available sedatives and their effects can often relieve some of these concerns. Regardless of the type of anesthetic chosen, patients must be assured of adequate analgesia and relief of their anxiety from induction to recovery. The anesthetist must also be sure to include in the discussion the potential side effects of anesthetic medications and subsequent options available to the patient.

Intraoperative Period

5. Choose the monitoring modalities that you would employ during surgery.

Monitoring should include all routine vital sign measurements such as ECG, noninvasive blood pressure monitoring, pulse oximetry, and body temperature. In patients that are physiologically unstable or those with severe comorbid diseases, continuous intra-arterial blood pressure monitoring may be indicated. However, an arterial line may be placed after the patient is anesthetized because there is no conclusive evidence that intra-arterial blood pressure monitoring during the induction of anesthesia prevents intraoperative complications. Central venous pressure monitoring may also be considered in patients scheduled for general anesthesia to determine filling pressures and left ventricular performance if high fluid shifts are anticipated. This patient will benefit from the use of simultaneous leads II, V_5, and multiple-lead ST analysis to monitor ventricular ectopy because patients with hypertension may be at increased risk of developing myocardial ischemia. Aberrant conduction in the ventricles of this patient should be further investigated with blood gas sampling and diagnostic attention to cause and effect with correction of factors contributing to the ectopy before the addition of more invasive procedures.

6. Which anesthetic techniques would be appropriate for this procedure?

The anesthetic technique that is most appropriate for this procedure would consider the patient's comorbid factors and acceptance after the informed consent process. General endotracheal anesthesia and regional anesthesia are both appropriate choices for this patient. With general anesthesia, the lateral position and her obesity necessitate the need for endotracheal intubation for airway management. Aggravation of cricoarytenoid arthritis in patients with rheumatoid arthritis can be minimized by using a smaller diameter endotracheal tube. Careful positioning of the head and neck are a primary concern during induction and intraoperative maintenance to avoid the potential for cervical spine or brachial plexus injury.

Regional techniques cause a sympathetectomy as a result of the inhibition of preganglionic B fiber transmission which extends from the thoracic to the first or second lumbar vertebrae. Vascular dilation leads to decreased blood pressure that can range from mild to severe. It is important for the anesthetist to realize that fluid volume loading and administering vasopressors might be necessary to avoid hypotension. This response may be more pronounced in the elderly

patient population. Initial positioning might be uncomfortable in patients who have sustained traumatic injuries to the hip, or have osteoarthritis and limited joint mobility.

7. Discuss the advantages of providing regional anesthesia for THA.

The advantages of using a regional anesthetic technique for THA includes decreased intraoperative blood loss, decreased perioperative DVT, and minimal need for airway manipulation or control. Lumbar epidural anesthesia can be performed even in the patient with rheumatoid arthritis because the lumbar spine is frequently unaffected in these patients. Single-dose spinal anesthesia placed at the L3-L4 level with 0.75% bupivacaine (15 mg) combined with 0.2 mg of morphine offers the patient a rapid onset of analgesia for up to 24 hours. A mixture of 2% lidocaine with 1:200,000 epinephrine administered over 13–17 minutes (approximately 15–20 ml) via an epidural technique provides a slow onset and gives the anesthetist more time to treat hypotension as compared to a spinal anesthetic. If epidural opioids are added to the solution, postoperative analgesia is also provided.

8. Discuss the physiologic manifestations of unintended (subarachnoid) intrathecal injection during the administration of local anesthesia with an epidural technique.

If an unintended intrathecal injection occurs, there will be a profound sensory and motor block shortly after injection. The brain is more susceptible than the heart to the effects of local anesthetic toxicity. Low plasma levels of local anesthetic result in minor neurologic symptoms which include numbness of the tongue, a metallic taste in the mouth, blurred vision, and circumoral numbness. As the plasma concentration increases, more severe neurologic signs such as decreased level of consciousness and seizures can occur. Other complaints may include dyspnea as a result of

| Table 49-2 | The Signs and Symptoms of Local Anesthetic Toxicity |

(Least severe to most severe signs and symptoms listed in descending order)

- Lightheadedness
- Numbness of the tongue
- Metallic taste in the mouth
- Circumoral numbness
- Visual impairment
- Altered level of consciousness
- Seizures
- Coma
- Myocardial depression

the blockade of proprioceptive afferent nerves of the abdominal and intercostals muscles progressing to respiratory arrest if the block continues to spread. Table 49-2 lists the signs and symptoms associated with local anesthetic toxicity.

9. Describe the anesthetic considerations regarding positioning during a THA procedure.

Positioning of the patient undergoing THA is extremely important to prevent neurovascular complications. The lateral decubitus position is most often used to facilitate exposure for the surgeon. Meticulous padding of the extremities and the maintenance of a neutral neck position are essential. Once the patient is anesthetized, an indwelling urinary catheter may be placed if the procedure is expected to be prolonged. Padded pegs are positioned at the level of the patient's rib cage and pubic areas when using the fracture table. A bean bag and axillary roll may be necessary to stabilize the patient, avoid compression of the brachial plexus and vascular structures, and relieve the pressure on the femoral triangle when placed in the lateral decubitus position. The dependent arm should be abducted and placed on a padded arm rest.

Care must be taken in the elderly and obese patients when positioned in lateral decubitus as pulmonary function can become compromised. This position results in increased perfusion in the dependent lung and increased ventilation in the nondependent lung. Hence, ventilation–perfusion mismatch will occur, resulting in shunting which may lead to a decrease in PaO_2. The degree of ventilation–perfusion mismatch is most pronounced in patients with underlying lung disease.

10. Discuss the importance of maintaining normothermia during THA.

Humans are *homeothermic*; as such, there are minimal variations in core body temperature. Unintentional perioperative hypothermia is one of the most common complications experienced by surgical patients because warming techniques are insufficient to counteract thermal redistribution resulting from the ablation of thermoregulatory vasoconstriction associated with anesthesia. Hypothermia can lead to metabolic acidosis as a result of the accumulation of acids (other than CO_2) or loss of base, resulting in a decreased pH and decreased HCO_3^-. The resulting central nervous system (CNS) effects of acidosis can greatly depress neuronal activity and increase the seizure threshold. Shivering-induced hypothermia can also increase oxygen consumption by as much as 600%, cause a leftward shift in the oxygen–hemoglobin dissociation curve (which decreases oxygen delivery to tissues), increase cardiac irritability, and reduce platelet function causing the potential for coagulopathy.

11. Discuss the anesthetic considerations for a patient with obstructive sleep apnea (OSA).

While this patient is moderately obese, OSA may be a concern because obesity is the most important independent risk factor for OSA. There is a relationship between obesity and decreases in the pharyngeal area as a result of adipose tissue deposition, causing a decrease in the patency of the pharynx and an increase in the likelihood of airway collapse.

Additionally, pharyngeal patency is determined by the difference between the extraluminal and intraluminal (transmural) pressure across its wall and the compliance of the wall. Obese patients have higher extraluminal pressure exerted on the pharyngeal wall as a result of superficial fat deposition.

12. Describe the concerns regarding blood and fluid requirements for this patient.

Blood and fluid requirements for this patient are of paramount importance because THA procedures are usually accompanied by major blood loss. Red blood cell (RBC) transfusion is one of the few treatments that adequately restore tissue oxygenation when oxygen demand exceeds supply. Securing two 14- to 16-gauge in intravenous catheters is ideal to ensure adequate vascular access. Lactated Ringers solution or normal saline may be started at 4–8 ml/kg/hr and adjusted as needed. While there continues to be controversy regarding the superiority of administering crystalloids as compared to colloid; crystalloid solutions are usually adequate to sustain normal hemodynamic parameters. Proponents of crystalloid therapy believe that hypovolemic shock causes both intravascular and interstitial fluid losses that can be easily replaced with crystalloids while proponents of colloid therapy state that resuscitation with colloids for hypovolemic shock requires less volume and maintains oncotic pressure which decreases extravasation to the extravascular space.

Intraoperative RBC scavenging can play an important role as an adjunct to autologous blood transfusion and help reduce total transfusion requirement. However, vigilance must be maintained to ensure that cells have been adequately washed to minimize drops in blood pressure upon reinfusion of scavenged blood. In cases when an infection is present, this modality is contraindicated. Another method of controlling blood loss is the use of deliberate hypotension in appropriately selected patients to decrease blood loss if mean arterial pressure is maintained between 50 and 60 mm Hg.

13. Identify the complications that are associated with cement fixation.

While the quality of the bone–cement interface helps to reduce bleeding and fixes the hardware to the bone during THA, profound hypotension and death may occur shortly after the cemented femoral prostheses is inserted. While this complication is not as common as in prior years, it can still be a factor in certain patient populations because methylmethacrylate can cause precipitous drops in blood pressure secondary to vasodilation and decrease PaO_2 secondary to embolization. It has also been theorized that methylmethacrylate has an inhibitory effect on myocardial excitation–contractile coupling resulting in direct cardiac depression. Embolization of fat, air, fragmented bone, and cement have all been shown to occur during THA. Providers must ensure that patients are adequately hydrated before the procedure and vasopressors are readily available if hypotension occurs.

Postoperative Period

14. Describe methods to enhance postoperative pain control after THA.

Postoperative pain management may be addressed in a number of ways. The use of patient controlled epidural opioids such as hydromorphone is extremely effective and can be accomplished via the epidural catheter placed for anesthesia. Likewise, a psoas compartment block (a single injection technique used with a nerve stimulator for anesthesia of the lumbar plexus) placed at the time of surgery provides postoperative analgesia for patients undergoing THA and significantly reduces narcotic requirements.

15. Discuss the methods to decrease the possibility of postoperative venous thromboembolism after THA.

Patients must be made aware of the potential for DVT and measures should be taken to prevent this complication. Due to her obesity, this

Table 49-3	Methods Used to Decrease the Incidence of Venous Thromboembolism

- Adequate oral hydration
- Compression stockings
- Ambulation
- Regional anesthesia
- Low–molecular weight heparin

patient is at increased risk of thromboembolism. Elastic compression stockings are used to facilitate venous return and improve circulation. Patients must be encouraged to actively exercise the lower extremities and continue to take their anticoagulants as prescribed. Table 49-3 lists intervention that can be used to decrease the incidence of thromboembolism.

REVIEW QUESTIONS

1. An advantage to providing regional anesthesia for hip arthroplasty includes:
   a. increased need for airway manipulation or control.
   b. decreased intraoperative blood loss.
   c. a more controlled environment for the patient to communicate discomfort.
   d. decreased need for prolonged recovery room stay.
2. Patients who have a body mass index of greater than _____ are at increased risk for developing postoperative complications.
   a. 30
   b. 40
   c. 50
   d. 60
3. Perioperative arrhythmias that occur during surgery are associated with:
   a. aggressive use of crystalloids.
   b. acute renal failure.
   c. antihypertensive agents.
   d. common peroneal nerve compression.

4. Regional techniques cause a sympathetectomy as a result of the inhibition of:
   a. preganglionic B fiber transmission.
   b. angiotensin-II release.
   c. decreased secretion of norepinephrine and epinephrine.
   d. postganglionic alpha-adrenergic blockade.
5. Shivering-induced hypothermia can:
   a. increase oxygen consumption by as much as 600%.
   b. increase platelet function.
   c. improve enzyme action of the coagulation cascade.
   d. cause a leftward shift in the oxygen–hemoglobin dissociation curve.

REVIEW ANSWERS

1. **Answer: b**
   Advantages to providing regional anesthesia include decreased intraoperative blood loss, decreased perioperative DVT and minimal need for airway manipulation or control.
2. **Answer: c**
   Patients who have a body mass index of greater than 50 are at increased risk for developing postoperative complications.
3. **Answer: c**
   Antihypertensive agents have different implications when anesthesia is administered. For instance, prolonged use of diuretics may lead to hypokalemia and hypomagnesemia and increase the risk of perioperative arrhythmias.
4. **Answer: a**
   Regional techniques cause a sympathetectomy as a result of the inhibition of preganglionic B fiber transmission which extends from the thoracic to the first or second lumbar vertebrae. Vascular dilation leads to decreased blood pressure that can range from mild to severe.
5. **Answer: d**
   Shivering-induced hypothermia can increase oxygen consumption by as much as 600%,

cause a leftward shift in the oxygen–hemoglobin dissociation curve, increase cardiac irritability, reduce platelet function, and impair enzymes of the coagulation cascade.

SUGGESTED READINGS

Bateman BT, Schumacher HC, Wang S, et al. Perioperative acute ischemic stroke in noncardiac and nonvascular surgery: incidence, risk factors, and outcomes. *Anesthesiology* 2009;110(2):231–238.

Batsis JA, Naessens JM, Keegan MT, et al. Impact of body mass on hospital resource use in total hip arthroplasty. *Public Health Nutr* 2009:1–11.

Dosanjh S, Matta JM, Bhandari M. The final straw: a qualitative study to explore patient decisions to undergo total hip arthroplasty. *Arch Orthop Trauma Surg* 2009;129(6):719–727.

Harkness M, Palmer JB, Watson D, et al. A questionnaire-based survey of perioperative blood conservation practice for revision hip arthroplasty in Scotland. *Transfus Med* 2008;18(5):296–301.

Hebl JR, Dilger JA, Byer DE, et al. A pre-emptive multimodal pathway featuring peripheral nerve block improves perioperative outcomes after major orthopedic surgery. *Reg Anesth Pain Med* 2008;33(6):510–517.

Ho MC, Beathe JC, Sharrock NE. Hypotensive epidural anesthesia in patients with aortic stenosis undergoing total hip replacement. *Reg Anesth Pain Med* 2008;33(2):129–133.

Kita T, Maki N, Song YS, et al. Caudal epidural anesthesia administered intraoperatively provides for effective postoperative analgesia after total hip arthroplasty. *J Clin Anesth* 2007;19(3):204–208.

Maurer SG, Chen AL, Hiebert R, et al. Comparison of outcomes of using spinal versus general anesthesia in total hip arthroplasty. *Am J Orthop* 2007;36(7):E101–E106.

Minville V, Lubrano V, Bounes V, et al. Postoperative analgesia after total hip arthroplasty: patient-controlled analgesia versus transdermal fentanyl patch. *J Clin Anesth* 2008;20(4):280–283.

Sathappan SS, Ginat D, Patel V, et al. Effect of anesthesia type on limb length discrepancy after total hip arthroplasty. *J Arthroplasty* 2008;23(2):203–209.

Above-the-Knee Amputation

50

Lisa Osborne

KEY POINTS

- The anesthetic management of the amputation patient depends largely on the coexisting diseases.
- Prevention of central sensitization and chronic pain requires a multimodal approach.
- The most frequent postoperative complication resulting from the procedure is phantom limb pain, with or without, accompanying stump pain.

CASE SYNOPSIS

A 25-year-old man was injured in a motorcycle accident. The patient has had three limb salvage surgeries in the past 6 months in an effort to save his affected leg. He is now scheduled for a right above-the-knee amputation (AKA).

PREOPERATIVE EVALUATION AND DEMOGRAPHIC DATA

Past Medical/Surgical History

- 5-year cigarette smoking history, but has not smoked in 3 months since accident
- 1998: appendectomy under general anesthesia, no complications
- 6 months ago: right lower extremity (RLE) open reduction internal fixation (ORIF) tibia/fibula, general anesthesia, no complications
- 1 month ago: revision to RLE general anesthesia, no complications
- 3 months ago: hardware exchange RLE general anesthesia, no complications

List of Medications

- Gabapentin
- Celecoxib
- Oxycodene (OxyContin)

Diagnostic Data

• Hemoglobin, 12.2 g/dl; hematocrit, 36.4 %

Height/Weight/Vital Signs

• 180 cm, 82 kg
• Blood pressure, 138/70; heart rate, 88 beats per minute; respiratory rate, 18 breaths per minute; room air oxygen saturation, 97%; temperature, 36.6°C

PATHOPHYSIOLOGY

Many patients who present for an AKA have significant coexisting diseases such as diabetes, peripheral vascular, and cardiovascular disease. However, there are also a significant number of patients who are otherwise healthy who present for amputation due to trauma to the lower extremity.

An understanding of the mechanisms that can lead to stimulation of the pain pathway is necessary in order to plan for this case. Pain is more complex than nociception; it is the experience of the sensation, which can be variable and is dependent on each individual. Psychologic and sociocultural factors influence the perception of pain. The primary afferent neurons have terminals that are stimulated by either heat, cold, or a mechanical event, such as pressure. There are many chemicals that are released, depending on the degree or type of tissue injury and include bradykinins, serotonin, and histamine, among others. This process activates the arachidonic acid cascade resulting in inflammation. The end products of the inflammatory process are also capable of stimulating the peripheral nerve, amplifying the pain stimulus. The process of conversion of the mechanical stimulation to the electrical activity, or an action potential, is a process known as transduction.

Primary afferent fibers have been classified by the type of stimulus and size; however, most nociceptive fibers can be stimulated by more than one modality. The afferent fibers are classified as A, B, or C. The speed of conduction is influenced by the amount of myelination that is present on the distinct fiber, which is present in A and B fibers. The A fibers transmit pain described as "sharp" and, because of the myelination, information is transmitted to the brain very rapidly. The C fibers are not myelinated and transmit pain signals more slowly which may be described by patients as "dull" or "aching." In normal physiologic conditions, the electrical impulse is conducted through a nerve by a process known as transmission.

Afferent nerves enter the dorsal horn and terminate in the lamina V or I. A branch of these nerves ends in the lamina II and III (substantia gelatinosa) where interneurons modulate pain by inhibitory neurons. Most axons ascend on the opposite side in the spinothalamic tract. These axons terminate in either the thalamus or the somatosensory cortex where pain is perceived. A diagrammatic description of central and peripheral pain transmission and medications used to treat pin is present in Figure 50-1.

SURGICAL PROCEDURE

During an AKA, the leg is completely excised at a point along the distal one third of the femur, preserving as much of the femur as possible. This procedure is generally performed due to chronic peripheral vascular disease and gangrene, uncontrolled infection, or traumatic injury. A stump is formed if there is no evidence of infection at the site by using the anterior and posterior musculature. The adductor tubercle is frequently removed, so the adductor muscle or tendon is repaired to the femur to prevent unopposed abduction. The procedure is most often performed with the patient in the supine position. Blood loss is not usually significant when a tourniquet is used. The most frequent postoperative complication resulting from the procedure is phantom limb pain, with or without, accompanying stump pain.

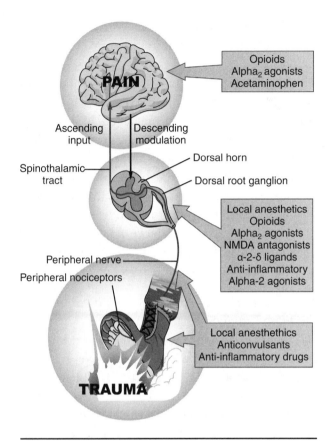

Figure 50-1 *Central and peripheral pain transmission.*

ANESTHETIC MANAGEMENT AND CONSIDERATIONS

Preoperative Period

1. Discuss the perioperative considerations for this patient.

The incidence of chronic pain resulting from amputation is reported to be as high as 80%. Therefore, a primary consideration for this case involves a treatment plan to prevent the development of this debilitating condition. Recent evidence suggests that the prevention of the wind-up phenomenon is important because, once this has occurred, it can result in intractable pain that is very difficult to treat, and may have long-lasting effects on many physiologic processes. Adequate treatment of the pain for this case involves a multimodal approach because the surgical trauma and

resultant inflammation creates significant afferent stimulation which leads to central sensitization.

2. Describe the process associated with central sensitization.

Acute pain, such as postoperative pain and the resultant inflammation, can have significantly long-lasting effects due to changes that occur in the peripheral and central nervous system. It has been well documented that the central nervous system has the capacity to be a dynamic system, a property known as plasticity. This dynamic system can result in a reduction of the threshold of peripheral neurons, and other changes in the characteristics of the afferent neuron. This is generally thought to be caused by the inflammatory process. The barrage of sensory input from the periphery leads to an increase in the spinal neurons excitability in the central nervous system. This peripheral and central sensitization has been called "wind up" and, once this has occurred, it can lead to intractable pain. Central sensitization involves physiologic changes in the nervous system that lead to symptoms such as allodynia, hyperalgesia, decreased pain threshold, and areas of referred pain. The underlying cause of these symptoms include:

- Changes in the N-methyl D-aspartate (NMDA) receptor
- Ectopic neuronal firing
- Changes in the gene expression of the sodium channel
- Sensitization of the nociceptive receptor

3. Explain the concept of multimodal analgesia.

Opioids are the mainstay for treating pain, but there are many undesirable side effects including nausea and vomiting, respiratory depression, sedation, pruritus, urinary retention, and sleep disturbances. The goal of multimodal analgesia is to improve analgesia and reduce the prevalence of opioid-related side effects. This strategy targets different aspects of the pain pathway, and utilizes the synergistic effects of combinations of medication to provide sufficient analgesia, while minimizing the side effects.

4. Identify the consequences associated with prolonged opioid therapy.

Prolonged use of opioids is associated with consequences above and beyond the side effects of the drug. Increasing dosages are often required to achieve the same level of analgesia—a process known as tolerance. Tolerance can be complicated by the fact that prolonged use of opioids is also associated with opioid-induced hypersensitivity. This phenomenon is not completely understood, but in animal studies the changes in the spinal cord after prolonged doses of opioids are similar to that of models of neuropathic pain. Prolonged use of opioids is also associated with hormonal changes and immunosuppression. Therefore, minimizing the dosages and length of opioid therapy is desirable.

5. What are the multimodal analgesic regimens for orthopedic surgery?

The multimodal analgesic regimens for orthopedic surgery include the use of local anesthetics, nonsteroidal anti-inflammatory drugs (NSAIDS), acetaminophen, NMDA receptor antagonists, and opioids.

6. Discuss the mechanism by which alpha-2 agonists facilitate analgesia.

Alpha-2 agonists have analgesic actions at peripheral, spinal, and brain stem sites where alpha-2 adrenoreceptors are located. However, the exact mechanism by which these medications reduce pain is not completely understood. Clonidine appears to enhance both peripheral and neuraxial blockade. Alpha-2 agonists are a valuable adjunct for treating sympathetically mediated pain by inhibiting the release of norepinephrine from the alpha-2 adrenoreceptors. When added to epidural infusion, clonidine has been shown to reduce the opioid requirement after orthopedic surgery. Dexmedetomidine is an alpha-2 agonist that has significant sedation associated with it, but administering this drug can be useful to decrease the physiologic stress response associated with surgery.

7. Discuss the mechanism by which ketamine or other NMDA receptor antagonists facilitate analgesia.

There has been great interest in ketamine as an adjunct for anesthesia after the mechanism of central sensitization has been elucidated. Although significant psychomimetic effects have been described with the use of ketamine, lower doses are not associated with these side effects and appear to provide excellent analgesic efficacy. Memantine is an alternative to ketamine that can be administered orally, and has a lower incidence of undesirable side effects. The NMDA receptors are located on primary afferents, interneurons, and projection neurons.

8. Discuss the mechanism by which gabapentin facilitates analgesia.

Gabapentin is an anticonvulsant that was developed to be a γ-aminobutyric acid (GABA) agonist, but it does not have an affinity for GABA. The binding site has been identified as the $\alpha2\delta$ subunit of voltage-gated calcium channels. Gabapentin inhibits the calcium current in sensory neurons and it is an important adjunct for preemptive analgesia. It is also thought to interact with the NMDA receptor complex but this mechanism is still poorly understood.

9. Discuss the mechanism of action of NSAIDs.

Tissue injury causes activation of the arachidonic acid cascade leading to the production of prostaglandins. These prostaglandins sensitize the nociceptors and can lead to hyperalgesia, or an increased response to stimuli. NSAIDS inhibit cyclooxygenase types 1 and 2 (COX 1 and COX 2) which decrease the production of prostaglandins. As shown in Figure 50-2, all NSAIDS with the exception of the COX 2–specific inhibitors such as celecoxib, which this patient is taking routinely, inhibit both COX 1 and COX 2 enzymes. The prostaglandins that are created by the COX 1 enzyme are necessary for homeostasis and contribute to adequate bronchial and renal vascular tone, normal platelet function, and gastric barrier. Therefore, when the prostaglandins necessary for physiologic

Figure 50-2 *Biologic formation of prostaglandins.*

functioning are inhibited, side effects such as bronchospasm, renal insufficiency, bleeding, and gastric ulceration can occur especially if NSAIDS are taken at high doses and on a routine basis. The prostaglandins that are created by the COX 2 enzyme mediate pain and have been implicated in increasing edema formation, resulting from surgical trauma. NSAIDS inhibit the production of prostaglandins in the periphery as well as in the spinal cord, resulting in a reduction in inflammation and pain after surgery.

10. Discuss the mechanism of action of acetaminophen.

Recent evidence suggests that acetaminophen may inhibit the production of prostaglandins in the central nervous system. Theoretically, this effect is mediated by inhibition of a COX 3 receptor; however, this concept remains controversial. However, multiple studies have demonstrated the efficacy of acetaminophen for decreasing pain and inflammation after surgery, without the side effects of the COX 2 inhibitors.

11. Discuss the anesthetic considerations for this patient in the preoperative period.

Administration of midazolam is recommended in the preoperative period because this procedure is associated with anxiety. It should be titrated to effect and an opioid may also be considered. The regularly scheduled medications for this patient should be continued. This patient is already taking gabapentin 600 mg and celecoxib 200 mg twice daily. Unless contraindicated, neuraxial anesthesia is recommended for anesthesia and analgesia. Recent evidence suggests that an epidural catheter insertion followed by a 48-hour continuous bupivacaine infusion should be placed before the amputation procedure to improve postoperative outcomes.

Intraoperative Period

12. Discuss the intraoperative considerations for this patient.

A multimodal technique should be utilized in order to meet the anesthetic goals for this patient. Titration of medications is paramount to a successful anesthetic because this patient has been requiring opioids for an extended period of time. As part of a balanced anesthetic, the following adjuncts may be considered:

- Ketamine infusion: 0.01–0.03 mg/kg/min intravenous (IV)
- Clonidine 30 mcg/hr in the epidural infusion
- Opioids: titrated to the observed analgesic effect

Postoperative Period

13. Discuss the postoperative considerations for this patient.

It is very important to meet the psychologic needs of the patient postoperatively. Providing a calm, quiet environment, especially if the patient exhibits signs of posttraumatic stress disorder, is vital. Multidisciplinary support as well as family support is optimal to aid the patient to deal with the significant emotional component of the loss of limb and loss of function.

The epidural infusion after surgery may contain a solution that will provide adequate sensory blockade, bupivacaine (0.125–0.25%) with or without adjuncts. Adjuncts to the epidural infusion include fentanyl 2 mcg/ml or hydromorphone 20 mcg/ml and/or clonidine 30 mcg/hr. The epidural infusion should be continued unless anticoagulation is required. If anticoagulation is planned and the epidural will be discontinued, a peripheral nerve catheter should be considered. A femoral nerve catheter and a sciatic catheter are required to provide adequate coverage for the amputee. The peripheral nerve catheters can be placed preoperatively, but if the epidural is to be used for the first 24 hours, the catheters can be placed on the first postoperative.

Multimodal therapy should be resumed as soon as possible after surgery, with attention to the time frame that the patient is tolerating oral medications. Intravenous agents should be utilized to maintain the multimodal therapy until

Table 50-1 Patient-Controlled Analgesia Settings			
	BOLUS (MG)	**LOCKOUT (MIN)**	**BASAL (MG/HR)**
Fentanyl	0.015–0.05	3–10	0.02–0.1
Hydromorphone	0.1–0.5	5–15	0.2–0.5
Morphine	0.5–3	5–20	1–10
Methadone	0.5–3	10–20	—

the patient can take oral medications. If there is breakthrough pain, a patient-controlled analgesia (PCA) may be necessary and Table 50-1 includes recommendations for PCA settings. If significant opioid side effects are present (nausea, respiratory depression), it is possible to add ketamine to the PCA.

REVIEW QUESTIONS

1. Which medication is not commonly used as a multimodal regimen for postoperative pain management?
    a. Clonidine
    b. Methadone
    c. Bupivacaine
    d. Celecoxib
2. Which is the primary pathway of the axons of second-order neurons on the contralateral side of the spinal cord?
    a. Spinothalamic tract
    b. Spinoreticular tract
    c. Spinomesencephalic tract
    d. Spinohypothalamic tract
3. Hydromorphone is _____ more potent than morphine.
    a. 2 times
    b. 3 times
    c. 5 times
    d. 10 times
4. Opioid induced hyperalgesia is caused by:
    a. improper dose escalation of opioids.
    b. inadequate treatment of depression.
    c. drug tolerance to the administration of opioids.
    d. abnormal sensitivity after repeated exposure to opioids.
5. Which receptor is involved in central sensitization causing persistent pain?
    a. NMDA
    b. Mu opioid
    c. Kappa opioid
    d. Alpha-2 adrenergic

REVIEW ANSWERS

1. **Answer: b**
    All of the medications with the exception of methadone are routinely used as a component part of a treatment plan utilizing various mechanisms of action for inhibiting the pain pathway. These agents target different points of transmission along the pain pathway.

2. **Answer: a**
    Most second-order axons form the spinothalamic tract and send projections to the thalamus, the reticular formation, the nucleus raphe magnus, and the periaqueductal gray area. Since there are projects to the hypothalamus and reticular formation, it is probably responsible for the arousal response to painful stimuli. This tract is divided into lateral and medial aspects, with the lateral sending projections containing the information about the location and intensity of the pain, while the medial aspect is responsible for the autonomic and unpleasant emotional response to pain.

3. **Answer: c**
    Hydromorphone is 5–7 times more potent than morphine. It is a useful alternative to morphine due to the potency, decreased incidence of nausea, pruritus, and sedation. It should be used with caution in patients with renal insufficiency due to the active metabolite hydromorphone-3-glucuronide that can produce neuroexcitation, including myoclonus and seizures.

4. **Answer: d**
    Opioid–induced hyperalgesia has been described in both humans and animals. It is characterized by increased pain from a noxious stimuli (hyperalgesia) and pain from a previously nonpainful stimuli (allodynia). The cellular mechanism of opioid–induced hyperalgesia is similar to neuropathic pain, which is caused by changes to the NMDA receptor.

5. **Answer: a**

The NMDA receptor is thought to be involved in central sensitization. Antagonists that block the receptor reduce the excitatory neurotransmitter glutamate and block the input from C fibers and prevent the wind up phenomenon.

SUGGESTED READINGS

Ballantyne JC, Mao J. Opioid therapy for chronic pain. *N Engl J Med* 2003;349:1943–1953.

Busse JW, Jacobs CL, Swiontkowski MF, et al. Complex limb salvage or early amputation for severe lower-limb surgery: a meta-analysis of observational studies. *J Ortho Trauma* 2007;21:70–76.

Buvanendran A, Kroin JS. Early use of memantine for neuropathic pain. *Anesth Analg* 2008;107: 1093–1094.

Hackworth RJ, Tokarz KA, Fowler IM, et al. Profound pain reduction after imduction of memantine treatment in two patients with severe phantom limb pain. *Anesth Analg* 2008;107:1377–1379.

Halbert J, Crotty M, Cameron ID. Evidence for the optimal management of acute and chronic phantom pain: a systematic review. *Clin J Pain* 2002; 18:84–92.

Nikolajsen L, Finnerup NB, Kramp S, et al. A randomized study of the effects of gabapentin on postamputation pain. *Anesthesiology* 2006;105:1008–1015.

Reuben SS, Buvanendran A. Preventing the development of chronic pain after orthopaedic surgery with preventive multimodal analgesic techniques. *J Bone Joint Surg* 2007;89:1343–1358.

Rosenblum A, Marsch LA, Joseph H. Opioids and the treatment of chronic pain: controversies, current status and future directions. *Exp Clin Psychopharmacol* 2008;16:405–416.

Schwartzman RJ, Grothusen J, Kiefer TR, et al. Neuropathic central pain. *Arch Neurol* 2001;58:1547–1550.

Wiech AK, Kiefer R, Topfner S, et al. A placebo-controlled randomized crossover trial of the N-Methyl-D-Aspartatic Acid Receptor Antagonist, Memantine in patients with chronic phantom limb pain. *Anesth Analg* 2004;98:408–413.

Pediatric Surgery

Bowel Resection for Necrotizing Enterocolitis

51

Shaun Mendel

KEY POINTS

- Necrotizing enterocolitis (NEC) is one of the most common neonatal gastrointestinal emergencies and it is a significant cause of morbidity and mortality in this group.
- The anesthetic management for these patients is often complicated by multiple comorbidities and congenital anomalies.
- Relatively large volumes of intravenous (IV) crystalloid, colloid, blood, and blood products may be required.

CASE SYNOPSIS

A 10-day-old infant, who is in the neonatal intensive care unit (NICU), is scheduled to have an emergent laparotomy and bowel resection due to an intestinal perforation resulting from NEC. Your patient was born at 27 weeks' gestational age and has been suffering from worsening abdominal distention over the last 3 days. This patient also has a patent ductus arteriosus (PDA).

PREOPERATIVE EVALUATION AND DEMOGRAPHIC DATA

Current Treatment and Medications

- Currently this patient is in the NICU receiving total parenteral nutrition, a broad spectrum antibiotic regimen, and oxygen via nasal prongs.

Diagnostic Data

- Hemoglobin, 9.8 g/dl; hematocrit, 29.4%; these values have been decreasing as compared to previous measurements.
- Sodium, 140 mEq/l; potassium, 4.2 mEq/l; chloride, 104 mEq/l; bicarbonate, 27 mEq/l
- Calcium, 7.9 mg/dl; glucose, 70 mg/dl

Weight and Vital Signs

- Birth weight, 1450 g
- Current weight, 1210 g

- Blood pressure, 47/18; heart rate, 168 beats per minute; respiratory rate, 55 breaths per minute; temperature, 36.6°C (radiant warming); oxygen saturation of 92% with supplemental oxygen via nasal prongs

PATHOPHYSIOLOGY

Although the exact causes of NEC are still the subject of debate, common predisposing factors include prematurity, sepsis, and formula feeding. The incidence of NEC is highest in low–birth-weight infants often defined as birth weight less than 1500 g. Some reviewers have supported the use of enteral supplementation of probiotics in premature infants who weigh greater than 1000 g to reduce the risk of severe NEC. Extreme prematurity which is defined as gestational age of 24–30 weeks, extraordinarily small size, and underdeveloped organ systems can provide a myriad of challenges independent of NEC that warrant consideration.

There are several factors that predispose low–birth-weight and premature neonates to developing NEC. Some of these causes include immune system and intestinal barrier immaturity which increases the patient's susceptibility to bacterial translocation from the gastrointestinal lumen into systemic circulation. This process can lead to sepsis, increased risk of nosocomial viral or bacterial exposure, and the presence of other anatomic and physiologic anomalies. Hemodynamic instability, respiratory failure, coagulopathy, perinatal hypoxia, and hypoperfusion may also be contributing factors.

The most frequent finding on assessment of the neonate with NEC is abdominal distention. Sometimes the abdominal wall can become so distended that respiratory compromise and failure occurs necessitating ventilatory support. Metabolic acidosis is common and it is believed to result from poor tissue perfusion. Thrombocytopenia and disseminated intravascular coagulation is present in a large number of these patients.

The abdominal radiographic findings that accompany NEC can include dilated loops of bowel, intraperitoneal fluid collection, and free air accompanying intestinal perforation as is shown in Figures 51-1 and 51-2. The hallmark sign of NEC is intramural gas collection. Currently, abdominal radiographs are used to determine the presence of intramural gas, portal venous gas, and free air within the abdomen. Sonography may improve the diagnostic ability of the surgeon as fluid in the abdomen, increased bowel thickness, and bowel perfusion are not always easily appreciated on abdominal radiographs. Figure 51-3 depicts the pathologic changes that occur to the bowel with NEC. Other findings may include poor skin turgor with a mottled appearance, diminished or absent peripheral pulses, and poor capillary refill. Decreasing blood pressure and urine output may indicate progressive intravascular hypovolemia.

SURGICAL TREATMENT

The effectiveness and survival rates of patients who are treated via laparotomy versus placement of a peritoneal drain at the bedside to decrease abdominal distention are comparable. Authorities have concluded that the type of operation (laparotomy versus peritoneal drainage) does not influence the survival or outcome of perforated NEC in low–birth-weight infants. Some have concluded that the difference in early mortality rate between cases of NEC treated with initial drain placement and laparotomy is not significant. The long-term outcomes in these groups are still under investigation.

Placement of a drain can be accomplished at the bedside by the surgeon in the NICU with minimal blood loss. Surgical exploration of these patients at the bedside or in the operating room is commonly accomplished via transverse laparotomy. After nonviable portions of bowel have been resected, a proximal stoma and distal mucus fistula are created which can be taken down at a later date after the patient's condition improves. The combined experience of the anesthesia care team, surgeon, and neonatologist should decide on the best course of

Figure 51-1   *An abdominal radiograph of a neonate with right lower quadrant pneumatosis partially obscured by the presence of a ventricular–peritoneal shunt.*

action. Additionally, communication among all of the team members is essential in order to facilitate high-quality patient care.

ANESTHETIC MANAGEMENT AND CONSIDERATIONS

Preoperative Period

1. Discuss the options that are available in order to optimize this patient for surgery.
Several interventions can be beneficial to optimize the patient's condition prior to the surgical

procedure. The operating room should be prepared by ensuring that the ambient temperature is increased, fluids are warmed, and forced-air warming devices are running prior to the arrival of the patient. Warming pads designed for use in neonates are available to minimize heat loss on the way to the operating room. Additionally, covering exposed body surface area with blankets or plastic will help maintain normothermia.

Ensuring adequate IV access can be extraordinarily difficult, especially during periods of hypovolemia and hypotension. Placing central lines, additional

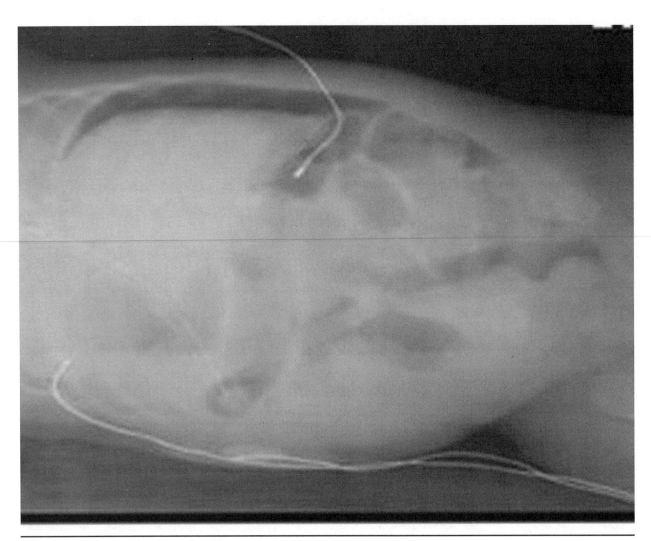

Figure 51-2   *An abdominal radiograph showing pneumoperitoneum.*

IV lines, or arterial lines as indicated by the patient's status prior to leaving the NICU, if time allows, can minimize operating room time while providing access for the infusion of fluids, blood products, or medications as needed during surgery. In situations where the patient is severely unstable or requires support difficult to maintain in the operating room such as an oscillating ventilator, bedside laparotomy can be undertaken in the NICU. Effective communication with transfusion services can ensure that blood and blood products are rapidly available if they are needed to decrease the incidence and severity of hypotension during anesthesia. An

attempt to correct electrolyte imbalances prior to surgery is imperative.

2. Describe the physiologic considerations affecting premature infants and their impact on anesthesia management.

There are many health problems that occur in premature infants independently of NEC, including the following.:

Intraventricular Hemorrhage   Premature infants are often at high risk for intraventricular hemorrhage from a variety of causes including

Inflammation
of the lining

Inflamed
bowel

Cross section of
inflamed bowel

Figure 51-3 *Pathologic changes that occur to the bowel with NEC.*

hypoxia, hemodynamic instability, and acidosis. Intraventricular hemorrhage occurs commonly in premature infants and many centers routinely screen extremely premature infants for this condition.

Cardiovascular Immaturity The patient in this scenario has a PDA and he is at increased risk for persistent left-to-right shunting and increased pulmonary blood flow resulting in pulmonary hypertension and congestive heart failure. Cardiovascular immaturity prevents effective compensation for blood loss and hypotension. Due to the functional immaturity of the heart, decreased ventricular elasticity limits contractility; therefore, increases in cardiac output are dependent on increases in the heart rate. Bradycardia is poorly tolerated because hypoperfusion occurs despite immense metabolic demands. Fluid shifts that are associated with NEC can lead to intravascular depletion requiring significant volume replacement. Persistent fetal circulation and congenital cardiac defects necessitate meticulous inspection of IV lines for air bubbles.

The ductus arteriosus (DA), an opening between the pulmonary artery and aorta, normally undergoes functional closure between 15 hours and 4 days after birth. The DA will remain patent if hypoxemia or sepsis is present. The process of continuous shunting through a PDA can be a continuous cycle resulting in systemic hypoperfusion and severe hypoxemia. Shunting of blood through the PDA makes the bowel more susceptible to developing ischemia via hypoperfusion which is thought to contribute to the incidence of NEC.

Hypothermia A large surface area to body weight ratio and diminished fat layer make premature infants prone to significant hypothermia, especially during laparotomy in the operating room. Many interventions can help maintain a relatively constant and warm environment and these methods are listed in Table 51-1. Hypothermia will cause nonshivering thermogenesis to occur in pediatric patients who are less than 3 months of age. Blood flow will be redistributed to brown fat and this process leads to the metabolism of triglycerides. Liberation of heat occurs as the

Table 51-1	Methods Used to Decrease Perioperative Hypothermia
Radiant warming or neonatal warming pad during transport	
Cover exposed body surfaces with plastic or blankets as appropriate	
Have a warm operating room waiting for the patient	
Warm the IV fluids and surgical irrigation	
Use the warming lights if available	
Utilize forced-air warming devices designed for this patient population	

triglycerides are broken into acetoacetic acid, B hydrobutyric acid, and ketones that results in metabolic acidosis.

Fluid and Electrolyte Management   Neonatal renal function is less efficient, predisposing them to sodium loss and less reliable reabsorption of sodium, glucose, bicarbonate, phosphates, and amino acids. During intraoperative management, neonates may require supplemental glucose; however, hyperglycemia should be avoided. These patients are frequently receiving total parenteral nutrition and this therapy should be continued throughout the perioperative period.

Respiratory Dynamics   Respiratory function of the premature neonate is immature. In the case of the patient with NEC, this immature system can be severely compromised by increased work of breathing due to worsening abdominal distention, fatigue, hypoxia, and increased metabolic rate which further decreases ventilatory reserves. Respiratory function also improves significantly if lung development is sufficient prior to birth. The younger the patient, the less viable the gas exchange mechanisms in the lungs, and more labile the intrinsic regulation of multiple physiologic processes like temperature management and blood sugar control.

High-frequency ventilation may be necessary to adequately oxygenate these patients during surgery. Effective means of providing additional supplemental oxygen, controlled ventilation, and intubation should be immediately available during transport to the operating room.

The effect of increased oxygen consumption and diminished functional residual capacity complicated by sepsis and severe abdominal distention on the oxygen reserve of these patients dramatically increases the potential for rapid desaturation, hypoxemia, and acidosis. Additional equipment and personnel experienced in securing the airway should be immediately available prior to induction. The neonatologist is a valuable resource in helping to secure the airway in the NICU prior to departure for the operating room.

Intraoperative Period

3. Discuss the factors that contribute to rapidly decreasing oxygen saturation during induction and intubation of a premature infant with NEC.
Neonatal hypermetabolism exacerbated by sepsis can combine to create a scenario where the patient is unable to compensate for periods of apnea or hypoxia. Additionally, respiratory compromise from lung immaturity and abdominal distention create a more fragile balance between oxygen supply and demand. These issues result in a state where the oxygen reserve of the patient is minimal and quickly exhausted. The oxygen exchange and reserve capacity of the lungs is diminished by the upward intrusion of abdominal distention and lung underdevelopment complicated by a lack of surfactant that facilitates alveolar collapse.

4. Identify interventions that will aid in the successful placement of an endotracheal tube for this patient.
There are several options for optimizing the airway management of this patient. Anesthetists and neonatologists familiar and experienced in intubating newborn patients should be present. Preoxygenation

of any patient prior to intubation is appropriate. The head of a child is proportionately larger than that of an adult compared to the rest of the body. A small pad or towel under the shoulders can help overcome the tendency of the chin to move toward the chest and optimize the position for successful laryngoscopy. Small variations in the position of an ETT result in proper placement, extubation, and endobronchial intubation. Careful verification of proper placement is vital.

Selecting the correct size endotracheal tube(s) and laryngoscope blade(s) for the patient is essential. If available, laryngoscope blades with the capacity to deliver in-line oxygen during laryngoscopy may help minimize the effect of apnea on oxygen saturation. Preoxygenation, immediately available help if needed, proper selection of equipment, and optimal positioning can all aid in providing an efficient and smooth induction and intubation.

5. Discuss the pharmacologic and physiologic consequences to consider when providing anesthesia to the premature neonate.

Inhalation anesthetic agents can be safely used in this patient population, although the exact minimum alveolar concentration for this group is unknown. Premature infants experience an exaggerated hypotensive response to inhalational anesthetics due to their myocardial depressant and vasodilating properties and their potential to cause bradycardia. Hemodynamic stability will de dependent on the titration of the inhalation agents to the individual's response.

If the operation is to be performed in the NICU or the patient requires the use of a neonatal ventilator, IV anesthesia must be provided. While many different IV agents have been used, opioid based anesthesia coupled with neuromuscular blockade has been determined to provide a more stable hemodynamic profile. However, IV agents including opioids and muscle relaxants have the potential to exhibit significant pharmacokinetic variability when administered to these young patients. Many

of these agents are metabolized by the liver by conjugation, hepatic function is immature, and medications can have a prolonged duration of effect. The choice of anesthetic agents that are to be used should be based on the individual patient's condition.

Opioid-based anesthesia often carries with it a prolonged respiratory depressant effect contributing to delayed emergence and a requirement for postoperative mechanical ventilation. Given the significant preoperative respiratory compromise of these patients, postoperative mechanical ventilation is often electively continued regardless of the anesthetic administered.

Immature metabolic processes and alterations in hepatic blood flow often contribute to the already wide variability in response to muscle relaxants. Neuromuscular transmission is immature, making titration of neuromuscular blockers difficult and can contribute to continued ventilatory support after surgery. The use of a nerve stimulator may be difficult and unreliable.

6. Discuss some issues that may affect the choice of gas mixture administered to this patient during surgery.

Continued administration of high concentrations of oxygen can contribute to visual impairment through the development of retinopathy of prematurity. Half of all low–birth-weight infants, less than 1500 g, experience some degree of retinopathy of prematurity. This percentage increases to greater than 90% in the smallest premature infants. Retinopathy of prematurity is thought to result from a combination of factors including hyperoxia. Experts suggest that titration of oxygen to maintain oxygen saturation between 87 and 92% is adequate. Maintenance of effective ventilation is challenging. Effective communication with the surgical team regarding the effects of abdominal packing and retraction can help balance the need for surgical exposure while minimizing ventilatory pressures.

The administration of nitrous oxide may contribute to further bowel distention; therefore, its use is generally avoided. A mixture of air and oxygen titrated to the needs of the patient supplemented with low-volume percentages of an inhalation anesthetic as tolerated is often used.

7. Discuss the fluid requirements of neonates undergoing laparotomy and bowel resection for NEC.

The presence of gangrenous, perforated bowel coupled with exposure of the abdominal viscera to the environment can cause large amounts of third-space and evaporative fluid loss. Relatively large amounts of surgical blood loss combined with the presence of underlying coagulation abnormalities may necessitate the transfusion of large amounts of crystalloid, colloid, blood, and blood products. Correction of coagulation defects may require packed red blood cells, platelets, fresh frozen plasma, and cryoprecipitate. Preoperative anemia is common in premature neonates due to decreased red blood cell production. The need for preemptive transfusion prior to surgery should be considered. Transfusion in neonates is administered per kilogram of body weight. In these small patients, portions of a single unit of blood can be preordered and delivered to the operating room in prefiltered syringes. This serves multiple purposes. First, more exact volumes can be delivered. Second, this practice of splitting a unit into several smaller doses can allow a neonate who will receive several transfusions to be exposed to a smaller number of blood donors. One standard unit can often be used for multiple transfusions for one neonate before the unit expires.

The criteria for the delivery of blood to a patient should include the underlying normal hemoglobin value of the patient according to age, the overall condition of the patient, most current lab values, and both current and anticipated surgical blood loss. Hypovolemia and a compromised tissue oxygenation capacity are two indications for red blood cell administration.

Determining the circulating blood volume and estimated allowable blood loss can guide the anesthetist in determining when transfusion is appropriate and the volume of blood that may be required. The estimated circulating blood volume of the premature infant is approximately 90–100 ml/kg of body weight. Determining the volume of blood that should be transfused can be estimated in relation to total blood volume and hematocrit.

In this example, the patient is 1210 g or 1.21 kg and hematocrit of 29.4%. An absolute hemoglobin or hematocrit value necessitating the transfusion of blood has not been determined and should be based on the individual's condition. Consultation with the neonatal and surgical service should be considered when contemplating transfusion to attempt to meet the overall treatment goals of the patient. For the sole purpose of demonstrating the relevant equations, we will use an example of a low hematocrit of 25%.

- Blood volume: 1.21 kg × 95 ml/kg = 114.95 ml
- Red blood cell mass (Hct 29.4%): 114.95 ml × 0.294 = 33.79 ml
- Red blood cell mass (Hct 25%): 114.95 ml × 0.25 = 28.73 ml
- Allowable blood loss: 33.79 ml − 28.73 ml = approximately 5 ml

This example demonstrates that a relatively small amount of blood loss can result in severe hypovolemia in these very small patients. The decision to transfuse must consider the overall situation, status of the patient, and surgical progress toward hemostasis. Transfusion of packed red blood cells is usually given in doses of 5 to 10 ml/kg of body weight per dose. These values provide only gross estimation because precise determination of surgical blood and fluid loss is difficult to ascertain. The effects of hemodilution by administration of crystalloid or colloid solutions must also be considered.

Laparotomy for bowel resection for NEC can require large blood volume transfusions and the need for other blood components. Preoperative low platelet counts coupled with large volume blood transfusions may indicate the need for platelet administration. Fresh frozen plasma is a blood product that can be considered when large amounts of packed red blood cells are transfused, as this can produce dilutional coagulopathy. Other information like coagulation studies can also guide transfusion decisions. Fresh frozen plasma, if indicated, is administered to improve plasma clotting factor availability and can be administered in 10 ml/kg infusions. The presentation of each patient and the operative course should be considered when the choice and volume of blood products is made.

Postoperative Period

8. Consider the postoperative care of this patient in the neonatal intensive care unit.

The choice of anesthetic administered will influence the need for postoperative mechanical ventilation. If neuromuscular blockade and opioid-based anesthesia are administered, it is likely than this patient will require a ventilator in the NICU. Massive volume transfusion and a difficult or prolonged surgical course may also lead the team to choose postoperative ventilatory support to aid in the care of the patient during the immediate postoperative period. If IV lines and ETT tubes are placed in the operating room, radiological confirmation of correct placement may be helpful to the neonatal care team.

REVIEW QUESTIONS

1. Which is the most common finding associated with necrotizing enterocolitis?
   a. Abdominal distention
   b. Hypotension
   c. Vomiting after feeding
   d. Lethargy

2. Which is a common radiographic finding associated with necrotizing enterocolitis?
   a. Poor bowel perfusion
   b. Pneumonia
   c. Pneumothorax
   d. Intramural gas

3. An intubated neonate that has NEC is at greatest risk for developing _____ during transportation to the operating room.
   a. blood loss
   b. third-space fluid loss
   c. hypothermia
   d. hypoxia

4. Which complication is most likely to occur during induction and intubation of a patient with NEC?
   a. Unrecognized difficult airway
   b. Esophageal intubation
   c. Dental injury
   d. Rapid desaturation

5. Which is a benefit to the patient of dividing one unit of blood into multiple transfusions for a patient with NEC?
   a. Cost containment
   b. Ease of dispensing
   c. Minimal donor exposures
   d. Conservation of scarce blood resources

REVIEW ANSWERS

1. **Answer: a**
   Abdominal distention is almost always present in cases of necrotizing enterocolitis.

2. **Answer: d**
   Intramural gas is a hallmark finding of necrotizing enterocolitis.

3. **Answer: c**
   Neonates are at increased risk of becoming hypothermic during transportation to the operating room.

4. **Answer: d**
   A rapid decline in oxygen saturation can occur during brief periods of apnea during laryngoscopy in the compromised neonate.

5. **Answer: c**

The division of one unit of packed blood cells by the blood bank per policy into small, weight-appropriate transfusions minimizes the number of donors to whom the patient is exposed. While cost containment, ease of dispensing, and conservation may be true and helpful to the hospital, minimal donor exposure can be of benefit to the patient.

SUGGESTED READINGS

Alfaleh K, Bassler D. Probiotics for prevention of necrotizing enterocolitis in preterm infants. *Cochrane Database Syst Rev* 2008;111(5):1202–1204.

Anand RJ, Leaphart CL, Mollen KP, et al. The role of the intestinal barrier in the pathogenesis of necrotizing enterocolitis. *Shock* 2007;27(2):124–133.

Blakely ML, Gupta H, Lally KP. Surgical management of necrotizing enterocolitis and isolated intestinal perforation in premature neonates. *Semin Perinatol* 2008; 32(2):122–126.

Brett CM, Davis PJ, Bikhazi G. Anesthesia for neonates and premature infants. In: Motoyama EK, Davis PJ. *Anesthesia for Infants and Children*, 7th ed. Philadelphia: Mosby Elsevier, 2006:552–555.

Epelman M, Daneman A, Navarro OM, et al. Necrotizing enterocolitis: review of state-of-the-art imaging findings with pathologic correlation. *Radiographics* 2007; 27(2):285–305.

Gregory GA. Anesthesia for premature infants. In: Gregory GA, ed. *Pediatric Anesthesia*, 4th ed. Philadelphia: Churchill Livingstone, 2002:345–368.

Hiller SC, Krishna G, Brasoveanu E. Neonatal anesthesia. *Semin Pediatr Surg* 2004;13(3):142–151.

Laussen PC, Wessel DL. Anesthesia for congenital heart disease. In: Gregory GA, ed. *Pediatric Anesthesia*, 4th ed. Philadelphia: Churchill Livingstone, 2002: 467–540.

Pierro A. The surgical management of necrotizing enterocolitis. *Early Hum Dev* 2005;81(1):79–85.

Smith BM, Mathes-Kofidis C, Golianu B, et al. Pediatric general surgery. In: Jaffe RA, Samuels SI, eds. *Anesthesiologist's Manual of Surgical Procedures*, 4th ed. Philadelphia: Lippincott Williams & Wilkins, 2009:1289–1292.

Stehling L. Blood transfusion and component therapy. In: Gregory GA, ed. *Pediatric Anesthesia*, 4th ed. Philadelphia: Churchill Livingstone, 2002:117–144.

Infantile Hypertrophic Pyloric Stenosis

Deborah T. Bergstein

52

KEY POINTS

- Infantile hypertrophic pyloric stenosis (IHPS) is the most common cause of gastrointestinal obstruction in newborns and infants.
- The classic presentation includes nonbilious repeated emesis that can progress to projectile vomiting.
- Infantile hypertrophic pyloric stenosis occurs in 3% of live births and it is more common among White men.
- Initial therapy for patients who have pyloric stenosis focuses on optimization of the patient's fluid volume and electrolyte status. Surgery is not performed on an emergency basis for pyloric stenosis.
- Preoperative management of fluid, electrolyte, and acid–base imbalances are imperative to the intraoperative and postoperative stability of the patient.

CASE SYNOPSIS

A 35-day-old infant boy is admitted for multiple episodes of projectile emesis after feedings, which began 48 hours ago. Diagnostic testing included an abdominal ultrasound which confirmed the presence of pyloric stenosis. Surgery is scheduled for the next morning. Appropriate fluid, electrolyte, and acid–base balance management is instituted.

PREOPERATIVE EVALUATION AND DEMOGRAPHIC DATA

Past Medical/Surgical History

- None

List of Medications

- None

Diagnostic Data

- Sodium, 127 mEq/l; potassium, 2.5 mEq/l; chloride, 78 mmol/l; carbon dioxide, 36 mEq/l

- Blood urea nitrogen, 12 mg/dl; creatinine, 0.6 mg/dl
- Glucose, 55 mg/dl
- Arterial blood gas (ABG): pH, 7.49; PaO_2, 91 mm Hg; PCO_2, 41 mm Hg; HCO_3, 32 mm Hg; base excess, −8.0
- Palpable solid mass upper abdomen
- Abdominal ultrasound: hypertrophic pyloric muscle measuring 4.8 mm
- Upper gastrointestinal imaging (UGI) barium series if ultrasound nondiagnostic

Height/Weight/Vital Signs

- 57 cm, 5.3 kg
- Blood pressure, 70/38; heart rate, 172 beats per minute; respiratory rate, 40 breaths per minute; room air oxygen saturation, 99%; rectal temperature, 37.3°C
- Urine output (OUP) < 1 ml/kg/hr

PATHOPHYSIOLOGY

Pyloric stenosis occurs due to thickening of the smooth muscle of the pyloric valve which is located at the junction between the stomach and small intestine as shown in Figure 52-1. This pathologic process is associated with a cleft palate and gastroesophageal reflux. Depending on the degree of gastric outlet obstruction, digestive contents are unable to move normally into the duodenum. This results in increased intragastric pressure which causes vomiting immediately after feeding. Newborns are predisposed to rapidly developing hypovolemia, gastric aspiration, and electrolyte abnormalities that most commonly results in *hypokalemic, hypochloremic,* and *metabolic alkalosis.* This occurs due to the persistent vomiting and resulting decrease in fluid volume intake. Also, there is a high concentration of hydrogen ion and chloride present in gastric

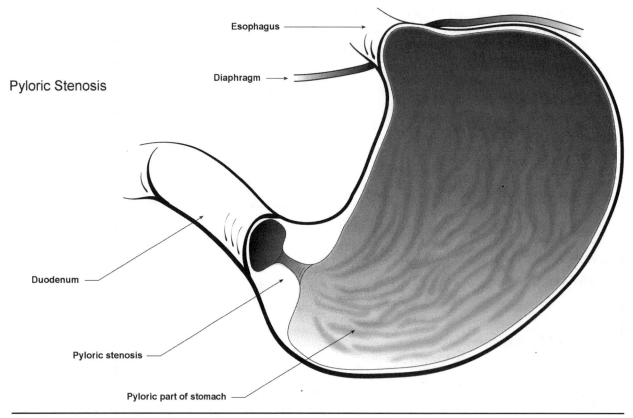

Pyloric Stenosis

Esophagus

Diaphragm

Duodenum

Pyloric stenosis

Pyloric part of stomach

Figure 52-1 *Anatomic abnormality associated with pyloric stenosis.*

fluid that is lost. Although the etiology of pyloric stenosis is unknown, there is a possible relationship that links thickening of the muscle of the pylorus to a deficiency in nitric oxide synthetase production.

SURGICAL PROCEDURE

Pyloromyotomy can be performed using various techniques: laparoscopic, endoscopic, or open via a periumbilical or right upper quadrant incision. The laparoscopic technique utilizes a periumbilical telescope and two incision sites. The surgeon may make the incision in the duodenum that extends toward the stomach or from the stomach toward the duodenum in order to adequately spread the pyloric muscle.

The open technique uses a small incision that is made in the skin on the anterior abdominal wall. The layer of thickened muscle is then separated. The avascular part of the pylorus is identified and a longitudinal incision is made to expose the mucosa. The separated muscle is brought up to the serous membrane at which point, closure of the area is initiated. The laparoscopic method allows quicker return to full feedings and has been associated with a more rapid hospital discharge as compared to the open technique.

ANESTHETIC MANAGEMENT AND CONSIDERATIONS

Preoperative Period

1. Describe the population that is most likely to be diagnosed with pyloric stenosis.
Infantile hypertrophic pyloric stenosis is the most common cause of gastrointestinal obstruction in newborns and infants. Pyloric stenosis most commonly occurs among first-born males. The ratio of males to females is 4:1. It occurs in 2–3 per 1000 live births and is predominant among Whites. The typical age that the diagnosis is confirmed is at 3–6 weeks of life but the pathologic process associated with pyloric stenosis can manifest as late as 12 weeks of age.

Table 52-1	Conditions Associated with Pyloric Stenosis
Intestinal malrotation	
Urinary tract obstruction	
Esophageal atresia	
Omphalocele	
Cleft palate	
Gastroesophageal reflux	

2. Discuss pathologic conditions that are associated with pyloric stenosis.
Over 90% of infants that have pyloric stenosis are not associated with pathologic conditions; however, a list of anatomic and physiologic abnormalities that may accompany pyloric stenosis is listed in Table 52-1.

3. Construct a preoperative strategy to optimize the patient condition prior to pyloromyotomy.
Pyloric stenosis may be a medical emergency due to the fluid loss, electrolyte, and acid–base imbalances caused by the repeated episodes of emesis over several days. Although it is well acknowledged that surgical repair is the definitive treatment, initial focus is placed on correction of the three areas mentioned previously.

- An initial fluid bolus with crystalloids between 10 and 20 ml/kg depending on severity of dehydration and the patient's preoperative medical condition.
- Fluids 1.5–2 times maintenance 5% dextrose and 0.25% normal saline with potassium chloride 2–4 mEq/100 ml only if UOP is greater than 1 ml/kg/hr.
- Repeat blood gas measurements to ensure improved metabolic alkalosis with pH between 7.30 and 7.50 and sodium bicarbonate less than 30 mmol/l.
- Repeat electrolytes to ensure stable sodium and potassium levels.

- Check urine dipstick to assess specific gravity to be less than 1.02.
- Ensure weighing of diapers for UOP greater than 1 ml/kg/hr.
- Metoclopramide 0.1 mg/kg 30–60 minutes before induction.
- Discuss antibiotic administration with surgeon; cefazolin, 25 mg/kg.

Intraoperative Period

4. Describe the induction plan most suitable for pyloric stenosis.

Rapid sequence induction (RSI) with cricoid pressure is the most suitable technique for this patient population. These patients have a gastric outlet obstruction and are at increased risk for aspiration. Stomach decompression with an orogastric tube is recommended in order to minimize the risk for aspiration.

Most of these patients have an intravenous catheter in place prior to surgery due to the need to balance their volume status. Typically, atropine 0.02 mg/kg (0.1 mg minimum) is administered before the induction of anesthesia to inhibit parasympathetic predominance resulting in bradycardia. Preoxygenation for several minutes followed by intravenous induction with propofol and rocuronium is indicated. Fentanyl may also be used to attenuate the response to laryngoscopy. If a difficult intubation is anticipated, then an awake intubation should be planned.

5. Construct a plan for maintenance and emergence.

The surgical time for pyloromyotomy regardless of technique is between 30 and 60 minutes. If the surgical time is greater than 30 minutes, muscle relaxation may be maintained. An inhalation agent such as sevoflurane and air/O_2 is an appropriate option. Small amounts of opiates are considered to minimize the risk for postoperative apnea. Communication with the surgeon in relation to wound infiltration with local anesthetic should be discussed to guide the plan for pain management.

The abdominal contents are suctioned prior to awakening. Ondansetron is administered to decrease the potential for postoperative nausea and vomiting. Neostigmine and atropine are administered on a per kilogram weight basis for reversal of the muscle relaxant. The patient should be extubated when they are fully awake and meets accepted extubation criteria.

6. Specify the primary intraoperative complications associated with pyloric stenosis.

- Increased risk for aspiration due to full stomach precautions. Preoperative medication to decrease gastric contents, gastric decompression, and placement of an endotracheal tube may decrease the risk, but do not prevent aspiration. Active inspiration and emesis may allow the passage of contents around endotracheal tube, especially because uncuffed tubes are commonly used in this population.
- Initiation of the celiac reflex results from mesenteric traction stimulating afferent vagal nerve endings. Parasympathetic nervous system predominance will lead to bradycardia, apnea, and hypotension. Since neonates are dependent on a rapid heart rate to establish cardiac output, bradycardia results in decreased tissue perfusion and potentially cardiac arrest. The response usually resolves when the surgeon is asked to release tension on the mesentery, pressure on the intra-abdominal organs, or peritoneal cavity. Atropine can also be administered to help extinguish this response or treat recurring episodes of bradycardia.
- Duodenal perforation occurs in less than 5% of cases performed by pediatric surgeons. If the procedure is performed laparoscopically, the surgeon may decide to convert the case to open for repair.

Postoperative Period

7. List the potential postoperative complications following pyloromyotomy.

Potential postoperative complications include:

- Respiratory distress
- Hypoxemia/hypercarbia
- Hypoglycemia
- Hypothermia
- Pain
- Recurrent vomiting
- Electrolyte abnormality
- Inadvertent bowel perforation resulting in septicemia

8. State two potential reasons for postoperative respiratory depression.

Hypothermia is common among neonates and infants due to their increased body surface area (large head and chest) and small amount of subcutaneous fat tissue. It is vital to maintain a warm environment (temperature 77–80°F), cover the head, and utilize forced warm air blankets intraoperatively and postoperatively. This patient population does not possess the concentration of muscle needed to shiver to increase heat production. If hypothermia exists in neonates and young infants, a process called nonshivering thermogenesis occurs as blood is shunted to anatomic areas where brown fat exists. The triglycerides that comprise the brown fat will be metabolized and this process liberates heat. However, metabolic acidosis can rapidly occur due to the formation of acetone, *B*-hydrobutyric acid and acetoacetic acid.

The presence of hypoglycemia should be ruled out if apnea is noted in the postoperative period. These patients should receive IV fluids with dextrose until they are advanced to full feedings. It is common to restart feedings 8 hours after surgery.

9. Discuss postoperative pain management for pyloromyotomy.

The estimated pain score that is associated with pyloromyotomy is 4–5 on a 10-point scale.

Acetaminophen 10–15 mg/kg every 4–6 hours either by mouth or per rectum is a common treatment for postoperative pain management. A caudal block can also be utilized.

REVIEW QUESTIONS

1. Which is the most appropriate initial intervention for a patient with pyloric stenosis?
   a. Continue feeding; observe type, volume, and frequency of emesis
   b. Prepare for an emergency surgical procedure
   c. Manage fluid and metabolic deficits
   d. Schedule surgery for 6 hours after last breast milk intake

2. Which acid–base abnormality is associated with pyloric stenosis?
   a. Respiratory acidosis
   b. Metabolic acidosis
   c. Respiratory alkalosis
   d. Metabolic alkalosis

3. Which laboratory tests are most valuable to diagnose pyloric stenosis?
   a. CBC, PT, PTT
   b. Chemistry panel, calcium, and glucose
   c. ABG
   d. Both b and c

4. If a difficult intubation is not anticipated, which is the best technique for induction on a patient with pyloric stenosis?
   a. Intravenous induction
   b. Mask induction
   c. Awake fiberoptic intubation
   d. Rapid sequence induction with cricoid pressure

5. Which intraoperative complication is most likely to occur during pyloromyotomy?
   a. Hemorrhage
   b. Hypervolemia
   c. Aspiration
   d. Duodenal perforation

REVIEW ANSWERS

1. **Answer: c**
   Medical management is best achieved prior to surgical treatment in these patients. Immediate management involves regulation of fluid status, electrolytes, and acid–base imbalances.

2. **Answer: d**
   Due to the repeated episodes of emesis, there is a deficit in hydrogen, chloride, sodium, and potassium. This results in hypovolemia and metabolic alkalosis.

3. **Answer: d**
   The degree of electrolyte and glucose imbalance as well as metabolic alkalosis must be assessed in order to appropriately and efficiently guide the medical management of these patients before surgical intervention.

4. **Answer: d**
   A rapid sequence induction is the best method because these patients are considered high risk for aspiration. Gastric decompression should be achieved prior to induction.

5. **Answer: c**
   Full stomach precautions including gastric decompression and endotracheal intubation are standard of practice for pyloric stenosis. Histamine-2 blocker, such as ranitidine, and a gastrokinetic, such as metoclopramide, are commonly used in pediatrics for aspiration precaution. However, these interventions do not guarantee total protection or prevention of aspiration.

SUGGESTED READINGS

Allan C. Determinants of good outcome in pyloric stenosis. *J Pediatr Child Health* 2006;42(3):86–88.

Golianu B, Hammer GB, Matthes-Kofidis C, et al. Pediatric general surgery. In: Jaffe RA, Samuels SI, eds. *Anesthesiologist's Manual of Surgical Procedures,* 3rd ed. Philadelphia: Lippincott Williams and Wilkins, 2004:1038–1040.

Hammer G, Hall S, Davis PJ. Anesthesia for general, abdominal, thoracic, urologic and bariatric surgery. In: Motoyama EK, Davis PJ, eds. *Anesthesia for Infants and Children*, 7th ed. Philadelphia: Mosby Elsevier, 2006:690–691.

Ibarguen-Secchia E. Endoscopic pyloromyotomy for congenital pyloric stenosis. *Gastrointest Endosc* 2005; 61(4):598–600.

Khan, K. High resolution EUS to differentiate hypertrophic pyloric stenosis. *Gastrointest Endosc* 2008;67(2): 375–376.

Kim SS, Lau ST, Lee SL, et al. Pyloromyotomy: a comparison of laparoscopic, circumumbilical, and right upper quadrant operative techniques. *J Am Coll Surg* 2005;201(1):66–70.

Leclair M, Plattner V, Mirallie E, et al. Laparoscopic pyloromyotomy for hypertrophic pyloric stenosis: a prospective, randomized controlled trial. *J Pediatr Surg* 2007;42(4):692–698.

Mullassery D, Perry D, Goyal A, et al. Surgical practice for infantile hypertrophic pyloric stenosis in the United Kingdom and Ireland–a survey of members of the British Association of Paediatric Surgeons. *J Pediatr Surg* 2008;43(6):1227–1229.

Naik-Mathuria B, Olutoye OO. Foregut abnormalities. *Surg Clin North Am* 2006;86:261–284.

Rix SW. Guidelines for the anesthetic management of pyloromyotomy. *AANA J* 1984;325–328.

Tracheoesophageal Fistula Repair

53

Travis Allen

KEY POINTS

- The hallmark signs associated with tracheoesophageal fistula (TEF) include coughing, choking, cyanosis during feeding, and the inability to pass an oral catheter into the stomach.
- Although there are several variations of TEF, the most common is esophageal atresia with distal fistula (Type C or IIIB).
- Positive pressure ventilation above the level of the fistula will inflate the stomach, increase the risk of aspiration, reduce the adequacy of ventilation, and can cause gastric rupture.
- Between 30 and 50% of patients with TEF have associated anomalies that must be evaluated prior to repair, most commonly VACTERL association.

CASE SYNOPSIS

A 2-day-old full term infant boy has demonstrated coughing, choking, and cyanosis during feeding. After an inability to pass an orogastric tube into the stomach, and radiologic evidence of air in the stomach, a diagnosis of TEF is made.

PREOPERATIVE EVALUATION AND DEMOGRAPHIC DATA

Past Medical/Surgical History

- Full-term 37 2/7 weeks male demonstrating polyhydramnios on ultrasound.

List of Medications

- Pantoprazole
- D10 1/4NS infusion rate 12 ml/hr

Diagnostic Data

- Hemoglobin, 16.4 g/dl; hematocrit, 47.1%
- Electrolytes: sodium, 141 mEq/l; potassium, 3.4 mEq/l; chloride, 110 mEq/l; bicarbonate, 24 mEq/l; glucose, 96 mg/dl

- Chest–abdominal radiograph: orogastric tube placed in blind esophageal pouch, air in stomach, right upper lobe atelectasis.
- Transthoracic echocardiography (ECG): Normal great vessels, small patent foramen ovale (PFO) with minimal left-to-right shunt, normal valves and function.

Height/Weight/Vital Signs

- 48 cm, 2.9 kg
- Blood pressure, 64/28; heart rate, 144 beats per minute; respiratory rate, 42 breaths per minute; room air oxygen saturation, 96%; temperature, 37.2°C

PATHOPHYSIOLOGY

TEF occurs in approximately 1 in 3500 live births. There are six primary anatomical variations of this congenital anomaly that have been described by two overlapping classification systems as shown in Figure 53-1. The most common type of TEF (Type C or IIIB) is represented by letter A in Figure 53-1 and accounts for almost 90% of all cases. The defect is an esophageal blind pouch (atresia) with a distal fistula connecting the stomach to the trachea. The lesion occurs because of incomplete separation of the trachea and esophagus that begins during the fourth to fifth week of embryo development. Survival of infants with TEF and no other congenital anomalies is greater than 95%. The presence of a TEF poses several severe risks to the infant: pulmonary aspiration is likely to occur, pneumonia and pneumonitis of the right upper lung are common, oral nutrition and fluids are not possible, and gastric distention with air can cause respiratory compromise.

SURGICAL PROCEDURE

Surgical management for TEF includes locating and ligating the fistula, and creating an anastomoses between the atretic segments of the esophagus. This is usually performed with the neonate in the left lateral decubitus position via a right thoracotomy. Thoracoscopic TEF repair is gaining popularity as surgeons become more adept with less invasive techniques. Thoracoscopic repair is usually performed in the prone position, and has similar complication rates as the traditional open technique. In cases of severe congenital cardiac defects, chromosomal abnormalities, or extreme prematurity and low birth weight, primary correction of the TEF is difficult

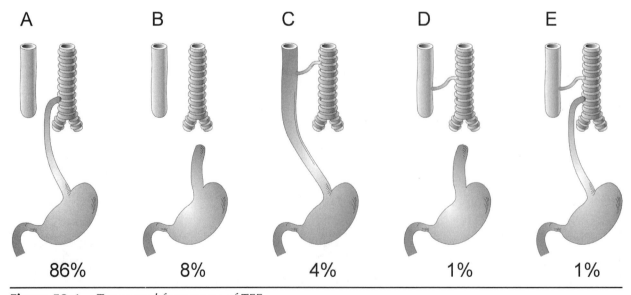

Figure 53-1 *Types and frequency of TEF.*

and is associated with significant risk. In high-risk cases, a gastrostomy is performed under local anesthesia and definitive surgical correction of the TEF is deferred. The surgical correction is completed in stages for babies who demonstrate signs and symptoms associated with severe aspiration pulmonitis, as adequate oxygenation and ventilation during a thoracic surgery may be unattainable.

ANESTHETIC MANAGEMENT AND CONSIDERATIONS

Preoperative Period

1. Discuss the clinical presentation of a neonate with a tracheoesophageal fistula.

TEF is most frequently diagnosed during the first day of life when the neonate is unable to tolerate oral feeds without coughing, choking, and cyanosis. The suspicion of TEF is then confirmed with a chest radiograph showing a nasogastric tube coiled in the proximal esophagus. Oral contrast studies are no longer routinely done because of the risk of aspiration and associated fatality. Due to the inability of the fetus to swallow, the prenatal ultrasound often reveals polyhydramnios.

2. Discuss the anatomic anomalies that are associated with TEF.

Over half of the babies born with TEF have other congenital anomalies or are born premature. Cardiac defects can be life threatening and must be ruled out with transthoracic echocardiography prior to TEF repair. Approximately 25% of those born with a TEF have cardiac defects, the most common being atrial or ventricular septal defects, coarctation of the aorta, and tetralogy of Fallot. TEF is also a component VACTERL, which are a combination of anomalies shown in Table 53-1. These defects were known as VATERL syndrome, but were modified to include the common cardiac and limb anomalies. The specific gene or set of genes that causes VACTERL has not yet been identified, which is why it is considered an association as opposed to a syndrome.

Table 53-1   Anomalies Associated with TEF
• VACTERL: Over 50% of patients with TEF have at least one additional anomaly
Vertebral defects
Anal atresia
Cardiac defects (25% have a ventricular septal defect, atrial septal defect, tetralogy of Fallot, atrioventricular canal, or coarctation of the aorta)
Tracheoesophageal fistula
Esophageal atresia
Radial or renal anomalies
Limb anomalies
• Prematurity: 20 to 40% are premature and weigh less than 2 kg
• Cleft lip and genital abnormalities: 5% have additional midline defects

3. Identify the anatomic and physiologic changes to the pulmonary system that can be present with TEF.

The anesthetist can expect that some degree of pulmonary compromise has occurred. Even after the patient is no longer ingesting fluid by mouth, the potential for pulmonary aspiration is still high due to the fistula between the stomach and the trachea and the inability of the patient to manage their oral secretions. Right upper lobe pneumonia and aspiration pneumonitis commonly occur in patients with TEF. Additionally, the stomach can become full of air, inhibit diaphragmatic expansion, and compress the lungs. Emergent gastrostomy and intubation with one lung ventilation could be lifesaving measures if extreme gastric insufflation of air occurs.

4. Discuss preoperative patient medical management for TEF.

TEFs must be repaired as soon as possible. Medical management of the patient focuses on prevention of aspiration pneumonitis that can preclude surgical correction. As soon as TEF is suspected, the child is given nothing by mouth and placed with their head elevated above their chest. The esophageal pouch is suctioned continuously via nasoesophageal tube. Intravenous (IV) fluids are given and metabolic acidosis is corrected prior to surgery. Preoperative lab evaluation should include arterial blood gases (ABG), complete blood count (CBC), chemistry panel, type and cross-match, and glucose. Transthoracic echocardiography and consultation from a pediatric cardiologist are also necessary prior to anesthesia. The presence of associated anomalies must be ruled out by examination, ultrasound, and radiography.

Intraoperative Period

5. Discuss options of securing the airway.

Correct placement of the endotracheal tube below the level of the fistula is crucial during endotracheal intubation and prior to ventilation. Maintaining spontaneous respirations during a mask induction with inhalation anesthetic agents prevents gastric insufflation from positive pressure. Alternately, a rapid sequence IV induction without positive pressure mask ventilation can also be accomplished safely. In both methods, the endotracheal tube is advanced into the right mainstem bronchus and withdrawn slowly until bilateral breath sounds are heard. A flexible fiberoptic bronchoscope can be used to verify placement of the endotracheal tube and fistula. To further prevent the chance of gastric insufflation, the fistula can be occluded with a Fogarty balloon-tipped catheter from the trachea, or from a gastrostomy. After confirmation of correct placement of the endotracheal tube, muscle relaxant can be used to assist with controlled ventilation. The endotracheal tube is in close proximity to the carina and fistula, and migration caudad can cause an endobronchial intubation; migration cephalad can cause insufflation of the stomach or inadvertent extubation. Therefore, constant vigilance and reassessment is required throughout the perioperative period in order to deliver competent care.

6. Describe appropriate monitoring and hemodynamic goals during TEF repair.

In addition to the standard monitoring, patients having a TEF require unique considerations. Arterial blood pressure monitoring gives the anesthetist the advantage of continuous beat-to-beat assessment and access for blood gas/glucose monitoring. A left-sided precordial stethoscope alerts the anesthetist to a right mainstem intubation either from endotracheal tube migration or from surgical manipulation of the trachea.

This surgery is most often associated with minimal blood loss; however, due to the proximity of the surgical site to great vessels and vital organs, blood products should be available for infusion prior to incision. These patients will be receiving an IV fluid that contains glucose prior to surgery. It is necessary to continue this infusion along with maintenance fluids. Stopping the glucose solution can result in rapidly occurring hypoglycemia. It is prudent to monitor the glucose values during the perioperative period. Additionally, surgical fluid loss should be replaced with lactated Ringers at a rate of 6 ml/kg/hr. Timely communication with the surgical team regarding the amount and speed of blood loss is essential. Consider replacing the blood loss 1:1 with 5% human albumin until the hematocrit falls below 30%.

The accuracy of end-tidal carbon dioxide monitoring as a reflection of arterial carbon dioxide levels can be compromised by surgical retraction of lung tissue, compression of bronchi, aspiration pneumonia, atelectasis, small endotracheal tube size, and fresh gas flow rates, among many other factors. Therefore, ABG should be routinely assessed at least every hour during surgical repair.

7. Discuss anesthetic maintenance and intraoperative considerations.

An adequate depth of anesthesia can be maintained with a combination of an inhalation anesthetic agent and opiates. The use of nitrous oxide for this surgical procedure and in this patient population is controversial. Nitrous oxide decreases the fraction of inspired oxygen, causes bowel distention, increases pulmonary vascular resistance, and inhibits methionine synthetase.

Muscle relaxation is usually required for surgical exposure and to facilitate in controlling ventilation. If vertebral defects are absent, a lumbar or caudal epidural can be used for intraoperative anesthesia and/or postoperative analgesia. Maintaining appropriate temperature with a forced-air blanket is imperative since the increased body surface area in pediatric patient predisposes them to developing hypothermia.

8. Discuss the challenge of maintaining adequate tissue oxygenation.

A common pitfall during TEF repair is difficulty maintaining adequate oxygenation. Oxygen should be diluted with air to prevent arterial hyperoxia because of the increase in risk of retinopathy of prematurity. Keeping the oxygen saturation between 95 and 99%, and confirming the values via an ABG values is prudent. Precipitous oxygen desaturation is not uncommon and can occur from a variety of reasons. Prior to surgery, there may be atelectasis and secretions that cause shunting of pulmonary blood that can result in hypoxia and hypercarbia. This problem is compounded during surgery with retraction on lung tissue, bleeding, tracheal and bronchial compression, or endotracheal tube

Table 53-2	Postoperative Complications Associated with Repair of TEF
Apnea	
Tracheal collapse or compression	
Pneumothorax	
Airway obstruction (blood or mucous)	
Anastomosis leak	
Hypoventilation	
Recurrent laryngeal nerve damage	
Atelectasis	
Aspiration pneumonia	

malposition. In the presence of arterial hypoxia, the surgeons may need to release traction and allow time for alveolar recruitment maneuvers. Frequent suctioning of blood and secretions may also be necessary to maintain satisfactory ventilation. Ventilator settings are frequently reassessed, as the peak inspiratory pressure and tidal volumes will vary during various stages of surgical repair.

Postoperative Period
9. Discuss extubation timing and options.
Extubation in the operating room at the conclusion of surgery is desirable if spontaneous respiration is sufficient. Respiratory depression in the newborn can originate from hypothermia, hypoglycemia, or anemia, all of which must be addressed prior to extubation. The presence of the endotracheal tube can cause excessive pressure on the newly created anastomosis and increase the possibility of wound dehiscence. Moreover, reintubation can disrupt the surgical repair. Therefore, the anesthetist must feel confident that the respiratory effort is sufficient prior to extubation. Although favorable, extubation is often precluded by poor pulmonary function, excessive secretions, and aspiration pneumonitis. Associated anomalies also complicate the clinical picture and the child may require prolonged mechanical ventilation in the intensive care unit. Other postoperative complications associated with TEF are listed in Table 53-2.

10. Discuss strategies that can be used to decrease postoperative pain.
TEF repair is performed via thoracotomy or thorascopy and adequate postoperative pain management is imperative. Opiate infusions are frequently used with close monitoring due to the potential for respiratory depression. Regional analgesia, in the form of lumbar or caudal epidural catheter, is particularly advantageous for postoperative pain control. Every TEF patient should be considered to have some degree of pulmonary insult, so avoiding the respiratory depressant effects of opiates is beneficial in the postoperative course.

11. Discuss the clinical course and outcomes for survivors.

Care of patients immediately following TEF repair should focus on the treatment of pulmonary insults and preventing pressure on the new anastomosis. During surgery, an orogastric tube is marked to the level of the anastomosis. Suction catheters should not be advanced past the TEF repair site. After surgery, every patient should be considered to have gastroesophageal reflux and be treated accordingly. A TEF is not a simple anomaly that can be completely treated by anastomosis and ligation. Upper gastrointestinal problems are chronic and corrective or palliative treatments in the form of esophageal stricture dilation or Nissen fundoplication are often performed later in life. These patients will have a decreased number and integrity of their tracheal cartilages that can result in acute tracheal collapse after extubation or progressive tracheal compression. This population exhibits recurrent respiratory infections, reactive airway disease, and chronic restrictive and obstructive lung disease. The presence of associated congenital anomalies significantly increases the morbidity and mortality following TEF repair, and can result in lifelong health problems.

REVIEW QUESTIONS

1. An advantage of maintaining spontaneous respirations during the anesthetic induction of a patient with a TEF includes:
   a. laryngeal muscles are relaxed for ease of endotracheal intubation.
   b. the need for positive pressure ventilation prior to securing the airway is reduced.
   c. fiberoptic placement of a balloon catheter in the distal fistula is facilitated.
   d. there are no advantages to maintaining spontaneous respiration in this population.
2. The hallmark sign(s) of a patient with a TEF include:
   a. impaired muscle tone and nasal flaring.
   b. arterial oxygen desaturation with clear lung sounds.

   c. coughing and choking during feeding.
   d. orogastric tube placement in stomach confirmed by x-ray.
3. _____ is the congenital anomaly most commonly associated with TEF.
   a. Trisomy 21
   b. Goldenhar syndrome
   c. Cleft lip and palate
   d. VACTERL association
4. Which situation is an indication for definitive correction of a TEF for a 3-day-old infant?
   a. Atelectasis and infiltrates of the right upper lobe
   b. Tetralogy of Fallot
   c. Premature infant weighing 850 g
   d. Severe aspiration pneumonitis
5. The most common type of TEF accounting for almost 90% of patients is:
   a. solitary esophageal blind pouch.
   b. double fistulas between esophagus and right mainstem bronchus.
   c. esophageal atresia with distal fistula.
   d. tracheal fistula with upper and lower esophagus.

REVIEW ANSWERS

1. **Answer: b**
   Positive pressure ventilation above the level of the fistula can cause gastric insufflation which increases the risk of aspiration, can compress the lungs, or cause the stomach to rupture. Maintaining spontaneous respiration during induction limits the need for positive pressure mask ventilation.

2. **Answer: c**
   The hallmark signs of a patient with a TEF are coughing, choking, and cyanosis during feeding; this is usually discovered in the first day of life. Lung sounds would not be clear due to recurrent aspiration.

3. **Answer: d**
   The VACTERL association is the most common congenital anomaly that occurs with TEF. Over

50% of babies have one associated anomaly, and 25% have three.

4. **Answer: a**

A patient with a TEF will frequently have atelectasis of the right upper lobe. Primary repair of the closure should be postponed for severe associated anomalies, pneumonitis, or prematurity and weight less than 1 kg. These patients will usually have a gastrostomy under local anesthesia and the thoracotomy is deferred until in can be performed safely.

5. **Answer: c**

The most common type of TEF is esophageal atresia with distal fistula, also known as Type C or IIIB.

SUGGESTED READINGS

Andropoulos DB, Rowe RW, Betts JM. Anaesthetic and surgical airway management during tracheo-oesophageal fistula repair. *Paediatr Anaesth* 1998; 8:313–319.

Diaz LK, Akpek EA, Dinaviahi R, et al. Tracheoesophageal fistula and associated congenital heart disease: Implications for anesthetic management and survival. *Pediatr Anesth* 2005;15(10):862–869.

Gopal M, Woodward M. Potential hazards of contrast study diagnosis of esophageal atresia. *J Pediat Surg* 2007;42(6):E9–E10.

Ho AM, Wong JCP, Chui PT, et al. Case Report: use of two balloon-tipped catheters during thoracoscopic repair of a type C tracheo-esophageal fistula in a neonate. *Can J Anesth* 2007;54(3):223–226.

Holcomb GW III, Rothenberg SS, Bax KM, et al. Thoracoscopic repair of esophageal atresia and tracheoesophageal fistula: a multi-institutional analysis. *Ann Surg* 2005;242(3):422–430.

Konkin DE, O'Hali WA, Webber EM, et al. Outcomes in esophageal atresia and tracheoesophageal fistula. *J Pediatr Surg* 2003;38(12):1726–1729.

Kovesi T, Rubin S. Long-term complications of congenital esophageal atresia and/or tracheoesophageal fistula. *Chest* 2004;126(3):915–925.

Krosnar S, Baxter A. Thoracoscopic repair of esophageal atresia with tracheoesophageal fistula: anesthetic and intensive care management of a series of eight neonates. *Pediatr Anesth* 2005;15(7):541–546.

Reeves ST, Burt N, Smith CD. Is it time to reevaluate the airway management of tracheoesophageal fistula? *Anesth Analg* 1995;81(4):866–869.

Tercan E, Sungun MB, Boyaci A, et al. One-lung ventilation of a preterm newborn during esophageal atresia and tracheoesophageal fistula repair. *Acta Anaesthesiol Scand* 2002;46:332–333.

Out of the Operating Suite Procedures

XVII

Electroconvulsive Therapy

54

Bernadette T. Higgins Roche

KEY POINTS

- Electroconvulsive therapy (ECT) is indicated for severe major depression and other psychiatric disorders that have no or a poor response to medical therapy.
- Approximately 100,000 patients receive ECT annually in the Unites States. The mortality rate is estimated to be 2 deaths per 100,000 treatments and usually occurs as a result of cardiovascular or pulmonary complications.
- General anesthesia is necessary to provide unconsciousness and muscle relaxation during the procedure.
- The major contraindications to providing ECT include pheochromocytoma, recent cerebrovascular accident (CVA), recent myocardial infarction (MI), increased intracranial pressure (ICP), and cervical spine instability.
- The disadvantages associated with ECT can include temporary or permanent cognitive impairment and memory loss.

CASE SYNOPSIS

A 68-year-old woman is scheduled for ECT. She has been treated for major depression for over 5 years and has become increasingly unresponsive to several psychotropic medications.

PREOPERATIVE EVALUATION AND DEMOGRAPHIC DATA

Past Medical/Surgical History

- Hypertension for 3 years
- Major depression for more than 10 years
- Cigarette smoking: 1 pack/day for over 25 years

List of Medications

- Sertraline (Zoloft)

Diagnostic Data

- Hemoglobin, 12.4 g/dl; hematocrit, 37%; glucose, 90 mg/dl
- Electrolytes: sodium, 140 mEq/l; potassium, 3.5 mEq/l; chloride, 106 mEq/l; carbon dioxide, 22 mEq/l
- Electrocardiogram (ECG): normal sinus rhythm; heart rate, 88 beats per minute, left ventricular hypertrophy, left anterior hemiblock

Height/Weight/Vital Signs

- 165 cm, 73 kg
- Blood pressure, 160/94; heart rate, 94 beats per minute; respiratory rate, 16 breaths per minute; temperature, 37.2°C; room air oxygen saturation, 97%

PATHOPHYSIOLOGY

There is no single cause of depression, rather a combination of genetic, biochemical, environmental, and psychologic factors have been implicated in the disorder. It is more common among women and it is theorized that the increased incidence of depression results from the variability of hormonal levels. Major depression is a chronic but treatable disorder and early intervention is associated with the best outcome. Bipolar disorder (manic depressive disorder) is characterized by episodes of major depression and abnormally elevated mood (mania) or hypomania (less severe). The symptoms associated with depression and bipolar disorder are included in Tables 54-1 and 54-2. The onset of depression typically presents during the late adolescent period or in early adulthood. However, it can occur in childhood as well as later in life.

Regardless of whether psychotherapy is instituted or not, the use of antidepressants is the primary intervention for treatment of depression. The most commonly used antidepressants are selective serotonin reuptake inhibitors (SSRIs) such as fluoxetine (Prozac), citalopram (Celexa), and sertraline (Zoloft). Serotonin and norepinephrine reuptake inhibitors (SNRIs) have similar effects as

Table 54-1 Symptoms of Depression
For a diagnosis of depression, five of the following symptoms must be present nearly every day for at least 2 weeks:
Feelings of sadness or emptiness
Decreased interest or pleasure in activities
Appetite change with weight loss or weight gain
Decreased or increased sleeping
Fatigue or loss of energy
Feelings of worthlessness or guilt
Agitation
Difficulty in thinking or concentrating
Recurrent thoughts of death or suicide

Table 54-2 Symptoms of Mania (or a Manic Episode) in a Patient with Bipolar Disorder
Increased energy and activity, restlessness
Euphoric mood
Extreme irritability
Fast speech patterns and flight of ideas
Inability to concentrate
Little need for sleep
Unrealistic beliefs in one's abilities and powers
Poor judgment
Spending sprees
A lasting change of behavior that is different from usual
Increased sexual drive
Drug abuse, especially cocaine, alcohol, and sedatives
Provocative and/or aggressive behavior
Denial
Symptoms of psychosis, such as hallucinations and delusions, may also be present

the SSRIs; examples include venlafaxine (Effexor) and duloxetine (Cymbalta). Both SSRIs and SNRIs have fewer side effects than older antidepressants such as the tricyclic antidepressants (TCA) and monoamine oxidase inhibitors (MAOIs). However, for some individuals, TCAs (such as desipramine [Norpramin], doxepin [Sinequan], imipramine [Tofranil] and nortriptyline [Pamelor]), or MAOIs (such as isocarboxazid [Marplan] and phenelzine [Nardil]) may be more effective than SSRIs or SNRIs. Regardless of the mechanism of action, antidepressants must be taken for 3 to 4 weeks before a full therapeutic effect is demonstrable. A relapse of the depression is possible if antidepressants are discontinued. For treatment of major depression, stimulants and antianxiety medications may be used in conjunction with an antidepressant. In addition to antidepressants, bipolar disorder is treated with mood stabilizers including lithium (Lithobid) and lamotrigine (Lamictal). Anticonvulsants such as valproate (Depakote) and carbamazepine (Tegretol) are beneficial for hard-to-treat bipolar episodes.

SURGICAL PROCEDURE

ECT was introduced in the 1930s after it was observed that psychiatric symptoms in a schizophrenic patient appeared to decrease after a spontaneous seizure. Shortly after, ECT was discovered to be an effective treatment for depression and bipolar disorder. After its widespread use in the 1940s through the 1960s when it was administered without the benefits of anesthesia, ECT fell out of favor because of the untoward physical side effects associated with the treatment such as awareness, bone fractures, broken teeth, myofascial pain, and memory loss. Indiscriminate use of the treatment, social stigma, and the introduction of antipsychotic and antidepressant drugs have also contributed to the decline. In the 1980s, there was renewed interest in ECT as an effective treatment for several psychiatric disorders, especially for those patients who did not respond to the new

pharmacologic agents. At the same time, the need for general anesthesia and muscle relaxation was recognized. Although often stigmatized as a last treatment resort, ECT is a very effective treatment and has several advantages for severe major (unipolar) depression, bipolar depression, acute mania, and catatonia. The response rate to ECT is greater and occurs much faster than the response rate to antidepressants, antipsychotics, or a combination of both antidepressants and antipsychotics. ECT is useful for treating schizophrenia that is unresponsive to medical antipsychotic therapy. It has also been used successfully to treat Parkinson disease and chronic pain, especially phantom limb pain. However, ECT is not an effective treatment for addiction, personality disorders, or somatization disorders. The majority of antipsychotic and antidepressant medications do not noticeably alter the patient's mood for 3 to 6 weeks. The rapid results obtained by ECT have been advantageous when treating patients who are acutely psychotic and suicidal. It is also considered a safe treatment alternative for mental illness during pregnancy. Older patients that have acute depression are the most likely group to benefit from ECT. The rate of reoccurring depression is high and patients will need to continue taking their antidepressant medications following a series of ECT treatments. Maintenance ECT treatments do not appear to offer any advantage to medical management in preventing relapse.

During ECT, a brief pulse current is delivered via transcutaneous electrodes to one or both cerebral hemispheres with the intent of producing a generalized seizure. Electrodes are placed above each temple in bilateral ECT. When performing a unilateral ECT, electrodes are placed over one temple, usually the right (nondominant hemisphere), and near the vertex on the same side, this is referred to as a right unilateral (RUL) ECT. Approximately 800 milliamps of electrical energy are delivered for 1–6 seconds, producing a grand mal seizure with 10–15 second tonic and 30–60 second clonic phases.

Three waveforms can be used for ECT: sine wave, brief pulse wave, or an ultra brief wave. Sine wave stimulus is associated with greater memory loss and is rarely used in the United States. The majority of ECT procedures utilize a brief pulse width of 0.5–1.0 msec. Regardless of the waveform that is administered, the strength of the stimulus must exceed the seizure threshold. Bilateral ECT delivers an electrical stimulus at 1.5 times the seizure threshold, whereas unilateral ECT may require a stimulus strength that is 6–12 times the seizure threshold. There is a significant increase in the seizure threshold with aging; to achieve a therapeutic seizure, a higher electrical stimulus may be required in elderly patients. In contrast to an RUL, bilateral ECT is associated with a rapid initial response and a longer remission of symptoms. RUL-ECT is associated with fewer cognitive side effects, especially for retention of verbal information, visual information, and autobiographical memory. When administered with an ultra brief pulse width (0.3 msec), RUL-ECT appears to have less negative cognitive effects, especially on the retention of verbal information, visual information, and retrograde autobiographical memory. Regardless of the delivery method, the mechanism of action for the therapeutic effects of ECT is still unknown. Seizure duration of 30 to 60 seconds is desirable. Treatment efficacy appears to be dependent upon a minimum seizure duration of 25 seconds. Seizures that last less than 25 seconds in duration provide little, if any, benefit. During ECT, seizure duration is monitored by an unprocessed electroencephalogram (EEG) or by observation of seizure activity in an isolated limb. To observe isolated seizure activity, a tourniquet is applied (or a blood pressure cuff is inflated) prior to the administration of succinylcholine to limit distribution of the drug to the limb. This allows direct observation of the intensity and duration of the resultant seizure. A positive response to ECT is usually seen after three to five treatments, and a therapeutic effect is generally observed after a total of 400–700 seizure seconds. A typical ECT series includes two or three treatments per week for approximately 6 weeks; twice-weekly procedures are associated with a lower incidence of cognitive impairment. ECT may be repeated monthly for an additional 6 months.

The electrocardiographic changes associated with ECT including atrioventricular dissociation may occur. The hyperdynamic response to the electrical stimulus occurs within 2 minutes and is usually self-limiting. ECT causes a 100 to 400% increase in cerebral blood flow caused by the seizure induced increase in cerebral metabolic rate and an increase in intracranial pressure. There is also an increase in intraocular and intragastric pressures during the procedure. The neuroendocrine response includes increased secretion of adrenocorticotropic hormone, cortisol, vasopressin, glucagon, epinephrine, and norepinephrine.

ANESTHETIC MANAGEMENT AND CONSIDERATIONS

Preoperative Period

1. Describe the mechanism of actions of antidepressants medications.

Patients who present for ECT are frequently taking oral antidepressants such as TCAs, MAOIs, SSRIs, SNRIs, and lithium carbonate. TCAs block presynaptic reuptake of norepinephrine and serotonin but have little effect on reuptake of dopamine. MAOIs block the presynaptic metabolism of norepinephrine, serotonin, and dopamine. The SSRIs block the reuptake of serotonin, whereas the SNRIs block the reuptake of both serotonin and norepinephrine. The exact mechanism of action for lithium is unknown. It has a narrow therapeutic index, and this drug should be discontinued before instituting ECT as it increases the risk of delirium and prolongs the seizure duration. Lithium also potentiates the action of depolarizing and nondepolarizing muscle relaxants. Salt restriction or thiazide diuretics decrease renal clearance of lithium.

2. List the contraindications to having ECT.

Major contraindications to ECT include pheochromocytoma, recent CVA, recent MI, increased intracranial pressure (ICP), and unstable cervical spine. Relative contraindications include angina, congestive heart failure (CHF), aortic aneurysm, cerebral aneurysm, pregnancy, thrombophlebitis, major bone fracture, severe osteoporosis, glaucoma, retinal detachment, and automatic implantable cardioverter defibrillators (AICD).

3. Discuss the preoperative testing indicated for patients undergoing ECT.

A baseline EKG is indicated for all patients having ECT. If the patient has a history of cardiovascular disease or a recent history of an acute cardiovascular event, a stress test or cardiac catheterization is indicated. Due to the potential increased risk of a second myocardial or cerebral ischemic event, ECT should be postponed for at least 6 to 8 weeks following an acute MI or CVA, respectively. Other preoperative tests are dependent on the individual patient and their medical history.

4. Discuss a typical ECT treatment plan.

ECT is administered two to three times per week for approximately 6 weeks. Maintenance ECT sessions may be continued monthly for an additional 6 months. Ideally, antidepressants and antipsychotics should be discontinued during the ECT treatments especially lithium which increases seizure duration and the incidence of postprocedure delirium. However, it is not always possible for antidepressants to be discontinued and ECT has been safely administered to patients taking a variety of antidepressants and mood elevators.

Intraoperative Period

5. Discuss the anesthetic requirements for a patient undergoing ECT.

General anesthesia is required to provide a rapid loss of consciousness (LOC), amnesia, and

Table 54-3   Anesthesia for ECT
Verify signed informed consent
Perform a preanesthetic assessment
Ensure presence of emergency airway equipment, suction, medications, and cardiac defibrillator
Establish IV access
Administer ketorolac to patients at risk for posttreatment headache or myalgia
Apply monitors: EKG, pulse oximeter, NIBP, precordial stereoscope
Apply tourniquet or second blood pressure cuff for observation of seizure activity
Administer glycopyrrolate for the antisialagogue effect. Consider pretreatment with esmolol or lidocaine.
Preoxygenate patient: administer induction agent (methohexital, 0.5–1 mg/kg; thiopental, 1.5–2.5 mg/kg; propofol, 0.75–1.5 mg/kg; or etomidate, 0.15–0.3 mg/kg) and a muscle relaxant (succinylcholine 0.5–1 mg/kg).
Insert bite block following loss of consciousness
Hyperventilate to decrease seizure threshold and prolong duration of seizure
Monitor duration seizure
Treat excessive sympathetic response with esmolol or labetalol
Treat emergence agitation with midazolam
Monitor recovery for ≥ 30 minutes

muscle relaxation during the procedure. Ideally, the anesthetic agents that are administered will also attenuate the hyperdynamic response caused by the electrical stimulus and allow for the prompt return of consciousness and spontaneous ventilation. Patients should be NPO (nothing by mouth) for 6–8 hours and patients who have cardiovascular disease should take their cardiovascular medication in the morning of the procedure.

Since the effectiveness of ECT is dependent on the duration of the seizure activity, drugs that increase the seizure threshold (anticonvulsants, benzodiazepines, lidocaine) should be discontinued prior to the treatment. Other drugs of concern include theophylline, which is associated with the development of status epilepticus during ECT and should be discontinued prior to treatment. Oral nonsteroidal anti-inflammatory drugs (NSAIDS) can be administered before therapy to prevent posttreatment myalgia or headache. Patients who have a history of severe posttreatment myalgia or headache, ketorolac 30 mg IV can be administered prior to induction. Anesthetic management typically involves the use of an induction dose of an IV anesthetic followed by a short-acting muscle relaxant. Tracheal intubation is not necessary except for patients with a full stomach or in the last trimester of pregnancy.

ECT is usually administered in the PACU or in a treatment room in a psychiatric treatment setting. Standard monitoring includes EKG, pulse oximetry, and NIBP measurement. Following assessment of the patient's baseline vital signs, preoxygenation, and pretreatment with glycopyrrolate 0.2 mg IV, an induction agent and muscle relaxant is administered. Following LOC, a bite block is inserted and the patient is ventilated by mask using 100% oxygen. Hyperventilation will decrease the seizure threshold but may increase the hemodynamic response to stimulation. Ventilation is discontinued during adminis-

tration of the electrical stimulus and the duration of the seizure noted by direct observation of the isolated limb. Following return of consciousness and spontaneous ventilation, the patient should be monitored for approximately 30 minutes. Midazolam can be administered to help treat emergence agitation.

6. Compare the effects of various induction agents on seizure activity.

Almost all IV anesthetics have anticonvulsant properties, and dosing is very important so as not to interfere with the therapeutic effect of the treatment. Larger than necessary dosages of IV anesthetics will shorten the seizure duration and reduce the efficacy of ECT, whereas inadequate dosing can result in awareness and recall.

Thiopental (1.5–2.5 mg/kg) was the first IV anesthetic to be used for ECT but methohexital (0.5–1 mg/kg) is the gold standard for ECT. Compared with methohexital, both thiopental and thiamylal (1.5–2.5 mg/kg) shorten the EEG seizure duration and increase the frequency of sinus bradycardia and premature ventricular contractions. Seizure duration with lower doses (0.75 mg/kg) of propofol is similar to the barbiturates. At higher doses (1–1.5 mg/kg), propofol can shorten the duration of seizure activity but does not appear to impact outcome of the treatment. Earlier recovery of cognitive function may be an advantage of propofol as an induction agent. Etomidate (0.15–0.3 mg/kg) prolongs the seizure duration, which may be beneficial in patients with seizure durations less than 25 seconds. However, it is associated with a greater hemodynamic response to electrical stimulation and a prolonged recovery period.

When used with lower doses of methohexital and propofol, both alfentanil (10–25 mcg/kg) and remifentanil (1 mcg/kg) are associated with a prolonged seizure duration and significant attenuation of the hyperdynamic cardiovascular response. With repeat ECTs, there appears to be a rise in seizure threshold during the treatment course when methohexital is used as the induction agent. Remifentanil can provide improved seizure response to ECT in patients who become refractory to seizure induction after a methohexital induction. As a sole agent or in combination with lower doses of methohexital or propofol, remifentanil is associated with lower seizure threshold, prolonged seizure duration, decreased hemodynamic response, and no increase in recovery time.

A pharmacodynamic property of benzodiazepines is prominent anticonvulsant activity. As a result, benzodiazepines significantly shorten the seizure duration and should be avoided before and during ECT. However, they may be required for termination of a prolonged ECT-induced seizure. The majority of ECT procedures are performed outside of the operating room and, therefore, inhalation anesthetics are rarely used. When used for ECT procedures, sevoflurane (1.7%) has a similar effect on seizure duration and hemodynamic response as thiopental and higher concentrations are more effective in blunting the hemodynamic response. Sevoflurane is considered useful for women requiring ECT in the late stages of pregnancy, as it may reduce the incidence of ECT-stimulated uterine contractions.

Ketamine has been used for ECT but concerns about increased intracranial pressure, increased sympathetic activity, and prolonged recovery has limited its use. However, ketamine is a racemic mixture and there are significant differences in potency and side effects between the two isomers; increased potency and decreased psychomimetic effects are seen with the S isomer. The intense seizure activity provoked by ECT may cause excitotoxic neuronal damage mediated by glutamate via the N-methyl-D-aspartate (NMDA) receptor. This damage that may account for the postoperative cognitive dysfunction associated with ECT. Ketamine is an NMDA antagonist and it

may offer protection against this neuronal damage. Repeated electrocortical stimulation is associated with mossy fiber sprouting in the hippocampus, which correlates with ECT-induced memory impairment; ketamine appears to block the development of mossy fiber sprouting. Compared to methohexital, ketamine is associated with shorter reorientation times, despite a longer elimination half-life.

7. Describe the role of muscle relaxants when providing anesthesia for ECT.

Muscle relaxants are used to prevent myalgia and other more serious musculoskeletal complications associated with ECT including dislocations and fractures. The most commonly used muscle relaxant is succinylcholine. It can produce post-treatment myalgia secondary to muscular fasciculations. NDMR can be used as an alternative to succinylcholine in certain patients but does not appear to be as effective as succinylcholine in preventing muscle contractions during ECT. The NDMRs require a prolonged period of ventilatory support during the recovery period.

8. Discuss the autonomic response to ECT.

A brief period of parasympathetic nervous system predominance, which lasts less than 20 seconds, is the initial response to the electrical stimulus. The result includes increased salivation, severe bradycardia, hypotension, and the potential for brief episodes of asystole. This is followed by intense sympathetic stimulation which can last for several minutes during which time tachycardia ($\geq$ 20% increase in heart rate), arrhythmias, and hypertension (30–40% increase in systolic pressure) will be present.

9. Discuss management of the hemodynamic effects of ECT.

The parasympathetic response to ECT can be limited or prevented by pretreatment with glycopyrrolate. It is effective as an antisialagogue and is associated with less tachycardia post-ECT than atropine. Atropine is used to treat bradycardia that persists during the procedure. Sympathetic effects such as tachycardia and hypertension are usually self-limiting. Lidocaine or Esmolol can be used to reduce the incidence of tachycardia and hypertension prior to initiating ECT. Labetalol can also be used to blunt the CV response but is associated with a prolonged period of hypotension immediately following the treatment and in the early recovery period. Nifedipine provides more effective control of the hyperdynamic response, especially in elderly patients. In hypertensive patients, pretreatment with sublingual nifedipine may prevent or limit an increase in systemic vascular resistance (SVR) in response to electrical stimulation.

10. Compare the different ECT techniques and their impact on cognitive function.

In comparison to a sine wave stimulus, the use of a brief pulse stimulus (0.5 to 2 msec) is associated with a less negative effect on cognition. Ultra brief pulse waveforms (less than 0.5 msec) may produce even fewer cognitive side effects. Although it requires the use of a higher dosage, RUL electrode placement is associated with a lower incidence of cognitive side effects. Treatments that occur twice a week are associated with a lower incidence of cognitive side effects as compared to when they are prescribed three times a week. Rather then using a standard electrical stimulus, titrating the stimulus strength to the individual patient will allow dosing to minimally exceed the threshold which is necessary to produce the therapeutic effect. When the electrical stimulus greatly exceeds the patient's seizure threshold, cognitive function is affected to a greater degree.

Postoperative Period

11. List potential postoperative complications associated with ECT.

During a standard course of ECT treatments, the overall mortality is 0.029%; the major causes of death are MI, CHF, and cardiac arrest. Complications include vertebral fracture, laryngospasm, myalgia, headache, confusion, memory loss, jaw pain, dental damage, and nausea and vomiting. Hemorrhagic and embolic stroke, prolonged seizure, postictal delirium, and brain stem herniation associated with a preexisting intracranial mass may also occur.

12. Discuss the cognitive changes associated with ECT.

Irrespective of the etiology, all seizures are associated with a period of cognitive impairment. Short-term effects include emergence agitation. Posttreatment disorientation (postictal confusion) lasting for minutes to hours is not uncommon; however, it occurs more frequently in the elderly population. Retrograde amnesia generally affects memories for weeks to months preceding the treatment. Memory loss gradually improves over time, usually within 7 months, but some patients complain of persistent or permanent memory loss. Antegrade amnesia can also occur immediately following the treatment, but these effects are short-lived and temporary as compared with retrograde amnesia. Cognitive side effects appear to be more frequent in patients taking lithium. To minimize cognitive dysfunction, ECT should be administered to the nondominant hemisphere. The degree of long-term memory loss increases as the number of treatments increases.

13. Describe the risk of awareness and recall during ECT.

During ECT, awareness under anesthesia, recall of paralysis, and seizures can occur as a result of an inadequate dosage of the induction agent and/or premature administration of the muscle relaxant. LOC should be assured before administering succinylcholine and the electrical stimulus. Awareness and recall during ECT may be underreported because bilateral ECT tends to obliterate the memory of the ECT procedure. RUL-ECT, which is associated with less memory loss, may increase the incidence of recall if an inadequate induction dose is used or succinylcholine is administered prior to LOC.

14: Discuss the long-term outcome of ECT.

ECT is a very effective short-term treatment for depression and other psychiatric disorders. However, relapse of symptoms is not uncommon. Patients who respond positively to a course of ECT will need to continue a treatment regimen with antidepressants following the prescribed series of ECT treatments. Some patients may require monthly maintenance ECT treatments for an extended period.

REVIEW QUESTIONS

1. An advantage of ECT as compared to antidepressant therapy for suicidal patients includes:
   a. faster relief of symptoms.
   b. retrograde amnesia of the suicidal thoughts.
   c. lower mortality rate.
   d. better patient compliance.
2. What electrical waveform is associated with the greatest degree of cognitive impairment?
   a. Ultra brief pulse width
   b. Sine wave
   c. Brief pulse wave
   d. Delta wave
3. Which is the first hemodynamic response that occurs after the administration of the electrical stimulus?
   a. Tachycardia
   b. Hypertension
   c. Bradycardia
   d. Decreased cerebral blood flow
4. Which is an absolute contraindication to having ECT?
   a. Increased intracranial pressure
   b. Angina
   c. Pregnancy
   d. Osteoporosis

5. Which induction agent represents the gold standard for patients having ECT?
   a. Propofol
   b. Etomidate
   c. Methohexital
   d. Diazepam

REVIEW ANSWERS

1. **Answer: a**
   A faster relief of symptoms is a definite advantage of ECT for suicidal patients. Antidepressant medication can take 3–6 weeks to reach full therapeutic effect.
2. **Answer: b**
   Sine wave ECT is associated with the greatest degree of cognitive impairment. Ultra brief pulse width is associated with the least effect on cognitive function.
3. **Answer: c**
   Parasympathetic activation, exhibited by bradycardia, is the initial response to electrical stimulation.
4. **Answer: a**
   Increased intracranial pressure is an absolute contraindication to ECT. Angina, pregnancy, and osteoporosis are relative contraindications.
5. **Answer: c**
   Methohexital is the gold standard for an induction agent for a patient undergoing ECT. With the exception of diazepam, etomidate and propofol can be used for ECT.

SUGGESTED READINGS

Abrams R. *Electroconvulsive Therapy*, 4th ed. New York: Oxford University Press, 2002.

American Psychiatric Association. *The Practice of Electroconvulsive Therapy: Recommendation for Treatment, Training, and Privileging*, 2nd ed. Washington, DC: American Psychiatric Press, 2001.

Andrad C. Thirthalli J, Gangadhar BN. Unilateral nondominant electrode placement as a risk factor for recall of awareness under anesthesia during electroconvulsive therapy. *J ECT* 2007;23(3):201–203.

Ding Z, White PF. Anesthesia for electroconvulsive therapy. *Anesth Analg* 2002;94(5):1351–1364.

Folk JW, Kellner CH, Beale MD, et al. Anesthesia for electroconvulsive therapy: a review. *J ECT* 2000; 16(2):157–170.

Geretsegger C, Nickel M, Judendorfer B, et al. Propofol and methohexital as anesthetic agents for electroconvulsive therapy: a randomized, double-blind comparison of electroconvulsive therapy seizure quality, therapeutic efficacy, and cognitive performance. *J ECT* 2007;23(4):239–243.

Litt L, Li D. Awareness without recall during anesthesia for electroconvulsive therapy. *Anesthesiology* 2007;106(4):871–872.

MacPherson RD, Loo,CK. Cognitive impairment following electroconvulsive therapy- Does the choice of anesthetic agent make a difference? *J ECT* 2008; 24(1):52–56.

Pierce K, Flynn P, Caudle M, et al. Electroconvulsive therapy: Current clinical standards. *Psychopharm Review* 2008;43(5):35–42.

Prudic J. Strategies to minimize cognitive side effects with ECT: aspects of ECT technique. *J ECT* 2008; 24(1):46–51.

Sawayama E, Takahashi M, Inoue A, et al. Moderate hyperventilation prolongs electroencephalogram seizure duration of the first electroconvulsive therapy. *J ECT* 2008; 24(3):195–198.

Anesthesia for Office-Based Pediatric Dental Surgery

55

Allan Schwartz

KEY POINTS

- Caries or dental cavities are the most prevalent chronic infection in early childhood, and are a major cause of school absenteeism.
- Caries in children can cause intense pain, severe infection, and aesthetic embarrassment, as well as difficulties in eating, swallowing, and chewing.
- It is estimated that 56% of children between 2 and 3 years of age have caries, and 80% of children have experienced caries by age 17. The presence of dental caries has reached epidemic proportions in lower income pediatric populations.
- Office-based anesthesia for dental surgery can be performed safely, conveniently, and cost effectively.

CASE SYNOPSIS

A 7-year-old girl presented to our dental office with complaints of pain in the teeth and jaw.

PREOPERATIVE EVALUATION AND DEMOGRAPHIC DATA

Past Medical/Surgical History

- Autism
- Obesity

List of Medications

- None

Diagnostic Data

- None

Height/Weight/Vital Signs

- 124.5 cm, 53 kg
- Blood pressure, 118/80; heart rate, 98 beats per minute; respiratory rate, 12 breaths per minute; room air oxygen saturation, 99%

PATHOPHYSIOLOGY

Dental caries is the most prevalent cause of chronic infections found in early childhood, and is a major reason of school absenteeism. It occurs 5 to 8 times more frequently than asthma. Caries in children can cause pain, aesthetic embarrassment, difficulties in eating, swallowing, chewing, and speaking. This intraoral disease process has reached epidemic proportions in lower income pediatric populations in North America. Early childhood caries has a lasting impact on both the child's primary dentition ("baby teeth") and their permanent dentition ("adult teeth"), because infection in the primary teeth disrupts the development of the permanent teeth. It is estimated that 56% of children between ages 2 and 3 have caries and 80% of children have experienced caries by age 17.

Dental caries cause the molecular destruction of a part or the entire calcified tooth structures (enamel, dentin, and cementum), which can progress into the dental pulp. Caries results in gradual loss of tooth structure, which can affect chewing, facial structure, and cause infection if left untreated, as shown in Figure 55-1. Caries are caused by the acidic metabolites (low pH) of oral bacteria, principally the bacterium *Streptococcus mutans*. The oral microbiologic flora combined with liquid saliva, salivary proteins, and food debris forms a thick sticky mass called *biofilm* or *dental plaque*.

Dental periodontal structures consist of the *gingiva* (gums), *oral mucosal tissue*, the *periodontal membrane*, and the *bones* of the maxilla or the mandible. Biofilm, which adheres to exposed tooth structures, causes caries, periodontal tissue inflammation, and permanently destructive periodontal disease. Bacterial endotoxins that originate from oral bacteria can enter the bloodstream.

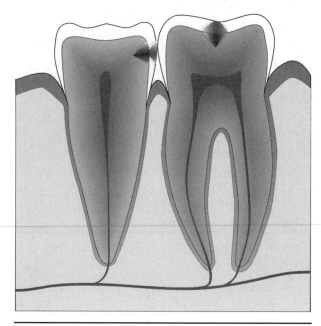

Figure 55-1 *Types of dental caries.*

These circulating endotoxins release inflammatory mediators that are transmitted to the coronary vasculature of the heart, causing coronary artery disease. Other long-term effects and serious illnesses resulting from untreated carious lesions include life-threatening systemic infections that can invade the fascial spaces of the head and neck, through the jawbones (osteomyelitis), and into the brain.

Fortunately, pediatric dental visits are increasing. Pediatric dentists and pediatricians recommend the first dental visit at the first year of age. The oral flora of the infant develops from oral and bodily contact with primary caregivers, so careful and thorough oral hygiene is important.

SURGICAL PROCEDURE

A dentist treats caries by careful and thorough excavation of caries from the tooth and then replaces the missing tooth structure with silver amalgam or glass-filled composite. Figure 55-1 shows common locations for dental caries. In more extensive caries with pulpal invasion, the caries is carefully excavated, the pulpal remnants in the crown of the tooth are removed, and the remaining pulpal tissue is mummified with formocresol. The tooth is then restored with a stainless steel crown. A root canal is not performed on primary teeth due to the potential for future exfoliation of the tooth with the eruption of the permanent adult teeth. The dental hand piece (drill) or dental laser uses copious amounts of water, which must be carefully suctioned by the dental assistant to prevent serious airway stimulation, which can cause coughing or laryngospasm.

ANESTHETIC MANAGEMENT AND CONSIDERATIONS

Preoperative period

1. Restate the importance of daily oral hygiene for the pediatric patient.

It is essential for parent(s) or guardian(s) to remove the child's biofilm each day, by brushing and flossing the teeth, since the child lacks the coordination to thoroughly cleanse their teeth with the needed proper and meticulous technique. Infants whose teeth have not yet erupted should have their mouth cleansed of biofilm at least daily with a clean wet washcloth—swabbing or wiping the entire inside of the mouth and the oral tissues. This process will have already been described and demonstrated by the dental team to the parent(s)/guardian(s), but can also be reinforced by the anesthesia provider.

2. Discuss the relationship between autism and dental pathology.

Autism is a neurologic developmental disorder that may result in severe impairment of language, social interaction, behavior, and cognitive function. The majority of autistic patients function with a moderate degree of mental retardation; however, autistic females often display severe mental retardation. Classic autism is prevalent in 10–20 cases per 10,000 births and the male-to-female ratio is 3:1.

The chronic pharmacologic treatment used to manage autism may have side effects that are of concern to dentists and anesthetists. Antipsychotic drugs may cause motor impairment affecting speech, swallowing, along with central nervous system depression, and orthostatic hypotension, sialorrhea (excessive salivation), or xerostomia (dry mouth). Other common symptoms are dysgeusia (altered taste), bruxism (teeth grinding along with clenching), stomatitis, and glossitis. Autistic patients can also present with gastroesophageal reflux disease (GERD), and a typical demand for low-textured foods which easily adhere to teeth, resulting in significant dental disease. As a result, autistic patients can be challenging yet manageable candidates for office-based dental anesthesia.

3. Identify indications and contraindications for office-based pediatric dental surgery.

Indications and contraindications for office-based anesthesia for pediatric dental surgery are listed in Tables 55-1 and 55-2, respectively. The anesthetist, along with the dentist, must weigh such factors as the medical condition of the patient, the behavior of the patient, and the capabilities of the dentist/supporting staff to deal with the challenging pediatric patient and ensure patient safety.

Table 55-1	Indications for Office-Based Anesthesia for Pediatric Dental Surgery
Uncooperative/unmanageable behavior	
Patient who requires immediate dental treatment	
Unable to thoroughly examine	
Unable to obtain intraoral dental radiographs	
Necessity for little or no patient movement or no swallowing	
Mentally challenged child or adult patients	
Hypersalivation	
Small mouth	
Large tongue	
Unable to attain intraoral local anesthesia	
Claustrophobia	
Need for comprehensive dental treatment needed in multiple quadrants	
Need for tooth extraction(s)	
Desire for convenience and significant cost savings	

Table 55-2	Contraindications to Providing Office-Based Anesthesia for Pediatric Dental Surgery
Severe allergies	
Severe asthma	
Severe cardiovascular pathology	
Need for invasive monitoring	
Inadequate facility or supporting staff	
Craniofacial deformities	
Aggressive or violent behavior	
Severe seizure disorder	
Severe claustrophobia	
Physical status III or greater	

4. Describe the necessity of a presurgical consultation appointment.

It is important to meet the patient, parent(s) or guardian(s), prior to the scheduled surgical appointment for a presurgical consultation. This gives the anesthetist the opportunity to perform a detailed examination of the patient's health history as is shown in Figure 55-2.

This appointment also allows the anesthetist to interact with the patient and gauge the temperament and challenges the patient could pose during the procedure. This meeting also gives the anesthetist time to discuss procedural rules such as strict nothing-by-mouth (NPO) policies, determine the need for physician consultation, and evaluate the risks and benefits of premedication.

5. Demonstrate importance of the day-of-surgery anesthesia assessment.

It is very helpful to interview the parent(s) or guardian(s) and assess the patient the day of the dental surgery. This valuable document as seen in Figure 55-3 demonstrates a preoperative anesthetic assessment.

There are times that the anesthetic and the dental surgical procedure may necessitate cancellation, as a result of the day-of-surgery anesthesia assessment. Table 55-3 lists some considerations that could postpone or cancel the dental surgical appointment due to a current medical condition(s) or an uncontrollable temperament of the patient. For patients with severe behavioral affect, the anesthetist should consider referral to a pediatric dentist (pedodontist) for treatment in an ambulatory surgical center or an operating room to be completed with general anesthesia.

6. Describe the process of oral premedication for office-based dental treatment for the pediatric patient.

Before administration of oral premedication, it is important to have the patient use the restroom to avoid patient movement after the onset of the premedication and to prevent soiling of the dental operatory. Preoperative sedation can be achieved using a variety of different medications; however, a common practice to administer oral midazolam mixed with either liquid ibuprofen or liquid acetaminophen. Dosing should be based on the patient's ideal body weight. Prior to the administration of oral or intravenous (IV) agents, a complete anesthesia setup is necessary and an example is included in Table 55-4. Any office-based anesthesia practice should comply with the Guidelines for Office-Based Anesthesia set forth by the American Association of Nurse Anesthetists.

Oral premedication is necessary to decrease a patient's separation anxiety from the caregiver(s), insertion of the IV line, and for its amnestic effects. Vivid memories of a difficult dental visit could affect future dental care the patient could seek as they mature. Some patients require no premedication and, thus, the anesthetist must decide whether premedication is beneficial to the individual patient.

The patient should rest only with the parent(s)/caregiver(s), in a quiet and nonstimulating room, away from the office reception area. Excessive stimulation could elicit unwanted behaviors and unnecessarily upset the patient. A warm blanket helps

ANESTHESIA HEALTH HISTORY

1. Patient Information

Today's date_____ Age_____ Birth date_____ Weight_____ Height_____ Sex M or F

Name_____ Home Phone_____

        Last   First   Middle Init.   Cell Phone_____

Home Address_____ City_____ State_____ Zip Code_____

Employer_____ Work Phone_____

Work Address_____ City_____ State_____ Zip Code_____

Spouse / Parent(s) / Guardian(s) Name(s)_____

Address_____ City_____ State_____ Home Phone_____

Person to contact in case of emergency_____ Phone_____

Address_____ City_____ State_____ Home Phone_____

2. Patient Medical History

Physician Name_____ Office Phone_____ Date of Last Exam_____

Reason for last visit_____

	Yes	No
1. Are you under the care of a physician?	❏	❏
2. Have you ever been hospitalized for any surgical operation or serious illness?	❏	❏
3. If yes, describe_____	❏	❏
4. Do you use tobacco?	❏	❏
5. Do you wear contact lenses?	❏	❏
6. Are you taking any medications, non-prescription medications, herbal medicines, vitamins?	❏	❏
Please list_____		

7. Are you allergic to or have you had any reaction to the following?

	Yes	No
Local Anesthetics	❏	❏
Penicillin or any antibiotics	❏	❏
Sulfa drugs	❏	❏
Aspirin	❏	❏
Codeine	❏	❏
Other_____		

8. Do you now, or have you had any of the following?

Respiratory/Lungs	Yes	No	Cardiovascular	Yes	No	Liver/Kidneys	Yes	No
Recent Cold	❏	❏	Rheumatic fever	❏	❏	Kidney diseases	❏	❏
Pneumonia/Cough/Flu	❏	❏	Mitral valve prolapse	❏	❏	Hepatitis/Jaundice	❏	❏
Asthma/Bronchitis	❏	❏	High/Low Blood pressure	❏	❏	Liver Disease	❏	❏
Emphysema Short of Breath	❏	❏	Abnormal Rhythm	❏	❏	**Other**		
Easily Winded	❏	❏	Peripheral Vascular Disease	❏	❏	Diabetes	❏	❏
Tuberculosis	❏	❏	Blood clots	❏	❏	AIDS/HIV/STD	❏	❏
Musculoskeletal			Leukemia or anemia	❏	❏	Thyroid disease	❏	❏
Arthritis/Back or Hip problem	❏	❏	Blood transfusion	❏	❏	Frequently tired	❏	❏
Joint replacement/Implant	❏	❏	Bleeding difficulty	❏	❏	Cancer	❏	❏
Muscle weakness/Paralysis	❏	❏	Heart disease	❏	❏	Stomach trouble/Nausea	❏	❏
Numbness/Tingling	❏	❏	Congestive Heart Failure	❏	❏	Hiatal hernia/Gastric reflux	❏	❏
Neurological			Swollen ankles	❏	❏	Hay fever/Seasonal allergies	❏	❏
Fainting	❏	❏	Cardiac Pacemaker/AICD	❏	❏	Radiation therapy	❏	❏
Epilepsy/Convulsions/Seizures	❏	❏	Heart murmur	❏	❏	Glaucoma	❏	❏
Psychiatric treatment/Nervous	❏	❏	Congenital heart lesions	❏	❏	Recent weight gain loss	❏	❏
Stroke/Transient ischemic attack	❏	❏	Cardiac Stent	❏	❏	Cold sores	❏	❏
			Heart Attack/Angina	❏	❏			
			Chest Pain	❏	❏			

9. Women only:

	Yes	No
a) Are you pregnant or do you think you may be pregnant?	❏	❏
b) Are you nursing?	❏	❏
c) Are you taking birth control pills?	❏	❏

Are you *now using* or have you *ever used* drugs such as: Cocaine, heroine, methamphetamine, marijuana or others?

❏ Yes   ❏ No

_____   _____

      Patient Signature   Date

_____   _____

Doctor Signature /Anesthesia Provider Signature   Date

Figure 55-2 *Anesthesia health history.*

DENTAL ANESTHESIA DAY-OF PREOPERATIVE ASSESSMENT

Patient Name_____ Date_____

ALLERGIES/ MEDICATION ALLERGIES:

NKDA _____ FOOD None Soy Eggs LATEX NO _____ YES _____

HISTORY OF ANESTHESIA COMPLICATIONS:

PT: **NO**_____ **YES**_____ BLOOD RELATIVES: **NO**_____ **YES**_____ If yes list:_____

SOCIAL:

ETOH USE: **NO**_____ **YES**_____ **#DRINKS** – FREQUENT_____ OCCASIONAL_____

ILLICIT DRUG USE: **NO**_____ **YES**_____

TOBACCO USE: **NO**_____ **YES**_____ Smokeless _____ **PPD** × _____ #YRS **QUIT**_____

PAIN:

ACUTE/CHRONIC_____ SCALE 0-10_____ LOCATION_____

OTHER:

LMP_____ / PREGNANT / NURSING / PATIENT STATES NOT PREGNANT

Bilateral Tubal Ligation / Hysterectomy / Vasectomy / Abstention

Pregnancy Test Name_____

Lot Number_____ **Result** (−) (+)

RECENT URI **NO**_____ **YES**_____ **DATE**_____ Expiration Date_____

HIATAL HERNIA/ GASTRIC REFLUX **NO**_____ **YES**_____

_____ OBESITY / LESS THAN 90% IDEAL BODY WEIGHT

_____ IMMUNOSUPPRESSED / STEROIDS

_____ PEDIATRIC PTS IMMUNIZATIONS UP-TO-DATE: **NO**_____ **YES**_____

_____ CANCER / CHEMO / RADIATION

_____ OTHER _____

_____ ANEMIA / BLEEDING DISORDERS

_____Swish with water. _____Contact lenses out.

_____ I have not had anything to eat or drink for 6 hours prior to my dental treatment.

_____ I have made arrangements for someone to drive me home after my dental treatment.

_____ There will be a responsible adult to take care of me for 24 hours after my dental surgery.

FOR ANESTHESIA USE ONLY

Sip of water with meds at_____

Lung Sounds_____ day of: **NPO STATUS**_____

Heart Sounds_____ Weight_____lbs./kg

MPC: I II III Height_____feet/inches; cm

AIRWAY / TEETH / NECK

CROWNS / BRIDGES / POOR REPAIR / PERIODONTAL DISEASE / LOOSE TEETH / CARIES/ THIRD MOLARS/ PULPITIS / DECREASED INTERMAXILLARY DISTANCE:

NECK: Short / Thick / Decreased ROM POTENTIAL DIFFICULT AIRWAY

REMARKS:_____

PHYSICAL STATUS: 1 2 3 4 5 E

ANESTHETIC PLAN / MONITORING **MAC GETA TIVA LOC**

❑ Anesthetic, possible complications, and alternatives to care were discussed with and accepted by Patient / Guardian

❑ All consents signed.

_____ _____ _____ _____
D.D.S. / C.R.N.A. Signature Date Time

POSTANESTHESIA NOTE

No apparent anesthetic complication or complaints ❑

Signed_____ Date_____ Time_____

Discharged to_____ Caregiver ❑ Yes ❑ No

and/or Other Caregiver _____

Figure 55-3 *Day-of patient preoperative assessment (some areas do not apply to children).*

Table 55-3	Considerations for Postponement or Cancellation of Pediatric Office-Based Dental Surgery

Patient is not within accepted guidelines of nothing by mouth (NPO)

Recent upper respiratory infection

Unwilling or unable to allow premedication

Systemic infection, other than due to dental causes

Inability to transfer or position the patient for dental surgery

Inability to obtain intravenous access

Inadequate number of needed assistants

Parental or caregiver interference

preserve body heat from the start, and provides a sense of security for the patient. The anesthetist should assess the physiologic effects of the premedication and reassure the parent(s)/caregiver(s) as necessary.

Intraoperative Period

7. Illustrate the anesthetic challenges that are present with an obese pediatric patient.
It is estimated that approximately 30% of the pediatric patient population within the United States is presently considered obese and the incidence is expected to increase in the future. Childhood obesity predisposes to a variety of pathologic disease processes in adulthood, which include type 2 diabetes mellitus, coronary artery disease, hypertension, cancer, joint disease, gallbladder disease, and pulmonary disease.

Calculating body mass index (BMI) for pediatric patients is based on data collected by the Centers for Disease Control and Prevention, and accounts for the child's age, height, and weight. These factors are then compared to children considered to have ideal BMI. This patient's height and weight are ≥ 95th percentile for her age which places her into the category of obesity.

Several physiologic factors that may complicate the anesthetic course include:

- ***Increased metabolic rate:*** Since the metabolic rate in school-aged children is greater as compared to an adult, short periods of hypoventilation or apnea will result in rapid desaturation.
- ***Decreased functional residual capacity (FRC):*** The FRC and specifically the residual volume (RV) are decreased in obesity. The RV acts a reservoir for oxygen during apnea. Patients with decreased FRC are prone to rapid desaturation during hypoventilation or apnea, therefore, preoxygenation is imperative.
- ***Redundant airway tissue:*** Obesity increases the possibility of developing redundant airway tissue that can cause complete airway obstruction when anesthetic agents are administered.
- ***Difficult ventilation/intubation:*** Due to the presence of redundant airway tissue and other physical characteristics associated with obesity such as thick neck and a large tongue, difficult ventilation and intubation can cause an airway emergency, necessitating rapid airway intervention.

8. Describe the anesthetic process for the office-based dental treatment for the pediatric dental patient.
Positioning The dental chair is adjusted to accommodate the needs of the dentist. Small patients can be cushioned on a standard dental chair with a large pillow placed horizontally on the dental chair, along with a small dog bone–shaped travel pillow under the neck. Foam pads or rolled towels may also be used for padding the bony prominences and properly positioning the arms. The use of a blanket can be used to maintain cleanliness and to decrease heat loss.

Monitoring Prior to administration of anesthesia, it is imperative to apply EKG leads, pulse oximetry, blood pressure cuff, precordial stethoscope, and a temperature monitor.

Table 55-4   Supplies Necessary for Pediatric Dental Surgery Anesthesia

UTILITIES

Back-up power (uninterruptible power system)

EQUIPMENT

• Patient monitor to include pulse oximeter, electrocardiogram, blood pressure monitor with a selection of adequate-sized cuffs

• Liquid crystal body temperature stickers

• Emergency E cylinder oxygen tanks

• Positive pressure ventilation sources including an ambu bag, with properly sized face masks, and a mouth-to-mask unit

• Defibrillator (charged) or AED

• Suction source or a suction machine, tubing, suction catheters, and Yankauer suctions; plan for emergency suction in the event of power failure

• Anesthesia cart to provide for organization of supplies including endotracheal equipment, laryngeal mask airways, combitubes, face masks, nasal cannulas, disposable face masks with oxygen tubing, oral and nasal airways, syringes (tuberculin, 3, 5, 10, 30, 60 ml), 18-gauge 1.5-inch needles, 20- and 22-gauge IV catheters, tourniquets, IV fluids and tubing, alcohol pads, adhesive tape, disposable gloves, stethoscope

• Battery powered flashlight for emergency lighting, along with extra batteries

• Medication syringe pump

• Warm blanket(s), large pillow, and dog bone–shaped travel pillow

• Emergency medications to include, at a minimum, atropine, glycopyrrolate, epinephrine, ephedrine, phenyl-ephrine, lidocaine, diphenhydramine, hydrocortisone, and a bronchial dilator inhaler such as albuterol

• Anesthetic medications: In addition to the emergency medications listed above (propofol, etomidate, ketamine):
  ▪ Narcotics: midazolam, fentanyl, alfentanil
  ▪ Muscle relaxants: succinylcholine
  ▪ Cardiovascular drugs: labetalol, esmolol, verapamil, hydralazine
  ▪ Narcotic reversal drugs: naloxone, flumazenil
  ▪ Antiemetic drugs: ondansetron, dolasetron

ADDITIONAL EMERGENCY EQUIPMENT AND SUPPLIES

Cricothyrotomy kit

Compression board

IV Line Insertion In order to decrease patient movement, inhalation of a nonhypoxic mixture of nitrous oxide and oxygen can be titrated to effect. Supporting the patient's head and face, and assessing for possible patient movement is important. The anesthetist should consider using a subcutaneous bolus of 2% plain Lidocaine, administered with a 29-gauge insulin syringe at the IV insertion site. The IV catheter is secured with tape and possibly gauze wrap to avoid inadvertent removal.

Induction Administration of an antisialagogue such as glycopyrrolate is used to decrease intraoral secretions. Suction must be available to evacuate

Table 55-5   Advantages of the Dental LMA for Office-Based Pediatric Anesthesia
Allows protection of the airway from dental debris, saliva, secretions, and blood
Provides a secure airway
Is easily placed
Is relatively atraumatic to the patient's mouth, throat, and airway
Can be adapted to work with dental nitrous oxide/oxygen machines
Can work with an anesthesia machine
Can be repositioned from side to side, to allow the dentist better access to the patient's mouth
Allows disconnection and reconnection at its mid-point to allow the dentist to check the occlusion (the bite) of the teeth

saliva from the floor of the mouth and from the buccal vestibules. At this time, nitrous oxide is discontinued and oxygen at flow at 3 l/min via mask is for at least 5 minutes to avoid diffusion hypoxia. Sedation is achieved and maintained by administering propofol by infusion. Both eyes are carefully taped to avoid corneal abrasions.

A special dental LMA will soon be available to assist the anesthesia provider to maintain and safeguard the airway. The dental LMA can be adapted to work with dental nitrous oxide/oxygen delivery systems, or attached to an anesthesia machine. Advantages associated with the dental LMA are listed in Table 55-5.

Maintenance Due to the increased metabolic rate that is characteristic of children, a propofol infusion is titrated to effect. Propofol infusion rates of 100–150 mcg/kg/min are frequently necessary to maintain unconsciousness. Patients experiencing stimulating dental procedures require noticeably higher maintenance infusion rates of propofol. Advantages to the use of propofol include ability to titrate, relatively short half-life, and potential antiemetic effects.

If the patient will require dental extractions, the anesthetist may consider administering incremental doses of fentanyl. Ketamine may also be titrated to help stabilize and control behaviorally agitated patients. Midazolam will help to decrease the possibility of postoperative emergence delirium. Due

to a synergistic anesthetic effect, the addition of these adjunctive agents will reduce the maintenance infusion rate of propofol. Dexamethasone is frequently administered to decrease postextraction swelling and inhibit nausea and vomiting. Additionally, a serotonin receptor antagonist such as ondansetron is also used as nausea and vomiting prophylaxis. Ketorolac can be used to decrease postoperative pain.

Postoperative Period

9. Explain the process of emergence from anesthesia after pediatric dental surgery.
Even without the use of narcotics, emergence after a propofol infusion is frequently prolonged. This can be explained by the concept of context-sensitive half-time. As a lipid-soluble medication is administered by infusion, over time the drug is sequestered in tissue and accounts for the prolonged sedative effects. This effect is dependent on the duration of drug administration and the total dose administered. Continuing support of the airway and leaving the oral bite block in place allows for access to the posterior pharynx for suctioning. Gently supporting and reorienting the patient upon emergence is vital. It is prudent to consider bringing only one caregiver/parent to the operatory, after the patient has nearly emerged and is stable. Explaining to the caregiver that there is a possibility that the patient may exhibit emergence delirium is important.

10. Correlate the Modified Aldrete signs to the assessment of the patient during recovery.

Recovery can be accomplished within the dental operatory or after transport of the patient to a well-equipped recovery area. The area should remain quiet and in the presence of a well-trained assistant. Hospital recovery room nurses commonly use modified Aldrete signs for postanesthetic assessment of the patient. The modified Aldrete score is obtained by assigning an objective score to assessment of the patient's activity, respirations, circulation, consciousness, and color. Discharge is appropriate when a patient is stable, and has attained a minimum modified Aldrete score of 10.

Pediatric patients anesthetized in an office-based setting typically are discharged after approximately 20–30 minutes. If narcotics are administered for analgesia, discharge times are frequently increased.

REVIEW QUESTIONS

1. Which is characteristic of advanced dental caries?
   a. Absence of intraoral inflammation and infection
   b. Minimal patient morbidity
   c. Pain and destruction of tooth structure
   d. Results from nonpreventable causes
2. Which patient should not be considered for office-based pediatric dentistry?
   a. ASA physical status classification III
   b. A cooperative 2-year-old patient
   c. An 11-year-old patient who refuses premedication
   d. A mentally challenged 55-year-old adult patient
3. The preoperative consultation and interview is:
   a. an unnecessary duplicity of the patient's health history.
   b. performed only by the anesthesia provider.
   c. completed several days prior to the patient's dental surgical appointment.
   d. highlights concerns that could interfere with the anesthetic plan.

4. Which is the most appropriate statement regarding premedication of a pediatric patient presenting for dental surgery?
   a. Prior to setup of the anesthesia equipment and supplies
   b. In a quiet, nonstimulating environment
   c. With the parent(s)/guardian(s) and siblings present
   d. All pediatric patients should receive premedication
5. Which is false regarding the recovery of a pediatric patient after dental surgery?
   a. Can be performed in the dental chair/operatory
   b. Should occur with parent(s) or caregiver(s) present immediately after dental surgery
   c. Can be performed after transport to a well-equipped recovery room
   d. Requires the availability of a well-trained assistant

REVIEW ANSWERS

1. **Answer: c**
   Initially, caries will cause almost unnoticeable destruction of tooth structure. The patient may not even feel the sensation of pain, but the patient will probably notice sensitivity to touch, temperature, and when eating sugary foods. As time progresses, more severe pain and oral tissue destruction will occur.

2. **Answer: a**
   Patients that present with compromised medical state, such as ASA physical status III or greater, are best treated in a hospital, where access to advanced medical personnel and equipment is present.

3. **Answer: d**
   This important assessment provides a timely assessment of the patient's health on the day of surgery and gives the anesthesia provider a highlight of concerns that could interfere with the anesthetic on that day.

4. **Answer: b**

It is optimal to provide premedication in a quiet, nonstimulating environment promoting sedation rather than causing activity and agitation.

5. **Answer: b**

Continuous vigilance is required during the recovery phase. As a result, a well-equipped and well-staffed environment is necessary. Due to the possibility of emergence delirium, it is necessary to be prepared to protect the patient from physical harm.

SUGGESTED READINGS

Aker J. Pediatric Anesthesia. In: Nagelhout JJ, Zaglaniczny KL, eds. *Nurse Anesthesia,* 3rd edition. St. Louis, MO: Elsevier Saunders, 2005:1120–1123.

American Academy of Pediatric Dentistry. Guideline on the use of anesthesia personnel in the administration of office-based deep sedation/general anesthesia to the pediatric dental patient. Available at http://www.aapd.org/media/Policies_Guidelines/G_AnesthesiaPersonnel.pdf. Accessed August 26, 2008.

American Academy of Pediatric Dentistry. Guideline for monitoring and management of pediatric patients during and after sedation for diagnostic and therapeutic procedures. Available at: http://www.aapd.org/media/Policies_Guidelines/G_Sedation.pdf. Accessed August 26, 2008.

American Association of Nurse Anesthetists. Standards for Office-Based Anesthesia Practice. Available at http://www.aana.com/resources.aspx. Accessed January 6, 2009.

Beauchamp J, Caufield P, Crall J, et al. Evidence-based clinical recommendations for the use of pit-and-fissure sealants. *J Am Dent Assoc* 2008;139:257–268.

Cannon M. Early childhood caries-taking treatment out of the hospital. *Dentistry Today* 2007;26:128,130–131.

Crall J. Improving oral health for individuals with special health care needs. *Pediat Denti* 2007;29:98–104.

Friedlander A, Yagiela J, Paterno V, et al. The neuropathology, medical management and dental implications of autism. *JADA.* 2006;137:1517–1527.

Jamieson W, Vargas K. Recall rates and caries experience of patients undergoing general anesthesia for dental treatment. *Pediat Dent* 2007;29:253–257.

Lalwani K, Kitchin J, Lax P. Office-based dental rehabilitation in children with special care needs using a pediatric sedation service model. *J Oral Maxillofac Surg* 2007;65:427–433.

Weinstein P, Harrison R, Benton T. Motivating parents to prevent caries in their young children one-year findings. *J Am Dent Assoc* 2004;135:731–738.

Yagiela J. Making patients safe and comfortable for a lifetime of dentistry: frontiers in office-based sedation. *J Dent Educ* 2001;65:1348–1356.

Figure Credits

Figure 1-1 *Source*: Adapted from Jaffe RA, Samuels SI. *Anesthesiologist's Manual of Surgical Procedures,* 3rd ed. Philadelphia: Lippincott Williams & Wilkins, 2004:143, Figure 3-1.

Figure 1-2 *Source*: Adapted from http://commons. wikimedia.org/wiki/File:Throat_with_Tonsils_ 0012J.jpeg, accessed February 17, 2009 and http://www.arthrocareent.com/wt/page/int_ tonsillectomy, accessed July 7, 2009.

Figure 4-1 *Source*: http://www.provoiceandmusic ed.com/resources/polypsVocalCords.gif, accessed November 23, 2009.

Figure 4-2 *Source*: http://www.provoiceandmusic ed.com/resources/polypsVocalCords.gif, accessed November 23, 2009.

Figure 4-3 *Source*: http://www.provoiceandmusic ed.com/resources/polypsVocalCords.gif, accessed November 23, 2009.

Figure 5-1 *Source*: Adapted from Coleman J. Oral and maxillofacial surgery for the management of obstructive sleep apnea syndrome. *Otolaryngol Clin North Am* 1999;32:235–241.

Figure 6-1 *Source*: Adapted from http://images. google.com/imgres?imgurl=https://www.nlm. nih.gov/medlineplus/ency/images/ency/full size/7171.jpg&imgrefurl=https://www.nlm.nih. gov/medlineplus/ency/presentations/100039_ 4.htm&usg=__c7Np4ibBzAljSxio7l5BWTJFR8c= &h=320&w=400&sz=26&hl=en&start=16&tb nid=wBlE6yhuwwdumM:&tbnh=99&tbnw=124 &prev=/images%3Fq%3Dbowel%2Bresection% 26gbv%3D2%26hl%3Den%26client%3Dfirefox- a%26rls%3Dorg.mozilla:en-US:official, accessed October 4, 2009.

Figure 6-2 *Source*: Adapted from http://www. healthline.com/images/staywell/82347.jpg, accessed October 4, 2009.

Figure 7-1 *Source*: Adapted from http://www. rochestergeneral.org/images/surgery/RNYGB.jpg, accessed October 13, 2009.

Figure 7-2 *Source*: Adapted from http://www.med students.com.br/.../proced5/intubat1.gif.

Figure 8-1 *Source*: Adapted from http://www.sjhsyr. org/.../graphics/images/en/7028.jpg.

Figure 8-2 *Source*: http://www.cgmh.org.tw/.../ c6700/OBGYN/F/LAVH/ap2.jpg.

Figure 9-1 *Source*: http://www.clevelandsurgical associates.com/yahoo_site_admin/assets/images/ lap1.136100715_std.jpg, accessed November 23, 2009.

Figure 9-2 *Source*: http://www.pwsurgery.com/ images/gallbladder_000.jpg, accessed November 23, 2009.

Figure 10-1 *Source*: Adapted from http://gigertive.niddk.nih.gov/ddiseases/pubs/nash/, accessed May 16, 2009.

Figure 11-1 *Source*: Adapted from http://www.niaaa.nih.gov/Resources/GraphicsGallery/Liver/lobulep295.htm, accessed October 2, 2008.

Figure 11-2 *Source*: Adapted from http://www.cpmc.org/images/liver/topics/liver_segments.jpg, accessed October 26, 2008.

Figure 12-1 *Source*: Adapted from synthesis.helsinki.fi/.../farma/vk/airio/fig22.gif.

Figure 12-2 *Source*: Roberts CP. Phaeochromocytoma: Recent progress in its management. *Br J Anesth* 2000;85(1):44–57.

Figure 13-1 *Source*: Adapted from Jaffe R. *Anesthesiologists manual of surgical procedures*, 4th ed. Philadelphia: Lippincott-Williams; 2009:659, Figure 7.11-4.

Figure 15-2 *Source*: Adapted from www.uic.edu/.../Final/scannedimages/7-4.gif.

Figure 16-1 *Source*: Adapted from http://images.google.com/imgres?imgurl=http://www.baja arizona.org/fklr/wund3000.gif&imgrefurl=http://www.bajaarizona.org/fklr/fklr.html&usg=__UBIndBshu_r7i85ldr2xZzRltsM=&h=375&w=640&sz=13&hl=en&start=21&tbnid=qCXGXqSw5wUszM:&tbnh=80&tbnw=137&prev=/images%3Fq%3Dbullet%2Byaw%26gbv%3D2%26hl%3Den. Accessed November 23, 2009.

Figure 18-3 *Source*: Adapted from Nagelhout JJ, Zaglaniczny KL. *Nurse anesthesia*, 3rd ed. St. Louis, MO: Elsevier Saunders; 2005:577, 578, Figures 25-2 and 25-5.

Figure 19-1 *Source*: Adapted from Baker RJ, Fisher JE. *Mastery of surgery*, 4th ed. Philadelphia: Lippincott, Williams, and Wilkins; 2001.

Figure 19-2 *Source*: Adapted from Petty C. Right radial artery pressure during mediastinoscopy. *Anesth Analg* 1979;58:428.

Figure 21-1 *Source*: Adapted from http://www.dana.org/uploadedImages/Images/Spotlight_Images/DanaGuide_CH16C52_P532_spot.jpg and http://www.daviddarling.info/images/thymus.jpg, accessed November 23, 2009.

Figure 21-2 *Source*: Adapted from http://totw.anaesthesiologists.org/wp-content/uploads/mg2mono.jpg, accessed November 23, 2009.

Figure 23-1 *Source*: Adapted from Morgan EG, Mikhail MS. Clinical anesthesiology. New York: McGraw Hill; 1992:429.

Figure 24-1 *Source*: Adapted from http://www.radiologyassistant.nl/images/thmb_441bd03469a54aorta.jpg, accessed November 23, 2009.

Figure 24-2 *Source*: Adapted from http://www.vcu.edu/hearts/images/aorta_dissection_repair.jpg, accessed November 23, 2009.

Figure 26-1 *Source*: Adapted from https://.../health-library/images/em_2383.gif.

Figure 26-3 *Source*: Adapted from Schermerhorn ML, O Malley JA, Jhaveri A, et al. Endovascular vs. open repair of abdominal aortic aneurysms in the medicare population. *N Engl J Med* 2008;358:464.

Figure 27-1 *Source*: Adapted from http://www.nhlbi.nih.gov/.../images/ather_lowres.gif, accessed October 13, 2009.

Figure 27-2 *Source*: Adapted from ccvsa.com/images/heart_img.jpg.

Figure 29-1 *Source*: Adapted from http://www.endotext.org/neuroendo/neuroendo3b/neuroendo3b_2.htm, accessed December 15, 2008, and Netter F. *Atlas of human anatomy*, 4th ed. Philadelphia: Saunders; 2006:104.

Figure 31-1 *Source*: Adapted from http://webvision. med.utah.edu/sretina.html, accessed October 25, 2009.

Figure 31-2 *Source*: Adapted from http://webvision. med.utah.edu/sretina.html, accessed October 25, 2009.

Figure 31-3 *Source*: Adapted from http://www.vrmny. com/pe/vitrectomy.html, accessed October 25, 2009.

Figure 31-4 *Source*: http://www.surgeryencyclo pedia.com/Pa-St/Scleral-Buckling.html, accessed October 25, 2009.

Figure 32-1 *Source*: http://media-2.web.britannica. com/eb-media/30/91430-004-828719A3.jpg, accessed September 24, 2008.

Figure 32-2 *Source*: http://img.medscape.com/pi/ emed/ckb/otolaryngology/834279-835401-23.jpg, accessed September 24, 2008.

Figure 33-1 *Source*: Adapted from http://medical-dictionary.thefreedictionary.com/Uterine + Fibroids, accessed October 8, 2008.

Figure 33-2 *Source*: Adapted from Jaffe RA, Samuels SI. *Anesthesiologist's Manual of Surgical Procedures*, 3rd ed. Philadelphia: Lippincott Williams & Wilkins, 2004:648, Figure 8.2-4.

Figure 33-3 *Source*: Adapted from Longnecker, Tinker, & Morgan, 1998, p. 1868.

Figure 34-1 *Source*: Adapted from http://www.acog. org/publications/patient_education/bp062.cfm, accessed November 23, 2009.

Figure 34-2 *Source*: Adapted from http://www.acog. org/publications/patient_education/bp062.cfm, accessed November 23, 2009.

Figure 34-3 *Source*: Adapted from The American College of Obstetricians and Gynecologists, 2004.

Figure 35-1 *Source*: Adapted from Stoelting RK, Miller RD. Basics of anesthesia, 5th ed. Philadelphia: Elsevier; 2007:478.

Figure 36-1 *Source*: Adapted from Chestnut D. *Obstetric anesthesia principles and practice*, 3rd ed. St. Louis, MO; Mosby; 2004:248, Figure 15-2.

Figure 41-1 *Source*: http://www.prostateuk.org/bph/ images/pic5-bph-p79, accessed October 19, 2009.

Figure 41-2 *Source*: Jaffe R. Anesthesiologist's man-ual of surgical procedures, 4th ed. Philadelphia: Lippincott, Williams and Wilkins; 2003:858.

Figure 41-3 *Source*: http://www.nature.com/.../v9/ n6/images/nrn2401-f1.jpg.

Figure 42-1 *Source*: Adapted from http://www. ecommunity.com/health/images/es_1885.gif, accessed October 20, 2009.

Figure 42-2 *Source*: Adapted from http://nihatuner. deltahospital.com.tr/eswl.jpg, accessed October 20, 2009.

Figure 47-1 *Source*: Adapted from Barash P. *Clinical anesthesia*, 5th ed. Philadelphia: Lippincott, Williams and Wilkins; 2006:1114.

Figure 47-2 *Source*: Yao FS. *Anesthesiology: Problem oriented patient management*, 6th ed. Philadelphia: Lippincott, Williams and Wilkins; 2008:1168.

Figure 47-3 *Source*: Barash P. *Clinical anesthe-sia*, 5th ed. Philadelphia: Lippincott, Williams and Wilkins; 2006:762.

Figure 47-4 *Source*: Cottrell JE, Smith DS. *Anesthesia for neurosurgery*, 4th ed. St. Louis: Mosby; 2001:188.

Figure 48-1 *Source*: http://www.southwest-ortho. com/.../rotator-cuff.html.

Figure 48-2 *Source*: wockhardthospitals.wordpress. com/.../.

Index

DATE DUE

Figure 2-1 *Apron incision along the posterior border of the sternocleidomastoid muscle, curving medially above the clavicles.*

Figure 2-2 *Neck dissection.*

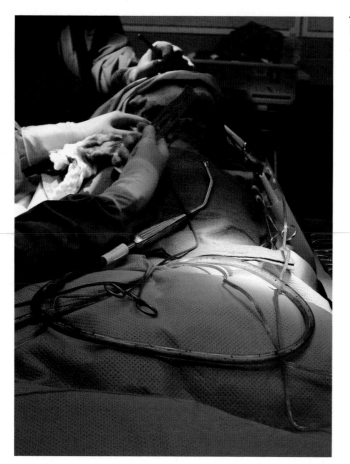

Figure 2-3 *Patient positioning 180 degrees away from the anesthesia provider.*

Figure 14-1 *Securing the airway in a trauma victim with suspected airway and cervical spine injuries using a rapid sequence induction with in-line manual axial stabilization.*

Figure 14-2 *Supraglottic edema and displacement of trachea.*

Figure 30-1 *Functional MRI scan of recurrent left frontal oligodendroglioma.*

Figure 30-2 *Ojemann cortical stimulator.*

Figure 30-3 *Anatomic areas are mapped that represent aphasia and anomia.*

Figure 30-4 *Use of the Ojemann cortical stimulator in concert with electrocorticography for identification of spike wave and seizure activity.*

Figure 37-1 *Classical uterine incision being repaired.*

Figure 43-1 *Capsulotomy before placement of the permanent breast implants.*

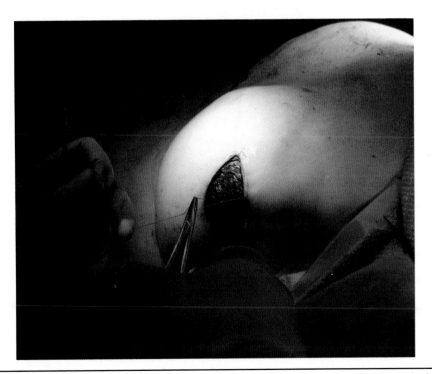

Figure 43-2 *The beginning of surgical closure of the wound. Note that the muscle layer is sutured over the breast implant to prevent implant exposure.*

Figure 43-3 *Preoperative marking prior to stage 2 breast reconstructive surgery.*